HIGH TECH UROLOGY

Technologic Innovations and Their Clinical Applications

JOSEPH A. SMITH, Jr., M.D., F.A.C.S

Professor and Chairman
Department of Urology
Vanderbilt University Medical Center
Nashville, Tennessee

HIGH TECH UROLOGY

Technologic Innovations and Their Clinical Applications

W.B. SAUNDERS COMPANY
Harcourt Brace Jovanovich, Inc.
Philadelphia • London • Toronto • Montreal • Sydney • Tokyo

W. B. SAUNDERS COMPANY
Harcourt Brace Jovanovich, Inc.

The Curtis Center
Independence Square West
Philadelphia, PA 19106

Library of Congress Cataloging-in-Publication Data

High tech urology : technologic innovations and their clinical applications / [edited by] Joseph A. Smith, Jr.
p. cm.
ISBN 0-7216-3053-7
1. Urology—Technological innovations. I. Smith, Joseph A.
[DNLM: 1. Technology, Medical. 2. Urology—methods. WJ 100 H638]
RC875.H54 1992 616.6′0028—dc20
DNLM/DLC 91-46822

HIGH TECH UROLOGY: Technologic Innovations and Their Clinical Applications ISBN 0-7216-3053-7

Printed in the United States of America

Last digit is the print number: 9 8 7 6 5 4 3 2 1

DEDICATION

TO

BARBARA, CAROLYN, BRAD, and CHRISTINE

CONTRIBUTORS

RICHARD K. BABAYAN, M.D.

Professor of Urology
Boston University School of Medicine
Boston, Massachusetts
Photography and Video Urology

MITCHELL C. BENSON, M.D.

Assistant Professor of Urology
Columbia University
College of Physicians & Surgeons;
Director, Urologic Oncology
Columbia Presbyterian Medical Center
New York, New York
Flow Cytometry in Urology

RALPH C. BENSON, Jr., M.D.

Co-Director
The Center for Urological Treatment and Research
Nashville, Tennessee
Lasers

PATRICK C. CARTWRIGHT, M.D.

Assistant Professor of Surgery/Pediatrics
University of Utah
Salt Lake City, Utah
Innovations in Pediatric Urology

ANITA N. CASSIS, M.D.

Fellow in Urology & Renal Transplantation
Virginia Mason Medical Center
Seattle, Washington
Stapling Devices in Urology

RALPH V. CLAYMAN, M.D.

Professor of Urology and Radiology
Washington University School of Medicine
St. Louis, Missouri
Ureteronephroscopy

JEFF E. FEGAN, M.D.

Fellow in Mineral Metabolism
University of Texas Southwestern Medical Center
Dallas, Texas
Extracorporeal Shock Wave Lithotripsy

H. BARTON GROSSMAN, M.D.

Professor, Department of Surgery,
Section of Urology
University of Michigan Medical School;
Director, Urologic Oncology Program
University of Michigan Cancer Center
Ann Arbor, Michigan
Recent Advances in Immunology and Molecular Biology

ALBERTO D. HERNANDEZ, M.D.

Fellow in Urology
University of Utah
Salt Lake City, Utah
Ultrasound in Urology

LAURENCE B. KANDEL, M.D.

Assistant Professor of Urology;
Director, The Long Island Kidney Stone Unit
SUNY at Stony Brook Health Sciences Center
Stony Brook, New York
Urologic Accessory Devices

LOUIS R. KAVOUSSI, M.D.

Assistant Professor of Urology
Harvard Medical School;
Head, Section of Endourology
Brigham and Women's Hospital
Boston, Massachusetts
Ureteronephroscopy

RICHARD C. LABASKY, M.D.

Assistant Professor of Surgery
Division of Urology
University of Utah Center for the Health Sciences
Salt Lake City, Utah
Urodynamics

MONICA LIEBERT, PhD

Assistant Research Scientist
Section of Urology
University of Michigan
Ann Arbor, Michigan
Recent Advances in Immunology and Molecular Biology

TERRENCE R. MALLOY, M.D.

Professor of Urology
University of Pennsylvania;
Chief of Urology
Pennsylvania Hospital
Philadelphia, Pennsylvania
Prosthetics

DOUGLAS F. MILAM, M.D.

Assistant Professor Department of Urology
Vanderbilt University School of Medicine;
Staff Urologist
Nashville Veterans Administration Medical Center
Nashville, Tennessee

Urologic Laparoscopy

JAY A. MOTOLA, M.D.

Chief Resident
Department of Urology
Long Island Jewish Medical Center
New Hyde Park, New York
Percutaneous Techniques

GLENN M. PREMINGER, M.D.

Associate Professor
Urology/Radiology/Internal Medicine
University of Texas Southwestern Medical Center
Dallas, Texas
Extracorporeal Shock Wave Lithotripsy

T. RAND PRITCHETT, M.D.

Staff Urologist
Urology and Renal Transplantation
Virginia Mason Medical Center
Seattle, Washington
Stapling Devices in Urology

ARTHUR D. SMITH, M.D.

Professor and Chairman Department of Urology
Long Island Jewish Medical Center
The Long Island Campus for the Albert Einstein College of Medicine
New Hyde Park, New York
Percutaneous Techniques

JOSEPH A. SMITH, Jr., M.D.

Professor and Chairman
Department of Urology
Vanderbilt University Medical Center;
Chief of Urologic Surgery
Vanderbilt University Hospital
Nashville, Tennessee
Ultrasound in Urology

BRENT W. SNOW, M.D.

Associate Professor
Department of Surgery and Pediatrics
University of Utah School of Medicine;
Primary Childrens Medical Center
University of Utah Hospital
Salt Lake City, Utah
Innovations in Pediatric Urology

PAUL TUREK, M.D.

Instructor in Surgery and Urology
University of Pennsylvania
Philadelphia, Pennsylvania
Prosthetics

RONALD L. URRY, Ph.D.

Professor of Surgery (Urology) and OB/GYN
University of Utah School of Medicine
Salt Lake City, Utah
Advances in Diagnosing and Treating Sperm Problems and Advanced Reproductive Techniques

IHN SEONG WHANG, M.D.

Resident in Urology
Columbia University
College of Physicians and Surgeons;
Resident in Urology
Columbia-Presbyterian Medical Center,
New York, New York
Flow Cytometry in Urology

PREFACE

Technologic innovations in modern society impact upon every aspect of life, including the practice of medicine. Technology driven changes have had a particularly dramatic influence upon the practice of urologic surgery. In many areas, urologic treatment and diagnosis bear little resemblance to the state-of-the-art of only a decade ago. Surely, even more profound changes are in store.

While often improving the care of our patients, the rapid technologic changes in medicine demand an active and ongoing educational effort by physicians. In order to provide contemporary treatment to patients, integration of new technology into clinical practice becomes mandatory. In fact, patients often demand the use of new technology about which they may have read in the newspaper or a magazine. Occasionally, it may be difficult to convince patients or other physicians that not all innovations represent an improvement over existing treatment. The expense of new technology sometimes limits its own use but also increases the pressure upon physicians to evaluate the practical clinical applicability of new devices.

By definition, technologic innovations and their clinical applications produce new information and physicians must search for appropriate educational sources. General urology texts tend to concentrate on proven and standard diagnostic and treatment methods. Publications devoted to a single new technologic advance are common but require collection of varied text books and other resources. This text provides a comprehensive reference of the technologic innovations which have affected the practice of urologic surgery.

Despite their sometimes innovative and creative aspects, not all technologic advances translate into practical clinical improvement in patient care. Why use a fancy, expensive machine when other methods work just as well? Often, new technology searches for a disease or application in which it can play a role. Any discussion which fails to recognize these considerations is of little practical relevance.

I am deeply indebted to the contributors to this work who have done an outstanding job in preparing the various chapters. Each author was chosen, not only because of his recognized expertise in a given area, but also because of his ability to make a balanced presentation. Often, "experts" in a new technology are so enamored with the technology that they fail to recognize their own biases and self-interests in promoting the technique. The contributors to this text have given a balanced practical discussion of the technology and its clinical utility.

Failure to acknowledge that proprietary concerns and self-interests frequently contribute to promotion of new techniques, either technologic or otherwise, would be naive. On the other hand, adoption of an inflexible stance which fails to recognize true advances and improvements can be equally inappropriate. Integration of technologic advances into urologic surgery should be driven by an attempt to improve the care of patients. I hope that publication of this text contributes to that effort.

Joseph A. Smith, Jr., M.D.

CONTENTS

CHAPTER 1

EXTRACORPOREAL SHOCK WAVE LITHOTRIPSY

JEFF E. FEGAN and GLENN M. PREMINGER

Surgical therapy for urinary tract calculi has changed significantly over the past 10 years. Formerly, removal of stones that caused symptoms required an open surgical procedure. However, advances in fiberoptics and the development of flexible instruments have led to the subspecialty of endourology. More recently, extracorporeal shock wave lithotripsy has allowed noninvasive destruction of renal and ureteral calculi. With this therapeutic modality, many patients can be rendered stone free without surgical access or even transurethral instrumentation.

Since 1980, when the first patient was treated successfully with extracorporeal shock wave lithotripsy, rapid acceptance and widespread use have made this therapy the treatment of choice for more than 80% of renal and ureteral calculi. Although the basic principles of shock wave lithotripsy remain unchanged, a myriad of technologic advances and modifications in lithotripters have significantly expanded the clinical applications of this treatment.

HISTORY

Physicists at Dornier Systems, Ltd., and Friedrich Shafen in West Germany began experimenting with shock waves and their travel through water and tissue in 1963. They discovered that shock waves could be generated under water and could travel through the body without appreciable energy loss. Brittle material such as renal calculi demonstrates a high accoustical impedance in comparison with the surrounding tissue. The difference in tissue "density" causes the energy from the shock wave to be absorbed by the stone, resulting in fragmentation. This finding was demonstrated initially in vitro in 1972.

Throughout the 1970s numerous experimental lithotripters were developed that used new methods of transmitting shock waves and different techniques of stone localization. In addition, experimental studies performed in vitro and in animal models examined the effects of shock waves on organs and tissues.

In 1980 Chaussy and associates first successfully treated a patient for a renal calculus with extracorporeal shock wave lithotripsy. They reported on the first series of 72 patients in 1982.[1] The Dornier Human Model 3 (HM-3) lithotripters arrived in the United States for clinical trials in the spring of 1984, and the U.S. Food and Drug Administration (FDA) approved the device in December of that year. Approximately 250 Dornier HM-3 lithotripters are now in use across the United States. In addition, many second-generation devices are undergoing clinical trials or have received FDA approval, and several manufacturers are nearing release of their third-generation machines.

BASIC PRINCIPLES

Shock Wave Physics

A review of shock wave physics will afford a better understanding of lithotripter function. Shock waves, or acoustic waves, are high-energy amplitudes of pressure generated in the air or water by an abrupt release of energy in a small space. They travel as alternate waves of compression (positive pressure) and rarefaction (negative pressure). Negative or tensile pressures are the exact opposite of compressive pressures. If tensile forces are strong enough, they may even exceed the cohesive strength of a specific medium. In liquids, for example, tensile forces may cause a phenomenon termed cavitation, in which the liquid is pulled apart to create a bubble.[2,3] As the cavitation bubble collapses, significant energy is released (Figure 1–1).

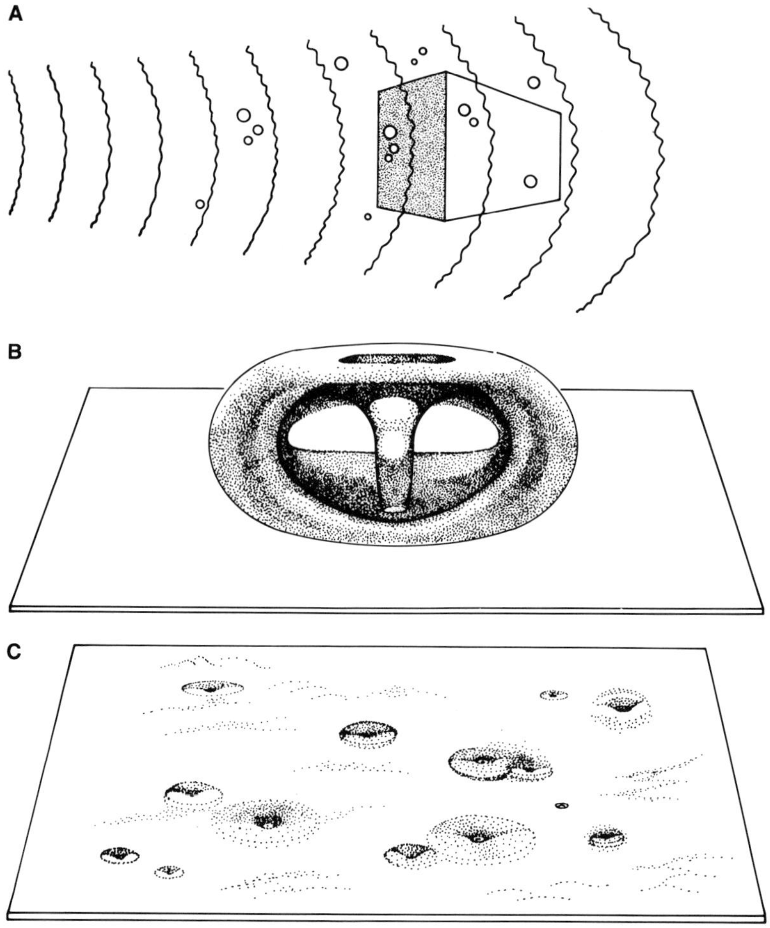

FIGURE 1–1. Cavitation. A, High-energy sound waves traveling through liquids generate cavitation bubbles. **B,** Imploding cavity (diameter approximately 150 μm) in a liquid. Since the cavity is formed near a solid surface, asymmetric implosion results, expelling a jet of liquid toward the solid surface. **C,** Pits on the surface of a solid, formed from high-velocity microjets.

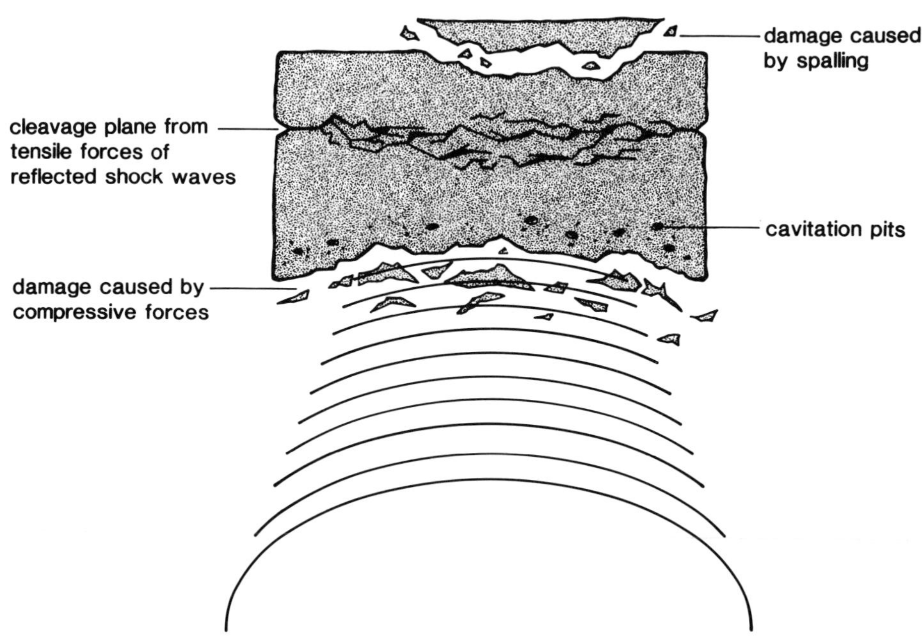

FIGURE 1–2. Mechanisms of Stone Fragmentation. Effects on a stone of the various forces generated by a focused, high-energy shock wave.

Sound waves transmitted through water and soft tissues show little attenuation (decrease in energy) because these materials have similar densities, or acoustic impedance. When a shock wave encounters a boundary between substances of different densities, however, the compressive stresses generated may overcome the tensile strength of the object that has greater density.

The speed of sound in stones is significantly different from that in normal tissue. Therefore, when a shock wave approaches the surface of a stone, energy is reflected, creating a compressive force on the front surface of the stone (Figure 1–2). At the back surface of the stone, reflection of the compression pulse creates a tensile wave that travels backward through the stone. Once the tensile force exceeds the cohesive strength of the stone, fragmentation occurs. The maximum tensile stress is theoretically created by an interaction between tensile and compressive shock waves near the back surface of the stone. These complex stresses generate crack patterns within the stone and eventually cause fragmentation. In addition, cavitation jets around the stone may cause erosive surface damage.[2,3] Although the exact characteristics of optimum stone fragmentation as caused by a particular shock wave have not yet been identified, peak shock wave pressures and rise time of the shock wave are assumed to play an important role in this equation.[4] These parameters differ among the types of clinical lithotripters.[5]

Repeated shock waves focused on a stone eventually reduce it to many small fragments that may be passed spontaneously. The obvious question is, what is the extent of damage to surrounding tissue generated by stone fragmentation? The compression-tensile wave phenomenon results in an implosion rather than an explosion of the fragments, and the total kinetic energy of all fragments can be minimized by using a large number of relatively low-energy shock waves rather than fewer shocks of higher energy. These findings, supported by extensive clinical research, explain the low incidence of adjacent tissue injury during stone fragmentation with high-energy shock waves.

Other investigators have defined two different modes of stone damage resulting from cavitation and spalling induced by piezoelectric shock waves.[6] At the stone's surface, directly facing the incident wave, damage of the cavitation type is identified as a deep crater surrounded by an annular zone of flake-off failure. Under magnification, pits can be seen at the flake-off region, apparently caused by the high-velocity penetration of microjets formed during cavitation bubble collapse.

On the back surface of the stone, spalling damage, characterized by the separation of a spherical cap from the stone surface, is observed. The incident compression wave is reflected as a tensile wave at the back surface of the stone material caused by an impedance mismatch between the stone and surrounding fluid medium. The separation occurs when the reflected wave exceeds the tensile strength of the stone. These findings suggest that the geometry of the stone, combined with the focal point of the shock wave, determines whether fragmentation will result from cavitation jets or from the spalling phenomenon and may predict the size of the stone fragments produced.

The same investigators used a standard stone phantom made of plaster of paris to compare stone damage after shock wave administration from electrohydraulic, electromagnetic, and piezoelectric lithotripters.[7] These three different types of shock wave generators produced distinctly different stone damage patterns. By altering shock wave configuration, intensity setting, and stone position in relation to the focal point, the investigators significantly changed the degree of stone fragmentation.

Lithotripsy Design

All lithotripters share four main features: an energy source, a focusing device, a coupling medium, and a stone localization system (Figure 1–3). In the original Dornier HM-3 design a sparkplug energy generator with an elliptical reflector is used to focus the shock waves. A water bath transmits the shock waves to the patient. Stone localization is provided by biplanar fluoroscopy. Modification of the four basic components of this first-generation lithotripter has provided a class of second-generation lithotripters, at least 10 of which are either available commercially or undergoing clinicl trials (Table 1–1).

Shock Wave Generation

While all lithotripters share the four main features of an energy source, a focusing device, a coupling medium, and a stone localization system, it is the mode of shock wave generation that determines the physical characteristics of a lithotripter. The objectives for using different types of energy sources are maximum efficacy (the overall stone-free rate) and maximum efficiency (cost-effectiveness or need for secondary treatments). The two basic types of energy sources for generating shock waves are point sources and extended sources. The electrohydraulic devices (Dornier, Direx, Medstone, Northgate, and Technomed) use point sources for energy generation, whereas extended sources are incoporated in the piezoelectric (Diasonics, EDAP, and Wolf) and electromagnetic (Siemens and Storz) devices.

The electrohydraulic generator is located at the base of a water bath and produces shock waves by an electric spark gap of 15,000 to 25,000 V lasting 1 μsec. This high-voltage spark discharge rapidly evaporates water, which generates a shock wave by expanding the surrounding fluid. The shock wave

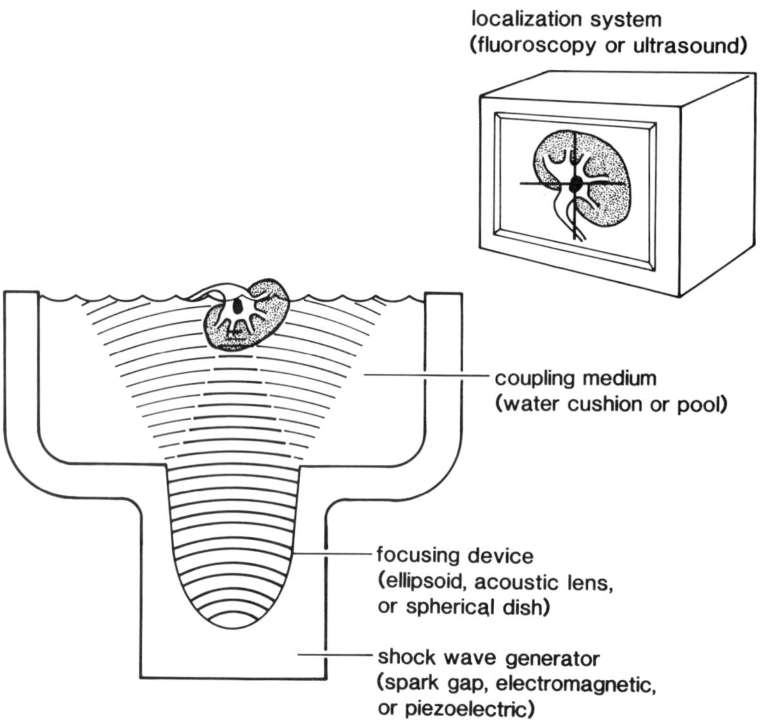

FIGURE 1–3. Basic Lithotripsy Design. The four main elements of an extracorporeal shock wave lithotripsy device, with the options for each element.

is propagated through the water bath in all directions. The generator is located in an ellipsoidal reflector that concentrates the reflected shock waves at a second focal point, F_2, with F_1 being the origin of the primary shock waves (Figure 1–4). The spark gap method of shock wave generation was pioneered by the first-generation Dornier HM-3 lithotripter and is also employed by the Direx, Medstone, Northgate, and Technomed machines.

Piezoelectric shock waves are generated by the sudden expansion of ceramic elements excited by a high-frequency, high-voltage pulse. Thousands of these tiny elements are placed along the inner surface of a hemisphere at the base of a pool of water. Although each element moves only slightly in response to a pulse of electrical energy, the simultaneous expansion of multiple elements results in a high-energy shock wave directed to the focal point at the center of the sphere. The shock wave is propagated through either a small water basin (Wolf) or a water-filled bag (EDAP, Diasonics) to the focal point, F_1 (Figure 1–5). The spherical focusing mechanism of the piezoelectric lithotripters provides a wide point of shock wave entry at the skin surface and a very small focal point. In the Siemens and Storz electromagnetic devices, shock waves are generated when an electrical impulse moves a thin, circular metallic membrane, which is housed in a cylindrical "shock tube" (Figure 1–6). The shock wave produced in the water-filled shock tube passes through an acoustic lens and is thereby directed to F_1. The shock wave is coupled to the body surface with a movable water cushion and coupling gel.

Shock Wave Focusing

Shock waves must be focused to concentrate their energy on a target, in this case a calculus. The type

TABLE 1–1. Second-Generation Lithotripters

Manufacturer	*Shock Wave Generation*	*Patient Focusing*	*Coupling*	*Localization*
Dornier HM-4	Spark gap	Ellipsoidal	Membrane	Biplane fluoroscopy
Direx	Spark gap	Ellipsoidal	Membrane	Fluoroscopy and ultrasound*
Medstone	Spark gap	Ellipsoidal	Membrane	Plain x-ray
Northgate	Spark gap	Ellipsoidal	Membrane	Ultrasound
Technomed	Spark gap	Ellipsoidal	Pool	Ultrasound
Diasonics	Piezoelectric	Spherical	Membrane	Fluoroscopy and ultrasound
EDAP	Piezoelectric	Spherical	Membrane	Ultrasound
Wolf	Piezoelectric	Spherical	Pool	Ultrasound
Siemens	Electromagnetic	Acoustic lens	Membrane	Biplane fluoroscopy

*This unit does not come with its own localization system; it must be used with separate ultrasound or fluoroscopy.

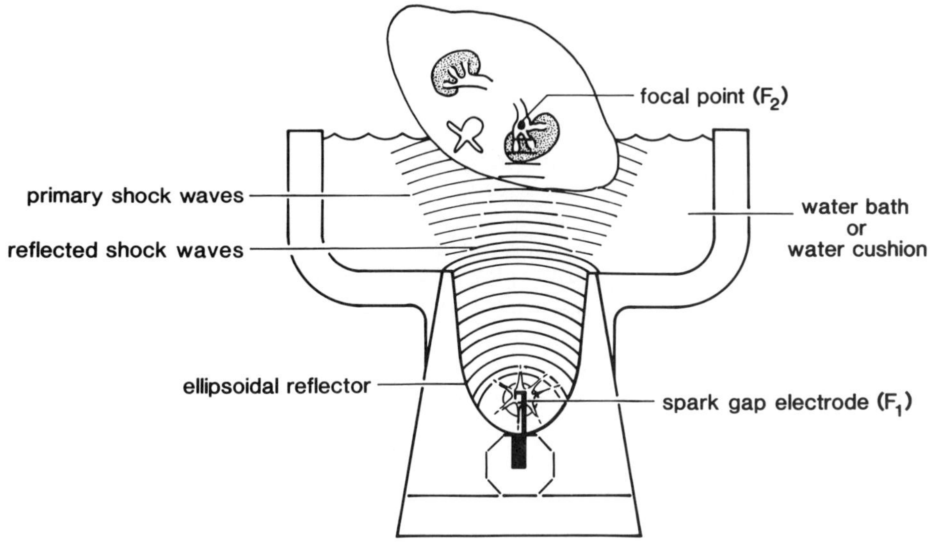

FIGURE 1–4. Spark Gap Shock Wave Generation. Ellipsoidal reflector focuses the shock waves, generated at F_1, to a focal point F_2, in which a kidney stone is positioned.

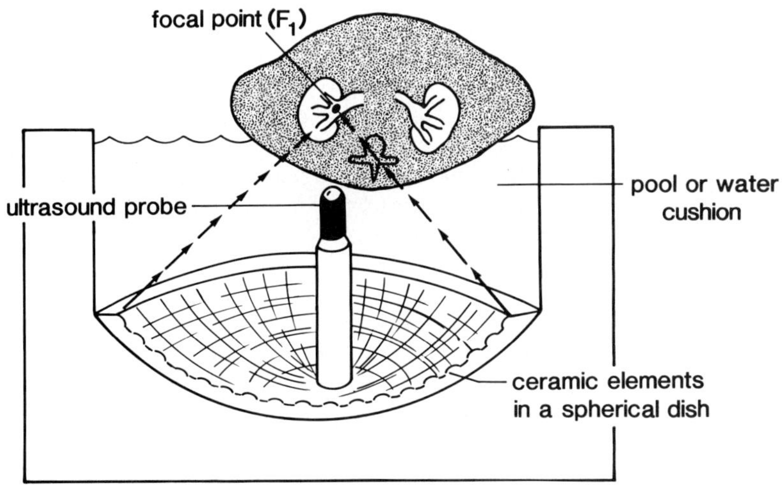

FIGURE 1–5. Piezoelectric Shock Wave Generation. Shock waves emanating from a wide spherical dish are concentrated at the focal point, F_1.

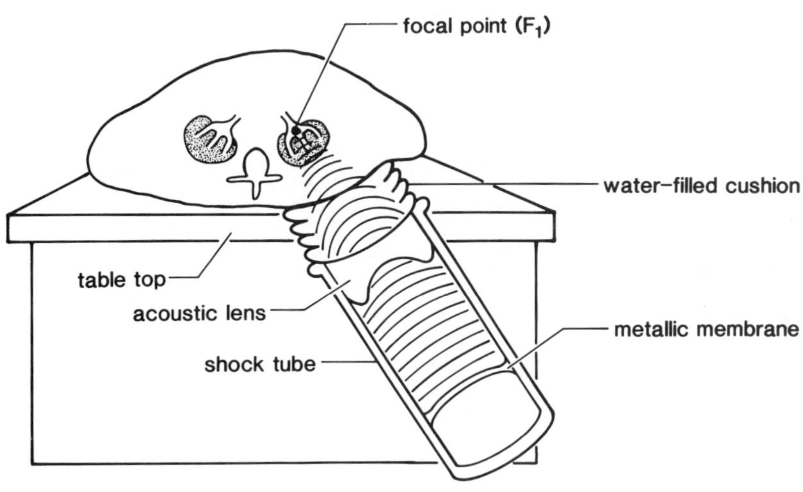

FIGURE 1–6. Electromagnetic Shock Wave Generation. Movable metallic membrane generates shock waves, which are focused to F_1 by an acoustic lens.

of shock wave generation dictates the method of focusing. Machines that use point sources, such as spark gap electrodes, generate shock waves that travel in an expanding circular pattern. All of these machines use ellipsoid reflectors for focusing the shock waves at the second focal point, F_2.

Since a single piezo element produces only a small amount of energy, piezoelectric lithotripters require larger transducers with multiple ceramic elements. The array of ceramic elements is positioned in a spherical dish that allows focusing in a very small focal region, F_1.

The vibrating metal membranes of the electromechanical lithotripters produce an acoustic plane wave that is focused at F_1 by use of an acoustic lens.

Coupling Medium

The original Dornier HM-3 machine used a 1000 L water bath to transmit the shock waves into the patient. This method of patient coupling requires careful positioning of the patient, since the anesthetized subject has to be lowered into the tub and the calculus accurately positioned at the second focal point. Remote monitoring and the physiologic effects of almost total body immersion produced new challenges for the anesthesiologist. Second-generation lithotripters were designed to overcome the physiologic, functional, and economic problems of the large water bath. Current models use an enclosed water cushion, a small exposed pool of water, or a totally contained shock tube. The water-filled cushions and shock tubes contain the shock wave source, conditioned water, and a coupling membrane to allow simplified positioning and "dry" lithotripsy. Two units (Technomed and Wolf) continue to use "wet" methods of patient coupling, however, because some believe that a water-skin interface permits better coupling of the shock wave to the patient than the membrane-skin design.

Stone Localization

During lithotripsy the stone is localized with either fluoroscopy or ultrasonography. Fluoroscopy provides the urologist with a familiar modality and is effective for ureteral stone localization. Moreover, the use of contrast material with fluoroscopy helps to delineate the anatomy of the collecting system. However, fluoroscopy requires more space, carries the risk of ionizing radiation to the patient and medical staff, and is not useful in localizing radiolucent calculi.

Ultrasonography is becoming an increasingly important modality for the urologist. Sonography-based lithotripters offer the advantages of stone localization with continuous monitoring and effective identification of radiolucent stones, without radiation exposure.[8] In addition, ultrasound can localize stone fragments as small as 2 mm and is as good as or better than routine radiography for detecting residual stone fragments following lithotripsy.[9] The ultrasound-based machines also have the important capability of gallstone localization for biliary lithotripsy (multipurpose lithotripters manufactured by Direx, EDAP, Technomed, Storz, and Wolf). The major disadvantages of ultrasound stone localization include the need to master the use of ultrasonic techniques and the difficulty in localizing ureteral stones.

To overcome the limitations of ultrasonography in localizing ureteral calculi, efforts are under way to improve the "echogenicity" of ureteral stents. Enhancement of sonographic stent localization will allow an operator to identify an internal ureteral stent within the renal collecting system and follow the stent and ureter down to the ureteral calculus.[10] Techniques to further enhance ultrasound localization of ureteral calculi include the development of an acoustic transponder[11] as well as integrated reflection C-scan ultrasound imaging.[12] Both of these modalities are still in development.

Anesthesia Requirements

Three factors contribute to the need for anesthesia during extracorporeal shock wave lithotripsy: shock wave pressure (power); area of the shock wave at its skin entry site; and size of the shock wave focal point (Table 1–2). The intensity of the shock wave is determined by the type of generator

TABLE 1–2. Anesthesia Requirements Versus Lithotripter Efficiency

	Dornier HM-3	*Dornier HM-4*	*Technomed Sonolith*	*Siemens Lithostar*	*EDAP LT-01*	*Wolf Piezolith*
Aperture (mm)	156	170	205	120	NA	300
Focal size (mm)	12 × 50	10 × 40	NA	11 × 90	NA	4 × 8
Maximum pressures (bar)	500	NA	780	440	1050	1140
Anesthesia	General	75% sedation	Sedation/general	Sedation, local, or transcutaneous electrical nerve stimulation	Sedation	None
Average number of shock waves	1200	2100	3600	3200	NA	3600
Secondary treatment (%)	16	22	13	18	32	29

NA, Not available.

used and the amount of power (usually electrical charge) supplied to the shock wave generator. The original electrohydraulic design delivers the most powerful shock wave but also causes the greatest discomfort for the patient. Although a single shock wave generated by a spark gap electrode is usually well tolerated, the summation of impulses produces pain at the skin level and within the focal point. Therefore general anesthesia (most commonly), regional anesthesia (spinal or epidural), or local anesthesia (skin infiltration) is necessary when the original spark gap machines are used. Recent studies have demonstrated the ability to use less anesthesia with the first-generation electrohydraulic devices.[13-15]

The size of the focal point and the area of shock wave entry at the skin are determined by the configuration of the focusing device. For example, with the first-generation Dornier HM-3 device, the aperture of the elliptical reflector used for focusing measures 156 mm, which results in a fairly small skin entry site and a relatively large focal area (approximately 12 × 50 mm). In contrast, the Dornier HM-4 (with a modified ellipse) has an aperture of 170 mm, which produces a larger area of shock wave skin entry and a focal size measuring approximately 10 × 40 mm. The increased area of skin entry and diminished focal size have lessened the need for general or regional anesthesia in patients treated with the HM-4, yet approximately 75% of patients still require sedation during the lithotripsy procedure.

The variable-power electrohydraulic lithotripters currently in clinical use are the Dornier HM-5 (MFL-5000) and the Sonolith 2000 ((Diatron generator-Technomed). These machines provide the advantage of a wide range of shock wave intensity to allow either a reduction in anesthesia requirements or an increased fragmentation efficacy with higher power under general or regional anesthesia. Using the lower power setting decreases the overall stone-free rate but increases the number of shocks required per treatment and the retreatment rate.[16-18] Therefore achieving an anesthesia-free status requires an increase in the number of secondary treatments and therefore a diminished efficiency of the lithotripter.

Shock waves generated by a piezoelectric source tend to be less powerful than those from an electrohydraulic source. This leads to a higher retreatment rate, but when combined with other design modifications, allows treatment of stone disease without anesthesia.[8] The aperture of the treatment dish on the Wolf machine measures 300 mm, which results in a large area of skin entry and a very small focal point (approximately 4 × 8 mm). The wide aperture of the focusing sphere, the larger skin entry zone, the small focal point, and lower peak pressures make piezoelectric machines truly anesthesia free. Recent modifications of the piezoelectric generator in the Wolf lithotripter will allow an increase in the shock wave pressure at the focus of 50% (up to approximately 1500 bar). Although the majority of patients treated with this higher power piezoelectric generator require no anesthesia or analgesia, some patients may require sedation or local anesthesia.[19,20]

Design characteristics of the Siemens electromechanical lithotripter place it between the other two machine types in terms of anesthesia requirements. It has an aperture of only 120 mm, resulting in a relatively small skin entry site and a large focal area (approximately 11 × 90 mm). Electromagnetic lithotripsy is usually performed with intravenous or oral sedation, with or without the use of local anesthesia at the skin entry site. Recent studies have demonstrated that a transcutaneous electrical nerve stimulator provides adequate analgesia during lithotripsy with the Siemens device.[21]

The Storz Modulith SL10 electromagnetic generator uses a parabolic metal reflector with a 40 cm diameter to focus the shock wave toward the focal point. This wide aperture has reduced the need for general anesthesia. In a recent study 87% of the patients undergoing treatment with the Storz Modulith required intravenous sedation and 13% needed only orally administered analgesics.[22]

CLINICAL RESULTS

Indications for extracorporeal shock wave lithotripsy in urinary tract stone management are the same as those for surgical intervention (Table 1–3). They include renal colic, urinary obstruction, infection, and decreasing renal function. Clinical studies to evaluate the use of extracorporeal shock wave lithotripsy in gallstone therapy are still in progress.

Relative contraindications to extracorporeal shock wave lithotripsy include large stones, that

TABLE 1–3. Indications and Contraindications for Extracorporeal Shock Wave Lithotripsy

INDICATIONS
Renal colic
Urinary obstruction
Infection
Declining renal function
Significant hematuria
RELATIVE CONTRAINDICATIONS
Calcium oxalate stones >2.5 cm
Struvite stones > 5.0 cm
Cystine stones
Distal obstruction
Poorly informed patients
ABSOLUTE CONTRAINDICATION
Pregnancy

is, calcium oxalate stones greater than 2.5 cm in diameter and struvite stones greater than 5 cm in diameter; cystine stones; distal obstruction; and poorly informed patients. Pregnancy remains an absolute contraindication to this treatment. Theoretically, it might be considered a relative contraindication for piezoelectric lithotripsy because of the small focal zone and lower peak pressures of the piezoelectric devices. No prospective controlled studies are likely to be done to test this hypothesis, however.

Small Calculi

The first-generation Dornier HM-3 represents the "gold standard" in terms of efficacy (overall stone-free rate) in stone fragmentation. As the shock wave pressure (power) and focal region of the second-generation machines have been reduced, so has the requirement for anesthesia or analgesia. However, the price for anesthesia-free lithotripsy is an increase in the secondary treatment rate (reduction in efficiency). For stones less than 1.5 cm in maximal dimension, the Dornier HM-3 lithotripter averages 1200 shocks per treatment and results in a stone-free rate of approximately 85% and a retreatment rate of 16%.[23,24] However, as the shock wave configuration changes owing to widening of the aperture of the ellipsoid (modified Dornier HM-3 and HM-4), the average number of shock waves required increases to 2100 to maintain a stone-free rate of 56% to 82%. In addition, the retreatment rate has been reported to increase to between 22% and 37%.[17,25-30] The Dornier MLF 5000 and Sonolith 2000 variable-power electrohydraulic devices have reduced anesthesia requirements at low power settings. However, with the lower power setting, these machines have approximately a 70% stone-free rate, with a mean number of 2650 shocks at 20 kV and a 14% retreatment rate.[16-18]

Efficiency is also compromised with the piezoelectric lithotripters. Clinical studies with the Wolf Piezolith 2300 and the EDAP LT.01 have reported an 84% to 90% stone-free rate at 3 months for stones less than 1.5 cm in diameter. However, nearly 30% of patients require a second treatment, and the average number of shock waves increases to approximately 3500 shocks per treatment.[8,31-37] The decreased efficiency of the piezoelectric machines is balanced by the convenience of performing treatment as an office procedure, without anesthesia or analgesia.

Electromagnetic lithotripsy, usually performed with intravenous or oral sedation, has been found to require a mean of approximately 3600 shock waves per treatment, with stone-free rates of 69% to 80% and retreatment rates of 7% to 21%.

Large Calculi

With increased stone volume, the efficacy of all lithotripters decreases significantly. For example, with Dornier HM-3 monotherapy the stone-free rate is only 30% for patients with a dilated collecting system and a stone or group of stones with total volume greater than 3 cm.[38] Although the stone-free rate for large calculi is approximately 70% for patients with normal collecting system anatomy, many clinicians still advocate percutaneous nephrolithotripsy as the initial therapy for large renal calculi.[38,39] Studies have found the combination of percutaneous nephrolithotripsy and extracorporeal shock wave lithotripsy to be more effective than extracorporeal shock wave lithotripsy alone. With this type of combination therapy, stone-free rates approaching 85% to 90% have been reported for large renal calculi.[40-44]

Efficiency Quotient

As can be seen from the previous discussion of clinical results for small and large calculi, the determination of lithotripter efficiency requires a delicate balance between the completeness of stone fragmentation and the ability to perform lithotripsy procedures without the need for anesthesia or analgesia. As the shock wave intensity is diminished to permit anesthesia-free lithotripsy, the ability to fragment stones adequately is also reduced, decreasing lithotripter efficiency. Diminished efficiency can be represented by an increase in the number of treatments needed to render a patient stone free, as well as the increased need for auxiliary procedures following lithotripsy, again to attain a stone-free status. Auxiliary procedures include placement of a percutaneous nephrostomy tube, formal percutaneous nephrostolithotomy, ureterorenoscopy, and placement of a ureteral stent to aid in fragment passage.

One can calculate an "efficiency quotient" by determining the stone-free rate obtained by various lithotripters in relation to the need for repeat lithotripsy, as well as the number of auxiliary procedures performed to render patients stone free.[45]

$$\text{Efficiency quotient} = \frac{\text{Percent of patients stone free}}{\text{100\% initial lithotripsy treatments} + \text{\% Repeat lithotripsy treatments} + \text{\% Secondary procedures}}$$

This efficiency quotient can be used to make more valid comparisons between the different types of first- and second-generation lithotripters.

Reports for many second-generation lithotripters have revealed stone-free rates similar to those obtained with the original electrohydraulic lithotripsy devices. If the need for repeat lithotripsy and

TABLE 1–4. Efficiency Quotient for Various Lithotripters

	Stone Fragmentation (%)	Retreatment Rate (%)	Auxiliary Procedures (%)	Efficiency Quotient (%)
FOR STONES LESS THAN 1 CM				
Dornier HM-3	77	5	12	66
Dornier HM-4	85	22	4	60
Direx	75	24	7	57
EDAP	72	29	2	55
Siemens	75	7	11	64
Technomed	81	13	7	68
Wolf	85	16	9	68
FOR STONES 1-2 CM				
Dornier HM-3	75	10	11	62
EDAP	64	68	6	37
Siemens	66	14	24	48
Wolf	69	27	8	51

the number of auxiliary procedures performed were also considered, however, the efficiency quotient of the lower power, second-generation devices and the original electrohydraulic machines would not be equivalent (Table 1–4).

The efficiency quotient is a more reliable gauge than the stone-free rate for comparing the effectiveness of individual lithotripters. For smaller calculi (measuring less than 1 cm), stone-free rates ranging from 77% to 85% have been reported for the Dornier HM-3. Combining these stone-free rates with retreatment rates of 5% to 8% and auxiliary procedure rates of 7% to 12% gives an efficiency quotient of 60% to 66%. For the most part, the lower power, second-generation lithotripters, which require less anesthesia, produce comparable stone-free rates of 72% to 85% for stones less than 1 cm. The efficiency quotients for these devices are also comparable to those of the electrohydraulic machines, which range from 55% to 68%.

The major change in efficiency quotient determination appears with the treatment of larger calculi (Table 1–4). Following treatment for stones between 1 and 2 cm in diameter, the stone-free rates for the first-generation electrohydraulic lithotripters average approximately 75%. With continued low retreatment rates, the efficiency quotient is maintained at 62%. Although the second-generation devices can also obtain stone-free rates between 64% and 69% for stones between 1 and 2 cm, their efficiency rates are only 37% to 51%. This reduced efficiency is due mainly to the significant increase in retreatments necessary for adequate stone fragmentation when these devices are used (Table 1–5).

With their higher retreatment rate, second-generation lithotripters increase the time commitments necessary from both patients and physicians. However, the decrease in stone fragmentation efficiency may be compensated by the fact that many of the second-generation lithotripters can be used in the physician's office, requiring no hospitalization, no intravenous lines, no anesthesia or analgesia, and no recovery room charges. Therefore some physicians and patients may accept the inconvenience of repeat treatment, since the safety and ease of operation of the second-generation machines outweigh the disadvantage of slightly diminished efficiency.

It appears that it is not possible to have true anesthesia-free capabilities with a lithotripsy device that has a high efficiency quotient. To eliminate the need for anesthesia, one has to expect the number of secondary treatments to increase and therefore the efficiency quotient of the lithotripter to be diminished. This trend is likely to continue as manufacturers of electrohydraulic lithotripters modify their shock wave generators to make them anesthesia free.

Stone Location

Stone location in the collecting system is an important determinant of the outcome of extracorporeal shock wave lithotripsy. Stone-free rates for patients with lower calyceal calculi are less than 60%, versus 75% to 80% for middle and upper cal-

TABLE 1–5. Efficiency of Extracorporeal Shock Wave Lithotripsy in Relation to Stone Size

	Stone Size		
	<1.5 cm	1.5-2.9 cm	>3.0 cm
Multiple ESWL (%)	5	10	15-30
Stone-free rate (%)	>90	60	50
Auxiliary procedures (%)	2	5-7	5-15
Repeat hospitalization (%)	1-2	10-15	15-20

yceal stones.[39] Treatment of renal pelvic and upper ureteral stones may result in stone-free rates of 85% to 92%. The success rate is slightly higher with manipulation of proximal ureteral stones into the renal pelvis or with bypass of the stone with a ureteral catheter.[46,47] Stone-free rates of 65% to 70% for lower ureteral calculi (below the pelvic brim) have been achieved through modifications in patient positioning,[47] but ureteroscopy for similar calculi is successful in 95% to 100% of patients. Ureteroscopic extraction is probably still the first choice of therapy for stones in this location.[42,48]

Treatment of stones in calyceal diverticula has long been a source of controversy. Extracorporeal shock wave lithotripsy provided improvement in or resolution of symptoms in 70% of patients in one series but generally renders such patients stone free in only 20% to 30% of cases.[49] Percutaneous management of these stones, by contrast, produces stone-free rates ranging from 87% to 95%.[50,51] These data suggest that calyceal diverticula should be managed with percutaneous techniques, since extracorporeal shock wave lithotripsy is unlikely to produce a stone-free state.

Stone Composition

As the stone composition changes, so does the efficacy of extracorporeal shock wave lithotripsy monotherapy. Harder stones such as calcium oxalate monohydrate require more shocks of higher intensity to achieve adequate fragmentation. Even at these higher settings, however, results with cystine calculi have been inferior to those with calcium oxalate stones.[52] This resistance to fragmentation is believed to be due to the uniform crystal structure of cystine calculi, but as yet is not completely understood. Some investigators advocate the use of combination therapy for large cystine calculi: initial percutaneous nephrolithotripsy followed by extracorporeal shock wave lithotripsy.[40,41,53]

Auxiliary Procedures

An additional controversy has been the efficacy of and indications for the use of ureteral stenting before extracorporeal shock wave lithotripsy. Although results in some clinical series suggest that liberal use of ureteral stents before lithotripsy would be advantageous, the benefits of anesthesia-free lithotripsy would be diminished if anesthesia or analgesia were required for stent placement. In fact, a recent large clinical series evaluating the use of ureteral stents with lithotripsy found no improvement in stone-free rates or increase in post-lithotripsy complications in patients with ureteral stents. However, the incidence of patient morbidity (discomfort, frequency, urgency, hematuria) was significantly higher in patients with ureteral stents.[54] Physicians must exercise judgment regarding the merit of ureteral stenting in individual patients. Patients with large calculi or those requiring general or regional anesthesia for lithotripsy are more likely to need stent placement.

BIOEFFECTS

Complications of extracorporeal shock wave lithotripsy include insufficient stone disintegration and incomplete stone fragment passage. Both problems usually necessitate additional procedures. Symptoms of obstruction such as nausea, vomiting, pain, and even obstructive pyelonephritis may occur during passage of fragments. From 10% to 25% of patients require auxiliary procedures such as ureteroscopy or placement of a percutaneous nephrostomy tube to aid in passage of their stone fragments. Other potentially significant side effects of extracorporeal shock wave lithotripsy have been reported.

In Vitro Studies

Several investigators have used tissue cultures and other in vitro methods as a model for cellular injury induced by extracorporeal shock wave lithotripsy.[55-61] McAteer and associates directed shock waves from the Dornier HM-3 device toward cultured cell lines of proximal and distal renal tubular cells and found the viability of dissociated cells to be influenced by the number of shocks but not the power level.[62] In contrast, Long and associates, studying human renal cancer cells in vitro, found that kilovoltage was a more important determinant of cell damage than the number of shock waves administered.[63]

In an in vitro comparison of cellular effects of the three forms of generated shock waves, Clayman and associates found that electrohydraulic, electromagnetic, and piezoelectric lithotripsy of cell suspensions immediately decreased cell viability. The viable cells did recover and eventually produced near normal growth curves following electromechanical and piezoelectric lithotripsy, but recovery following electrohydraulic lithotripsy was significantly diminished.[64]

High-energy shock waves have been found to kill 60% to 70% of clonogenic rat prostate cells and to have at least a cumulative effect with cisplatin therapy.[65,66] Another study examined the cytotoxic effect of high-energy shock waves on human prostate carcinoma cells in vitro and found a significant reduction in cell survival (<50%) at relatively low doses of shock waves (400 at 18 kV). This study also found that shock wave intensity (kilovoltage) had a greater effect on cell death than did number of shock waves. The investigators noted a correlation between cell damage and the position of the cells along the blast path.[67]

Animal Studies

Gross hematuria is the most consistent sign of renal injury following extracorporeal shock wave lithotripsy. Jaeger and associates have attributed the hematuria to focal renal parenchymal damage found in histologic sections of canine kidneys obtained soon after electrohydraulic lithotripsy.[68] This study documented bleeding foci in the corticomedullary transition area, which appeared to correlate with radiographic changes seen in this region. At 24 to 36 hours after treatment the investigators noted intracapsular and intratubular blood, with vacuolated tubule cells at the edge of these foci, signifying early tubular necrosis. After 3 months following lithotripsy the principal histologic finding was streaky interstitial fibrosis at the site of previously hemorrhagic foci.

In the swine model, where the ion transport, size, and anatomy of the collecting system most closely resemble those of the human kidney, several studies have been performed to investigate the bioeffects of extracorporeal shock wave lithotripsy. Evan and associates evaluated the functional and histologic changes following Dornier HM-3 lithotripsy.[69] They noted two patterns of histologic renal injury: (1) subcapsular hematomas and (2) focal parenchymal changes, including epithelial cell vacuolization, cell necrosis, disruption of the tubular wall, luminal casts, and most consistently, disruption of the peritubular capillary walls. They found no alterations in the glomerular filtration rate (measured by inulin clearance) or the renal blood flow (measured by para-aminohippurate [PAH] clearance), indicating no significant change in the overall renal function.

Many animal studies evaluating the potential deleterious effects of extracorporeal shock wave lithotripsy on renal morphology and function have been performed without stones in the renal collecting system. Although some investigators believe that shock wave energy may be partially absorbed by a stone in the focal region and thus produce less renal injury than a direct insult to the kidney, others suggest that a stone within the collecting system may increase renal damage because of fragmentation or cavitation phenomena. Wilson and associates evaluated the renal changes in swine following piezoelectric lithotripsy with and without a stone in the treated kidney.[70] They were unable to demonstrate any long-term functional or morphologic differences between kidneys treated with and those without a stone in the intrarenal collecting system, suggesting that the key determinants of renal injury are the applied shock wave pressure and the size of the focal region, not the presence or absence of a stone in the treated kidney.

A swine model was also used to compare the renal parenchymal damage and functional impairment for different modes of stone removal.[71] Interestingly, a comparison of pyelotomy incision, nephrotomy incision, extracorporeal piezoelectric lithotripsy, and percutaneous nephrolithotomy showed that none of these significantly reduced renal function as measured by creatinine and PAH clearances. All four modes of renal stone removal produced minimal histologic renal injury and did not significantly impair renal function.

Additional studies have documented histologic changes in rabbits. Immediate changes included subcapsular hematomas and intrarenal and perinephric hemorrhage, while long-term changes were primarily subcapsular and focal parenchymal fibrosis.[72-74] Investigators have found that multiple treatments with a lower number of shock waves may be less damaging than a single treatment with a higher number of shock waves.[75,76] Moreover, Morris and colleagues demonstrated that the different forms of shock wave generation (electrohydraulic, electromechanical, and piezoelectric) produce different types of acute and chronic morphologic changes in rabbits.[77] It appears that the piezoelectric machines produce the least renal tissue injury.

Animal studies have also been performed to evaluate the effects of extracorporeal shock wave lithotripsy on tissue other than renal parenchyma. Damage to other organ systems includes injury to lung parenchyma, pancreatitis, and shock wave–dependent arrhythmias, but these have rarely been clinically significant.[24,78-80] Administration of high-energy shock waves to rat ovaries and growing bone produced only minor changes in bone growth and no significant effect on ovarian tissue or subsequent fertility at clinically relevant shock wave intensity levels.[81,82] These and other clinical studies suggest that extracorporeal shock wave lithotripsy is relatively safe for children and females of reproductive age.[83,84]

Recent studies in young animals, however, have demonstrated increased renal injury with long-term sequelae in developing kidneys. Investigations in rabbits, swine, and primates have demonstrated significant long-term diminution of renal function and renal plasma flow, as well as significant increases in blood pressure and peripheral renin levels, suggesting that immature renal tissue may be at higher risk of significant damage than normal adult renal tissue.[85-87] These data imply that extracorporeal shock wave lithotripsy should be used with caution in children, as well as in patients with renal impairment or limited renal tissue.

Moran and colleagues investigated the effects of high-energy shock waves on rapidly proliferating fetal tissues by exposing chick embryos to shock waves from a Dornier XL-1 experimental lithotripter at a 13 kV power setting.[88] Exposure was immediately lethal to 15% of the embryos because of massive hemorrhaging from both intraembryonic and extraembryonic vessels. Those that survived showed disruption of renal organogenesis. Pregnancy therefore remains an absolute contraindication to extracorporeal shock wave lithotripsy because of teratogenic potential and risk of fetal demise.

Clinical Studies

The immediate postlithotripsy period is marked by a significant increase in levels of serum and urine enzymes, including creatine phosphokinase, lactic dehydrogenase (LDH), aspartate aminotransferace (AST), *N*-acetyl-β-glucoaminidase, β-galactosidase, γ-glutamyltransferase (GGT), as well as transient nephrotic-range proteinuria.[89-91] Recent studies have sought to localize the site of the cellular injury following lithotripsy. Smith and associates found an increase in both brush border enzymes (angiotensin-converting enzyme, GGT) and lysosomal enzymes (α-*N*-acetyl-D-glucosaminidase, β-galactosidase) in the urine of 20 patients 1 day after Sonolith 2000 lithotripsy, although all levels returned to baseline within 1 week.[91] Jaeger also noted an immediate increase in serum LDH, AST, and alanine aminotransferase (ALT), and a delayed increase in alkaline phosphatase in his canine studies. In this series, serum levels of blood urea nitrogen, creatinine, sodium, potassium, and amylase remained normal, but urinary creatinine and glucose excretion decreased sharply, indicating that the proximal tubule was the primary site of injury.[90]

Clinical studies using sonography, computed tomography, and magnetic resonance imaging (MRI) have documented acute morphologic renal changes following electrohydraulic shock wave lithotripsy. Radiographic changes include perinephric edema and hemorrhage, subcapsular and intrarenal hematomas, loss of the corticomedullary demarcation, cystic hemorrhage, and renal enlargement.[92-96] Such changes have been found in up to 85% of patients following electrohydraulic lithotripsy.[97] However, in one recent study MRI scans documented acute morphologic changes in only 5% of patients following piezoelectric lithotripsy.[96] Fortunately, all of these lithotripsy-induced subclinical morphologic renal changes resolved spontaneously.

Clinically significant subcapsular hematomas have been noted in up to 2.5% of patients treated with electrohydraulic lithotripsy. The risk of subcapsular hematoma appears to be greatest in patients with uncontrolled hypertension but also is increased in patients with pretreatment urinary tract infections and those who undergo simultaneous bilateral lithotripsy.[97-99] In one large study that looked at the incidence of subcapsular hematomas following lithotripsy, one third of the patients required blood transfusions.[94] Preexisting blood dyscrasias should also be considered a high risk factor for the development of intrarenal or subcapsular hematomas, and thus physicians should attempt to correct hematologic abnormalities before lithotripsy or should even consider alternative forms of stone therapy.

Hypertension may be the most important possible side effect of extracorporeal shock wave lithotripsy. In 1987 Lingeman and associates reported the results of a retrospective study of 295 patients, in which they discovered an 8.2% incidence of new-onset hypertension requiring drug therapy 1 or more years following stone treatment.[100] They also noted a 15.2% incidence of increased diastolic blood pressure not requiring therapy. These findings were similar to those of Kaude and colleagues, which also suggested an 8% incidence of new-onset hypertension.[93] However, several recent animal and human studies have failed to demonstrate any cause-and-effect relationship between extracorporeal shock wave lithotripsy and the development of hypertension when lithotripsy patients were compared with age-matched control subjects.[23,101-104] Lingeman and colleagues recently performed a large retrospective clinical trial in which they found that the annual incidence of hypertension in patients undergoing extracorporeal shock wave lithotripsy did not differ significantly from that in control patients.[105] Among patients who received extracorporeal shock wave lithotripsy, they found no correlation between the incidence of hypertension and whether treatments were unilateral or bilateral, the number of shock waves administered, the kilovoltage applied, or the power of the shock waves.

Recent work in animals has suggested an increase risk of hypertension in immature kidneys, as well as in normal adult kidneys that receive excessive shock wave energy.[85,87,106] Therefore most investigators still agree that a well-designed, long-term clinical trial must be performed to answer important questions about the potential deleterious clinical effects of extracorporeal shock wave lithotripsy (hypertension, diminished renal function, alterations in ion transport, etc.).

BILIARY LITHOTRIPSY

The principles of stone fragmentation with extracorporeal shock wave lithotripsy have also been applied to the biliary tract.[107,108] Goals of this program are twofold: to find a less expensive treatment for cholelithiasis than cholecystectomy and to reduce the small, but present, morbidity and mortality of biliary tract surgery and general anesthesia.[109,110] Studies have shown that human gallstones implanted into canine gallbladders can be fragmented by means of extracorporeal lithotripsy and that stone fragments of up to 2 mm can pass from the gallbladder through the cystic duct and the ampulla of Vater. In fact, glass beads up to 5 mm in diameter implanted into canine gallbladders pass from the gallbladder to the duodenum within 1 month in 11% of cases.[111]

The first reported series of humans undergoing extracorporeal biliary lithotripsy included 14 patients treated in Munich with a Dornier HM-3 lithotripter.[112] Nine patients had functioning gallbladders containing symptomatic gallstones, and five patients had common bile duct stones that could not be removed endoscopically. Six of the nine patients with cholelithiasis had complete stone disappearance within 25 weeks. In four of the five patients with common bile duct stones, extracorporeal lithotripsy achieved stone disintegration, permitting successful transampullary endoscopic extraction or spontaneous passage of stone fragments. The only side effects detected during a follow-up period of 34 weeks were transient biliary pain in two patients and mild pancreatitis in one patient.

In the Munich study all patients received a combination of chenodiol and ursodiol to dissolve stone fragments that did not pass into the intestine spontaneously. Both drugs were administered 1 week before lithotripsy, and these drugs were continued up to 6 months after complete disappearance of stones.[112]

The Munich group recently reported the results of extracorporeal biliary lithotripsy in 175 patients.[113] Successful stone fragmentation was achieved in all but one of the patients. In 91% of patients followed up for 12 to 18 months, no gallstones were detected. The only side effects of lithotripsy were cutaneous petechiae (14%) and transient gross hematuria (3%). One third of the patients had biliary colic after fragmentation. Two patients had pancreatitis, requiring endoscopic sphincterotomy in one case.

In vitro and animal experiments with piezoelectric lithotripters have demonstrated gallstone fragmentation with minimal damage to surrounding tissues. In canine studies 4000 pulses from a piezoelectric device focused on the gallbladder caused small subcapsular and parenchymal hepatic and gallbladder hematomas, but these resolved completely within 6 weeks.[111]

Clinical experience from Europe suggests that piezoelectric lithotripsy is effective for the treatment of biliary tract calculi. Studies from London, Erlangen, and Vienna have demonstrated that this second-generation machine fragments gallstones and common bile duct stones adequately without the need for anesthesia or analgesia.[114-116]

The extracorporeal biliary lithotripsy trials conducted in the United States have generally incorporated patient selection criteria derived from the European experience. As with the initial studies, the current clinical trials have restrictive inclusion and exclusion criteria (Table 1–6). Patients who have symptoms or signs of extrahepatic biliary obstruction and those whose common bile ducts are greater than 8 mm in diameter when measured by ultrasound undergo cholangiography before entrance into the protocol.

TABLE 1–6. Inclusion and Exclusion Criteria for Recent Clinical Trials of Biliary Lithotripsy

INCLUSION CRITERIA

- Gallbladder imaging by oral, transampullary, or transhepatic cholecystograms
- Specific symptoms attributable to biliary calculi
- Calculi noncalcified
- Calculi demonstrable by ultrasonography
- No stone larger than 2 cm in maximal diameter
- Three or fewer stones
- Stone mass no larger than 3 cm in maximal diameter
- One stone at least 5 mm in diameter

EXCLUSION CRITERIA

- Requirement for bile acid–sequestering agent such as cholestyramine and colestipol, as well as aluminum-based antacids
- Age less than 18 years
- Allergies or intolerance to oral bile acids
- Pregnant patients and nursing mothers
- Hepatic lesions or vascular calcifications in the lithotripsy pulse wave path
- Acute cholecystitis, cholangitis, pancreatitis, or hepatitis
- Recurrent gallstones and previous successful biliary lithotripsy
- Liver enzyme levels greater than three times normal
- Uncorrectable bleeding disorder
- Patient cannot undergo cholecystography because of allergies or intolerances

Although biliary lithotripsy is technically feasible, the differences between the biliary and urinary tracts must be considered in evaluating the overall impact of biliary lithotripsy. Gallstones are significantly softer than most renal calculi, and in vitro studies suggest that gallstones do not fragment as well as renal calculi. Most gallstones float within the gallbladder, making continuous targeting more difficult. Moreover, access to the biliary tract is more difficult than routine access to the urinary tract. Endoscopic access can be gained either through a percutaneous approach or via esophagogastroduodenoscopy with direct cannulation of the common bile duct.[117,118]

Although long-term follow-up is not yet available, preliminary results from the U.S. clinical trials have demonstrated stone-free rates of approximately 47% for solitary gallstones.[119] The stone-free rate drops to approximately 20% when multiple gallstones are treated, yielding an overall stone-free rate of approximately 30%.[120] These results are not as good as those reported from Europe, probably because the entrance criteria of the initial European studies were more restrictive.

Questions have been raised about the long-term consequences of biliary lithotripsy. These include the stone recurrence rate following successful removal of stone fragments, the fate of a "diseased" gallbladder after the removal of gallstones via lithotripsy, and the potential for lithotripsy to alter gallbladder function. Although the incidence of symptomatic cholelithiasis is nearly ten times that of symptomatic nephrolithiasis, a major problem in identifying appropriate patients for biliary lithotripsy has been the rigid selection criteria of the current clinical trials. Surprisingly, the most common contraindication to biliary lithotripsy is lack of patient interest, mainly because they must take oral chemolytic medication for a minimum of 1 to 2 years after lithotripsy.[121,122] The inconvenience and cost (over $100 per month) have caused many candidates to select other therapy. Only approximately 10% to 20% of patients referred for biliary lithotripsy have been enrolled in the clinical trials.

As in the early days of extracorporeal shock wave lithotripsy for renal calculi, the absolute indications and contraindications for biliary lithotripsy have yet to be determined. Only after the completion of long-term clinical trials will the true impact of biliary lithotripsy on the management of symptomatic cholelithiasis be known.

NEW DEVELOPMENTS

Limitations of Current Lithotripters

In the decade since the first clinical application of extracorporeal shock wave lithotripsy by Chaussy and associates, technical refinements have produced more than 10 second-generation devices. These designs concentrated on altering the methods of shock wave generation, focusing, coupling, and localization, with the primary goal of equaling the stone-free rate of the Dornier HM-3 while increasing the safety, convenience, and cost-effectiveness of treatment. The new devices are designed to improve stone fragmentation, to decrease or eliminate anesthesia requirements, and to decrease radiation exposure from x rays. Despite great technical progress, however, these new machines have specific shortcomings.

In general, second-generation lithotripters can be divided into a higher power electrohydraulic and electromagnetic group and a lower power piezoelectric group. Disadvantages of the first group include pain necessitating anesthesia and renal tissue damage. Disadvantages of the second group include a small focal size of the shock wave, the need for a greater total number of shock waves, and a higher retreatment rate.

Because the apertures of the electrohydraulic and electromechanical lithotripters are relatively small, the skin entry site is smaller and the focal zone is larger. The large focal zone creates the need for general or regional anesthesia or heavy intravenous sedation in most cases. The larger aperture of the treatment dish of the piezoelectric lithotripters results in a large area of skin entry and a small focal zone. The discomfort produced by treatments with these machines is minimal enough to allow anesthesia-free lithotripsy.[8]

The relatively large focal region of the electrohydraulic lithotripters exposes a larger amount of normal renal tissue to maximal shock wave pressures. The aforementioned animal and clinical studies have demonstrated more acute renal parenchymal injury from electrohydraulic and electromagnetic lithotripers than from piezoelectric shock wave administration.

The drawback of the small focal region in the piezoelectric machines is that it mandates constant monitoring of the effects of treatment on the fragmenting calculus. Accurate focusing of the shock wave is mandatory, since pressure drops off rapidly outside the small focal zone. The requirement of exact focusing is not necessary with the electrohydraulic or electromagnetic machines, which have a much larger area of maximal shock wave energy. As noted previously, the advantage gained by performing anesthesia-free lithotripsy must be weighed against less efficient stone fragmentation. Apparently it is not possible to have both anesthesia-free capabilities and a very "efficient" lithotripter that has only a minimal secondary treatment rate (less than 10%).

Additional limitations of current lithotripsy devices relate to the method of stone localization. Although the lithotripters using fluoroscopy can visualize the entire urinary system, they expose the patient to significant radiation. In addition, identifying small calculi within the kidney or ureter, as well as radiolucent stones, is nearly impossible. Furthermore, fluoroscopy is not useful for the visualization of most biliary stones.

The devices that use sonography for stone localization potentially can be used for both renal and biliary lithotripsy and pose no risk of radiation exposure. Their main disadvantage is that they offer poor visualization of stones in the middle and lower ureter. As noted previously, efforts to develop echogenic ureteral stents, as well as new modes of sonography for ureteral stone localization, are in progress.

The Ideal Lithotripter

Extracorporeal shock wave lithotripsy can be used effectively to treat most renal and ureteral calculi with minimal morbidity and convalescence. Research in lithotripter design is ongoing, however, with attempts to improve performance and ultimately to design the "ideal lithotripter" (Table 1–7). Such a device should be compact and portable, so that it can be transported or shared between small institutions. In fact, mobile lithotripsy units are in operation across the United States. The ideal lithotripter should also be adaptable for other pro-

TABLE 1–7. The Ideal Lithotripter

Low cost (purchase and operation)
Portable and compact
Powerful
Adjustable energy source
Adaptable for other procedures (endourology)
Multipurpose (renal and biliary)
Anesthesia-free capability
Reliable
Easy to use

cedures such as endourology and biliary lithotripsy. Some of the machines that use fluoroscopic stone localization can be used for percutaneous stone removal, as well as ureteroscopic procedures. Moreover, the ultrasound-based machines can be used for both urinary and biliary calculi.

By having an adjustable energy source, the ideal lithotripter would permit anesthesia-free treatments of smaller or "routine" calculi, yet would have the power required to fragment hard or large renal or ureteral stones. This capability would lead to effective and efficient lithotripsy treatments, with the knowledge that in some cases sedation or anesthesia will be necessary to allow the use of more powerful shock wave energy.

Finally, the ideal lithotripter would be economical to install and operate. Minimal site renovations would be needed before installation of the lithotripter, and daily operating costs would be low.

Third Generation Lithotripters

Designers of a number of third-generation lithotripters have tried to incorporate many of the characteristics of the ideal lithotripter (Table 1–8). The basic design of the third-generation machines includes dual imaging capabilities and variable shock wave power. Four third-generation lithotripters are currently undergoing clinical trials in both the United States and Western Europe. These include the Dornier MFL 5000 (HM-5), Siemens Lithostar Plus, Storz Modulith SL20, and Wolf Piezolith 2500.[19,20,123-125]

Dual Imaging

Dual imaging capability entails having both fluoroscopic and sonographic localization systems in the same machine. Such a design has the advantage of using fluoroscopy for imaging stones within the kidney and ureter, with the option of sonography for the identification of radiolucent or biliary tract calculi. Another advantage of a sonographic localization system is that the operator can use fluoroscopy to target a stone and then switch to sonography to avoid excessive ionizing radiation. Moreover, having fluoroscopy capabilities may aid in the learning process for many urologists who are unfamiliar with sonographic stone localization procedures.

Interestingly, although the Dornier, Siemens, and Storz machines all have ultrasound capabilities to provide dual imaging, none of these systems provides "in-line" imaging for both the fluoroscopic and sonographic localization devices. For example, with the Dornier and Siemens devices the operator can use sonography to target a radiolucent or biliary tract calculus, yet the patient must be moved "blindly" to the fluoroscopy unit, which is in-line with the shock wave generator. With the Storz machine the operator can use the fluoroscopic localization system, yet only the ultrasound is in-line with the shock wave generator.

The Wolf Piezolith 2500 is the only third-generation device that has both the fluoroscopy and the sonography in-line with the piezoelectric shock wave generator. This permits a rapid change from fluoroscopic to sonographic stone localization, without moving the patient off the treatment dish.

Variable Power

All four of the third-generation devices mentioned previously have variable power shock wave generators. This capability allows the shock wave energy to be tailored to the requirements of a particular stone. The operator can turn down the generator power to significantly reduce anesthesia and analgesia requirements with the Dornier, Siemens, and Storz machines, as well as to provide totally anesthesia- and analgesia-free lithotripsy with the Wolf device. Moreover, with all four machines the shock wave intensity can be increased to allow adequate fragmentation of extremely hard or large calculi. However, when used in the "high-power mode," these lithotripters require various forms of anesthesia or analgesia.

Clearly the "ultimate shock wave" that allows

TABLE 1–8. Third-Generation Lithotripters

Manufacturer	*Shock Wave Generation*	*Focusing*	*Patient Coupling*	*In-Line Localization**
Dornier HM-5	Spark gap	Ellipsoid	Membrane	Fluoroscopy
Siemens Lithostar Plus	Electromagnetic	Acoustic lens	Membrane	Two fluoroscopic tubes
Storz Modulith SL 20	Electromagnetic	Parabolic reflector	Membrane	Ultrasound
Wolf Piezolith 2500	Piezoelectric	Spherical	Membrane	Ultrasound and fluoroscopy

*Describes which of the localization systems is "in-line" with the shock wave generator.

anesthesia-free lithotripsy with maximum efficiency is still in the future. Yet, by varying the shock wave energy, the operator can administer a highly efficient shock wave, recognizing the need for anesthesia or analgesia when high shock wave pressures are indicated.

Although the industry has pushed for anesthesia-free capabilities in recent years, many physicians have perhaps not been aware of or have ignored the potentially deleterious effect of excessive administration of the higher power electrohydraulic shock waves. Now, with the availability of variable-power lithotripters that use electrohydraulic, electromagnetic, and piezoelectric energy sources, the operator must continue to monitor the amount of energy delivered to limit the incidence of significant renal injury.

CONCLUSION

Extracorporeal shock wave lithotripsy has revolutionized the treatment of urinary calculi. It should be considered the treatment of choice for all renal calculi smaller than 2 cm and for most nonimpacted ureteral calculi. Under these circumstances, stone-free rates approaching 90% can be expected. For larger renal stones or impacted ureteral calculi, endoscopic techniques, with or without adjunctive intracorporeal lithotripsy (ultrasonic, electrohydraulic, or laser fragmentation) should probably be used.

Potential complications of extracorporeal shock wave lithotripsy must be kept in mind. Known complications include incomplete stone fragmentation and obstruction resulting from incomplete passage of stone fragments. Potential complications, especially in patients with immature kidneys or impaired renal function, include hypertension and chronic loss of renal function. Long-term clinical studies to investigate these deleterious effects have yet to be completed.

Biliary lithotripsy showed great promise in early European studies. Stone-free rates in German studies approach 90%. Probably owing to less restrictive entrance criteria in this country, however, U.S. clinical trials have not been as successful. In addition, the cost and inconvenience of posttreatment medication have limited the enrollment of patients in clinical trials to 10% to 20% of those referred. Because of the recent successful introduction of laparoscopic cholecystectomy, the future of biliary lithotripsy in the United States is questionable.

Whereas the original lithotripter design necessitated general anesthesia and a 1000 L water bath and subjected patients to fairly high doses of ionizing radiation, technical refinements in the second-generation devices have increased the safety and convenience of lithotripsy. Although decreasing the shock wave pressure and focal size has diminished or eliminated anesthesia requirements, the price has been a rise in the retreatment rate. An "efficiency quotient" can be used to compare the relative benefits and disadvantages of various second-generation machines. Current lithotripters do not rate high on the efficiency quotient scale while maintaining anesthesia-free capabilities. Third-generation machines, however, with modifications to allow variable shock wave power, use for auxiliary procedures, and dual imaging capabilities, should achieve this goal. As research continues and new devices become adaptable to multiple tasks, we will come closer to making the "ideal lithotripter" a reality.

REFERENCES

1. Chaussy C, Schmiedt E, Jocham D, et al: First clinical experience with extracorporeally induced destruction of kidney stones by shock waves. J Urol 127:417, 1982.
2. Coleman AJ, Saunders JE, Crum LA, Dyson M: Acoustic cavitation generated by an extracorporeal shockwave lithotripter. Ultrasound Med Biol 13:69, 1987.
3. Williams AR, Delius M, Miller DL, Schwarze W: Investigation of cavitation in flowing media by lithotripter shock waves both in vitro and in vivo. Ultrasound Med Biol 15:53, 1989.
4. Hunter PT, Finlayson B, Hirko RJ, et al: Measurement of shock wave pressures used for lithotripsy. J Urol 136:733, 1986.
5. Coleman AJ, Saunders JE: A survey of the acoustic output of commercial extracorporeal shock wave lithotripters. Ultrasound Med Biol 15:213, 1989.
6. Chuong CJC, Zhong P, Preminger GM: Stone damage modes during piezoelectric shock wave delivery. J Urol 141:341A, 1989.
7. Zhong P, Chuong CJC, Preminger JM: Stone damage modes from three different lithotripters. J Urol 143:229A, 1990.
8. Preminger GM: Sonographic, piezoelectric lithotripsy: more bang for your buck. J Endourol 3:321, 1989.
9. Abernathy BB, Morris JS, Wilson WT, et al: Evaluation of residual stone fragments following lithotripsy: sonography versus KUB. In Lingeman JE, Newman DM (eds): Shock wave lithotripsy II: urinary and biliary lithotripsy. New York: Plenum Press, 1989, Chapter 47, p 247.
10. Wilson WT, Feagins BA, Preminger GM: Development of an echogenic stent to aid in sonographic stone localization. J Urol 143:260A, 1990.
11. Laungani JB, Grunberger I, Marich KW, Stein A: Acoustic transponder improves ureteral stone localization. J Endourol 4:S158, 1990.
12. Marich KW, Stein A, Jensen JF, et al: Improved ultrasound localization and characterization of calculi for lithotripsy using reflex transmission imaging. J Endourol 4:S159, 1990.
13. Fried FA, Anderson J: Experiences with conscious sedation in ESWL. J Endourol 4:S102, 1990.
14. Lazica M, Thuroff J, Hausler E: High-pass filtering, a new development in ESWL. J Endourol 4:S102, 1990.
15. Monk TG, White PF, Meretyk S, Clayman RV: Anesthesia for shock wave lithotripsy: a comparison of epidural and intravenous sedative-analgesic techniques using an unmodified HM-3 lithotripter. J Endourol 4:S103, 1990.
16. Benkert S, Graff J, Pastor J, Senge Th: Experience with a new multi-functional lithotripter MFL 5000: results of 300 treatments. In Lingeman JE, Newman DM (eds): Shock wave lithotripsy II: urinary and biliary. New York: Plenum Press, 1989, Chapter 79, p 431.
17. Jocham D, Liedl B, Schuster C, et al: New techniques and

developments in ESWL: Dornier HM4 and MPL 9000. Urol Res 16:255A, 1988.
18. Tomera KM, Benson RC, Martin X: Sonolith 2000: Technomed International. In Copcoat MJ, Miller RA, Wickham JEA (eds): Lithotripsy II. London: BDI Publishing, 1987.
19. Turk C, Steinkogler I, Krings F, Marberger M: First experience with a lithotripter with in-line ultrasonic and fluoroscopic stone localization. J Endourol 4:S90, 1990.
20. Neisius D, Zwergel TH, Jung P, Ziegler M: Extracorporeal piezoelectric lithotripsy (EPL) with the new Piezolith 2500: first clinical experiences. J Endourol 4:S92, 1990.
21. Fernandez J, Clayman RV, Gray D, McClennan BL: Transcutaneous electrical nerve stimulator: an approach to anesthesia-free shock wave lithotripsy with the Lithostar unit. In Lingeman JE, Newman DM (eds): Shock wave lithotripsy. New York: Plenum Press, 1988, Chapter 34, p 181.
22. Rassweiler J, Cohrmann U, Heini G, et al: Modulith SL10/20: first clinical experience with a new interdisciplinary lithotripter. Z Urol Poster 2:75, 1990.
23. Graff J, Diederichs W, Schulze H: Long-term follow up in 1003 extracorporeal shock wave lithotripsy patients. J Urol 140:479, 1988.
24. Lingeman JE, Newman DM, Hertz JHO, et al: Extracorporeal shock wave lithotripsy: the Methodist Hospital experience. J Urol 135:1134, 1986.
25. Graff J, Schmidt A, Pastor J, et al: New generator for low pressure lithotripsy with the Dornier HM-3: preliminary experience of two centers. J Urol 139:904, 1988.
26. Newman D, Lingeman H, Mossbaugh P, et al: ESWL treatment using IV analgesia alone with an "unmodified" Dornier HM-3 lithotripter. In Lingeman JE, Newman DM (eds): Shock wave lithotripsy II: urinary and biliary. New York: Plenum Press, 1989, Chapter 75, p 411.
27. Marks J, Leiter E, Fruchtman B: Experience with Medstone second generation lithotripter. In Lingeman JE, Newman DM (eds): Shock wave lithotripsy II: urinary and biliary. New York: Plenum Press, 1989, Chapter 72, p 393.
28. Rassweiler J, Gumpinger R, Mayer R, et al: Extracorporeal piezoelectric lithotripsy using the Wolf-Lithotripter versus low energy lithotripsy with the modified Dornier HM-3: a cooperative study. World J Urol 5:218, 1987.
29. Voegeli T, Mellin HE, Ackermann R: High dose ESWL with modified HM-3 lithotripter. In Lingeman JE, Newman DM (eds): Shock wave lithotripsy II: urinary and biliary. New York: Plenum Press, 1989, Chapter 13, p 67.
30. Wilbert DM, Bichler KH, Strohmaier WL, Fluchter SH: Initial experience with the second generation lithotripter Dornier HM4. Urol Res 16:262A, 1988.
31. Kiely EA, Ryan PC, McDermont TE, et al: EDAP piezoelectric shock wave lithotripsy: experience in 511 patients. In Lingeman JE, Newman DM (eds): Shock wave lithotripsy II: urinary and biliary. New York: Plenum Press, 1989, Chapter 68, p 371.
32. Marberger M, Turk C, Steinkogler I: Painless piezo-electric extracorporeal lithotripsy. J Urol 139:695, 1988.
33. McNicholas TA, Carter ST, Wickham JEA: One year of lithotripsy with the Wolf Piezolith 2300. In Lingeman JE, Newman DM (eds): Shock wave lithotripsy II: urinary and biliary. New York: Plenum Press, 1989, Chapter 70, p 381.
34. Philip T, Kellett MJ, Whitfield HN, Wickham JEA: Painless lithotripsy: experience with 100 patients. Lancet 2:41, 1988.
35. Preminger GM, Ewing JH: Piezoelectric lithotripsy: initial experience with the Wolf 2200. In Lingeman JE, Newman DM (eds): Shock wave lithotripsy: state of the art. New York: Plenum Press, 1988, Chapter 57, pp 281-284.
36. Vallancien G, Aviles J, Munoz R, et al: Piezoelectric extracorporeal lithotripsy by ultrashort waves with the EDAP LT01 device. J Urol 139:689, 1988.
37. Zwergel U, Neisius D, Zwergel T, Ziegler M: Results and clinical management of extracorporeal piezoelectric lithotripsy (EPL) in 1321 consecutive treatments. World J Urol 5:213, 1987.
38. Winfield HN, Clayman RV, Chaussy CG, et al: Monotherapy of staghorn renal calculi: comparative study between percutaneous nephrolithotomy and extracorporeal shock wave lithotripsy. J Urol 139:895, 1988.
39. McDougall EM, Denstedt JD, Clayman RV, et al: Lower pole calyceal calculi: extracorporeal shock wave lithotripsy (ESWL) vs. percutaneous nephrostolithotomy (PCN). J Endourol 3:265, 1989.
40. Brown RD, Preminger GM: Changing surgical aspects in urinary stone disease. In Resnick MI (ed): Surgery clinics of North America. Philadelphia: Saunders, 1988, pp 1085-1104.
41. Chang CR, Webb DR, Payne SR, Wichhara JE: Comparison of treatment of renal calculi; by open surgery, percutaneous nephrolithotomy and extracorporeal shock wave lithotripsy. Br Med J 292:879, 1986.
42. Eisenberger F, Fuchs G, Miller K: Extracorporeal shock wave lithotripsy and endourology: an ideal combination for the treatment of kidney stones. World J Urol 3:41, 1985.
43. Kahnoski RJ, Lingeman JE, Lowry TA, et al: Combined percutaneous and extracorporeal shock wave lithotripsy for staghorn calculi: an alternative to anatrophic nephrolithotomy. J Urol 135:679, 1986.
44. Schultz H, Hertu L, Graff J, et al: Combined treatment of branched calculi by percutaneous nephrostolithotomy and extracorporeal shock wave lithotripsy. J Urol 135:1138, 1986.
45. Denstedt JD, Clayman RV, Preminger GM: Efficiency quotient as a means of comparing lithotripters. J Urol 143:376A, 1990.
46. Fetner CD, Preminger GM, Seger JA, Lea TA: Treatment of ureteral calculi by extracorporeal shockwave lithotripsy at a multi-use center. J Urol 139:1192-1194, 1988.
47. Muller SC, Wilbert D, Thuroff JW, et al: Extracorporeal shock wave lithotripsy of ureteral stones: clinical experience and experimental findings. J Urol 135:831, 1986.
48. Fuchs GJ, Chaussy CG, Bender L, Stenzl A: Current management concepts in the treatment of ureteral stones. In Lingeman JE, Newman DM (eds): Shock wave lithotripsy. New York: Plenum Press, 1988, Chapter 10, p 55.
49. Psihramis KG, Dretler SP: Extracorporeal shock wave lithotripsy of calyceal diverticula calculi. J Urol 138:707, 1987.
50. Hulbert JC, Reddy PK, Hunter DW: Percutaneous techniques for the management of caliceal diverticula containing calculi. J Urol 135:225, 1986.
51. Lingeman JE, Jones JA, Steidle CP: ESWL versus percutaneous management of calyceal diverticula. J Endourol 4:S140, 1990.
52. Bhatta KM, Prien E, Dretler SP: Cystine calculi: two types. In Lingeman JE, Newman DM (eds): Shock wave lithotripsy II: urinary and biliary. New York: Plenum Press, 1989, Chapter 11, p 55.
53. Hockley N, Lingeman J, Hutchison C: The relative efficacy of extracorporeal shock wave lithotripsy and percutaneous nephrostolithotomy in the management of cystine calculi. In Lingeman JE, Newman DM (eds): Shock wave lithotripsy II: urinary and biliary. New York: Plenum Press, 1989, Chapter 52, p 277.
54. Preminger GM, Kettelhut MC, Elkins SL, et al: Ureteral stenting during extracorporeal shock wave lithotripsy: help or hindrance? J Urol 142:32-36, 1989.
55. Chaussy CG, Randazzo RF, Fuchs GJ: The effects of extracorporeal shock waves on FANFT bladder tumors in C3H/He mice. J Urol 135:289A, 1986.
56. Chaussy CG, Randazzo RF, Fuchs JG: The effects of extracorporeal shock waves on human renal carcinoma cells and normal human embryonic kidney cells. J Urol 135:320A, 1986.
57. Drach GW: Effects of shock waves on cells and tissues—

critical factors in the conduct of research. J Urol 141:964, 1989.
58. Laudone VP, Morgan TR, Huryk RF, et al: Cytotoxicity of high energy shock waves: methodologic considerations. J Urol 141:965, 1989.
59. McCullough DL, Holmes RP, Li WJ, et al: The effect of shock waves and cisplatin therapy on rat prostate tumor growth. In Lingeman JE, Newman DM (eds): Shock wave lithotripsy II: urinary and biliary. New York: Plenum Press, 1989, Chapter 22, p 111.
60. Russo P, Stephenson R, Heston W, Fair W: The in vitro effect of high energy shock waves on human prostate cancer cell line PC-3. Proc Am Assoc Cancer Res 26:267, 1985.
61. Russo P, Stephenson RA, Mies C, et al: High energy shock waves suppress tumor growth in vitro and in vivo. J Urol 135:626, 1986.
62. McAteer JA, Evan AP, Haak R, Lingeman JE: Cell culture and in vitro to assess the bioeffects of ESWL. J Urol 141:228A, 1989.
63. Marcus M, Long S, Denstedt J, Clayman RV: Bioeffects of extracorporeal shock wave lithotripsy: the relationship of applied voltage and shock wave number to cell viability. J Urol 143:230A, 1990.
64. Clayman RV, Preminger GM, Long S, et al: A comparison of the in vitro cellular effects of shock waves generated by electrohydraulic, electromagnetic and piezoelectric sources. J Urol 141:228A, 1989.
65. Behrens MI, Welander CE, Griffith AS, McCullough DL: High energy shock waves (HESW) inhibit tumor cell proliferation and potentiate efficacy of cytotoxic agents. J Urol 137:228A, 1987.
66. McCullough DL, Holmes RP, Li WJ, et al: The effect of shock waves and cisplatin therapy on rat prostate tumor growth. In Lingeman JE, Newman DM (eds): Shock wave lithotripsy II: urinary and biliary. New York: Plenum Press, 1989, Chapter 17, p 91.
67. Kaver I, Koontz WW, Wilson JD, et al: The effect of shock waves on human prostatic carcinoma cells in vitro. In Lingeman JE, Newman DM (eds): Shock wave lithotripsy II: urinary and biliary. New York: Plenum Press, 1989, Chapter 22, p 111.
68. Jaeger P, Redha F, Uhlschmid G, Hauri D: Morphologic changes after shock wave treatment of canine kidneys. In Lingeman JE, Newman DM (eds): Shock wave lithotripsy. New York: Plenum Press, 1988, Chapter 70, p 341.
69. Evan AP, McAteer JA, Steidle LP, et al: Acute renal changes induced by ESWL in the minipig. J Urol 141:228A, 1989.
70. Wilson WT, Morris JS, Hussman DA, et al: Evaluation of stone-shock wave interaction during piezoelectric lithotripsy. J Urol 143:230A, 1990.
71. Wilson WT, Miller GL, Hussman DS, et al: Deleterious effects of four modes of renal stone removal: how does lithotripsy fare? J Urol 143:361A, 1990.
72. Abrahams C, Lipson S, Ross L: Pathologic changes in the kidney and other organs of dogs undergoing extracorporeal shock wave lithotripsy with a tubless lithotripter. J Urol 140:391, 1988.
73. Donovan JM, Weber C, Farjardo LL, et al: The effects of ESWL on rabbit and rat microvasculature. J Urol 141:227A, 1989.
74. Gunasekaran S, Donovan JM, Chuapil M, Drach GW: Effects of extracorporeal shock wave lithotripsy on the structure and function of rabbit kidney. J Urol 141:1250, 1989.
75. Fuchs AM, Coulson W, Fuchs GJ: The effect of extracorporeally induced high energy shock waves on the rabbit kidney and ureter: a morphologic and functional study. J Endourol 2:341, 1988.
76. Morris JS, Hussman DA, Wilson WT, Preminger GM: Temporal effects of shock wave lithotripsy. J Urol 143:131A, 1990.
77. Morris JS, Hussman DA, Wilson WT, et al: Piezoelectric versus spark-gap lithotripsy: a comparison of morphologic and functional alterations. J Urol vol 141, 1989.
78. Chaussy C: Extracorporeal shock wave lithotripsy: new aspects in the treatment of kidney stone disease. Basel: Karger, 1982.
79. Drach GW, Dretler S, Fair W, et al: Report of the United States Cooperative Study of Extracorporeal Shock Wave Lithotripsy. J Urol 135:1127, 1986.
80. Lingeman J, Evan A: Bioeffects of extracorporeal shock wave lithotripsy. J Endourol 1:89, 1987.
81. McCullough DL, Yeaman LD, Bo WJ, et al: Effects of shock waves on the rat ovary. J Urol 142:666, 1989.
82. Yeaman LD, Jerome CP, McCullough DL: Effects of shock waves on the structure and growth of the immature rat epiphysis. J Urol 142:670, 1989.
83. Adams MC, Newman DM, Lingeman JE: Pediatric extracorporeal shock wave lithotripsy: long-termed results and effects on renal growth. In Lingeman JE, Newman DM (eds): Shock wave lithotripsy II: urinary and biliary. New York: Plenum Press, 1989, Chapter 45, p 223.
84. Newman DM, Kulb T, Lingeman JE, et al: Extracorporeal shock wave lithotripsy experience in children. J Urol 136:238, 1986.
85. Kaji D, Xing WW, Hardy B, Huffman J: The effects of ESWL on renal growth and function in a rabbit model. J Endourol 4:S55, 1990.
86. Evan AP, Willis LR, Conors B, et al: SWL induces more severe renal structural and function changes in juvenile versus adult mini-pig kidney. J Endourol 4:S58, 1990.
87. Neal DE, Harmon EP, Kaack B, et al: Renin production after experimental ESWL. J Endourol 4:S49, 1990.
88. Moran ME, Sandock D, Drach GW: Effects of high energy shock waves on chick embryo development. J Urol 143:230A, 1990.
89. Gilbert B, Riehle R, Vaughan D: Extracorporeal shock wave lithotripsy and its effect on renal function. J Urol 139:482, 1988.
90. Jaeger P: Changes of blood and urine chemical parameters after extracorporeal shock wave exposure on canine kidneys. In Lingeman JE, Newman DM (eds): Shock wave lithotripsy II: urinary and biliary. New York: Plenum Press, 1989, Chapter 2, p 7.
91. Smith AD, Karlin GS: Enzymuria evaluation of renal tubular injury following extracorporeal shock wave lithotripsy treatment with the Sonolith 200. In Lingeman JE, Newman DM (eds): Shock wave lithotripsy II: urinary and biliary. New York: Plenum Press, 1989, Chapter 1, p 3.
92. Dyer RB, Karstaedt N, McCullough DL, et al: MRI evaluation of intermediate changes in kidneys treated with extracorporeal shock wave lithotripsy. In Lingeman JE, Newman DM (eds): Shock wave lithotripsy II: urinary and biliary. New York: Plenum Press, 1989, Chapter 38, p 203.
93. Kaude J, Williams C, et al: Renal morphology and function immediately after extracorporeal shock wave lithotripsy. AJR 145:305, 1987.
94. Knapp P, Lingeman JE: MRI following ESWL with the Dornier HM-3 lithotripter. J Urol 137:287A, 1987.
95. Rubin J, Arger P, et al: Kidney changes after extracorporeal shock wave lithotripsy: CT evaluation. Radiology 162:21, 1987.
96. Wilson WT, Miller G, Morris JS, et al: Morphologic renal changes following piezoelectric and spark-gap lithotripsy. In Lingeman JE, Newman DM (eds): Shock wave lithotripsy II: urinary and biliary. New York: Plenum Press, 1989, Chapter 5, p 19.
97. Knapp P, Lingeman J: ESWL-induced perirenal hematomas. J Urol 139:700, 1988.
98. Littleton RH, Melser M, Kupin W: Acute renal failure following bilateral extracorporeal shock wave lithotripsy without ureteral obstruction. In Lingeman JE, Newman DM (eds): Shock wave lithotripsy II: urinary and biliary. New York: Plenum Press, 1989, Chapter 37, p 197.
99. Newman LH, Saltzman B: Identification of risk factors in

the development of clinically significantly subcapsular hematomas following shock wave lithotripsy. In Lingeman JE, Newman DM (eds): Shock wave lithotripsy II: urinary and biliary. New York: Plenum Press, 1989, Chapter 39, p 207.

100. Lingeman J, Kulb T: Hypertension following extracorporeal shock wave lithotripsy. J Urol 137:142A, 1987.
101. Lingeman JE, Woods JR, Toth PD: Blood pressure changes following extracorporeal shock wave lithotripsy and other forms of treatment for urolithiasis. In Lingeman JE, Newman DM (eds): Shock wave lithotripsy II: urinary and biliary. New York: Plenum Press, 1989, Chapter 40, p 211.
102. Montgomery BSI, Cole RS: Is there an association between ESWL and hypertension: A study of 1000 patients. In Lingeman JE, Newman DM (eds): Shock wave lithotripsy II: urinary and biliary. New York: Plenum Press, 1989, Chapter 41, p 217.
103. Puppo P, Bottino P: ESWL and hypertension: no evidence for causal relationship. J Urol 141:241A, 1989.
104. Zwergel T, Neisius D, Zwergel U: Hypertension after extracorporeal shock wave lithotripsy: incidents in Dornier HM-3 and Wolf Piezolith 2300 lithotripter treatment. In Lingeman JE, Newman DM (eds): Shock wave lithotripsy II: urinary and biliary. New York: Plenum Press, 1989, Chapter 42, p 223.
105. Lingeman JE, Woods JR, Toth PD: Blood pressure changes following extracorporeal shock wave lithotripsy and other forms of treatment for nephrolithiasis. JAMA 263:1789, 1990.
106. Fuchs GJ, Wolfson B, David R, Barbaric Z: In-vivo model to investigate the risk of hypertension following high energy shock wave application to the kidney. J Endourol 4:S59, 1990.
107. Ell C, Hochberger J, Oux G, Demling L: Laser lithotripsy of gallstones by means of pulsed Nd:YAG lasers. Gastroenterology 94:A113, 1988.
108. Gelfand DW, McCullough DL, Myers RT, et al: Choledocholithiasis: successful treatment with extracorporeal lithotripsy. Am J Radiol 148:1114, 1987.
109. Garibaldi RA, Sholurich D, et al: Post cholecystectomy wound infection. Ann Surg 204:650, 1986.
110. Vernava A, Andrews C, et al: Pancreatitis after biliary tract surgery. Arch Surg 122:575, 1987.
111. Brendel W, Enders G: Shock waves for gallstones, animal studies. Lancet 1(8332):1054, 1983.
112. Sauerbruch T, Delius M, Baumgartner G, et al: Fragmentation of gallstones by extracorporeal shock waves. N Engl J Med 314:818, 1986.
113. Sackman M, Delius M, Sauerbruch T, et al: Shock-wave lithotripsy of gallbladder stones: the first 175 patients. N Engl J Med 318:393, 1988.
114. Ell C, Kerzel W, Heyder N, et al: Piezoelectric lithotripsy of gallstones. Lancet 2:1149, 1987.
115. Hood K, Kneightly A, Dowling R, et al: Piezo-ceramic lithotripsy of gallbladder stones: initial experience in 38 patients. Lancet 1:1322, 1988.
116. Weiss W, Turk C, Brownstone E, et al: Extracorporeal piezoelectric shock wave lithotripsy, a new pain-free therapy for biliary stones. Endoscopy 20:75, 1988.
117. Kellett MJ, Wickham JAE, Russell RCG: Percutaneous cholecystolithotomy. Br Med J 296:453, 1988.
118. Shaver RW, Hawkins IF, Soong J: Percutaneous cholecystostomies. AJR 138:1133, 1982.
119. Becker CD, Fache JS, Gibney RA, et al: Treatment of retained cystic duct stones using extracorporeal shock wave lithotripsy. Am J Radiol 148:1121, 1987.
120. Turner WW: Personal communication, 1989.
121. Allen MJ, Borody TJ, Bugliosi, et al: Rapid dissolution of gallstones by methyl tertbutyl ether: preliminary observations. N Engl J Med 312:217, 1985.
122. Schoenfield LJ, Lachin JM, et al: Chenodiol (chenodeoxycholic acid) for dissolution of gallstones: the National Cooperative Gallstone Study; a controlled test of efficacy and safety. Ann Intern Med 95:257, 1981.
123. Haupt G, Benkert S, Graff J, Senge T: Results of more than 1500 ESWL treatments with the MFL 5000. J Endourol 4:S151, 1990.
124. Schlick R, Rodenbeck D, Gonnermann O, Jonas U: Experience in ESWL using the Modulith SL20: cost reduction by multifunctionality. J Endourol 4:S89, 1990.
125. Rassweiler J, Kohrmann KU, Wess O, Alken P: Modulith SL20: its clinical establishment. J Endourol 4:S90, 1990.

CHAPTER 2

URETERONEPHROSCOPY

LOUIS R. KAVOUSSI and RALPH V. CLAYMAN

Endoscopy constitutes a major part of the foundation of urologic practice. With the aid of the cystoscope, urologists have been diagnosing and treating diseases of the lower urinary tract for over a century. More recently, advances in endoscope design and fiberoptic technology have given birth to ureteronephroscopy, which allows the urologic surgeon to inspect the entire upper urinary tract via the urethra. Furthermore, with the development of small accessory instruments to use through these endoscopes, many disease entities once managed only by open surgery can be successfully treated with less morbidity through an endosurgical approach.

HISTORY

Although endoscopic inspection and treatment of disease in the lower urinary tract have been performed for decades, endoscopy of the upper urinary tract has become accepted only in the past 10 years. Transurethral endoscopic visualization of the ureter was first reported by Hugh Hampton Young in 1929.[1] He reported on passing a pediatric cystoscope into the renal pelvis of a 2-week-old child who had a massively dilated upper collecting system resulting from posterior urethral valves. Ureteroscopy was not reported again until 50 years later, when Tobias Goodman described the use of an 11F pediatric cystoscope to visualize the distal ureter in three patients.[2] Furthermore, in one of these patients, a small, superficial distal ureteral tumor was endoscopically fulgurated, marking the first completely endoscopic treatment of a pathologic condition of the upper collecting system. One year later Lyon and associates reported that they had dilated the distal ureteral tunnel to 16F with rigid Jewett sounds to perform ureteroscopy with a 14F resectoscope for the purpose of endoscopically resecting a distal ureteral tumor.[3] This group later used the first purposely built 13F ureteroscope to examine the distal ureter in males.[4] In 1980 Perez-Castro Ellendt and Martinez-Pineiro developed a longer rigid ureteroscope that enabled visualization of the entire ureter, renal pelvis, and upper calyces.[5] Over the ensuing years, further refinements have made available a variety of practical and useful rigid ureteroscopes.

Parallel with the development of the rigid instruments was the evolution of fiberoptic flexible endoscopy. The gastroduodenoscope was the first endoscope using fiberoptic technology to be employed clinically.[6] McGovern and Walzak are credited with the earliest use of the flexible instrument in the urinary tract: in 1964 they reported using a flexible passively deflectable ureteronephroscope for transurethral visualization of a ureteral calculus.[7] Subsequently, Takagi and associates designed a passively deflectable fiberoptic pyeloureteroscope for inspection of the upper urinary collecting system.[8] These early instruments lacked an irrigation channel and active deflection, which made visualization and passage somewhat difficult. During the following two decades, smaller endoscopes with irrigation/working channels and actively deflectable tips were developed. The irrigation/working channel allowed irrigant to clear the visual field and permitted passage of instruments for a variety of diagnostic and therapeutic procedures. The actively deflecting tip enabled the urologist to direct the endoscope, which provided easier passage and manipulation of instruments passed through the working channel.

The evolution of the ureteronephroscopes has been accompanied by advances in transurethral ureteral access. Ureteral dilation to facilitate calculus passage was first reported in the early 1900s.[9,10] Bransford Lewis is credited with using a two-blade dilator for stone extraction in 1904.[9] Three years later Nitze designed the first balloon catheter for ureteral dilation.[9] Dilating techniques were further popularized in the 1920s by Ralph Dourmashkin, who devised metallic dilators and later an inflatable rubber bag to dilate the ureter.[10] Over the ensuing 50 years several refinements in the early dilating systems were made. Interest in these techniques as an adjunct in performing ureteronephroscopy has led to guidelines (outlined later in this chapter) for performing safe and effective ureteral dilation.

Endoscopic diagnosis of pathologic conditions of the entire upper urinary tract is possible with currently available actively deflectable ureteronephroscopes. These instruments permit inspection of the majority of the intrarenal collecting system in most patients.[11,12] Furthermore, they allow treatment of a variety of upper urinary tract pathologic conditions with minimal morbidity: ureteral calculi, essential hematuria, ureteropelvic junction obstruction, ureteral strictures, and, in carefully selected patients, transitional cell cancer.[11-14]

ANATOMY OF THE UPPER URINARY COLLECTING SYSTEM

When performing ureteroscopy for diagnostic or therapeutic purposes, the endoscopist must thoroughly understand the anatomy of the kidney, intrarenal collecting system, and ureter. Although the anatomic configuration varies from patient to patient, certain morphologic relationships remain constant.

The kidneys and ureters are retroperitoneal organs surrounded by a layer of fat (Figure 2–1). Each kidney is surrounded by a distinct fascial layer, Gerota's fascia. This fascia surrounds both the kidneys and the adrenal glands, but separates these organs by a thin membranous sheath. The fascia fuses medially and adheres closely to the tissue of the vena cava and aorta to prevent communication between the spaces of the kidneys bilaterally. Inferomedially Gerota's fascia extends along the ureter as the periureteric fascia. Gerota's fascia, along with the renal hilum, is fixed to the kidney within the retroperitoneum; however, they are both relatively mobile in this space.

The ureter is a tortuous tubelike structure that varies in diameter as it passes between the bladder and the renal pelvis (Figure 2–1). When the ureter's path is followed from the bladder, the distal third travels posteriorly and laterally along the pelvic side wall. It then bows anteriorly at the bifurcation of the iliac vessels and continues to move anteriorly as it crosses over the psoas muscle. The ureter again travels slightly posteriorly just as it reaches the renal hilum.

The diameter of the ureter varies along its length from 1 to 5 mm. The upper two thirds has an average diameter of 3.8 mm, and the lower portion averages 3.7 mm.[15,16] The ureter has three physiologic areas of narrowing: the ureterovesical tunnel (i.e., ureterovesical junction to ureteral os) with a diameter of 1 to 5 mm, the point where the urethra crosses the iliac vessels with an average diameter of 4 mm, and the ureteropelvic junction with an average diameter of 2 mm.

The intrarenal collecting system is made up of the renal pelvis and the multiple infundibula leading from it to the upper, middle, and lower pole calyces (Figure 2–2). Adults have 4 to 14 minor calyces (average 8), and these empty into two or three major calyces that drain into the renal pelvis.

The upper ureter derives its blood supply from multiple arteries medially along its path. The main

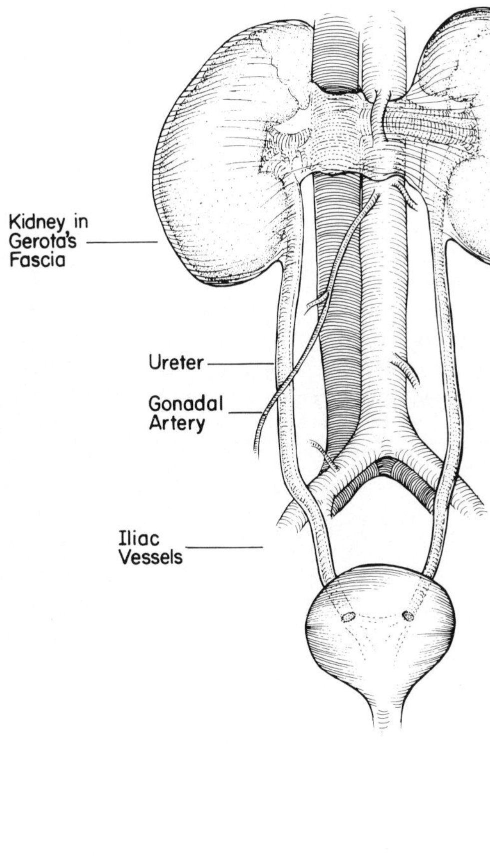

FIGURE 2–1. Diagram of peritoneal coverings of the urinary collecting system, illustrating the renal fascia and its extensions. Note the course of the ureter as it passes into the retroperitoneum. The distal third of the ureter passes posterolaterally. The proximal two thirds of the ureter passes anteriorly and medially over the psoas muscle. The gonadal vessels cross the ureter in its midportion. The superior vesical artery and the uterine artery in females pass anteriorly over the distal ureter.

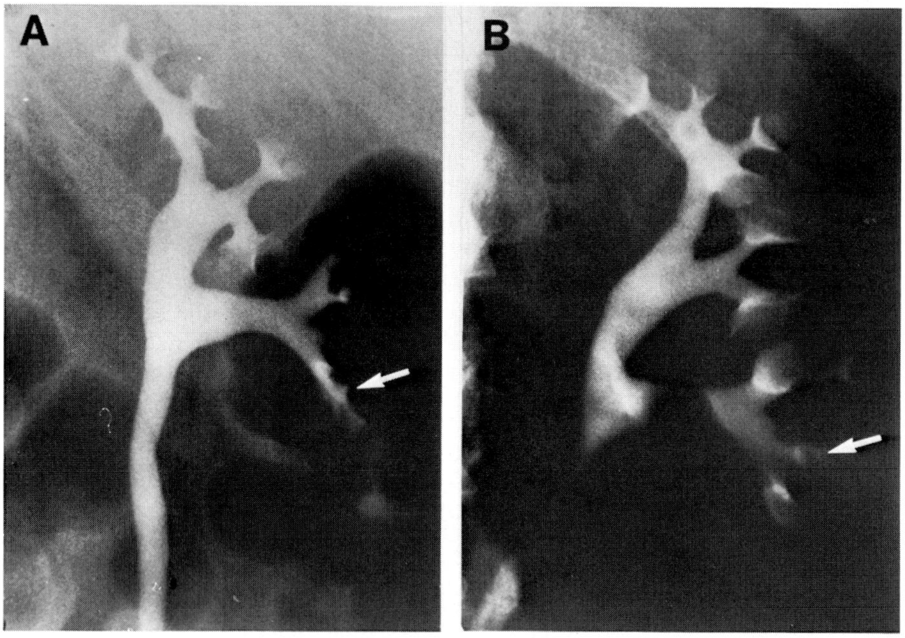

FIGURE 2–2. **A,** Anteroposterior and, **B,** oblique radiographic views of the renal pelvis, calyces, and infundibula. The arrow demonstrates a calyx not visible on the initial anteroposterior view.

supply to the upper ureter is from the main renal artery, and through its upper course the ureter also receives branches from the aorta and the gonadal and common iliac arteries. Once it passes into the pelvis, it derives its main blood supply laterally from branches of the internal iliac, gluteal, deferential, uterine, and vesical arteries. Venous drainage follows the arterial routes.

The ureter consists of three layers: urothelium, the muscular layer, and fibrous adventitia (Figure 2–3). The smooth muscle layer has two distinct arrangements of fibers, longitudinally in the outer layer and circumferential in the middle layer.

ANATOMIC LANDMARKS FOR ENDOSCOPY

Several landmarks can be observed during ureteroscopy. Once the distal ureter is entered, the smooth urothelium can be identified. The distal ureteral tunnel is thicker than the upper ureter; therefore, the lower ureter takes on a characteristic star-shaped appearance when the ureteroscope is advanced. When the pelvic brim is reached, the ureter appears more circular; narrowing over the common iliac vessels may be noted. As the ureter crosses this region, the common iliac artery can

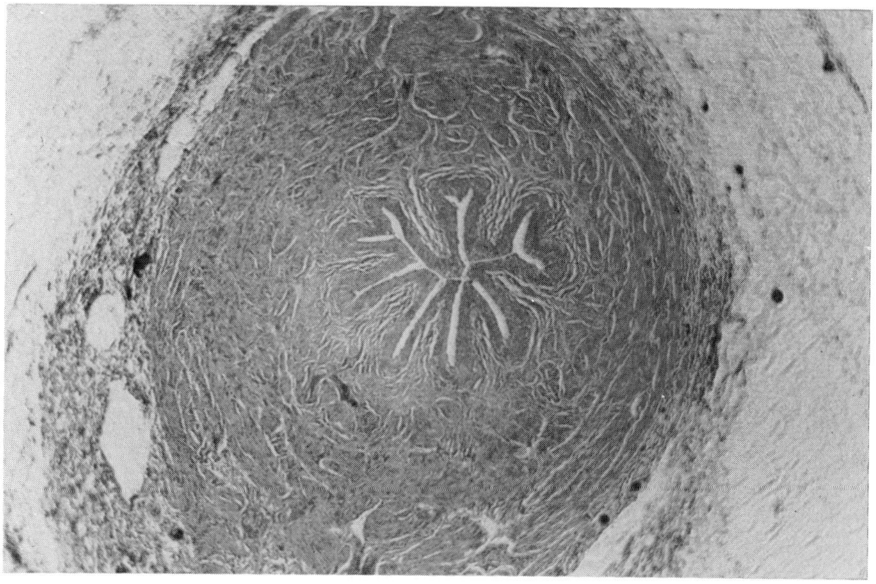

FIGURE 2–3. Histologic cross section of a ureter, demonstrating the three separate layers: urothelium, smooth muscle, and fibrous adventitia. (Magnification 100×.)

often be seen pulsating posteriorly. Once the proximal ureter is entered above the common iliac vessels, motion of the ureter with the patient's respiration can be appreciated. Inspiration leads to caudad movement of the renal pelvis and proximal ureter, whereas expiration results in cephalad movement. Because the ureteropelvic junction dips posteriorly, the endoscope is easier to advance during expiration, which straightens the junction.

The renal pelvis is easily identifiable as a markedly capacious space after the instrument exits the relative narrower ureter. When the endoscope enters the renal pelvis, the openings to the major calyces leading to the upper, middle, and lower pole of the kidney are visible (Figure 2–4). Arterial pulsation from the renal arteries can sometimes be noted anteriorly along the renal pelvis.

When a major calyx is entered, from one to three infundibula can be visualized leading to a minor calyx. In the calyces, renal papillae appear as rounded cones of pink mucosa (Figure 2–5). In the upper and lower pole calyces more than one papilla may be seen projecting into a single calyx; these papillae are often fused, forming a compound papilla. In the middle calyces the papillae remain as separate entities because of the embryologic lack of calyceal fusion in that portion of the kidney.

INSTRUMENTATION FOR URETERONEPHROSCOPY

A wide variety of ureteronephroscopes and accessories are available to the urologist. Ureteronephroscopes fall into two basic categories: rigid ureterscopes and flexible ureteronephroscopes.

Rigid Ureteroscopes

Several rigid ureteroscopes are currently on the market (Table 2–1). These instruments all contain a rigid shaft housing the optical, illumination, and working systems. The sheaths range in length from 25 to 45 cm. The shorter instruments are useful for inspecting the distal ureter, while the longer ones may be advanced to visualize the upper ureter and portions of the renal pelvis and upper calyces. The diameters of these instruments range from 6.9 to 13.5F. The smaller diameter instruments can often be passed without the need for dilating the distal ureter; however, the field of view is smaller than with the larger ureteroscopes.

Two lens systems are available with rigid ureteroscopes: the traditional rigid rod lens system and the combination rod lens fiberoptic system. The rigid rod lens is the same as that used in rigid cystoscopes and gives excellent optics for visualizing the upper urinary tract. The lenses for these instruments can often be interchanged (e.g. 0 to 70 degrees) within the working sheath to allow visualization of the major infundibula in the middle and occasionally the lower pole.

More recently, instruments have become available that use a combination of a rigid integral rod lens and fiberoptic image bundle. This allows a much smaller lens system, resulting in a smaller endoscope. The fiberoptic system permits the endoscope to be somewhat flexible, with approximately 2.5 cm deflection at the tip. However, because of the fiberoptic design the image is less sharp than with the rigid lens system, although it is sufficient for most therapeutic and diagnostic procedures in the ureter.

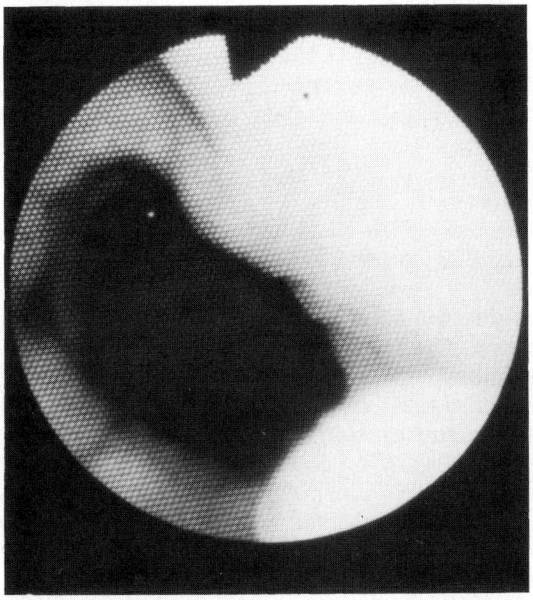

FIGURE 2–4. Endoscopic view through the ureteroscope, demonstrating the opening into the major and minor calyces (air bubble in the distance).

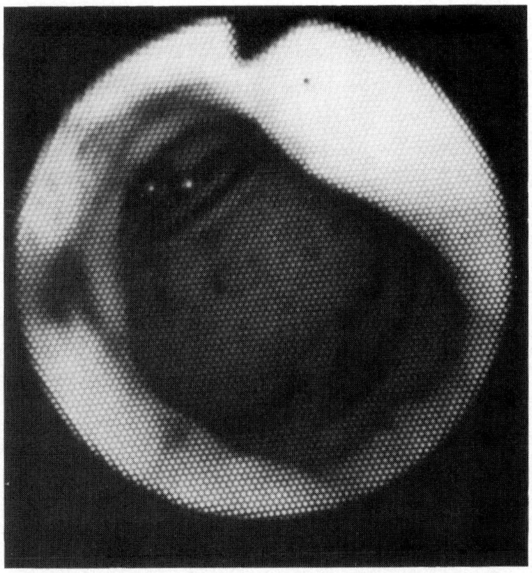

FIGURE 2–5. Simple papillae as they are usually found in the middle calyces.

TABLE 2–1. Rigid Ureteronephroscopes*

Company	*Size of Sheath (Tip) (F)*	*Length of Endoscope (cm)*	*Accessory Channel (F)*	*Lens (Degree)*	*Other Features*
Storz	11.5	15	4	6	
		41	4	6, 70	
	12.5	38.5	5	6	Angled eyepiece
Olympus	11.0	34	3		
	54	5 and 4	0 or 70	Available with 13.5	Angled eyepiece
	11	45	5	5	Offset eyepiece
Wolf	7.5		3.3	0	Fiberoptic integral lens system
	9.5	43	5	5	
	11.5	28	6 or 5 and 3	5, 25, 70	Angled eyepiece available
	13.5	43	6	5	
Circon	6.9	33/41	3.4 and 2.3	5	Focusing ocular
ACMI	10	43	5	5, 90	
	13	27/43	5	5	Eyepiece can be deflected
Candela	7.2	41	2.1 and 2.1	0	Semirigid shaft; fiberoptic; integrated
Applied Medical Resources	6.9	33	3.4	0	Semirigid shaft; fiberoptic; integrated
	5.5	33	2.3	0	

*This is a sampling in which the variety of endoscopes is displayed.
Some data from Weinberg, 1988.

All ureteroscopes have one or two irrigation/working channels. Some of the larger diameter ureteroscopes have a separate insulated sheath and working element, which allows both cold knife and hot knife incision or loop resection. Also, some of the larger instruments have an offset lens to allow passage of a solid ultrasound probe for calculus fragmentation. The smaller ureteroscopes, which use a combination of rigid or fiberoptic imaging with a fiberoptic light bundle, have one common channel (≤3.4F) or two channels, one for irrigation and one for auxiliary instruments. The latter working channels are small (2.1 to 3.4F), allowing passage of laser fibers (<600 μm), 1.9F electrohydraulic probes, 2F electrocautery probes, 2F grasping forceps, or 2F stone baskets.

Despite the refinements in rigid instruments, several drawbacks remain. First, in passage, the rigid instruments force the ureter to conform to the straight shape of the endoscope. In many patients, especially males, the anatomic configuration causes difficulty in passage, particularly when the operator tries to get the instrument above the level of the iliac vessels. Also, the rigid endoscope may be impossible to pass because of a lack of ureteral compliance (resulting from prior surgery, radiation, spasm, or trauma) or other iatrogenic anatomic factors (e.g., ureteral reimplantation, urinary diversion). Attempts at forcing the ureter to conform to the endoscope can result in ureteral injury or instrument damage. Furthermore, passage of the rigid instruments is painful, necessitating a general or regional anesthetic. In addition, separate lenses (0, 30, and 70 degrees) are needed to inspect the renal pelvis, and therefore the entire intrarenal collecting system cannot be visualized easily. Lastly, the lithotomy position is necessary for introduction and manipulation of the rigid ureteroscope. This position may be impossible for some patients to achieve and awkward for the endoscopist.

Flexible Ureteronephroscopes

Because of the shortcomings of the rigid instruments, flexible ureteronephroscopes were developed. The flexible ureteronephroscopes permit complete closed access to the entire upper urinary tract. They are much easier to pass above the pelvic brim than their rigid counterparts because they conform to the anatomy of the upper urinary tract; thus the flexible endoscopes can be used to traverse even very tortuous ureters.

A variety of flexible ureteronephroscopes are on the market, and their specifications are given in Table 2–2. A number of accessory instruments are available for use in both rigid and flexible ureteronephroscopes (Table 2–3).

All flexible ureterscopes are constructed of four basic elements: an optical system (i.e., image bundle), an illumination system (i.e., light bundle), an irrigation/working channel, and a deflecting mechanism (Figure 2–6). The optical system carries light from the interior of the collecting system to the endoscopist and consists of a coherent fiberoptic bundle (i.e., fibers aligned parallel) fitted to a lens system that magnifies and focuses the image. Thousands of coated and wrapped 10 to 20 μm optical fibers make up the image bundle. The coating is of

TABLE 2–2. Instrument Specifications for Flexible Ureteronephroscopes

	Company							
	Baxter	*Bard*	*Surgitek*		*Storz*		*Wolf*	
PASSIVELY DEFLECTABLE FLEXIBLE URETERONEPHROSCOPE								
Model number	GU77	2000	SU-7	SU-9	11270A	11271A	7320.01	7320.03
Weight (g)	90	303	89.6	89.6	110	110	200	200
Length (mm)								
Overall	850	904	980	980	815	815	840	840
Working unit	680	804	860	860	640	640	600	600
Outer diameter (F)	7	7	7	9	9	7	6	7.5
Working port diameter (F)	5	3.5	1.2	3.5	3.6	1.2	2.0	3.3
Depth of field (mm)	5-12	2-00	5-15	5-15	2-20	2-20	2-50	2-50
Field of view (air/water); (degrees)	62/52	72/54	100/65	100/65	110/65	110/65	85/60	85/60
Modular	No	Yes	No	No	No	No	Yes	Yes
Tip shape	Oval, tapered	Oval, tapered	Round, tapered	Round, flush	Round, flush	Round, flush	Round, tapered	Round, tapered
Light bundles	2	2	2	2	1	1	2	2

	Company							
	ACMI		*Bard*	*Olympus*		*Storz*	*Surgitek*	*Wolf*
ACTIVELY DEFLECTABLE FLEXIBLE URETERONEPHROSCOPE								
Model number	AUR-8	AUR-9	2000	URFP	URF-P2	11276B	MSU11	7317
Weight (g)	340	340	320	566	560	410	249	300
Length (mm)								
Overall	980	980	904	101	990	930	990	910
Working unit	700	700	804	700	700	700	710	600
Outer diameter (F) (shaft)	8.5	9.8	9	10.8	9.3	10.5	11.9	10.5
Flexibility (two ways); (degrees)	160	160	180	160/100	160/100	180/130	160/100	180/90
Lock	No	No	No	Yes	Yes	No	No	Yes
Channel diameter (F)	2.5	3.6	3.2	3.6	3.6	3.6	4	3.3
Working channel exit relative to field marker (o'clock)	9:00	11:00	6:00	2:00	11:00	5:00	8:00	6:00
Depth of field (mm)	2-40	2-40	2-00	3-50	1-50	3-50	5-50	2-50
Field of view (air/water); (degrees)	82/62	82/62	72/54	72/54	90/69	160/76	70/65	85/60
Tip shape	Round, beveled	Round, flush	Oval, beveled	Round, beveled	Round, beveled	Round, flush	Round, tapered	Round, tapered
Secondary deflection	Yes	Yes	No	Yes	Yes	Yes	No	Yes
Light bundles	1	1	2	1	1	2	6	2

a lower refractive index than the glass fiber, thus acting as an interference where light is internally reflected. This allows the fiber to transmit light when bent at any angle (Figure 2–7). Unfortunately, the coating and packing of the fibers produce spaces between the fibers, giving the final image a granular appearance. This limits the optical resolution and results in an image quality that is only fair compared with that of the rigid lens system. However, the image is sufficient for a wide range of diagnostic and therapeutic procedures. With rough handling the optical imaging fibers may break. Each broken fiber results in a black dot appearing in the visual field (Figure 2–8). The optical system also contains a field marker at the 12 o'clock position to aid in orientation during endoscopy.

The illumination system transmits light from an external source to the tip of the endoscope. It is constructed of a noncoherent (i.e., fibers aligned in a nonparallel manner) larger fiberoptic bundle (20 to 25 μm). As with the optical fibers, rough handling can break the fibers and lead to decreased illumination.

The irrigation-working channel is a hollow circular tube that runs the length of the endoscope and allows irrigation and passage of instruments. When instruments are passed down the channel, irrigant flow is decreased and increasing the inflow pressure by manual (syringe) or mechanical (pressure bag or roller pump) means may be necessary to allow sufficient flow for visualization.

The location of the irrigation/working port's entrance into the visual field varies among endoscopes (Figure 2–8). The endoscopist must have knowledge of this location in order to easily maneuver instruments and perform therapeutic procedures.

There are two categories of flexible ureteronephroscopes based on the deflecting mechanism: passively deflectable and actively deflectable. The passively deflectable endoscopes rely on their intrinsic flexiblity to conform to the upper urinary collecting system. They do not contain a mechanism to direct the tip. The passively deflectable endoscopes are less expensive and smaller than their actively deflectable counterparts. Because of this, they often can be passed over a guidewire without the need for dilating the ureteral orifice. Unfortunately, they cannot be directed by the surgeon, which precludes visualization or treatment of lesions affecting the majority of the intrarenal collecting system. They are used primarily to study the ureter and portions of the renal pelvis. These instruments can be directed into a calyx only by first passing a guidewire into the area of interest and then attempting to manipulate the endoscope over this wire. This can be tedious and in many instances is unsuccessful. Therapeutic maneuvers through the passive flexible endoscope are also difficult.

The actively deflectable ureteronephroscopes have both intrinsic shaft flexibility and a deflection mechanism in the handle that allows the endoscopist to manipulate the tip. The active deflecting mechanism consists of interlocking metal plates in the distal portion of the instrument, which are attached to guidewires in the shaft. These guidewires run the length of the instrument and are connected to a deflecting mechanism in the handle near the eyepiece. Movement of the deflecting lever is translated into controlled tip deflection. Furthermore, some manufacturers have hinged a portion of the shaft a few centimeters proximal to the actively deflecting tip to allow extensive secondary passive deflection. Secondary deflection permits the endoscope to be bent back on itself when the urologist is attempting to access the lower pole collecting system or to maneuver through a tortuous ureter (Figure 2–9).

TABLE 2–3. Available Instruments for Use in the Flexible Ureteronephroscope

Laser fiber	200-600 μm (0.6-1.8F)
Guidewire	0.025-0.038 inch (1.9-3F)
Electrosurgical probes	2-3F
Electrohydraulic lithotripter probes	1.6-3F
Graspers	2-3F
Baskets	2-3F
Biopsy forceps	2-3F
Grasping forceps	2-3F
Snares	2-3F

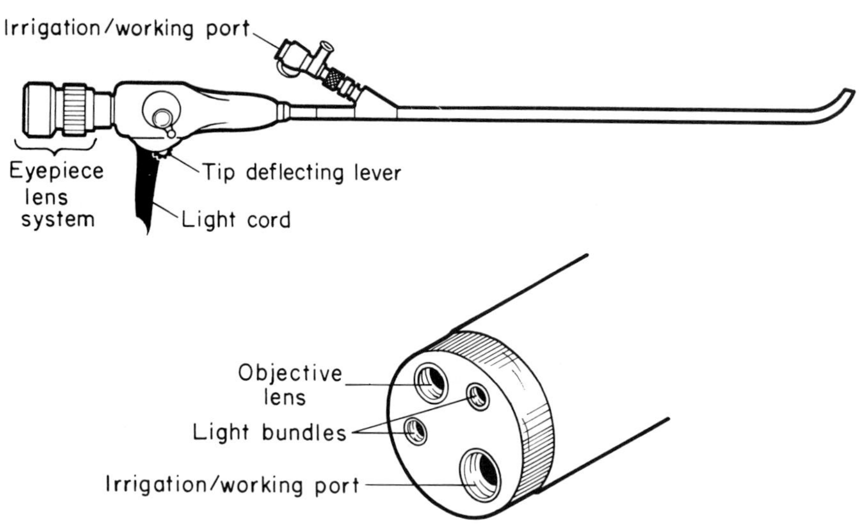

FIGURE 2–6. Diagramatic representation of the body and tip of a flexible ureteronephroscope.

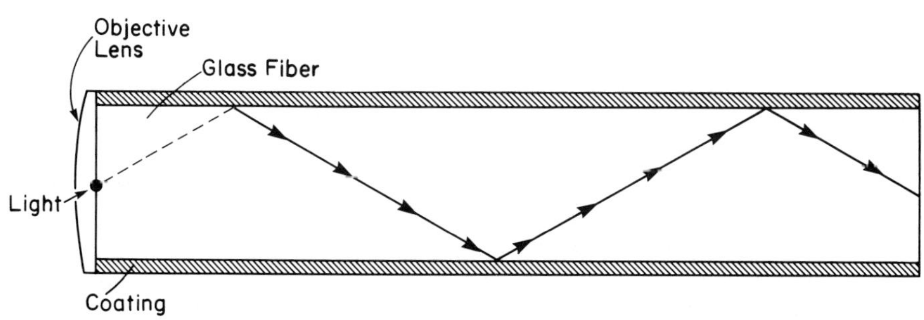

FIGURE 2–7. Light transmission within the coated (high refractive index) glass fiber by total internal inflection. There are approximately 15,000 reflections per meter.

Because of the intricate deflecting mechanism, these ureteronephroscopes are more expensive, larger, and more delicate than their passively deflecting counterparts. Dilation of the ureteral orifice is necessary for passage of most of the actively deflectable endoscopes.

TECHNIQUE FOR PASSING THE URETERONEPHROSCOPE

The endoscopic approach to diseases affecting the urinary tract differs markedly from traditional open surgery. During incisional exploration the urologist has the benefit of three-dimensional vision and direct tactile perception to locate and treat disease. In contrast, while performing ureteroscopy, the surgeon must rely on real-time fluoroscopy, monocular endoscopy, and tactile impressions transmitted through instruments to achieve the diagnostic or therapeutic goals. During ureteroscopy the three-dimensional picture is derived from a thorough knowledge of the patient's anatomy depicted on preoperative radiographs and from intraprocedural dynamic fluoroscopic and endoscopic monitoring.

Before any ureteroscopic procedure a detailed radiographic study of the affected collecting system, including anteroposterior and oblique views, is mandatory. When these radiographs are not available, retrograde pyelography should be performed before any ureteral manipulation to better define the anatomy and abnormalities of the intrarenal collecting system. Intraoperatively, fluoroscopy aids in maneuvering instruments along the ureter. Injection of contrast medium through the irrigation

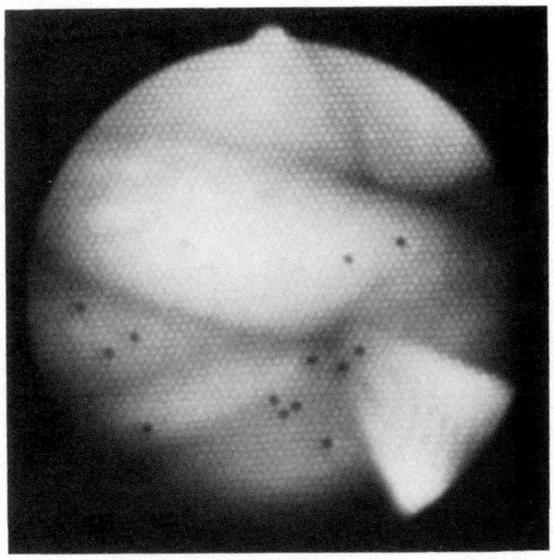

FIGURE 2–8. View through the flexible ureteronephroscope. A field marker is located at the 12 o'clock position and a probe exits the working channel at the 5 o'clock position. The black spots represent broken optical fibers. (From Kavoussi LR, Dierks SM: Flexible ureteronephroscopy: New avenue to the upper tract. In Oradell NJ: Contemporary Urology. Medical Economics, 1990.)

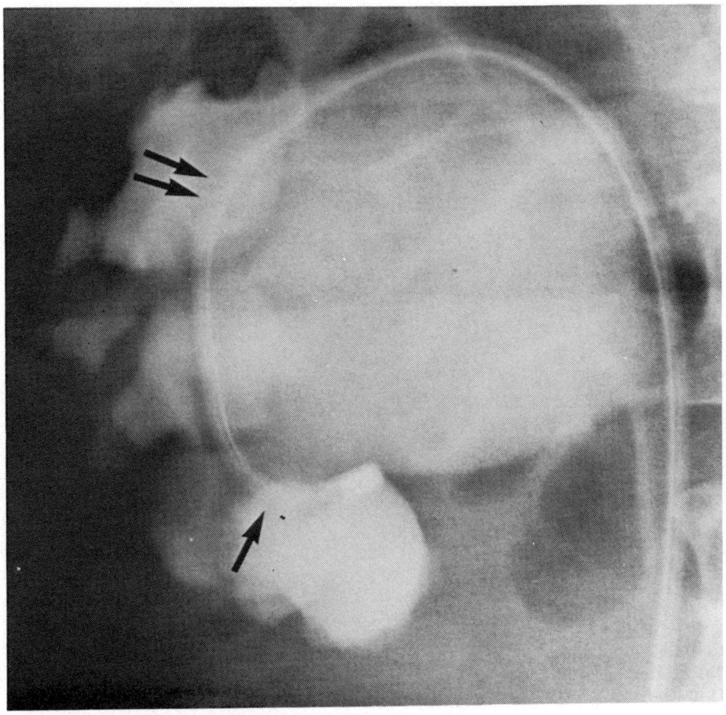

FIGURE 2–9. Radiograph demonstrating both primary active *(single arrow)* and secondary passive *(double arrow)* deflection.

port of the ureteroscope is helpful in outlining the course of the ureter during passage of the ureteronephroscope.

Visual control is necessary during the entire ureteroscopic procedure. The location of the tip of the ureteronephroscope should be continually monitored endoscopically and checked radiographically; the endoscope should be advanced only under visual control. During ureteronephroscopy, continuous visualization of the lumen of the collecting system is crucial. If a bright white reflection is seen, the operator is pushing against the ureteral wall and should slowly retract the endoscope until the lumen is identified. If continued forward force is applied, disruption of the urothelium and bleeding (red field) will occur. Further pressure will result in perforation into the retroperitoneum; if this occurs, wispy yellow fat (yellow field) may be identified and the endoscopic field becomes very large without identifiable walls.

Tactile information received during ureteroscopy is as crucial as visual and radiographic monitoring. All wires, catheters, and instruments should be passed without force. If difficulty is encountered, the operator must stop and reevaluate the situation endoscopically and radiographically to prevent instrument breakage or ureteral perforation.

Ureteral Access

The first step in performing ureteroscopy is obtaining ureteral access. Cystoscopy is performed to determine the location of the ureteral orifice and to rule out any other lower urinary tract disorder. Through the cystoscope a guidewire (preferably a floppy tip wire) is advanced through the orifice up to the renal pelvis (Figure 2–10). A coaxial 8F/10F dilator and sheath combination is passed over the wire, after which the 8F dilator is removed. Through the 10F sheath a second guidewire can be introduced into the ureter, providing the surgeon with both "working" and "safety" guidewires. After removal of the 10F sheath the "safety" guidewire is secured to the drape with a clamp or sewn to the glans penis or labia minora to prevent its being dislodged during the procedure.

Several points concerning passage of the initial

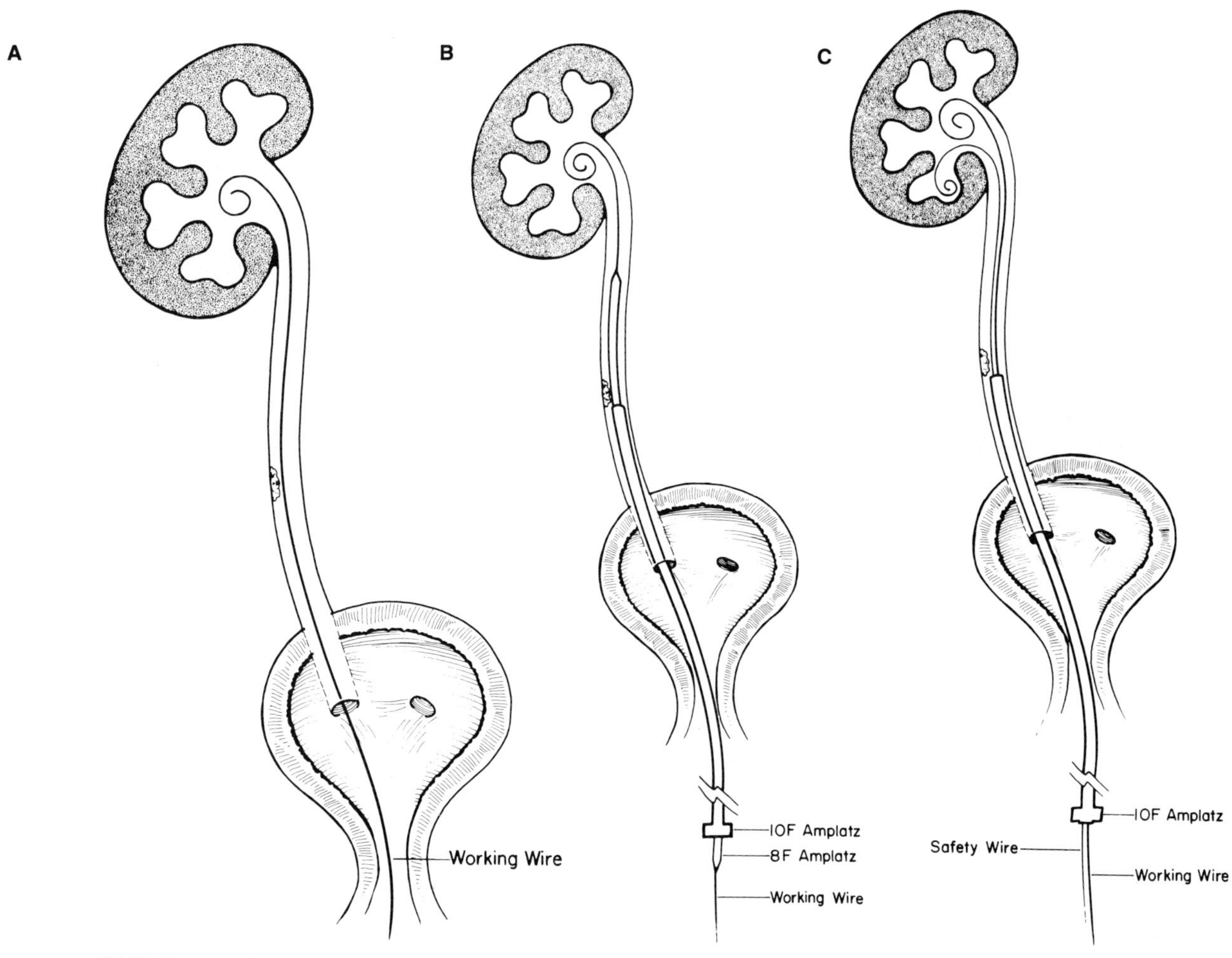

FIGURE 2–10. Steps in gaining access. **A,** The guidewire is advanced and coiled in the renal pelvis. **B,** A coaxial Armplatz 8 F/10F dilator/sheath is passed, and the 8F dilator is removed. **C,** Via the 10F sheath, a second 0.035-inch ("safety") guidewire can be introduced beyond the stone and secured in place; the 10F sheath is then removed.

access guidewire merit emphasis. In the treatment of calculi, if a wire cannot be manipulated above the level of the stone, the wire should be positioned as close to the stone as possible. This wire acts as a guide to allow dilation up to the level of the calculus. Also, when distal ureteral stones are treated, a working wire may not be needed if one of the smaller (6.9F to 7.2F) rigid endoscopes can be passed directly into the ureteral orifice and used to fragment the calculus without ureteral dilation; however, a "safety" guidewire must always be in place. Finally, when the upper urinary tract is inspected for benign essential hematuria, it is important not to abrade the urothelium while passing a guidewire. Blind intubation of the ureter may result in an iatrogenic petechial lesion that can be mistaken for the source of the bleeding. To minimize this risk, the urologist first clears the distal ureter by passing a short diagnostic rigid instrument. After the distal ureter has been thoroughly inspected, the guidewire should be passed only to the area previously examined by the short rigid ureteroscope. The tunnel can then be dilated, and with careful visualization of the ureter, flexible ureteronephroscopy can be performed in a retrograde manner. After the endoscope enters the intrarenal collecting system, the pelvis and the upper, middle, and lower calyces should be inspected in that order, taking care not to produce any iatrogenic lesions (Figure 2–11). In this instance, the entire upper collecting system is visualized by the surgeon prior to its being intubated with a guidewire.

Dilation of the Distal Ureter

The distal ureter must be dilated for the safe passage of most larger rigid and flexible ureteronephroscopes. In general, the distal ureter should be dilated to 2F or 3F larger than the ureteroscope that will be used. The currently available methods for ureteral dilation are listed in Table 2–4. Both nonguided (no ureteral guidewire) and guided (performed over a ureteral guidewire) methods are available.

In a few instances dilation of the ureteral tunnel is unnecessary. The new diminutive rigid endoscopes can routinely be passed into the orifice without prior dilation. Also, dilation is seldom necessary when an indwelling stent has been present for several days, since the ureter usually expands passively. Finally, dilation may not be needed in patients with a patulous refluxing or previously resected ureteral orifice and associated hydroureter.

Nonguided dilation can be performed by passing successively larger semirigid catheters or metal bougies under endoscopic and fluoroscopic control. However, the risk of perforation on passage is high, and with the availability of wire-guided dilation these techniques are less favored.

Hydrodilation of the ureteral orifice using high-flow irrigation through the ureteroscope can be classified as a nonguided method for ureteral dilation. In 1986, Perez-Castro Ellendt introduced a roller pump to pressurize the irrigant flowing through the ureteroscope.[17] With this technique the ureteroscope is placed flush against the ureteral orifice and the irrigant pressure is increased to 180 mm Hg (maximum: 200 mm Hg).[18] A flow of 300 to 350 ml/min (maximum: 400 ml/min) is used to expand the ureteral orifice and the intramural portion of the ureter. The ureter slowly opens, and the endoscope can be advanced through the tunnel. Once access is achieved through the ureterovesical junction, the pressure and flow rate should be decreased until flow is just sufficient to keep the ureteral luman patent. With this form of dilation, normal saline must be used as the irrigant to avoid problems with systemic absorption of irrigant, especially in the event of ureteral perforation or forniceal rupture. Furthermore, so that renal injury will be prevented, high pressures should be used for only a brief period (less than 30 minutes) while the orifice is entered. Studies by Eshghi and associates have revealed that prolonged exposure of the renal pelvis to pressures greater than 200 cm H_2O can result in renal damage.[19]

The most common forms of ureteral dilation are guided (i.e., performed over a guidewire). Dilating in this manner is accurate and controlled. By careful positioning of the working guidewire and avoidance of force when passing dilators, ureteral perforation and the creation of false passages can be prevented.

The graduated individual dilators or graduated coaxial dilators can be used to dilate the ureteral orifice to 2F or 3F larger than the outer diameter of the endoscope. They also have the advantage of being reusable. However, their larger sizes will not fit through the sidearm of the cystoscope, and thus they must be passed with fluoroscopic control alone. Furthermore, multiple passes are necessary, increasing the potential risk of ureteral injury.

Balloon dilating catheters are easy to pass over a guidewire under either radiographic or endoscopic control. Dilation can be performed more rapidly with this technique than with sequential dilators. The major disadvantage of balloon catheters is their expense because of one-time use directives.

Several 5 or 6 mm diameter balloons of 4 to 10 cm in length are available to achieve ureteral dilation. The inflation of the balloon is monitored fluoroscopically by filling the balloon with dilute radiographic contrast medium; the balloon is filled by a syringe, which is always connected to a reliable pressure gauge. High-pressure balloons capable of maintaining 12 atm of pressure should be used, since Huffman has shown that 22% of normal ureters require 10 atm or more to achieve adequate dilation.[20] The balloon must not be inflated over its

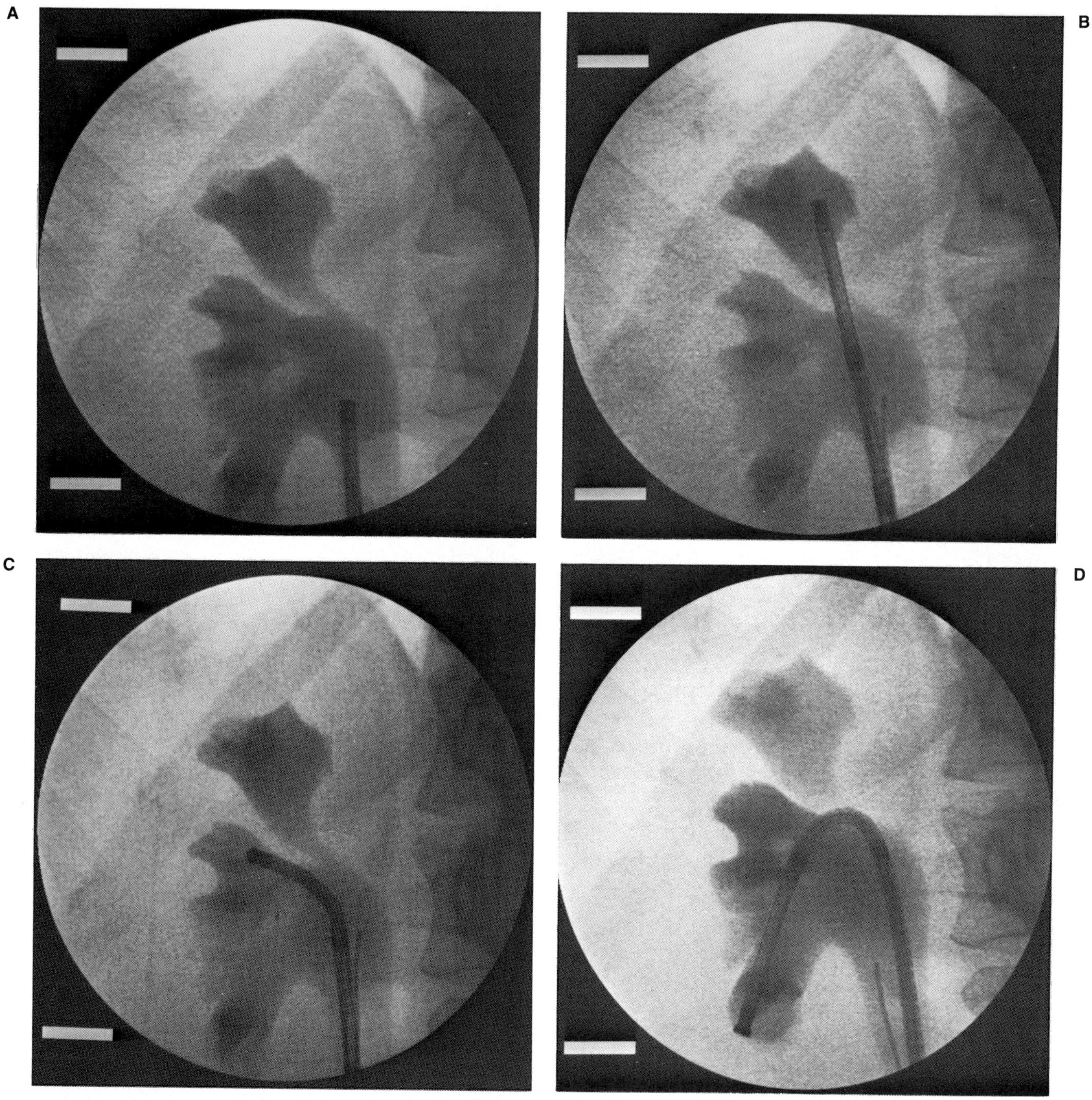

FIGURE 2–11. The collecting system should be inspected with the actively deflectable flexible ureteronephroscope in a systematic fashion: **A,** the renal pelvis, **B,** the upper pole calyces, **C,** the middle calyces, and, **D,** the lower pole calyces.

rated pressure to avoid balloon rupture and ureteral injury.

The dilating balloons have metal markers on either end to allow accurate positioning under radiographic control. They should be positioned fluoroscopically so that the cylindrical portion of the balloon is centered over the ureteral tunnel. As the ureter is dilated, a waist develops at the site of the ureterovesical junction, which usually fills out when the pressure is increased (Figure 2–12). Once the waist has been overcome, the balloon can be left inflated for 5 minutes to stabilize dilation and allow hemostasis of any small vessels that have been torn during the dilation process.

Occasionally the ureteral tunnel cannot be dilated. In these instances forceful dilation will only tear the ureter and frustrate attempts at ureteroscopy. Instead the urologist is encouraged to place an indwelling ureteral stent and terminate the procedure. The stent allows gradual dilation of the ureter over 72 hours, after which ureteroscopy can usually be performed without difficulty.

TABLE 2–4. Available Instruments for Ureteral Dilation

NONGUIDED SYSTEMS

Metal bougie dilators
Hydrodilation of the ureteral orifice via a high-pressure irrigation pump (Ureteromat)

GUIDED SYSTEMS

Graduated ureteral dilators (e.g., Nottingham type)
Graduated flexible coaxial dilators (e.g., Amplatz type)
Dilating balloon catheters
Ureteral access system (e.g., Finlayson type)
Passive dilation with indwelling ureteral stent

Semirigid ureteral access sheaths have recently become available. These permit repeated access to the upper collecting system, which can be useful for therapeutic procedures with flexible ureteronephroscopes. The sheath provides a direct conduit from the urethral meatus to the distal ureter. Several types of sheaths are available, but all have in common a central rigid dilator and a coaxial sheath (Figure 2–13). The dilator is tapered to pass over the guidewire, and the sheath is usually thin walled. The major difficulty with the sheath is that it tends to kink in the urethra of male patients, causing difficulty in passing the ureteronephroscope (Figure 2–14). In some sheaths the urethral portion is reinforced and enlarged to prevent this problem. Kinking may also occur as the sheath passes over the iliac vessels. Therefore, the access sheath should be advanced only until it is slightly beyond the ureterovesical junction.

As the ureteroscope is passed, ureteral spasm may preclude endoscopic access. The two general methods of alleviating this problem are pharmacologic dilation and mechanical dilation.

Pharmacologic dilation can be attempted topically or systemically. Lidocaine jelly (2%) and aminophylline (3ml of a 5mg/ml solution) have been injected through the working port of the ureteroscope to facilitate ureteral relaxation, with limited success.[21,22] Too rapid injection may cause perforation. Some authors have recommended systemic agents, including glucagon, halothane, and meperidine (Demerol), to induce ureteral relaxation. Unfortunately, definitive studies demonstrating the efficacy of local or systemic pharmacologic dilation are lacking.

Mechanical means of dealing with spasm are more successful and most commonly accomplished with a 5 mm dilating balloon catheter. After a guidewire is passed beyond the area of the spasm, a balloon is placed and inflated over the desired area. The balloon should be left inflated for 5 to 10 minutes before removal to allow the ureter to accommodate. Balloon dilation may be performed through the rigid ureteroscope and monitored fluoroscopically. The ureteroscope can then usually be passed beyond the area of narrowing. However, caution must be observed when the upper ureter is dilated, since long ureteral tears can occur and lead to extravasation of irrigant.

If the preceding methods of alleviating ureteral spasm are unsuccessful, the best course of action is to place an indwelling ureteral stent and terminate the procedure. The stent allows the ureter to dilate passively and facilitates subsequent ureteroscopy. Forcing the endoscope to pass an area of spasm might cause instrument damage or ureteral perforation.

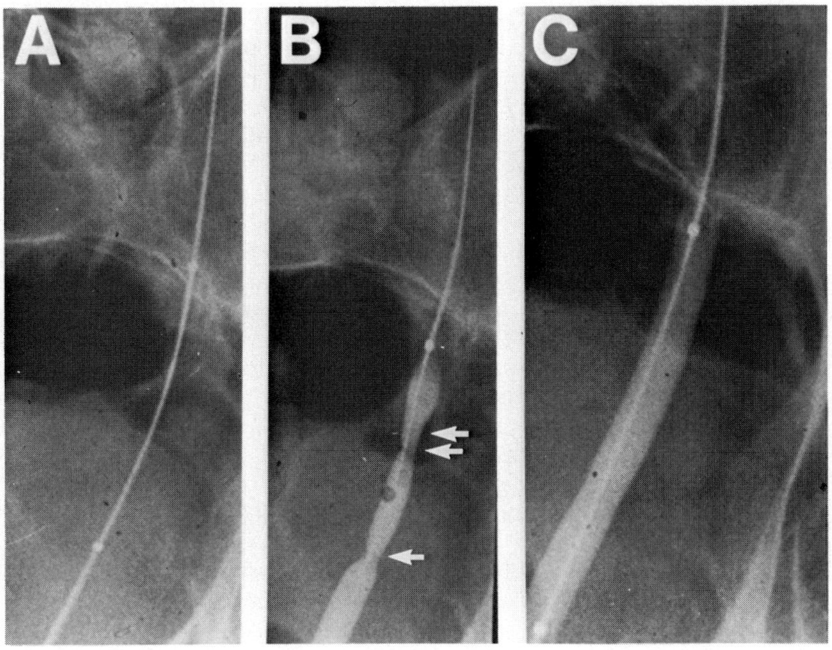

FIGURE 2–12. Radiograph demonstrating a 6 mm ureteral dilating balloon. **A,** Two metal markers can be seen on fluoroscopy. They lie at either end of the balloon. **B,** After the balloon is dilated, a waist is seen over the ureteral orifice *(single arrow)* and ureterovesical junction *(double arrow)*. **C,** After complete inflation the waist has disappeared.

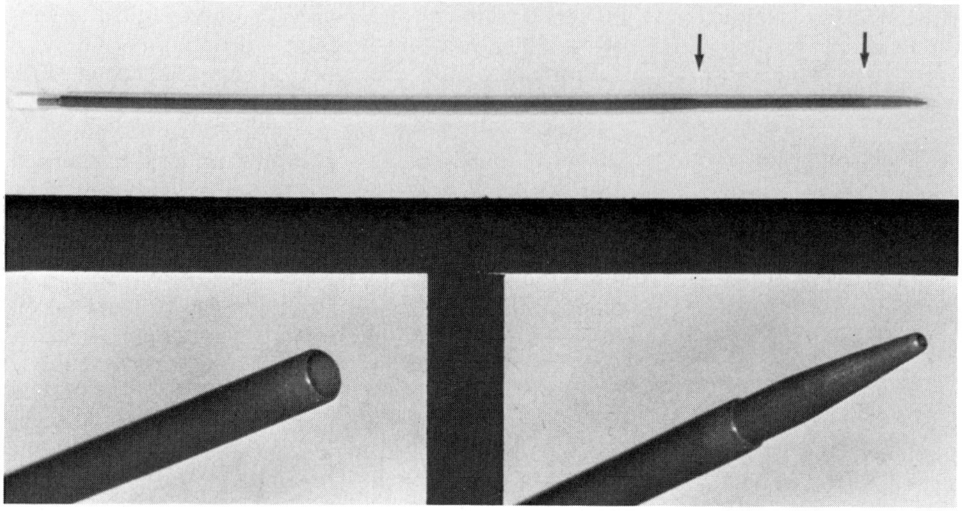

FIGURE 2–13. Ureteral access sheath system demonstrating tapered 12F dilator and coaxial thin-walled sheath. The arrows indicate the tapered segments (14F and 18F) of the sheath.

Rigid Ureteronephroscopy

When rigid ureteroscopy is performed, the working wire may be removed after adequate dilation of the tunnel. Alternatively, the ureteroscope can be passed directly over the working wire. The safety wire is left in place as a guide into the ureteral orifice and provides ready access for placement of a ureteral stent. The ureteroscope is advanced under direct vision through the urethra and bladder. The smaller therapeutic and diagnostic ureteroscopes have rounded tips, allowing the examiner to pass them directly into the ureteral orifice without additional manipulation. The therapeutic rigid ureteroscopes usually have a beveled tip. Before inserting the tip into the ureteral orifice, the operator must rotate the endoscope 180 degrees until the beveled tip is directed posteriorly (Figure 2–15). In that position the tip of the endoscope can engage the posterior lip of the ureteral orifice and be advanced along the ureteral tunnel. After the ureterovesical junction is passed, the endoscope is turned upright (i.e., bevel down). Alternatively, the tip of the endoscope can be passed under the safety guidewire, which can be used to lift open the orifice.

When traversing the ureter at the level of the iliac vessels, the tip of the endoscope must be raised gently at the pelvic inlet to prevent ureteral perforation. A guidewire or ureteral catheter can be passed through the working channel of the therapeutic endoscope to help straighten this part of the ureter and facilitate passage. An additional aid in straightening the ureter is to place the patient in the Trendelenburg position and have an associate manually push on the upper abdomen toward the patient's head to further displace the kidney upward (Mertz maneuver) and possibly straighten the ureter.

Inspection of the ureter above the iliac vessels with a rigid ureteroscope is usually more difficult than in the lower ureter, and flexible ureteroscopy is recommended when working above the level of the iliac vessels. In male patients urethral angulation caused by the suspensory ligament of the penis may preclude adequate passage of the rigid endoscope. A perineal urethrostomy may be helpful in overcoming this problem, especially if a therapeutic maneuver is necessary.[24]

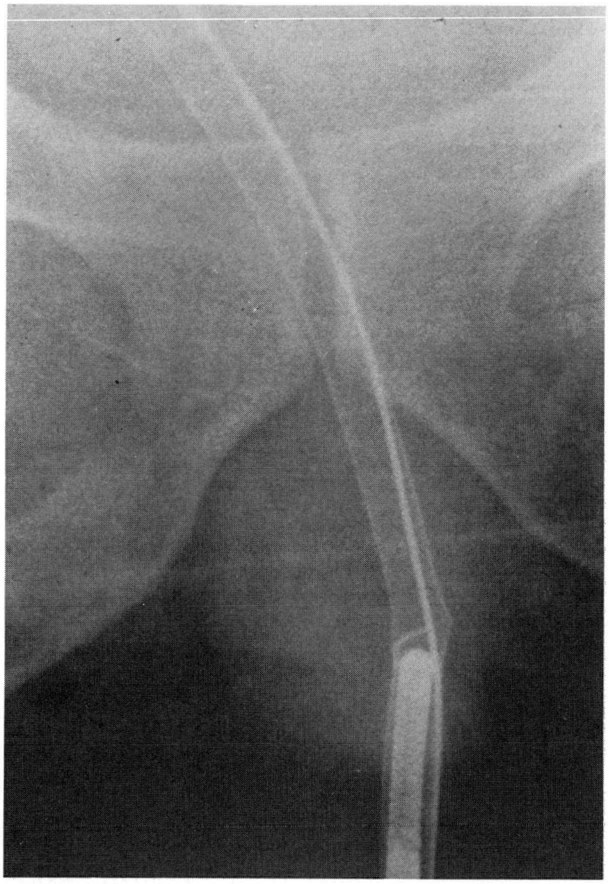

FIGURE 2–14. Radiograph demonstrating kinking of the ureteral access sheath in the urethra of a male patient, precluding passage of the ureteronephroscope.

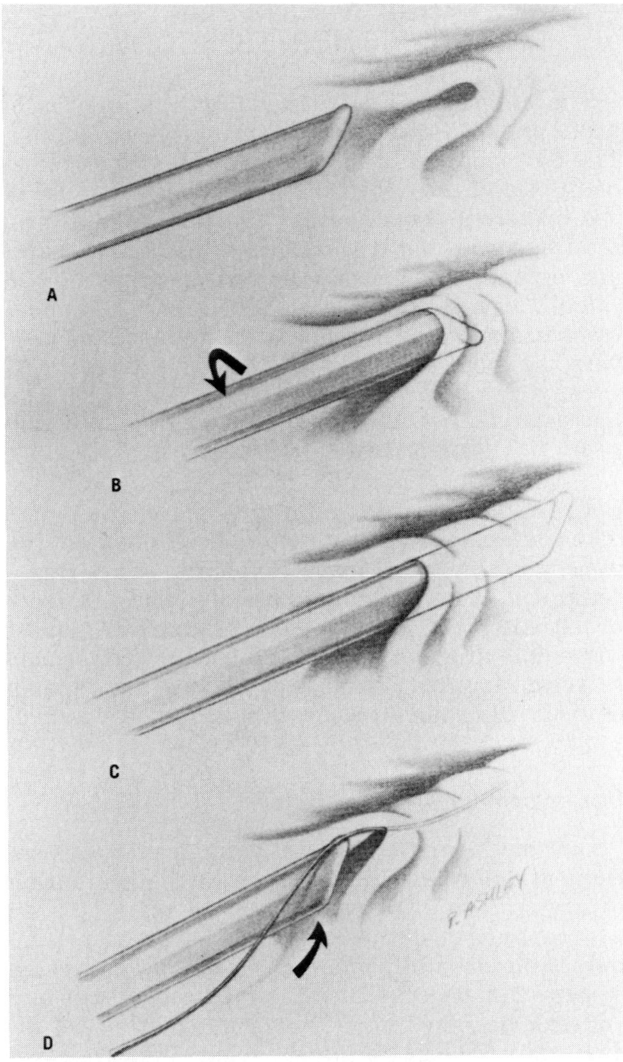

FIGURE 2–15. Technique for advancing the rigid ureteronephroscope into the ureteral orifice. **A,** The instrument is advanced to the orifice. **B,** It is rotated 180 degrees, enabling the beak to slide under the lip of the orifice. **C,** Once inside the ureter, it is turned upright. **D,** If a guidewire has been placed, the beak may be used to elevate the orifice and allow for direct introduction and advancement of the ureteroscope. (From Sosa E, Huffman JL: Complications of uretereopyeloscopy. In Huffman JL, Bagley DH, Lyon ES (eds): Ureteroscopy. Philadelphia: W.B. Saunders Co., 1987).

With the rigid endoscope the examiner can obtain an excellent view of the entire ureter and portions of the renal pelvis and upper pole calyces. With a 70-degree-angle lens, part of the midcalyces may be visualized. However, a flexible actively deflectable ureteronephroscope is necessary for a thorough inspection of the entire renal collecting system.

Flexible Ureteronephroscopy

Passage of the flexible ureteronephroscope is quite different from that of its rigid counterpart. The intrinsic flexibility of the shaft often causes the endoscope to buckle as it is advanced through the urethra and bladder into the ureter, especially in males. Two people are often needed to advance these instruments.

Most commonly the flexible ureteronephroscope is passed over the working guidewire that was used to dilate the orifice. Because the working channel is eccentrically located at the tip of the instrument, the endoscope may catch at the ureteral orifice. By turning the instrument so that the working channel is anterior, the endoscopist can usually pass the instrument without difficulty (Figure 2–16).

Several methods have been devised to facilitate passage. Threading a wire through the irrigation channel stiffens the ureteronephroscope and may allow direct passage. Alternatively, the sheath of a cystoscope can act as a guide to prevent buckling of the ureteroscope within the bladder. The sheath must be held near the ureteral orifice throughout the procedure. Unfortunately, this may be unwieldy because the rigid sheath cannot be removed, and the ureteronephroscope may be damaged. Recently an Olympus introducer endoscope became

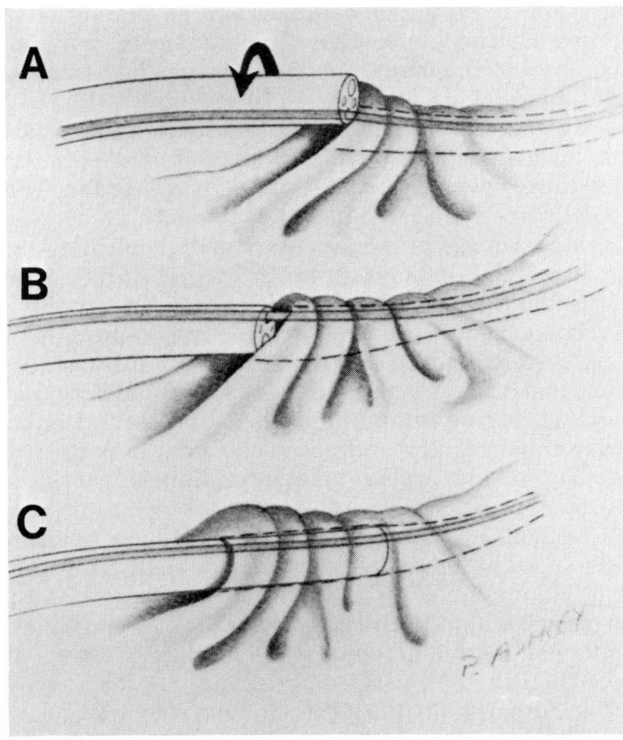

FIGURE 2–16. Method for advancing the flexible ureteronephroscope over a guidewire. The irrigation channel is located eccentrically on the shaft. **A,** Once the ureteronephroscope has reached the orifice, it should be rotated so that the guidewire is anterior. **B,** This allows the guidewire to elevate the orifice. **C,** The instrument can then be passed into the lumen under the anterior lip of the ureteral orifice. (From Sosa E, Huffman JL: Complications of uretereopyeloscopy. In Huffman JL, Bagley DH, Lyon ES (eds): Ureteroscopy. Philadelphia: W.B. Saunders Co., 1987).

available. This endoscope can be used to access the distal ureter and then be divided into halves so that the introducing endoscope can be removed after passage of the flexible ureteronephroscope. Finally, as discussed in the section on ureteral dilation, an ureteral access sheath can be passed to just below the level of the iliac vessel. This is useful when several insertions of the endoscope are expected.

As with the rigid endoscopes, combined fluoroscopic and visual control should be used during manipulation. If the ureteronephroscope meets resistance during passage, further advancement may cause buckling in the bladder, which may be detected fluoroscopically. By injecting radiographic contrast material through the working channel during fluoroscopic visualization, the endoscopist can view the anatomy of the ureter and deflect the tip as necessary to aid in its passage. When areas of tortuosity are encountered, tip manipulation to keep the lumen in the center of the visual field can be helpful. High-pressure (<200 mm Hg) irrigation via the working channel of the ureteronephroscope causes ureteral distention, which can also facilitate passage. Alternatively, the ureteronephroscope may be passed up a tortuous part of the ureter by passing a super-stiff guidewire via the ureteroscope into the renal pelvis. Care should be taken not to perforate the upper collecting system or working channel of the ureteronephroscope with the heavy duty wire.

Once the renal pelvis is entered, fluoroscopic monitoring with injection of contrast media via the ureteroscope is essential to provide orientation. The position of the instrument can be more accurately located radiographically than endoscopically. Inspection should begin in the pelvis, followed by the upper, middle, and lower pole infundibula and calyces, respectively. To enter the lower pole collecting system, the tip of the endoscope is fully flexed. The instrument is then passed further, and the secondary, more proximally located passive deflection system within the endoscope causes it to passively deflect as the upper pole infundibulum (Figure 2–9).

Several points are important when manipulating instruments passed through the irrigation/working channel. Significant tip flexibility can be lost when instruments are passed via the working channel. The degree of loss depends on the stiffness of the instrument and the make of the endoscope. Furthermore, the working instruments may impede irrigant delivery, making gravity-dependent flow of irrigant inadequate to keep the visual field clear. Increasing the inflow pressure by pressurizing the irrigant (with a pressure cuff or roller pump) or by manual syringe irrigation may be helpful. The former methods are preferable because manual syringe infusion can generate intrarenal pressures in excess of 400 mm Hg.

INDICATIONS FOR URETERONEPHROSCOPY

The diagnostic and therapeutic applications of ureteronephroscopy are continually expanding. The development of newer endoscopes and refinement of accessory instruments are allowing use of the ureteronephroscope for a wider range of procedures, including evaluation of upper tract lesions and essential hematuria, as well as treatment of calculi, ureteral obstruction, and on occasion upper tract tumors. Diagnostic and therapeutic maneuvers are successful in 79% to 84% of patients.[11,25]

Diagnostic Indications

The major power of ureteronephroscopy is that it potentially allows transurethral access to all of the upper urinary tract. Inspection of the entire intrarenal collecting system is possible in 65% to 85% of patients.[11,25,26] Incomplete visualization is most commonly due to inability to access the lower pole calyces. Moreover, these instruments are capable of visualizing the area of urothelial disease in 92% to 96% of patients.[11,25]

Upper Urinary Tract Lesions

One of the most important diagnostic applications of ureteroneophroscopy is in the evaluation of ureteral or intrarenal filling defects noted on urography. With these techniques greater than 90% of disease in the upper urinary tract collecting system can be evaluated.[11,25-27] These results are superior to conventional diagnostic methods of radiography with retrograde cytology and brush biopsy. Gittes analyzed 68 patients in whom upper collecting system filling defects were evaluated by conventional retrograde methods.[28] He reported a 6% false positive and a 16% false negative rate. Streem and associates studied 12 patients with upper urinary tract filling defects via standard techniques of cytology and brushings and compared these with ureteronephroscopic findings.[29] They found the standard evaluation to be accurate in only 58% of the patients, whereas ureteronephroscopy provided a diagnosis in 83%. These studies indicate that ureteronephroscopy is more accurate than nonendoscopic methods for evaluating upper urinary tract filling defects.

To avoid altering the true pathologic condition, the physician must not pass a guidewire or catheter to or beyond the lesion being investigated. Guidewires and the endoscope should be passed just beneath the level of the suspected filling defect before inspection.

When a lesion is encountered, cytologic examination and biopsy may be performed. Cytologic specimens may be obtained by placing the tip of the ureteroscope on the lesion and irrigating directly through the endoscope with saline solution to wash off cells for analysis. If contrast material is used to perform a retrograde pyelogram, it is important to use nonionic, low-osmolar contrast agents (i.e., Optiray 320: Ioversol 68%) as this will minimize cytologic artifacts.[30]

When possible, tissue should be obtained from all patients for diagnosis. Because samples obtained with the 3F biopsy forceps through the flexible ureteronephroscope are very small, a conclusive diagnosis is often difficult. Grasping tissue and pulling the forceps through the endoscope permits a diagnosis in only 30% of patients.[11] However, if a ureteroscope access sheath is used, larger biopsy specimens can be obtained by grabbing the lesion and pulling the entire endoscope out of the sheath with the forceps still protruding from the tip. With this technique adequate pathologic material for diagnosis can be obtained in 80% of patients.

A stone is the most common lesion encountered when ureteronephroscopy is used for diagnosis of an upper urinary tract filling defect.[11] A low-grade transitional cell carcinoma is discovered in 20% of patients. However, if the filling defect is associated with macroscopic hematuria, a tumor is more likely.[25] Additional findings include papillary necrosis, peripelvic cysts, pyelitis cystica, fungus ball, blood clots, or a segmental crossing renal vessel.[11,25] The last can be diagnosed when a pulsatile extrinsic mass is visualized endoscopically in the area where the filling defect was previously noted. On fluoroscopy the lesion should become less obvious during intraluminal distention and more prominent when the renal pelvis is decompressed through the ureteroscope.

If upper tract urinary cytologic tests show abnormalities in the presence of a filling defect, a high-grade transitional cell carcinoma should be suspected. In this situation it is reasonable to avoid ureteronephroscopy and proceed directly with nephroureterectomy or segmental ureterectomy, as necessary, if a normal contralateral kidney is present.

Essential Hematuria

Evaluation of patients with benign essential lateralizing hematuria can represent a major diagnostic challenge. Laboratory studies, including hemoglobin electrophoresis, sickle cell preparation, cytologic examination of urine, urinalysis, and urine culture, can be helpful in differentiating a medical from a surgical cause of hematuria. In patients with benign essential hematuria, conventional radiographic studies, including intravenous pyelography, retrograde ureterography, computerized tomography, ultrasonography, and arteriography, are usually inconclusive and thus ureteronephroscopy is indicated.

Cystoscopy is performed to rule out a lower tract source of bleeding. Cytologic analysis is performed on bladder washings, and both ureteral orifices are observed for upper tract bleeding.

In general, ureteroscopy should be performed when the patient is actively bleeding to increase the yield of the diagnostic procedure. If ureteronephroscopy is performed after the bleeding episode has ceased, a definitive diagnosis may be more difficult.

The method of performing ureteronephroscopy for benign essential hematuria is described earlier in this chapter (p. 29). The ureter and renal collecting system must be inspected carefully and systematically. Every effort should be made to avoid producing an iatrogenic guidewire lesion, which could be mistaken for the source of hematuria.

A definitive source of bleeding can be determined in 50% to 90% of patients.[11,12] Bagley and Allen reported finding discrete lesions in 16 of 32 patients with benign essential hematuria.[12] The majority of these lesions were small vascular abnormalities that were amenable to fulguration. Six were in the middle calyces, five in the lower pole calyces, two in the upper pole calyces, and two in the renal pelvis. The majority of the vascular lesions appeared as prominent vessels traversing the top of the papilla or as a mulberry collection of small vessels on the papilla. Other, rarer causes of hematuria are transitional cell carcinoma (5%) and urolithiasis (2%).[11,12]

Other Diagnostic Applications

Careful evaluation is mandatory when studying patients with persistent urinary cytologic abnormalities. If upper tract localization studies reveal that abnormal cells originated in the upper tract, ureteronephroscopy can be performed. The ureteroscopic approach in these patients should be identical to that described for benign essential hematuria. The short rigid ureteroscope is used to examine the distal ureter, and the flexible ureteronephroscope is used for systematic study of the intrarenal collecting system, with care taken not to produce iatrogenic lesions. If no disease is identified, brushings or random cold cup biopsies may be performed to find the source of malignant cells.

Unfortunately, there is little data regarding the utility of ureteronephroscopy in this setting. From our experience and from that reported by Fuchs, no cause of malignant cells in the upper tract has been found in the absence of a radiographic abnormality.[11,31] Moreover, to date, no case of carcinoma in situ of the upper collecting system has been identified with ureteronephroscopy. Continued surveillance of this group of patients is warranted for the earliest possible detection of any subsequent macroscopic tumor.

Another diagnostic application of ureteronephroscopy, albeit infrequently used, is the evaluation of the ureteropelvic junction (UPJ) before and after pyeloplasty or endopyelotomy. This may be a helpful adjunct in assessing the presence or degree of obstruction in the face of an equivocal Whittaker test or diuretic renogram. Postoperatively, endoscopic evaluation of the UPJ may give helpful information regarding patency.

Therapeutic Indications

With the development of ≤5F accessory instruments that can be passed through the ureteronephroscope, a variety of therapeutic procedures can now be performed. The main impact of these instruments has been in the area of calculus retrieval and lithotripsy. Other successful therapeutic applications with these instruments include the fulguration of bleeding vessels, retrograde endopyelotomy, treatment of ureteral strictures, and, in carefully selected patients, the treatment of low-grade transitional cell carcinomas of the upper tract.

Ureteral Calculi

The predominant therapeutic application of ureteronephroscopy is in treating urolithiasis. Along with the development of extracorporeal shock wave lithotripsy, endosurgical techniques have revolutionized the treatment of upper urinary calculi. Urolithiasis can be approached in three ways with the ureteronephroscope: primary removal, intracorporeal shock wave lithotripsy, or manipulation of the stone in preparation for extracorporeal shock wave lithotripsy.

Smaller calculi can usually be removed with primary endoscopy; however, this requires dilation of the ureteral tunnel to extract the stone. If the stone is in the distal ureter near the orifice, a 15F or 18F balloon dilator can be positioned alongside or beneath the stone and inflated. This opens the tunnel and, if the dilator is placed beside the stone, simultaneously pushes the stone into (not through) the wall of the ureter. Ureteroscopy can then be performed to gently tease the stone away from the wall of the ureter with a grasping forceps. If the dilator is beneath the stone, the stone lies directly in front of the ureteroscope and can be directly grasped for removal. Occasionally, significant ureteral spasm below a calculus precludes access. In this situation, passing a dilating balloon catheter alongside the stone is recommended.

The maximum size stone that can be removed intact is usually 6 mm. However, Garvin and associates have reported on successful balloon dilation of the distal tunnel to 8 mm for the removal of distal ureteral calculi up to 8 mm in diameter.[32] This dilation resulted in successful stone removal in all 131 patients; however, asymptomatic low-grade reflux developed in 20% of patients. Interestingly, none of 86 patients returning for a follow-up urogram developed a ureteral stricture. Nonetheless, presently, large ureteral calculi are preferentially fragmented in situ with one of the intracorporeal lithotripters.

A variety of graspers and baskets are available for removing calculi under direct vision. We prefer using a 3F, 4F, or 5F three- or four-prong wire grasper with a retractable sheath rather than a basket. In this way, if the calculus is too large to remove primarily, it can be released. If a basket is used, release of the calculus may not be possible; furthermore, excessive force to remove the basket and stone can result in ureteral avulsion or delayed ureteral stricture formation.

Intracorporeal shock wave lithotripsy is a relatively new modality for the endoscopic treatment of ureteral stones. Currently three methods are in use: ultrasonic lithotripsy, electrohydraulic lithotripsy, and laser lithotripsy.[33-35] With these techniques the ureteroscope is passed to the level of the stone, the stone is fragmented to particles less than 2 mm in situ, and the fragments are allowed to pass spontaneously. Intracorporeal shock wave lithotripsy is useful in treating impacted stones, larger stones that cannot be removed intact, and stones that are trapped in a basket.

Ultrasonic lithotripsy converts electrical energy into ultrasonic energy to fragment urinary calculi.[34] The ultrasonic lithotripter is composed of a handle containing a transducer with a long solid (2.5F) or hollow (4.5F) metal probe that is placed on the stone for fragmentation (Figure 2–17). The hollow probe has the capability of aspirating the stone particles as they are created. A piezoceramic element in the transducer is activated electrically and produces an ultrasound wave that is transmitted along the solid tube. This creates a mechanical vibration at the tip of the probe, which when placed on the stone can fragment it into small pieces. The probe is rigid and thus can be passed only through a rigid endoscope.

Electrohydraulic lithotripsy fragments stones by

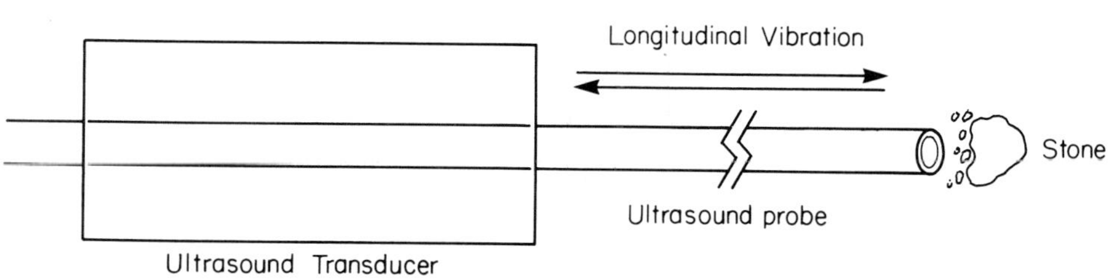

FIGURE 2–17. Diagram of a solid ultrasonic lithotripter probe. Electrical energy generates an ultrasonic wave that is transmitted along the solid tube. The tip of the probe vibrates at high speed and grinds the stone into small fragments.

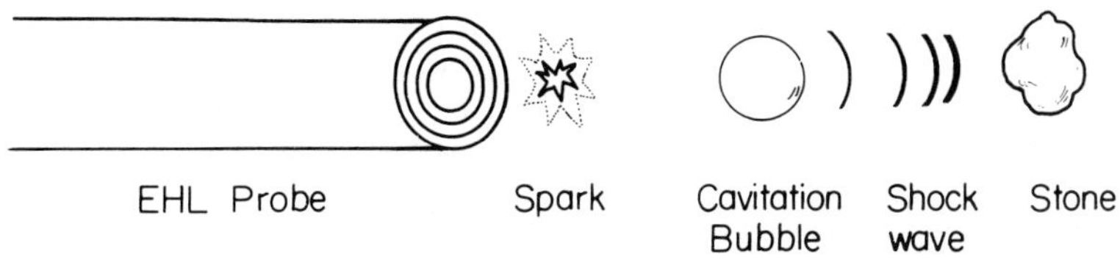

FIGURE 2–18. The electrohydraulic lithotripsy (EHL) probe generates a shock wave when an electrical current is sent down the central core. This produces a spark at the tip. The heated fluid produces a gas bubble, which in turn causes a hydraulic shock wave that strikes the stone.

the electrical production of a hydraulic shock wave.[35,36] The probe consists of an outer layer of insulation surrounding a layer of metal, another layer of insulation, and a central metal core (Figure 2–18). When an electrical charge is sent down the central metal core, a spark is produced at the tip of the probe. The spark rapidly heats the fluid media around the tip, causing vaporization of a small amount of irrigant. A gas bubble forms and pushes fluid in front of it at a speed of 4900 feet/sec. The expanding bubble produces a shock wave that is sufficient to fragment a stone.[37] As the irrigant cools at the probe tip, the gas bubble collapses and a second shock wave is produced. This entire sequence occurs in 1/800 second.

The electrohydraulic lithotripsy probe should be discharged at room temperature; hence the irrigant should be prewarmed. The manufacturer suggests using a 1/6 normal saline solution as the irrigant, but satisfactory probe discharge has been noted with normal saline. The tip of the probe should be placed within 1 mm of or directly upon the stone's surface but must protrude 5 mm from the endoscope to avoid damaging the lens.

Electrohydraulic lithotripsy probes as small as 1.9F are available and are very effective in fragmenting ureteral and intrarenal calculi. Care must be taken to avoid placing the probe on the ureteral mucosa, which would cause ureteral perforation.[36,38] If used as suggested and under direct endoscopic control, electrohydraulic lithotripsy is an efficient, economical, and safe means of performing intraureteral lithotripsy.[35,39]

Laser lithotripsy is also safe and effective for most ureteral and intrarenal stone fragmentation.[33,40-47] Two laser systems are capable of performing lithotripsy: the pulsed flashlamp pumped-dye laser and the pulsed Q-switched neodymium: yttrium aluminum garnet (Nd:YAG) laser. The bulk of clinical data concerns the former; however, the latter operates in the infrared spectrum and therefore does not impair visualization during lithotripsy. This potential advantage of the Q-switched Nd:YAG laser needs to be borne out clinically.

The dye lasers provide energy at wavelengths (514 nm) that are absorbed by calculi but not by normal tissue or hemoglobin. Thus they cause minimal tissue damage; however, they are extremely expensive to purchase and maintain. Fragmentation occurs when laser light energy is taken up by the stone, creating a microscopic heated focus (Figure 2–19). Materials in the stone such as calcium are vaporized into a cloud of colliding electrons called plasma. The plasma expands, dissipating the heat by creating an acoustic pressure wave, and then collapses. These events generate sufficient pressure to fragment the stone.

The pulsed-dye lasers have fibers as small as 200 μm with a 50 μm cladding. The lasers can be fired up to 10 times per second. The laser fiber must be placed directly on the stone for efficient fragmentation.

Stone composition can affect the efficiency of laser lithotripsy. Calcium oxalate dihydrate, struvite, and uric acid stones fragment easily, whereas the harder calcium oxalate monohydrate and calcium phosphate stones are resistant to laser lithotripsy at 60 mJ.[42,43] However, the newer 120 to 140 mJ pulsed dye lasers have been effective against these harder calculi. Cystine stones are resistant to laser lithotripsy.

Stones that cannot be manually extracted or fragmented may be manipulated with the ureteronephroscope into the renal pelvis in preparation for extracorporeal shock wave lithotripsy.[48] Stones may be pushed up with a grasper, or alternatively a stent may be placed to relieve obstruction.

The success rate for ureteroscopic stone extrac-

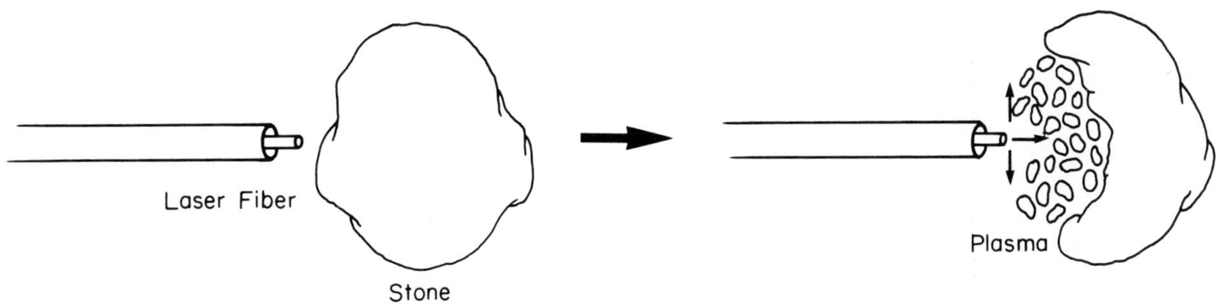

FIGURE 2–19. Laser energy creates a microscopic heated focus on the surface of the stone. The resulting expanding plasma of electrons creates an acoustic shock wave that fragments the stone.

tion is high. Therapeutic success varies with the location of the calculus within the collecting system and the type of ureteronephroscope (rigid versus flexible) used. Although the flexible endoscopes can be used in the distal ureter, their length and flexiblity make them cumbersome to manipulate. Thus the rigid ureteroscopes are most effective for extracting calculi in the lower ureter, whereas the flexible ureteroscopes perform better than the rigid ureteroscopes in the upper ureter (i.e., at or above the iliac vessels).

Lower ureteral stones can be removed with the rigid ureteroscope in 93% to 99% of patients.[49-51] The success rate with the rigid ureteroscope in the upper ureter diminishes to 50% to 78%.[49,52] The deflectable ureteronephroscope is more effective in this area, with a success rate of 70% to 85%.[11,53]

Intracorporeal shock wave lithotripsy has greatly increased the efficacy of treating ureteral calculi. For most distal ureteral stones, this can be accomplished with a small-diameter ureteroscope (6.9F to 7.2F) and a 250 μm tunable dye laser probe or 1.9F electrohydraulic lithotripsy probe, obviating the need for ureteral dilation. Alternatively, for upper ureteral calculi, the laser or electrohydraulic lithotripsy probe can be used with the flexible ureteronephroscope. In contrast, the rigid ultrasound probe is limited to the larger off-angle viewing rigid ureteroscopes, and ureteral dilation is thus usually necessary.

Results with all types of intracorporeal lithotripters are excellent. Huffman and Fuchs reported successful ultrasonic disintegration of ureteral stones with hollow or solid wire probes in 95% of patients[34,54]; the majority of patients in these series had distal ureteral stones. In contrast, success with electrohydraulic lithotripsy in fragmenting ureteral calculi regardless of their location is 90%.[35,55,56] Complications have been limited to small ureteral perforations in 6% to 18% of patients and are apparently due to ureteral dilation rather than to the lithotripsy itself. To date, with intraureteral EHL, no series has noted delayed ureteral stricture formation, perforation at the lithotripsy site, or other adverse side effects.[35,36,55,56] The pulsed-dye laser and the Q-switched pulsed Nd:YAG laser have completely disintegrated ureteral calculi in 73% to 100% of patients.[44-47]

Benign Essential Hematuria

When a benign vascular lesion is the cause of hematuria in the upper urinary tract, endoscopic fulguration is effective.[11,12] If the lesion is not a vascular abnormality, a biopsy is recommended. Fulguration is performed with either an Nd:YAG laser or a small (2F or 3F) electrosurgical probe. When fulguration is performed with electrocautery, 2% glycine or 3% sorbitol should be used. This technique is successful in alleviating the hematuria in 68% to 100% of patients.[11,12,57]

Ureteropelvic Junction Obstruction

Percutaneous endopyelotomy has been effective in treating ureteropelvic junction obstruction in 70% to 87% of patients.[58,59] Performing this procedure retrograde, completely through the ureteroscope, avoids the morbidity associated with a percutaneous procedure.[60,61] Both the flexible, actively deflectable and the rigid endoscopes have been used to perform the incision. The easiest method is usually to pass the flexible instrument to the ureteropelvic junction and cut with the electrosurgical probe or a contact tip (Nd:YAG or KTP) laser fiber. However, the rigid endoscope makes cutting with a cold knife easier to control.

Before retrograde endopyelotomy, a small nephrostomy tube may be placed at the time of a Whitaker pressure study, which is performed to confirm the presence of functional obstruction. A pressure differential (renal pelvis versus bladder) of greater than 22 cm H_2O at a flow of 10 ml/min is indicative of obstruction.[62] The nephrostomy tube allows continuous flow during ureteroscopy to keep the surgical field clear, while at the same time decreasing the risk of irrigant absorption from pyelovenous backflow and retroperitoneal extravasation. Alternatively, if an indwelling stent was placed preoperatively, no neephrostomy tube is placed.

Retrograde endopyelotomy is accomplished by first passing a guidewire beyond the area of obstruction (Figure 2–20). An 8F/10F Amplatz dilator and sheath assembly is passed over the guidewire. The 8F catheter is removed, and a second guidewire is passed. The 10F catheter is removed. A 6 mm balloon catheter is advanced over the first guidewire to the area of obstruction. The balloon is expanded to 1 atm of pressure to calibrate and define the area of obstruction. This is marked on the fluoroscopy screen. The balloon dilator is removed. The ureteronephroscope is advanced over the first guidewire, and when it reaches the ureteropelvic junction, the guidewire is removed. The ureter is cut along its posterolateral portion, 1 cm on either side of the ureteropelvic junction, until retroperitoneal fat is seen. The incision must extend through the full thickness of the ureter. When electrosurgery is used to make the incision, the metal guidewire should be insulated with a 5F angiographic catheter or the metal guideline should be exchanged for a plastic (i.e., Terumo) guidewire. When a cold knife or Nd:YAG laser is used to complete the cut, covering the metal guidewire is unnecessary. Indeed, the laser might melt any catheter placed over the guidewire.

After the incision an 8 mm balloon catheter is inflated to further separate the edges of the ureter; no waist should develop, and the balloon should be

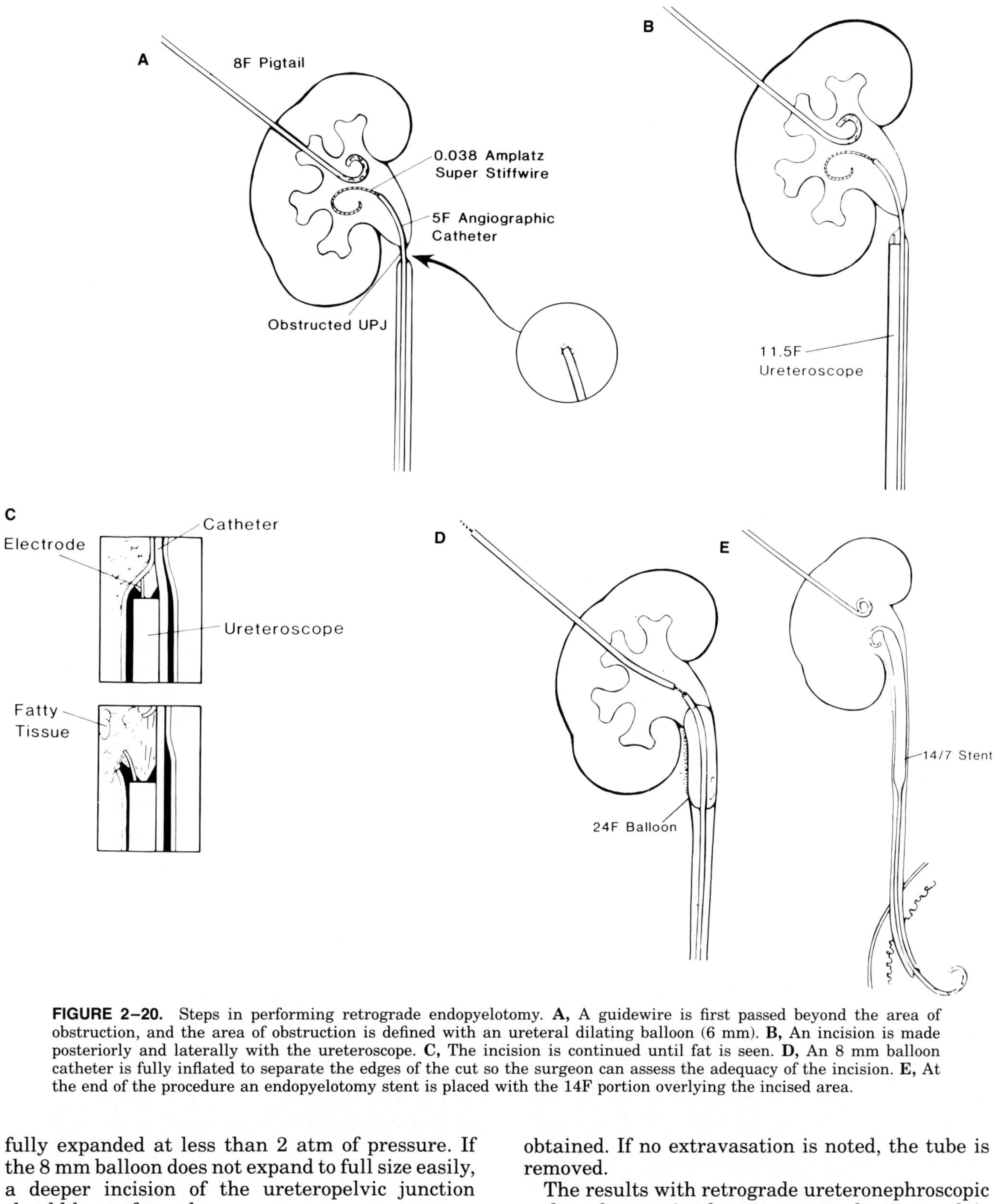

FIGURE 2–20. Steps in performing retrograde endopyelotomy. **A,** A guidewire is first passed beyond the area of obstruction, and the area of obstruction is defined with an ureteral dilating balloon (6 mm). **B,** An incision is made posteriorly and laterally with the ureteroscope. **C,** The incision is continued until fat is seen. **D,** An 8 mm balloon catheter is fully inflated to separate the edges of the cut so the surgeon can assess the adequacy of the incision. **E,** At the end of the procedure an endopyelotomy stent is placed with the 14F portion overlying the incised area.

fully expanded at less than 2 atm of pressure. If the 8 mm balloon does not expand to full size easily, a deeper incision of the ureteropelvic junction should be performed.

At the conclusion of the procedure an endopyelotomy stent (7F/14F) is placed with the 14F section positioned over the incised area; this stent is left in place for 3 to 6 weeks. The nephrostomy tube is left for 48 hours, after which a nephrostogram is obtained. If no extravasation is noted, the tube is removed.

The results with retrograde ureteronephroscopic endopyelotomy in the treatment of ureteropelvic junction obstruction are equivalent to those reported with antegrade percutaneous techniques. The success rates in small series range from 83% to 100%.[60,61,63] Unfortunately, when performing this technique with electrosurgery in 20 patients, Clayman and associates found a 20% incidence of delayed distal ureteral strictures requiring endoureterotomy in 3 patients and a nephrectomy in 1 patient (greater than 12-month follow-up in all patients).[63] This was not noted by Thomas and Cherry, who used both cold knife and electrosurgery to perform their incisions.[61] However, their series had a briefer follow-up (minimum of 6 months) and all patients had an indwelling stent placed several days before endopyelotomy. Longer follow-up and larger series will be needed before the place of the retrograde approach can be ascertained.

Ureteral Strictures

Ureteral strictures can be successfully treated with the ureteronephroscope.[64,65] A cold knife incision through the rigid ureteroscope is the treatment of choice for distal ureteral strictures. For completely obstructing strictures or upper ureteral strictures, a combined antegrade and retrograde approach may be necessary. The same cutting modalities are available for performing an endoscopic incision as for endopyelotomy; however, in the vast majority of cases the cold knife and a rigid endoscope are used.

In the treatment of proximal ureteral strictures the method of incision is similar to that described for endopyelotomy. The main goal is to marsupialize the stricture into the renal pelvis. It is always easier to approach these strictures via the percutaneous nephrostomy tract, especially when they are dense. A posterior and lateral incision is routinely made.

For distal ureteral strictures the goal is to marsupialize the stricture into the bladder. In this situation a guidewire is first passed and coiled into the renal pelvis. The stricture may be approached directly with the cold knife urethrotome and the ureter opened from the inside outward by cutting anteriorly at the ureteral tunnel and medially between the ureterovesical junction and a point just below the iliac vessels. In female patients the surgeon must be aware of the uterine artery, which crosses the distal ureter anteriorly. Inadvertent injury may result in significant hemorrhaging. After the incision a 7F/14F endopyelotomy stent should be placed in an inverted fashion so that the 14F portion traverses the incised distal ureter. A Foley catheter is inserted. A cystogram should be obtained 1 week after the procedure to be sure that no extravasation is present before the Foley catheter is removed. As with an endopyelotomy, the stent is left in place for 3 to 6 weeks.

Midureteral strictures are the most difficult type to treat. Using the rigid ureteroscope is easier if the midureteral stricture is below the level of the iliac vessels and the flexible ureteronephroscope is preferred when the stricture is at or above this level. In these cases normal caliber ureter borders both ends of the incised stricture. A 7F/14F stent with the 14F portion overlying the incised stricture is left in place for 6 weeks. No urethral catheter is placed postoperatively.

For total ureteral occlusion a cut-to-the-light or guidewire puncture procedure may be performed with use of a combined antegrade and retrograde approach (Figure 2–21).[64,65] A flexible antegrade ureteronephroscope is passed down to the level of the stricture. The light from the antegrade endoscope is disconnected, and the light from the ureteroscope is sought. When light is observed from the retrograde ureteroscope and fluoroscopy demonstrates that the tips of the two endoscopes are aligned in two planes, a stiff guidewire can be used to perforate the stricture. Alternatively, a direct cold knife or electrosurgery incision to the light can be made. An exchange guidewire is then passed to establish a through-and-through access from the flank to the urethral meatus. The incision can then be made and the 7F/14F stent placed again with the 14F portion traversing the incised area.

Triamcinolone may prevent stricture recurrence, especially if the scar tissue is particularly dense. Transurethral steroid injection is of some benefit in preventing recurrent bladder neck strictures following surgical resection.[66] We have injected triamcinolone (10 mg/ml) with a 3F Greenwald needle directly into the bed of an incised ureteral stricture. A LeVeen or other type of pressure syringe is useful to forcibly inject the triamcinolone into the scar tissue that lines either side of the endoureterotomy. Controlled studies are needed to assess the efficacy of steroid injection in this situation.

The results with endoscopic incision of ureteral strictures are promising. Success rates of 57% to 82% have been noted.[64,65,67] The success of the procedure is affected by the stricture length and density, the cause of the stricture, and prior surgery. Patency rates are much lower in patients with long (>1 cm) or completely obstructing strictures. Likewise, a prior history of radiation therapy, ischemic injury, or a radical hysterectomy augur poorly. Follow-up beyond a year is needed to establish the efficacy and indications for this procedure.

Upper Urinary Tract Transitional Cell Carcinoma

The role of ureteroscopy in the treatment of upper urinary tract transitional cell carcinoma is controversial. Unquestionably this technique is valuable in diagnosing transitional cell tumors; however, many concerns exist when treating cancer in this manner.

First, local and systemic seeding may result from ureteronephroscopic manipulation. If the ureter is perforated during the procedure, tumor cells might be washed into the retroperitoneum. Also, increased intrapelvic pressure during irrigation can lead to pyelovenous and pyelolymphatic backflow, potentially transporting tumor cells into the sys-

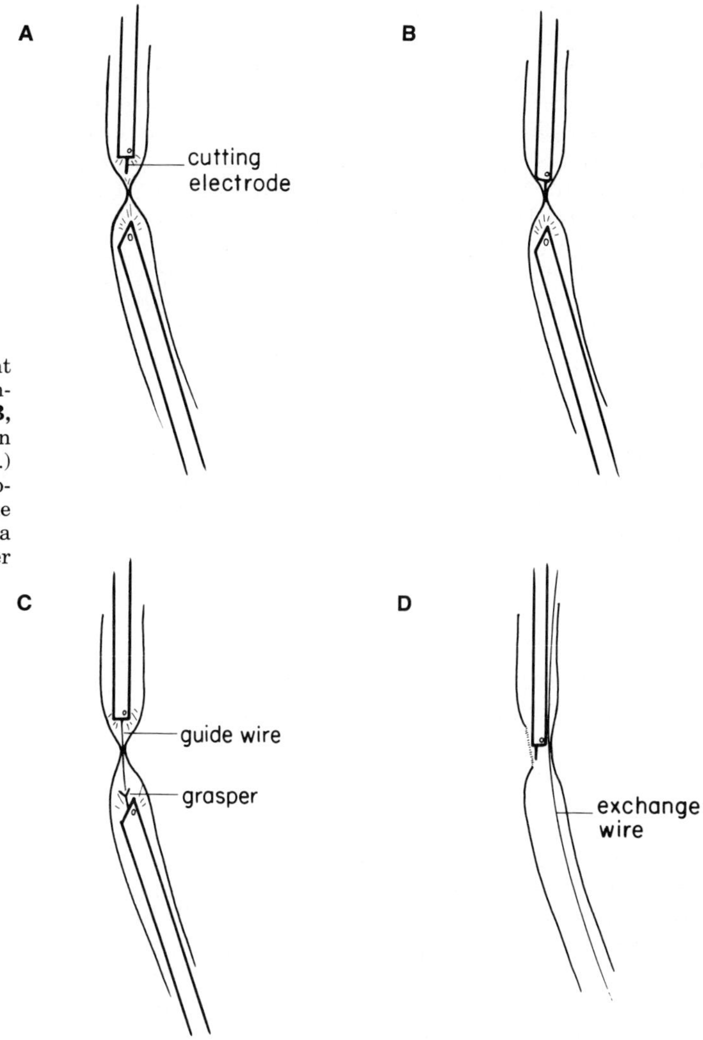

FIGURE 2–21. For total ureteral occlusion a cut-to-the-light procedure is performed. **A,** A retrograde endoscope and an antegrade endoscope are aligned on either side of the stricture. **B,** A wire is poked through the stricture. (Alternatively, a cut can be made with an electrosurgical probe or a cold knife.) **C,** An exchange guidewire is passed through the area of obstruction and retrieved via the retrograde endoscope. **D,** The incision is completed, and a balloon is used to calibrate the area of incision. At the conclusion a 7F/14F double pigtail catheter is placed with the 14F portion traversing the incised area.

temic circulation. Furthermore, scuffing of the mucosa with instrument passage may provide a bed for the implantation of tumor cells. Each of these problems is a significant, albeit hypothetical, concern.

The technique for ureteronephroscopic treatment of upper urothelial tumors depends on the size and location of the lesion. Irrigant flow is kept at 40 cm H_2O during diagnostic ureteroscopy. Small lesions (<5 mm) can be removed completely with a cold cup biopsy forceps, and the base of the tumor can be lightly fulgurated (Nd:YAG laser and 2F or 3F electrosurgery probe). Larger lesions (5 to 10 mm) can be resected with the rigid ureteroresectoscope. The cutting current should be at the lowest possible setting to minimize tissue injury. Only the tumor within the ureteral or renal pelvic lumen is resected. No deep cuts in the ureter or pelvis should be attempted, since they would likely perforate the thin wall. The resectoscope loop should be extended beyond the tumor and then pulled into the instrument to cut the tissue. Each cut of tissue should be retrieved separately. The base of the lesion can then be coagulated at a low current. Alternatively, the lesion can be treated completely with the Nd:YAG laser.

No effective cutting loop is available for the flexible ureteronephroscope, and the small biopsy forceps is not suitable for removing even a small tumor. The only effective means of treating tumors with the flexible ureteronephroscope is by using a Nd:YAG laser or an electrosurgery probe to ablate the tumor.

Accuracy in ureteroscopic assessment of the local extent of disease, especially for renal pelvic tumors, has not been demonstrated in the literature.[68-71] Although biopsy specimens of the tumor can be obtained through the ureteronephroscope, the tissue obtained may be insufficient for proper staging. Huffman and associates reviewed ureteroscopic staging in six patients with renal pelvic tumors who subsequently underwent nephroureterectomy.[68] In only two of the patients (33%) was the cancer properly staged with rigid ureteroscopy. In the remainder it was understaged. In another study examining staging of renal pelvic tumors with the flexible deflectable ureteronephroscope, Huffman found that only 65% of pelvocalyceal tumors could be correctly staged.[69] Thomas and associates found ureteroscopy superior to traditional methods for diagnosing upper tract transitional carcinoma; however, only 10% of biopsies led to the correct assessment of tumor stage and grade.[70] Furthermore, carcinoma in situ may be difficult or impossible to detect with routine ureteronephroscopy.[69]

The effectiveness of ureteronephroscopic treatment of upper urinary tract transitional cell carcinoma is unknown. In a limited series the local recurrence rate appeared to be similar to that after conventional open surgery; however, longer follow-up with a larger number of patients is necessary.[68-71] The local recurrence rate at 2 years appears to be only 15% in the ureter and 30% in the renal pelvis; bladder failure rate is not increased.

In patients treated conservatively for upper tract transitional carcinoma, follow-up ureteroscopy is helpful in detecting local recurrences, often before they can be demonstrated radiographically.[68] However, ureteroscopic surveillance subjects patients to the morbidity of a repeat anesthetic procedure and is relatively expensive and time consuming.

Because of the possibility of understaging and the unknown effectiveness of ureteronephroscopic treatment of upper urinary tract urothelial tumors, therapeutic ureteroscopy should be reserved for patients who are high surgical risks, with a solitary kidney or compromised renal function. Moreover, candidates for therapeutic ureteroscopy should have a low-grade (preferably grade 1) tumor and low tumor volume (<1.5 cm). Patients treated by ureteronephroscopy should be carefully followed with cystoscopic and ureteroscopic surveillance at 3-month intervals for at least 2 years after tumor resection, biannual examinations for another 2 years, and annual checkups thereafter. The examinations should be supplemented with radiographic and cytologic screening.

Other Therapeutic Indications

Other reported uses of the ureteronephroscope include treatment of calyceal diverticula, peripelvic cysts, and ureteroenteric strictures. In a series of six patients with calyceal diverticula reported by Mikkelsen and associates, only two were successfully treated with ureteronephroscopy.[14] The difficulty was related to problems in identifying and incising the neck of the diverticulum. A percutaneous approach is still probably the most effective method of treating calyceal diverticula.

We have had experience with retrograde ureteroscopic incision of peripelvic renal cysts in three patients, one of whom had a large cyst obstructing the ureteropelvic junction. Ureteronephroscopy allowed the marsupialization of each cyst into the renal pelvis while permitting inspection and biopsy of the cyst. No cyst recurred in any of these patients on follow-up (>1½ years) radiographic studies.

The flexible actively deflectable ureteronephroscope has been used via a percutaneous nephrostomy tract to incise ureteroenteric anastomotic strictures. Meretyk and associates reported on 19 strictures in 15 patients followed up for 9 to 54 months after treatment with this modality.[72] The overall patency rate was 64%. A permanent external stent was left in five strictures because of metastatic disease. In only one patient in the study was open surgical correction subsequently indicated.

As noted above, ureteroscopes can be used in other than a retrograde manner. Both the short, rigid and the flexible actively deflectable ureteronephroscopes can be used to perform antegrade inspection and treatment of the urinary collecting system during percutaneous procedures (e.g., calculus removal, endopyelotomy). Furthermore, these endoscopes can be helpful in performing endoscopy through a variety of urinary diversions: ileal conduits, continent diversions, and cutaneous ureterostomies.

GUIDELINES TO MINIMIZE COMPLICATIONS

Several guidelines can be followed to mimimize complications during ureteronephroscopy (Table 2–5). Endoscopy is at best a clean, not a sterile, procedure. Thus the upper urinary tract may be contaminated during ureteroscopy. A sterile urine culture must be obtained before manipulation to avoid sepsis. Moreover, parenteral antibiotics (cephalosporin or penicillin and an aminoglycoside) should be administered preoperatively. Antibiotics are also given postoperatively, and oral antibiotics are continued until 2 days after stent removal.

The pyelogram must be adequate to define the upper collecting system and serve as a roadmap to areas of disease. Fluoroscopic, as well as endoscopic, control during the procedure is mandatory to prevent ureteral injury. A safety guidewire should be placed before manipulation of the upper collecting system to act as a guide and a means of placing a ureteral stent if the procedure must be terminated for technical or medical reasons. Excessive force in passing guidewires or endoscopes

TABLE 2–5. Guidelines for Minimizing Complications During Ureteronephroscopy

Preoperative sterile urine culture
Perioperative antibiotics
Adequate preoperative pyelography
Placement of a safety guidewire
Fluoroscopic monitoring
Maintenance of endoscopic control
Avoidance of excessive force
Postoperative ureteral stents

should be avoided, since it only leads to ureteral injury or equipment breakage.

Most ureteral manipulations cause transient ureteral edema. A ureteral stent should be inserted at the end of the procedure and left in place for at least 72 hours to prevent postoperative obstruction.

COMPLICATIONS OF URETERONEPHROSCOPY

Complications of ureteronephroscopy can be divided into intraoperative, early postoperative, and late postoperative.

Intraoperative Complications

The most common complication of ureteroscopy is ureteral perforation.[11,73-75] Perforations are usually detected fluoroscopically and are minor, but if they are noted, the procedure should be terminated. The injury usually occurs during ureteral dilation and can be successfully managed by leaving a ureteral stent in place for 72 hours. An intravenous pyelogram or cystogram should be obtained before removal of the stent to ensure adequate healing. For large perforations an external ureteral stent is usually left in place and a stent injection is done 72 hours later. If no extravasation is noted, the external stent is replaced by an indwelling ureteral stent, which is left in place for 3 to 6 weeks.

Loss of ureteral access can occur if the safety guidewire is not used or not secured in place. The safety guidewire should be sutured to either the labia minora or the glans penis or carefully clipped to the perineal area of the drapes for a female patient. If a ureteral perforation occurs and access is lost, indigo carmine and furosemide (Lasix) may be given intravenously in an attempt to locate the true ureteral lumen endoscopically. If this is not possible, a percutaneous nephrostomy may need to be placed and the ureter stinted via an antegrade approach.

Care should be taken not to create a submucosal false passage with the guidewire (Figure 2–22). This occurs when a guidewire perforates the ureteral urothelium and travels within the mucosa between the urothelium and muscular layer of the collecting system. Some initial resistance to passage of the guidewire is encountered. Then, as force is applied, the guidewire is felt to move suddenly across a short area of resistance. The guidewire then passes up the ureter easily. However, it does not form a broad curl in the renal pelvis. Instead, multiple tight coils are noted in the upper ureter. If a ureteral stent is placed, the proximal coil of the stent never forms properly. Ureteroscopy reveals rough tissue everywhere and no smooth mucosa. Although the guidewire can be clearly seen, the stone or other pathologic condition is never visualized. Retrograde injection of contrast material (through the ureteroscope) fails to fill the renal pelvis. If a submucosal guidewire is suspected, at-

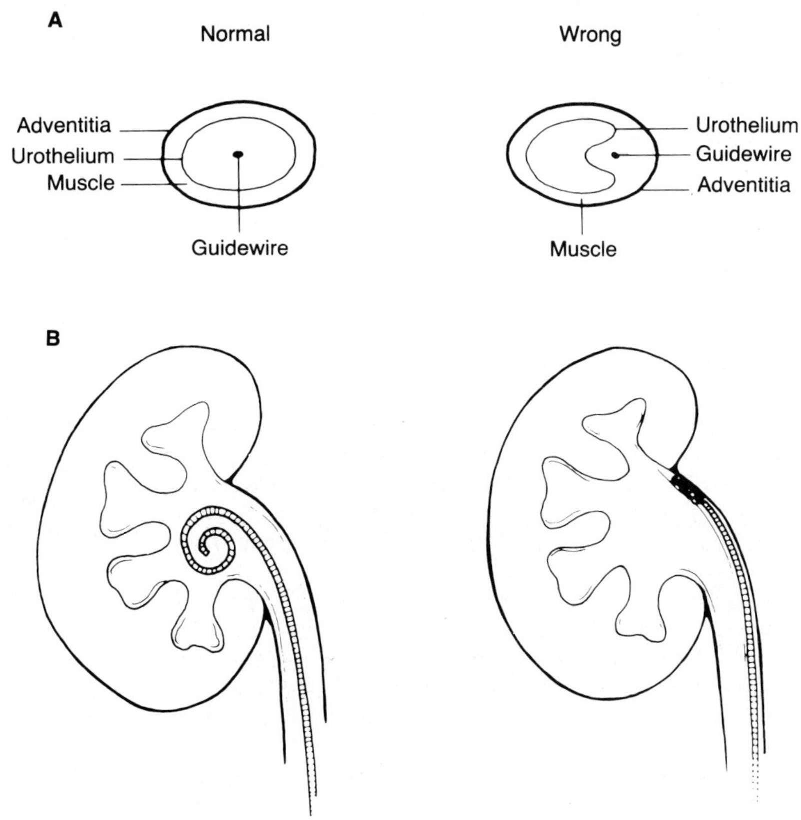

FIGURE 2–22. Submucosal guidewire. **A,** The guidewire travels between the urothelium and muscle. **B,** The guidewire coils tightly in the upper ureter when a submucosal false pass is made. It does not form the broad coil that is normally seen.

tempts should be made to find the true lumen (after intravenous injection of indigo carmine and furosemide) and to pass a retrograde stent. If these efforts fail, a percutaneous nephrostomy and antegrade stent should be placed.

Instruments can break if undue force is applied. All instruments should be checked before use, and any rigid ureteroscope that is bent should be returned to the factory for repair. If during rigid ureteroscopy the visual field changes from oval to elliptical, undue force is being placed on the shaft of the ureteroscope and further force could result in fracture of the endoscope with injury to the patient. The newer, small fiberoptic short rigid ureteroscopes are easily broken; in general, they are most safely used below the iliac vessel crossing. The accessory items are also fragile. Biopsy forceps can be snapped, baskets permanently disfigured, and laser, electrohydraulic lithotripsy, or electrosurgery probes fragmented, possibly resulting in a foreign body left in the patient.

Hematuria commonly occurs during and shortly after ureteronephroscopy. Severe bleeding is unusual and is the basis for terminating the procedure, especially since visualization is impaired. Hematuria usually clears within 3 days postoperatively but may last longer if intrarenal surgery has been performed. On occasion, repeat ureteroscopy to fulgurate a bleeding site may be necessary. To date, no problems of postoperative bleeding caused by arterial or venous malformations or of bleeding necessitating embolization have been reported.

Extravasation of irrigant during ureteroscopy may cause fluid overload and, if the irrigant is glycine or sorbitol, may result in hyponatremia. These problems can be avoided by using normal saline as the irrigant for ureteronephroscopy. If a ureteral perforation is noted, the procedure is terminated, a pharmacologic diuresis is maintained during and after the procedure, and the fluid status during the postoperative period is carefully monitored. Hypotonic solutions should be used only during electrosurgery and not during diagnostic inspection.

Early Postoperative Complications

Postoperative infection is rare (<1%). Postoperative fever, despite a sterile urine culture, occurs in 3% of patients.[11,73,74] Therefore parenteral and then oral postoperative antibiotics during the period of stinting and for 48 hours after stent removal are recommended.

Transient ureteral obstruction and colic can follow ureteronephroscopy. They usually last 72 hours. The problem can be avoided by placement of an indwelling ureteral stent at the conclusion of ureteronephroscopy; the stent can be removed after 3 days.

Persistent severe postoperative flank pain, despite a stent, is usually due to obstruction of the stent or stent migration. An abdominal radiograph is necessary to assess the location of the stent, and hydronephrosis or a perinephric fluid collection should be sought with renal ultrasound. A cystogram can document stent patency if reflux is present; however, absence of reflux does not necessarily indicate stent obstruction. If the stent fails to show reflux, an intravenous pyelogram should be obtained. The stent should be changed if it migrates or becomes blocked.

A perinephric urinoma may occur postoperatively. This is associated with flank pain and can best be diagnosed by computed tomography. Once adequate drainage of the intrarenal collecting system is established (i.e., ureteral stent plus urethral catheter), the problem usually resolves. In some instances, however, percutaneous drainage of the urinoma may be necessary and the urinoma tube is left in place until drainage ceases. If the drainage continues beyond 2 weeks, the communication must be identified and severed, either endourologically or with open surgery.

Occasionally a retroperitoneal hematoma develops. This is monitored with serial hematocrits and periodic radiographic examination. With bed rest, the bleeding is usually self-limiting and a transfusion is rarely needed. If active bleeding is suspected, embolization or, more rarely, surgical exploration (angiography) may be necessary.

Long-Term Postoperative Complications

Ureteral stricture formation follows ureteroscopy in 0.5% to 3% of patients.[73-75] Most strictures occur within 6 months of ureteroscopy. They usually develop at the site of a prior ureteral injury or an impacted stone. When noted early, they can often be treated with simple balloon dilation to 24F and placement of an indwelling ureteral stent (7F/14F or 10F) for 6 weeks. If the stricture is discovered late, an endoscopic incision may be necessary. Because of the possibility of stricture formation, follow-up intravenous pyelography or renal scanning is recommended 4 to 6 weeks after ureteroscopy to detect asymptomatic early obstruction.

Ureteral reflux occurs in 6% of patients and is related to the degree of ureteral dilation.[32,73] Reflux is usually of minimal clinical significance. Garvin and Clayman noted asymptomatic grade 1 or 2 reflux at 3-month follow-up in 5% of patients whose ureters were dilated to 18F and in 20% of those with 24F dilation.[32]

CONCLUSION

Ureteronephroscopy has dramatically changed the surgical approach to the upper urinary tract. Currently available rigid and flexible endoscopes allow accurate diagnosis of pathologic conditions in the upper urinary collecting system. Furthermore, the development of myriad accessory instruments permits the urologist to perform a wide variety of therapeutic procedures in a closed controlled manner. The decreased morbidity and shorter convalescence associated with ureteronephroscopy have made its use increasingly popular. Further advances in technology and improvements in instrument design are occurring rapidly. Already, videoimage flexible actively deflectable ureteronephroscopes as small as 6F in diameter are being developed.[76] Both the application and the margin of safety of ureteronephroscopy will certainly continue to expand over the next several years.

REFERENCES

1. Young HH, McKay RW: Congenital valvular obstruction of the prostatic urethra. Surg Gynecol Obstet 48:509, 1929.
2. Goodman TM: Ureteroscopy with pediatric cystoscope in adults. Urology 9:394, 1977.
3. Lyon ES, Kyker JS, Schoenberg HW: Transurethral ureteroscopy in women: a ready addition to the urological armamentarium. J Urol 199:35, 1978.
4. Lyon ES, Banno JJ, Schoenberg HW: Transurethral ureteroscopy in men using juvenile cystoscopy equipment. J Urol 122:152, 1979.
5. Perez-Castro Ellendt E, Martinez-Pineiro JA: Transurethral ureteroscopy—a current urological procedure. Arch Exp Urol 33:445, 1980.
6. Hirschowitz BI, Curtiss LE, Peters CW, Pollard HM: Demonstration of a new gastroscope, the fiberscope. Gastroenterology 35:50, 1958.
7. Marshall VF: Fiberoptics in urology, J Urol 91:110, 1964.
8. Takagi T, Go T, Takayasu H, Hioki R: Small caliber fiberscope for visualization of the urinary tract, biliary tract, and spinal canal. Surgery 64:1033, 1968.
9. Eshghi M: Dilatation of ureteral orifice for ureterorenoscopy. Urol Clin North Am 15:301, 1988.
10. Dourmashkin RL: Cystoscopic treatment of stones in the ureter with special reference to large calculi: based on the study of 1550 cases. J Urol 54:245, 1945.
11. Kavoussi LR, Clayman RV, Basler JW: Flexible actively deflectable fiberoptic ureteronephroscopy. J Urol 142:949, 1989.
12. Bagley DH, Allen J: Flexible ureteropyeloscopy in the diagnosis of benign essential hematuria. J Urol 143:549, 1990.
13. Higashihara E, Horie S, Takeuchi T, et al: Laser ureterolithotripsy with combined rigid and flexible ureterorenoscopy. J Urol 143:273, 1990.
14. Mikkelsen DJ, Kavoussi LR, Clayman RV, Picus DD: Advances in flexible deflectable ureteronephroscopy (FDU): intrarenal surgery. J Urol 141:192A, 1989.
15. Hunter III PT, Newman RC, Finlayson B: Acute mechanical dilation of the ureter: an experimental study. J Urol 138:161, 1987.
16. Gal D, Buchsbaum HJ: A cinefluoroscopic study of ureteral function following radical hysterectomy. Obstet Gynecol 61:82, 1983.
17. Perez-Castro Ellendt E, Mancebo Gomez JM, Massarra J: Dilatacion hidraulica con bomba impulsora de liquido irrigante: nuevo aparataje en ureterorenoscopia. Arch Exp Urol 39(suppl 1):3, 1986.
18. Eshghi M: Pressure-controlled hydraulic dilation of the ureter: "one-step ureteroscopy." J Urol 140:950, 1988.
19. Eshghi M, Schwalb D, Davison M, et al: Morphological changes in the urinary tract associated with ureteropyeloscopy: an experimental study. J Urol 141:208A, 1989.
20. Huffman JL, Bagley DH: Balloon dilation of the ureter for ureteroscopy. J Urol 140:954, 1988.
21. Green DF, Glickman MG, Weiss RM: Preliminary results with aminophylline as smooth-muscle relaxant in percutaneous renal surgery. J Endourol 1:243, 1987.
22. Ellis WJ, Graham JB: Lidocaine jelly dislodgement of ureteral calculi before ESWL. In Proceedings of the 5th Symposium on Shock Wave Lithotripsy: Urinary and Biliary. March 10-12, 1989, p 117.
23. Ryan PC, Jones BJ, Hargaden KM, et al: Pharmacological dilatation of the human ureter for ureteroscopy: an in vitro experimental study. J Urol 143:363A, 1990.
24. Marchuk JM: Transperineal placement of ureteroscope in males. Urology 27:526, 1986.
25. Bagley DH, Huffman JL, Lyon ES: Flexible ureteropyeloscopy: diagnosis and treatment in the upper urinary tract. J Urol 138:280, 1987.
26. Bagley DH: Active versus passive deflection in flexible ureteroscopy. J Endourol 1:15, 1987.
27. Bagley DH, Rivas D: Flexible ureteroscopic diagnosis of filling defects in the upper urinary tract. J Urol 141:470A, 1989.
28. Gittes RF: Retrograde brushing and nephroscopy in the diagnosis of upper-tract urothelial cancer. Urol Clin North Am 11:617, 1984.
29. Streem SB, Pontes JE, Novick AC, Montie JE: Ureteropyeloscopy in the evaluation of upper tract filling defects. J Urol 136:383, 1986.
30. Andriole GL, McClennan BL, Picus D, Becich MJ: The effect of low-osmolar contrast material on the interpretation of urinary cytology specimens. J Urol 139:177A, 1988.
31. Fuchs G, David R, Fuchs A: Retrograde ureteroscopic intrarenal surgery (RIRS): a minimally invasive alternative to percutaneous and open surgery. J Urol 143:361A, 1990.
32. Garvin JT, Clayman RV: Balloon dilation of the distal ureter to 24F: an effective method for ureteroscopic stone retrieval. J Urol 130:280A, 1988.
33. Dretler SP: Laser photofragmentation of ureteral calculi: analysis of 75 cases. Endourology 1:9, 1987.
34. Huffman JL, Bagley DH, Schoenberg HW, Lyon ES: Transurethral removal of large ureteral and renal pelvic calculi using ureteroscopic ultrasonic lithotripsy. J Urol 130:31, 1983.
35. Denstedt JD, Clayman RV: Electrohydraulic lithotripsy of renal and ureteral calculi. J Urol 143:13, 1989.
36. Green DF, Lytton B: Early experience with electrohydraulic lithotripsy of ureteral calculi using direct vision ureteroscopy. J Urol 133:767, 1985.
37. Naser ME: Studies on the fracture mechanism in urinary test concretions by lithotriptor devices. Master of Science Thesis, University of Florida, Gainesville, 1982.
38. Goodfriend R: Ultrasonic and electrohydraulic lithotripsy of ureteral calculi. Urology 23:5, 1984.
39. Lamont JS, Birkett DH, O'Keane JC, Babayan RK: Tissue effects of a pulsed dye laser and electrohydraulic lithotriptor on porcine urothelium. J Endourol 4:586, 1990.
40. Dretler SP: An evaluation of ureteral laser lithotripsy: 225 consecutive patients. J Urol 143:267, 1989.
41. Higashihara E, Horie S, Takeuchi T, et al: Laser ureterolithotripsy with combined rigid and flexible ureterorenoscopy. J Urol 143:273, 1989.
42. Dretler SP: Stone fragility—a new therapeutic distinction. J Urol 139:1124, 1988.
43. Dretler SP: Techniques of laser lithotripsy. J Endourol 2:123, 1988.
44. Bagley DH, Grasso M, Shalaby M, El-Akkad MA: Ureteral laser lithotripsy using the Pulsolith. J Endourol 3:91, 1989.
45. Maghraby H, Knipper A, Muschter R, Hofstetter AG: Laser lithotripsy: further experience with Nd:YAG laser. J Endourol 4:161, 1990.
46. Hofmann R, Hartung R, Schmidt-Kloiber H, Reichel E: Laser-induced shock wave ureteral lithotripsy using Q-switched Nd:YAG laser. J Endourol 4:169, 1990.
47. Grasso M, Bagley DH: Flexible ureteroscopic lithotripsy using pulsed-dye laser. J Endourol 4:155, 1990.
48. Liong ML, Clayman RV, Gittes RF, et al: Treatment op-

tions for proximal ureteral urolithiasis: review and recommendations. J Urol 143:504, 1988.
49. Seeger AR, Rittenberg MH, Bagley DH: Ureteropyeloscopic removal of ureteral calculi. J Urol 139:1180, 1988.
50. Lingeman JE, Sonda P, Kahnoski RJ, et al: Ureteral stone management: emerging concepts. J Urol 135:1172, 1986.
51. Blute ML, Segura JW, Patterson DE: Ureteroscopy. J Urol 139:510, 1987.
52. Thomas R: Rigid ureteroscopy: pitfalls and remedies. Urology 32:328, 1988.
53. Aso Y, Ohta H, Nakano M, et al: Retrograde removal of upper ureteral and renal calculi under fiberoptic control. J Urol 141:188A, 1988.
54. Fuchs GJ, Lupu AN, Chaussy CG: Ultrasonic lithotripsy for ureteral calculi. Endourology 1:5, 1986.
55. Willscher MK, Conway JF Jr, Babayan RK, et al: Safety and efficacy of electrohydraulic lithotripsy by ureteroscopy. J Urol 140:957, 1988.
56. Begun FP, Stephen CJ, Lawson RK: Use of a prototype 3F electrohydraulic electrode with ureteroscopy for treatment of ureteral calculus disease. J Urol 139:1188, 1988.
57. Kumon H, Tsugawa M, Matsumura Y, Ohmori H: Endoscopic diagnosis and treatment of chronic unilateral hematuria of uncertain etiology. J Urol 143:554, 1989.
58. Badlani G, Eshighi M, Smith AD: Percutaneous surgery for ureteropelvic junction obstruction (endopyelotomy): technique and early results. J Urol 135:26, 1986.
59. Van Cangh PJ, Jorion JL, Wese FX, Opsomer RJ: Endoureteropyelotomy: percutaneous treatment of ureteropelvic junction obstruction. J Urol 141:1317, 1989.
60. Clayman RV, Basler JW, Kavoussi LR, Pincus DD: Ureteronephroscopic endopyelotomy. J Urol 144:246, 1990.
61. Thomas R, Cherry R: Ureteroscopic endopyelotomy for management of ureteropelvic junction obstruction. J Endourol 4:S141, 1990.
62. Whitaker RH: An evaluation of 170 diagnostic pressure flow studies of the upper urinary tract. J Urol 121:602, 1978.
63. Meretyk S, Meretyk I, Kavoussi LR, Clayman RV: Ureteronephroscopic vs antegrade endopyelotomy for treatment of ureteropelvic junction obstruction. J Endourol 4:S141, 1990.
64. Bagley DH: Endoscopic ureteroureterostomy. J Urol 143:234A, 1990.
65. Clayman RV, Meretyk S, Denstedt J: Endoureterotomy: ureteronephroscopic treatment of ureteral strictures. J Urol 143:235A, 1990.
66. Farah RN, DiLoreto RR, Cerny JC: Transurethral resection combined with steroid injection in treatment of recurrent vesical neck contractures. Urology 13:395, 1979.
67. Netto NR, Ferreira U, Lemos GC, Claro JFA: Endourological management of ureteral strictures. J Urol 144:631, 1990.
68. Huffman JL, Morse MJ, Bagley DH: Endoscopic diagnosis and treatment of upper tract urothelial tumors—a preliminary report. Cancer 55:1422, 1985.
69. Huffman JL: Endoscopic management of upper urinary tract urothelial cancer. J Endourol 4:S141, 1990.
70. Thomas SP, Knipper A, Bohle A: Endourologic diagnosis and therapy of upper urinary tract carcinoma. J Endourol 4:S108, 1990.
71. Blute ML, Segura JW, Patterson DE, et al: Impact of endourology on the diagnosis and management of upper urinary tract urothelial cancer. J Urol 141:1298, 1989.
72. Meretyk S, Clayman RV, Picus D, Kramolowsky G: Endourological treatment of uretero-enteric anastomotic strictures: long term follow-up. J Urol 143:233A, 1990.
73. Stackl W, Marberger M: Late sequelae of the management of ureteral calculi with the ureterorenoscope. J Urol 136:386, 1986.
74. Weinberg JJ, Snyder JA, Smith AD: Mechanical extraction of stones with rigid ureteroscopes. Urol Clin North Am 15:339, 1988.
75. Sosa E, Huffman JL: Complications of ureteropyeloscopy. In Huffman JL, Bagley DH, Lyon ES (eds): Ureteroscopy. Philadelphia: Saunders, 1987, pp 159-168.
76. Yoshida K, Nishimura T, Kawamura N, et al: Videoimage ureteroscope, J Nippon Med Sch 57:192, 1990.

CHAPTER 3

LASERS

RALPH C. BENSON, JR.

Laser is an acronym for light amplification by stimulated emission of radiation. A laser is a source of optical radiation having four special properties: the radiation is intense, monochromatic, coherent, and unidirectional. All significant laser applications are a direct result of one or more of these special properties. The principles necessary for the concept of the laser were firmly established as early as the nineteenth century with the advent of Bohr's theory and optical resonators. In 1917 Einstein proposed the concept of stimulated emission, thus laying the foundation for Schwalow and Townes and Prokhorov Basov to describe independently the physical principles of maser (microwave amplification by stimulated emission of radiation) several decades later.[1] In 1960 Maiman first observed stimulated emission in the visible portion of the spectrum by exciting a ruby rod with intense pulses of light from a flashlamp, generating the first laser beam.[2] The first gas laser, a helium-neon laser, was developed by Javan, Bennett, and Herriott (1961)[3]; the neodymium:yttrium aluminum garnet (Nd:YAG) laser by Johnson (1961)[4]; and the carbon dioxide laser by Patel, McFarlane, and Faust (1964).[5]

PHYSICAL PRINCIPLES

The energy in an atom depends on the motion and distribution of its orbiting electrons. Electrons close to the nucleus have a low energy level known as the ground state (E_o). Absorption of energy (thermal, electrical, chemical, and radiation) moves electrons to orbits farther from the nucleus, resulting in an excited or singlet state (E_n) (Figure 3–1). An electron in an excited state (E_n) tends to return spontaneously to the ground state (E_o) and therefore to release energy in the form of photons of light (spontaneous emission) (Figure 3–2). For example, the light from a tungsten bulb results from the absorption of electrical energy and spontaneous emission of light of various wavelengths, that is, white light.

When certain atoms are in the singlet state, they quickly drop to an intermediate energy level called the metastable state. This partially explains why some materials can go through the process called lasing whereas others cannot. Only certain types of atoms are capable of the lasing process; those atoms characteristically have a metastable state in their energy structure. This metastable state is unique in that these atoms may stay at this energy level for as long as a couple of seconds. A couple of seconds may not seem long, but in photobiology, where most reactions occur in nanoseconds (10^{-9}) or picoseconds (10^{-12}), 1 second is considered a long time.

What happens next is a spontaneous event. According to the laws of thermodynamics, atoms are always moving. Atoms that exist in the metastable state spontaneously, by random action, return to the ground state with the loss of some energy. This energy loss is in the form of light: the release of a photon. If the photon is close to another atom that is in the metastable state (remember that the metastable state is long lived, so many atoms are at that energy level), it actually strikes or collides with the other atom. This interaction stimulates the second atom to return to its ground state and in the process to emit another photon. According to the basic principles of physics, since both photons come from identical energy levels, they are of the same wavelength (color) and move parallel to and in phase with each other. What is termed a population inversion occurs when a disproportionate number of atoms are in the excited or metastable state (E_n) as compared with the lower energy ground state (E_o). If an atom in the excited state (E_n) collides with a photon of light energy with a wavelength identical to the energy characteristics of the energized atom, this atom in the E_n state releases an identical photon that travels in the same plane and phase as the stimulating photon and the atom returns to the ground state energy level (E_o). This is termed stimulated emission (Figure 3–3).

In such an atomic or molecular system, when the number of atoms in excited states (E_n) is sufficiently large (a population inversion) for an incident wave-

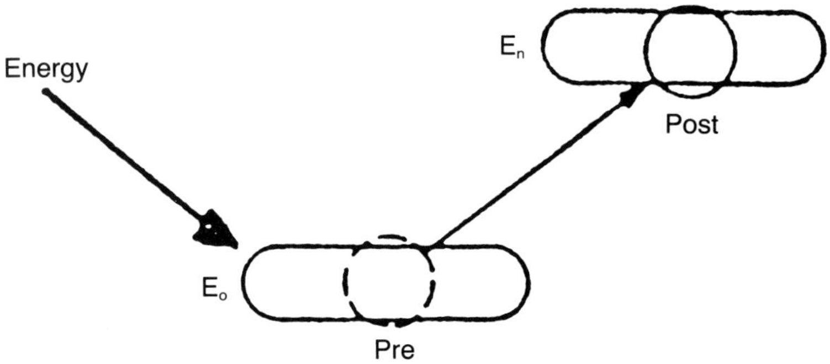

FIGURE 3–1. Absorption of energy. Energy, usually in the form of a photon, is transferred to an atom in the resting state (E_o). The E_o atom absorbs this energy, resulting in a higher energy state (E_n).

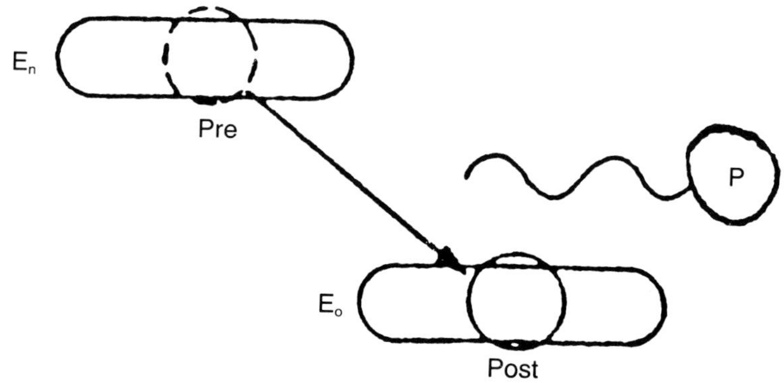

FIGURE 3–2. Spontaneous emission of energy. An atom at a higher energy level (E_n) spontaneously discharges a photon of energy (P) and drops down to the ground state (E_o).

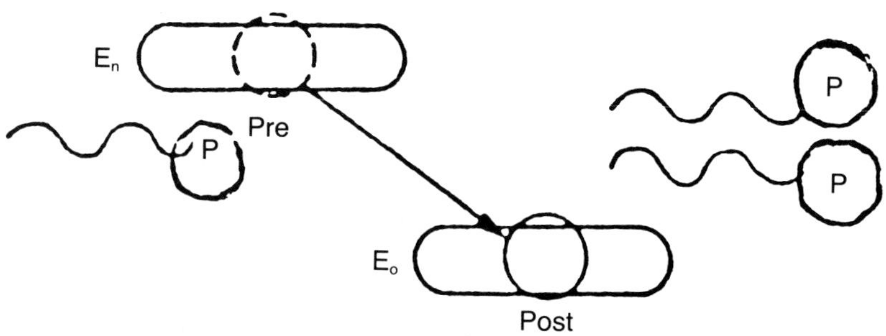

FIGURE 3–3. Stimulated emission. When an atom of a higher energy state (E_n) is struck by another photon, it drops down to the ground state (E_o), giving off two photons of energy that are identical.

length to produce more stimulated emissions than absorption, the energy released amplifies the beam (amplification by stimulated emission).

A laser consists of a pumping system, a laser cavity with the lasing medium and two mirrors, one fully reflecting and one partially reflecting with a small aperture in the center (Figure 3–4). The pumping mechanism is usually electrical or optical in the medical laser systems. It is used to raise the energy state of the laser medium atoms within the laser. As the atoms are raised to higher energy states, some photons are given off by spontaneous emission and light begins to travel in all directions within the laser cavity. The light that is directed exactly parallel to the laser cavity continues to be reflected back and forth between the mirrors at the ends of the cavity. The light that is not completely parallel to the laser cavity is lost, and the energy is dissipated into the area surrounding the laser cavity. As the beam continues to be reflected back and forth between the mirrors, the principle of stimulated emission begins to take place. Eventually the light is amplified greatly as it travels between the mirrors and can be released through the aperture as the foot pedal is operated.

The output may be varied depending on the method of opening and closing the aperture in the partially reflecting mirror. If the aperture is continuously open, the laser delivery will be steady, in what is called a continuous wave. The beam may be emitted in discrete pulses, in what is known as a pulsed laser, or can be allowed to achieve great power ranges and discharged in extremely short bursts in a process known as being Q-switched.

A medical laser is referred to in terms of its wavelength in nanometers (nm), micrometers (μm), or millimeters (mm). At present, lasers occupy a relatively small portion of the electromagnetic spectrum.

Different kinds of lasers are identified by the type of material inside the device that is going through the lasing process. Liquid, solid, and gas lasers are available. Lasing action can be obtained from any of these materials, provided their atomic structures

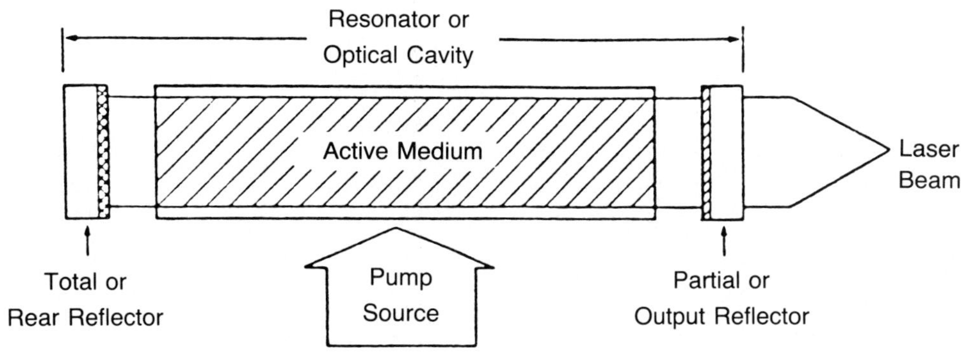

FIGURE 3–4. Basic components of a laser. The active medium is a collection of atoms or molecules (solid, liquid, or gas).

have a metastable state that permits the stimulated emission process.

The wavelengths obtainable from lasers may be modified. Certain crystals, called nonlinear asymmetric crystals, take photons from very intense light and, through an interaction of these photons with the crystal lattice, generate laser light with twice the frequency (half the wavelength) of the incident radiation. This is known as frequency doubling or harmonic generation. Using these crystals in conjunction with lasers makes it possible to double, triple, or quadruple the wavelengths from the primary laser source. It is also possible to use one laser to excite another and, by using liquid dyes that can go into many different metastable states, to obtain a variety of wavelengths from a single laser device.

Laser-Tissue Interactions

Light from lasers generally follows the basic laws of photobiology. The one exception is extremely short, intense laser pulses, which may produce so-called nonlinear events. These effects, such as multiphoton absorption, plasma generation, and ionization, occur as a function of photon intensity; they were not possible until extremely short (nanosecond or picosecond) laser pulses were generated. If a laser beam is directed at a tissue, it may be reflected back to the source or to another undesired surface. Since tissues reflect light, their reflectant properties (reflectance) are important considerations.

When reflectance is adequately controlled and the laser light enters the tissue, the goal is absorption of light energy to change the tissue. Two complications other than absorption in the tissue can occur. The tissue itself can scatter the light, which literally bounces off particles and structures within the tissue and "scatters" to places where it is not wanted. Furthermore, the light may be transmitted right through the tissue and only a minimal amount may be absorbed. Since every tissue has reflective, scattering, and transmissive properties, understanding these characteristics is important in knowing how to use the laser.

The process of absorption is the key to laser use. When photons enter the tissue, those that are not reflected, scattered, or transmitted are absorbed. Their energy is transferred to other molecules and groups of atoms within the tissue that is to be altered or changed. Once this photon energy is absorbed, it produces different tissue changes. Where and how is this energy dissipated? Normally we think of lasers as producing heat. Probably 90% of the clinical procedures for which lasers are used involve the production of a local thermal event. Heat, however, is only one way the photon energy can be dissipated. It can also be dissipated as photochemistry, photoablation (photodisruption, "bond breaking"), fluorescence or phosphorescence, or ionization. The point to remember is that when photons are absorbed, the absorbing structure or tissue must get rid of that energy. The way the energy is dissipated causes the different biological effects seen clinically.

Before light energy can be absorbed, some absorbing molecule must be present in the tissue. These molecules are generally referred to as pigments. Figure 3–5 plots the absorption spectrum of two common body constituents that can function as pigments: hemoglobin and water.

Hemoglobin has a high absorption in the violet and blue-green portions of the visible spectrum. This is the rationale for using an argon laser, which emits blue-green light, as the primary treatment for vascular lesions such as hemangiomas and port-wine stains.

Water, on the other hand, does not absorb in the visible, and very minimally in the near infrared, portions of the spectrum. In the far infrared regions, water absorbs maximally. This is why a CO_2 laser has a direct effect on any tissue in the body; water is a major constituent of every body tissue. Therefore CO_2 energy is absorbed on the surface of tissue and causes a direct ablative effect. In a third laser, the Nd:YAG, the light energy is poorly absorbed by hemoglobin, water, and other body pigments. This is why the Nd:YAG laser penetrates much more deeply into tissue.

The selection of the correct laser for a particular clinical procedure requires an understanding of the absorptive, as well as the reflective, scattering, and transmissive, properties of the target tissue.

The control of tissue heating is important. Figure

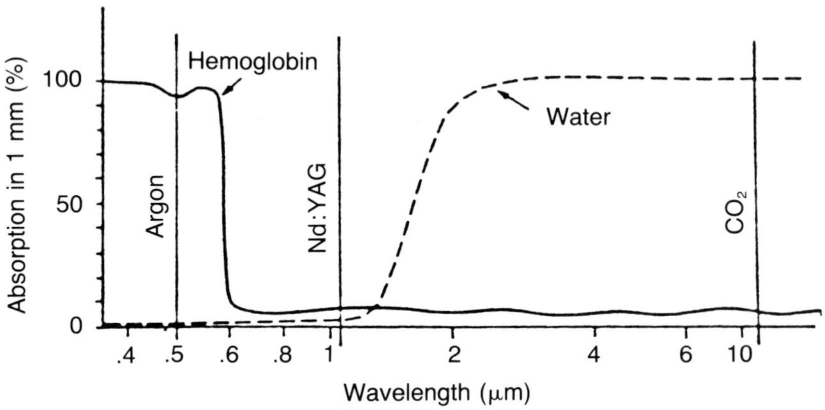

FIGURE 3–5. The absorption of hemoglobin and water as a function of wavelength of three common medical lasers.

3–6 shows the effect of temperature rise in the tissue under irradiation. As the temperature rises to between 37° and 60° C, protein denaturation and coagulation occur. From 90° to 100° C, carbonization and tissue burning occur. Above 100° C the tissue is vaporized and ablated. Ideally, the physician can stop the heating process at any one of these thermal ranges to produce the desired clinical result. Physicians experienced in laser therapy acquire the ability to discern tissue changes visually, so that they can stop the heating process at the desired point. Therefore physicians who plan to use lasers should complete a preceptorship with an instructor who has considerable experience in this field and can help them develop the requisite skills.

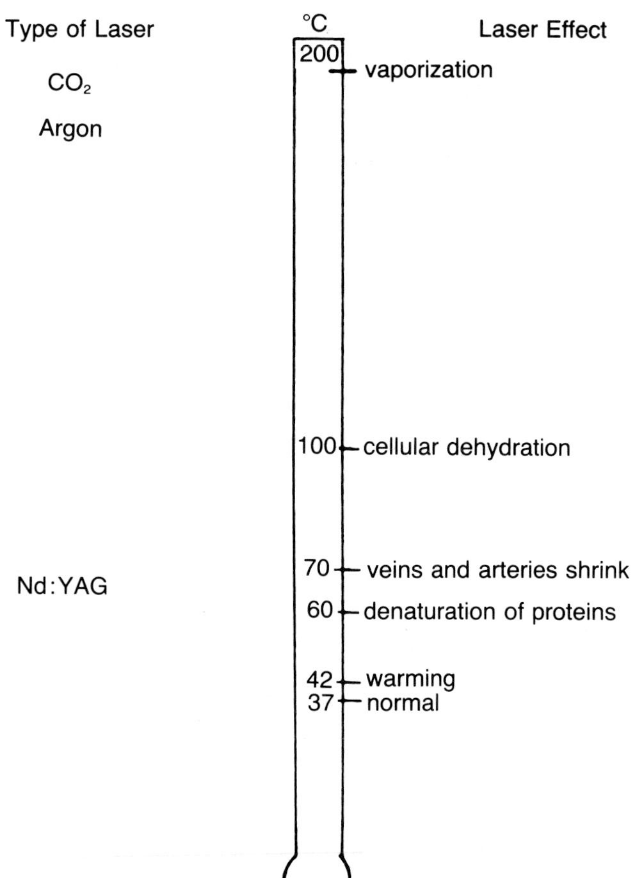

FIGURE 3–6. Thermal effects of lasers.

Another point that must be emphasized is dosimetry. Obviously, 1 watt of power (1 watt = 1 joule of energy delivered in 1 second) delivered over 1 cm^2 is very different from 1 watt delivered over 1 m^2. As the spot size decreases while the power remains constant, the power density (power per unit area) must necessarily increase. Conversely, as spot size grows from small to large, the power density diminishes. If the clinical objective is to make a quick incision, the surgeon should use a very small spot with a high power density because the laser will penetrate deep into the tissues. If the intent is to ablate gently from the surface, however, a larger spot size with a lower power density should be used. The operator can therefore control the effect produced in tissue by manipulating either the spot size or the power settings on the laser. This ability is important to recognize, so that the operator will be able to get the most out of the device and produce the best clinical results for the patient. Thus far the generation of heat within the target tissue has been the most important use of lasers. Interactions between the photon energy and tissue are necessarily complex and depend on many factors (Figure 3–7).

Photon energy may also be dissipated by photochemistry. The basic concept of photochemistry is that certain molecules can function as photosensitizers. The presence of these photosensitizers in certain cells makes these cells vulnerable to light of an appropriate wavelength and intensity. The photosensitizers act by absorbing sufficient photons to elevate the sensitizer to an excited state. The excited photosensitizer subsequently reacts with a molecular substrate, such as oxygen, to produce singlet oxygen, which causes irreversible oxidation of some essential cellular components. All of this occurs without the generation of heat.

Photon energy may be dissipated as the reemission of light. If this happens within 10^{-6} seconds after absorption, it is called fluorescence.

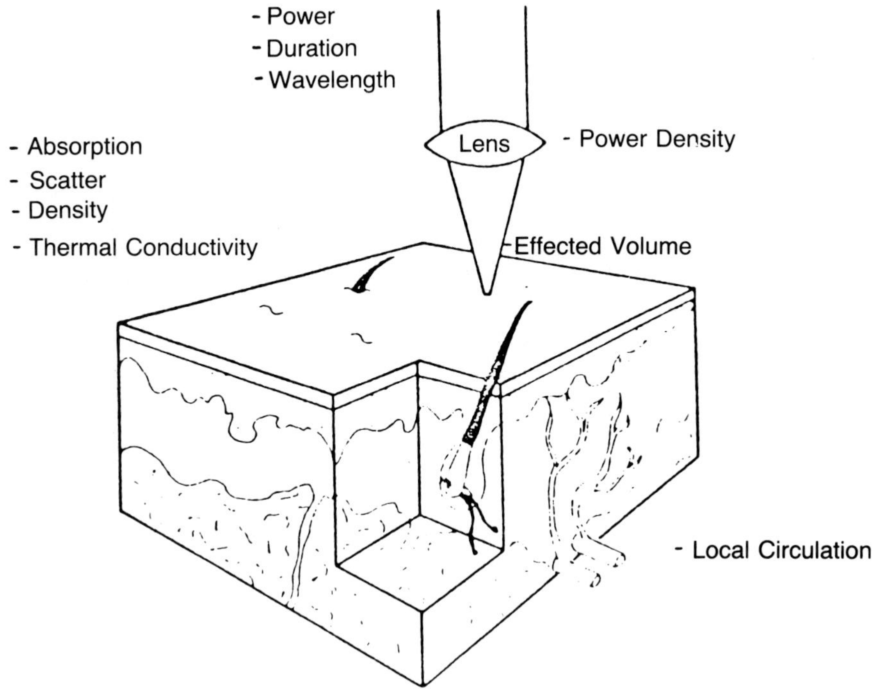

FIGURE 3–7. Factors that determine the effect of a laser on tissue.

The fluorescent photon is emitted as the excited atom returns to the ground state. Because excess vibrational energy in the singlet state is dissipated as heat by collisions with other atoms in the excited state, the energy of the fluorescent photon is lower (therefore the wavelength is longer) than that of the absorbed photon.

How can the fluorescence phenomenon be used diagnostically? Many of the photosensitizing dyes used to induce photochemistry detection of fluorescence can demonstrate the presence of occult neoplasms. Laser-stimulated fluorescence can also be used analytically to scan large populations of cells that flow through a laser beam in a cytofluorometer. In addition, lasers may be used to excite small microscopic regions of single cells to study the binding and movement of biologically important molecules.

The photoablative process consists of photodissociation or the direct breaking of intramolecular bonds in polymeric chains caused by the absorption of high-energy ultraviolet photons that are produced by the excimer laser. The lasing material of excimer lasers is excited dimers of unstable gases, usually a halogen and some rare element.

The ultraviolet photons generated by excimer lasers possess so much energy that they break apart molecular bonds before their energy can be dissipated as heat, reducing the tissue to its atomic constituents. Since ultraviolet radiation from 200 to 360 nm is well absorbed by most biological molecules, the penetration depths are only a few microns. This feature has recently been exploited experimentally to produce well-defined, nonthermal cuts of very small width by excimer lasers at several ultraviolet wavelengths (argon fluoride 193 nm, krypton fluoride 248 nm, xenon fluoride 308 nm). When validated, this experimental surgical technique may prove unique in its ability to produce sharp incisions with minimal thermal damage to adjacent normal structures.

Ionization is the ejection of an electron from an atom. The individual photons generated from existing lasers do not have enough energy to cause the absorbing molecule to lose an electron; however, it is possible for a molecule to absorb more than one photon simultaneously in a "multiphoton process." This process has been observed in solutions and theorized in living cells but does not occur in most present clinical situations. With an x-ray laser (under development by the military) the photon energy would be sufficient to cause the ejection of an electron.

Plasma formation is one of the laser-tissue interactions that does not obey the basic laws of photobiology. With the advent of Q-switched (nanosecond) and short-pulsed, mode-locked (picosecond) lasers, it is now possible to generate very high power densities (gigawatts/cm^2) in focal spots of 25 to 50 μm. When these lasers are precisely focused on a small spot of tissue, events occur that obviate the classic laws of physics and photobiology. It is possible to generate a plasma, a gaseous cloud rich in free electrons. This plasma has sometimes been called the fourth state of matter because its properties are very different from those of solids, liquids, or gases. The sudden production of an electrical field in 10^{-9} to 10^{-12} seconds generates an intense acoustical shock wave in the medium. This acoustic wave, which emanates from the focus, carries potentially damaging kinetic energy and has been used clinically.

Instrumentation

All of the major laser wavelengths (CO_2, argon, KTP, and Nd:YAG) that are commercially available for urologic applications have been employed in open and endoscopic urologic procedures. Their use is dictated by their unique absorption characteristics.

CO_2 lasers with a wavelength of 10,600 nm are useful as cutting tools because this wavelength is strongly absorbed by cellular water, resulting in tissue vaporization achieved by cellular dehydration at high temperature levels.[6,7] The depth of penetration of CO_2 laser energy is not more than 0.1 mm. Limited heat dissipation from the point of laser impact results in a discrete area of tissue injury and minimizes injury to adjacent tissues with little resultant tissue fibrosis and scarring. The CO_2 laser has often been referred to as a laser knife; however, light of this wavelength is capable of coagulating blood vessels only of approximately 0.1 to 0.5 mm in diameter, which may limit its usefulness in transurethral procedures where many of the vessels are significantly larger. At present, CO_2 laser energy is delivered either by coupling to an operating microscope or with the aid of an articulating arm with multiple reflective mirrors that direct the beam through a hand-held probe, which can often be cumbersome in the operating room (Figure 3–8). Nontoxic, flexible fibers for transmission of CO_2 laser energy are not currently available for clinical use. This factor, plus the strong absorption of CO_2 laser energy by water, has limited the endoscopic use of the CO_2 laser in urology. Experimental CO_2 laser fibers have been developed, however, and prototype laser cystoscopes that direct the CO_2 laser beam by means of reflective mirrors are being investigated. In the future, such advances may enable the urologist to take advantage of the precise tissue effects and cutting properties of the CO_2 laser for selected endoscopic applications.

The emission spectrum of an argon laser (488 to 515 nm) is close to the maximal absorption of hemoglobin and melanin (Figure 3–5). Thus the energy is selectively absorbed by pigmented lesions and by tissues with high blood perfusion. Argon energy penetrates to a depth of 1 mm and is capable of coagulating blood vessels with a diameter of 1.5 mm. When active bleeding is present, however, the energy is rapidly absorbed by the blood, and effective delivery of the laser beam to the underlying tissues and blood vessels is impossible. Although an argon beam can be passed down a flexible quartz fiber, it is less effective for cutting than the CO_2 laser because of deeper tissue penetration and less intense surface vaporization. The absorption and penetration characteristics of argon laser energy limit its transurethral use to small or pigmented lesions and its open use to the treatment of pigmented or erythematous skin lesions. The argon laser fiber can be either used in contact with tissue (cutting) or held a short distance from the lesion in a noncontact manner (tissue coagulation).

The KTP laser has a wavelength (532 W) close to that of the argon laser and has similar properties. One unique feature of the KTP laser is that both Nd:YAG energy and KTP energy can be produced by the same machine. The KTP laser can also be used in a contact or noncontact manner, depending on the desired tissue effect.

The Nd:YAG laser emits light with a wavelength of 1060 nm, which is not strongly absorbed by either water or body pigments (Figure 3–5). Thus the tissue effect may penetrate to more than 1 cm, depending on the power density, exposure time, and medium employed. Because of the heterogeneous nature of various tissues, a 20% to 30% forward scatter of Nd:YAG energy occurs, which heats a relatively large volume of tissue around the point of impact. Application of Nd:YAG energy results in a cone-shaped zone of coagulation, with the depth of penetration a function of the total dose delivered. Visible carbonization and vaporization can occur at very high dosages, but the depth of penetration causing cellular death after Nd:YAG irradiation can be as great as 1 cm in the absence of easily

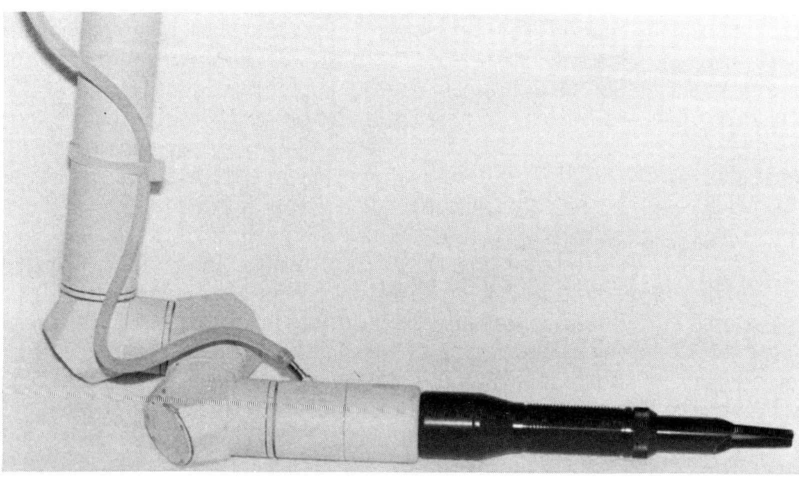

FIGURE 3–8. Straight handpiece for CO_2 laser.

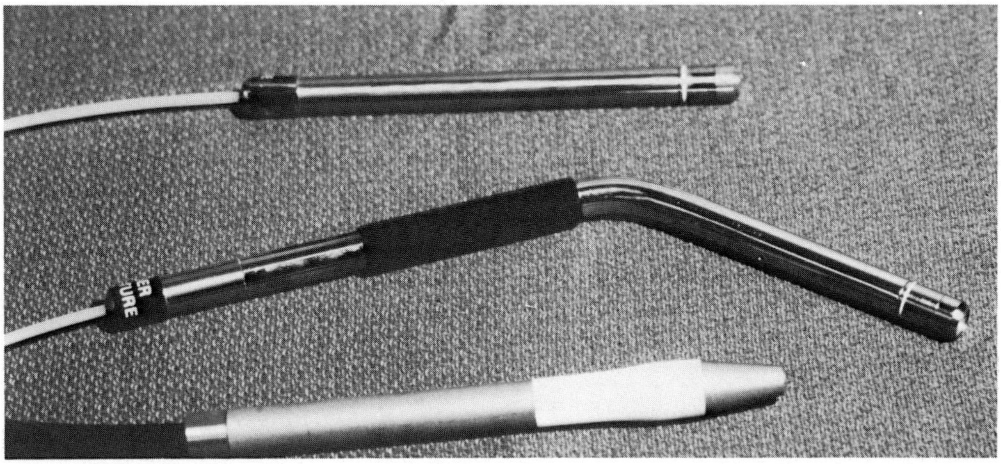

FIGURE 3–9. Straight and angled handpieces for the Nd:YAG laser.

visible vaporization effects. Therefore the Nd:YAG laser is an ineffective cutting device, although large volumes of tissue can be effectively coagulated and removed by secondary tissue slough. Adjacent organs may be damaged by heat conduction from the forward scatter of Nd:YAG energy. This fact, plus the different tissue properties (e.g., amount of collagen and reticulin) of various organs, makes some other organs more susceptible to significant damage (perforation) than the bladder.

The Nd:YAG laser is capable of coagulating blood vessels approximately 3 to 4 mm in diameter. In addition, the beam can be easily passed down a quartz fiber and used in a liquid medium. These characteristics make the Nd:YAG laser very effective for endoscopic use.

In open urologic surgery it is important to keep the fiber tip of the Nd:YAG laser free of tissue and blood, since accumulation will result in the absorption of energy at the fiber tip and destruction of the tip. For open application the use of a handpiece (Figure 3–9) with different focal lengths allows delivery of the laser beam from a safe distance and prevents tissue from adhering to the fiber tip. The focused distance for the handpiece is that distance from the tissue that provides the smallest spot size and therefore the highest energy density. As the beam is moved either closer to or farther from the focused position, the spot size enlarges or becomes unfocused. Defocusing the beam enhances its hemostatic capability.

The Nd:YAG laser has been used primarily in a noncontact manner. However, the tissue effects can be changed by altering the fiber tip to allow it to be used in contact with tissue. The tip modification is generally to contact tip laser probes, which increase the power density and improve use of the laser for cutting. Both quartz and synthetic sapphire contact tips have been developed. Interchangeable tips of various shapes can be selected to provide a variety of power densities for incision, coagulation, vaporization, and other uses (Figure 3–10).

The use of laser beams must be accompanied by

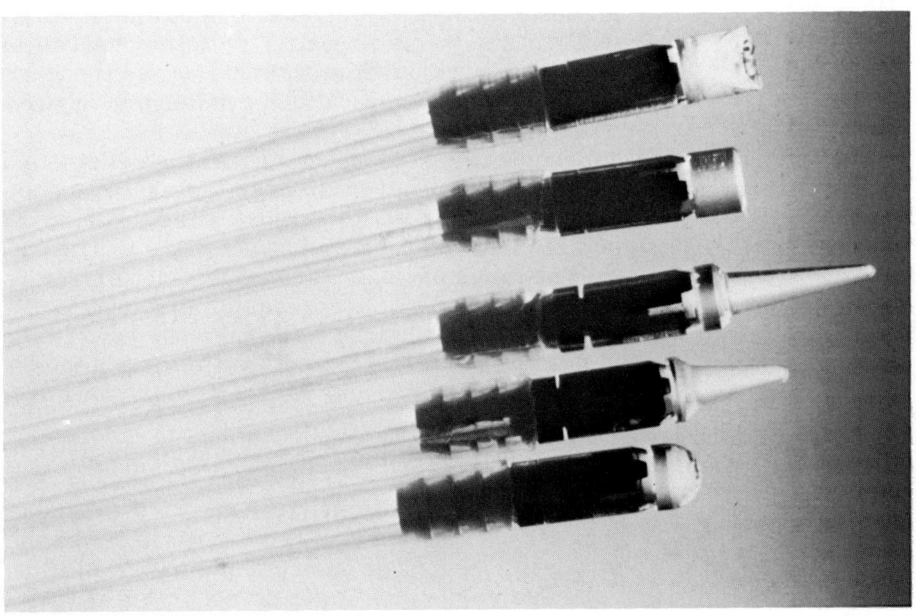

FIGURE 3–10. Contact tips made of artificial sapphire crystal for an Nd:YAG laser.

stringent safety precautions. Careless use of laser beams can damage skin and the cornea and retina of the eye. In addition, contact with materials such as catheters, stents, drapes, and sponges can result in dangerous fires. Laser beams are easily reflected by polished surfaces such as surgical instruments and guidewires, and therefore the operator should ensure that the fiber is protruding beyond the end of the endoscope and is not directed at any shiny metallic object before it is fired.

USES OF LASERS IN UROLOGY

Bladder

Malignancies

All laser wavelengths approved for urologic use have been used for the treatment of transitional cell carcinoma of the bladder.

Because CO_2 laser energy is rapidly absorbed by water, cannot be passed down a fiber, and has a depth of penetration of only 0.1 mm, its endoscopic use has been limited. Experimental studies of CO_2 laser treatment of bladder epithelium in animals have demonstrated the ability of this laser to ablate transitional epithelium, but minimal capability for penetration into the lamina propria. However, treated areas heal with minimal scarring.[8,9] Willscher and associates have devised prototype CO_2 cystoscopes that deliver laser energy by use of an articulating arm to the endoscope.[10] In their most recent model the beam is directed down the instrument by means of a "joy stick." Although CO_2 laser endoscopes have the apparent advantages of precise tissue effects and cutting properties, they have several important drawbacks. Significant amounts of laser energy are lost as heat as the beam passes through the small boom arm. In addition, CO_2 must be insufflated during the procedure to distend the bladder and keep the proximal lens free of blood and urine. Careful attention must be maintained to prevent overinsufflation and perforation of the bladder during CO_2 laser endoscopy because of the risk of fatal CO_2 gas embolization during the procedure.[11] Bulow and Lavene described a hand-held 20 W CO_2 laser small enough to allow direct connection to a cystoscope.[12] Although this instrument was cumbersome, incorporating the CO_2 laser directly into the endoscope may be the best way of eliminating beam alignment problems. If a fiber could be developed that would allow the efficient passage of CO_2 energy, many of the aforementioned problems of endoscopic application of CO_2 energy might be eliminated.

The published data regarding endoscopic use of CO_2 lasers are few, but the authors who have published preliminary results indicate that vaporization is slow. Even with significantly improved delivery systems, the CO_2 laser is unlikely to play an important role in the endoscopic treatment of bladder tumors.

The emission spectrum of the argon laser (488 to 515 nm) is in the visible portion of the electromagnetic spectrum and is close to the maximal absorption of hemoglobin and melanin. Argon laser energy can be transmitted easily to the bladder epithelium through an endoscope. A shallow coagulation effect and small amounts of tissue vaporization are noted. Even with increasing power densities, the zone of muscle penetration and necrosis increases little and the temperature of the outer bladder wall generally does not reach 60° C until obvious surface effects (vaporization) are visible. As energy is delivered, cratering increases and bleeding may occur with resultant absorption of the laser energy. When a power output of 5 W for as long as 30 seconds has been used, no bladder perforations have been observed. The risk of thermal damage to adjacent organs is low. Because argon energy is preferentially absorbed by pigments such as hemoglobin and melanin, the argon ion laser has been used successfully to treat small erythematous bladder lesions. Rothauge successfully used an argon laser to treat 38 patients with bladder tumors, but in an expanded series of patients he and his colleagues did not find that argon ion treatment was superior to conventional therapy.[13] Smith and Dixon treated 11 patients with superficial transitional cell bladder tumors and judged the treatment safe and effective.[14] There is little question that an argon ion laser can be used effectively to treat small superficial tumors and also carcinoma in situ, which is usually slightly erythematous. Because of the argon laser's limited power output and superficial depth of penetration, however, it is usually impractical for tumors larger than 1 cm. Most tumors are treated at power settings of 5 to 6 W and are assumed to be adequately treated when they blanch or when tissue shrinkage is noted. An argon ion laser is an extremely safe tool to use endoscopically in the bladder because its tissue penetration is minimal, which significantly reduces the possibility of bladder perforation or damage to adjacent bowel.

Because the KTP laser has a wavelength (532 nm) similar to that of an argon laser, their endoscopic uses are almost identical. The KTP laser can be used in a noncontact manner at 10 to 12 W for the treatment of small transitional cell carcinomas, or in a contact manner to cut small exophytic tumors from the bladder wall. Like the argon laser it is useful for the treatment of erythematous or pigmented lesions, and it has a high margin of safety.

For endoscopic laser treatment, regardless of whether the argon, KTP, or Nd:YAG laser is used, laser energy is delivered by means of a flexible fiber that can be inserted through the working channel of a cystoscope. Rigid instruments with a modified Albarran apparatus are used most often with 600 mm diameter fibers. Access to the bladder neck can often be difficult and is facilitated by a retrograde telescope with an exaggerated Albarran deflector or by flexible instruments (400 mm fibers).

Endoscopic treatment of transitional cell carcinoma of the bladder with the Nd:YAG laser is the area in which lasers have generated the most interest in the field of urology. The Nd:YAG laser was first used for the treatment of human bladder tumors by Hofstetter and Staehler and their associates, and a large clinical experience has subsequently been amassed in the United States and abroad.[15,16] The pioneering work of the German group established the effects of the Nd:YAG laser on bladder tissue and led to the establishment of guidelines for the safe and effective endoscopic use of this instrument in urology. Their work demonstrated the ability of the Nd:YAG laser to produce a sharply delineated band or cone-shaped area of coagulation necrosis that is much more regular and predictable than that produced by electrocoagulation.[17-19] In fresh human bladder preparations, they determined that a dose of 50 W maintained for 4 seconds produced a temperature of approximately 65° C at the serosal surface of the bladder, which would result in complete transmural coagulation of the bladder wall. An important finding was that adjacent intestine did not exceed 40° C and therefore would not be damaged.[20]

The efficacy of any new therapeutic modality should be evaluated by being critically compared with standard or conventional therapy. Transurethral resection (TUR) of bladder tumors is the "gold standard" to which laser photocoagulation must be compared. The potential advantages and disadvantages of both are shown in Table 3–1. Although many parameters remain incompletely defined, the rapidly expanding experience with laser treatment of bladder cancer indicates that lasers will have a lasting role in this area.

Three broad issues must be considered when evaluating laser versus TUR treatment of bladder tumors: (1) biologic, (2) patient risk, comfort, and convenience, and (3) economic. Included within the biologic category are the problems of tumor grading and staging and of tumor recurrence. Urologic endoscopists are comfortable with electrocautery resection of superficial bladder tumors because of their past experience with the technique and their ability to visualize tissue effects and judge the depth of tissue removed. Unfortunately, recurrence rates after TUR of superficial bladder tumors are disturbingly high. Although preexisting severe dysplasia or carcinoma in situ may contribute to this high recurrence rate, experimental and clinical evidence suggests that many of these recurrences may be due to implantation of tumor cells that became dislodged during tumor resection.[21] See and Chapman have demonstrated experimentally that the number of viable tumor cells liberated during ablation was 620% greater in a group of electrosurgically resected tumors than in a laser-irradiated group.[22] It is theoretically, although not always practically, possible to photocoagulate and devitalize tumor cells using the Nd:YAG laser without direct tissue contact. This "no touch" technique could conceivably reduce tumor recurrence. The only way to demonstrate this contention convincingly is to randomly assign patients with primary bladder tumors to laser or TUR therapy without preliminary biopsy. This difficult protocol has been initiated in Europe, but at the present writing the number of patients has been insufficient to allow statistical evaluation.[23]

TABLE 3–1. Advantages and Disadvantages of Transurethral Resection of Bladder Tumors Compared with Laser Photocoagulation

Advantages	*Disadvantages*
TRANSURETHRAL RESECTION	
Past experience and expertise	Bleeding
Direct visualization of effects of the current	Possible cell dissemination
Depth of perception	Intravesical
Specimens available for pathologic examination	Intravascular
	Perforation
	Inpatient usually
	Anesthetic needed
	Catheter postoperatively
	? Viable tumor at limits
	Difficult to have access to dome etc.
	Obturator nerve stimulation
LASER	
No-touch technique (? decreased seeding)	New tool, lack of experience
? Decreased recurrences	Cannot visualize depth
No visible perforation (bladder wall stabilized)	Specimen may not be available for pathologic examination
Local anesthesia (outpatient)	Possible late bowel injury
No bleeding (can use for hemostasis)	Increased expense
Seals lymphatics	Increased training
Most areas bladder essentially accessible	Danger to operating room personnel
No obturator reflex	Infancy: new equipment forthcoming
No catheter	Lesions ≥2.5 cm difficult to treat
Use in patients receiving anticoagulants	
Use over ureteral orifice	

In an attempt to determine the impact of various biologic factors on recurrence, Beisland and Seland compared results of the Nd:YAG laser and TUR in a prospective randomized study of 122 patients with T1 and T2 tumors.[24] When tumor recurrences were correlated with size, they found that small tumors did not recur in the treated area regardless of type of therapy, whereas large tumors were more likely to recur after TUR alone than after TUR followed by laser therapy. They could show no significant advantages for laser therapy in the number of out-of-field recurrences.

Another factor that may or may not be of importance in bladder cancer recurrence rates is the sealing of lymphatics. The Nd:YAG laser may be more effective than electrocautery in sealing lymphatics.[12] This observation is likely to be more pertinent to the treatment of invasive than of noninvasive bladder cancer.

An extremely important biologic issue is the pathologist's ability to grade and stage a tumor after laser irradiation. To provide the pathologist with adequate tissue for review, cold cup biopsy specimens may be taken from the tumor before laser therapy or the tumor may be resected with electrocautery followed by laser treatment of the tumor base. These procedures, however, could obviate many of the potential advantages of laser treatment, such as noncontact tumor destruction and possible decreased tumor seeding with resultant decreased tumor recurrence rates. Cytologic studies of voided urine can also be an accurate means for tumor identification and grading, but low-grade lesions often are cytologically normal and stage cannot be assessed.

It is possible to perform a biopsy after Nd:YAG laser therapy and to obtain adequate grade and stage assessment from an experienced pathologist. Laser photocoagulation may produce certain recognizable artifacts, but in general enough cytologic and architectural integrity is preserved to permit an accurate diagnosis. Laser therapy should not be so excessive as to result in tumor carbonization or vaporization, and biopsy after laser treatment is perhaps best performed with a resectoscope to provide the pathologist with adequate tissue for accurate staging. When the difficulty of grading and staging is considered, laser therapy does not appear to compromise treatment for the majority of patients with bladder tumors. It is also of significant interest that the bladder wall maintains its architectural integrity even after full-thickness laser photocoagulation. The risk of bladder perforation is therefore minimal. However, tissues vary in their tolerance to laser energy. The small bowel is an extremely laser-sensitive organ, and if treatment parameters or laser calibration is incorrect, it is possible to obtain a transmural bladder laser injury with the bladder remaining intact and a perforation of the adjacent small bowel from forward scatter of the beam.

A number of factors pertaining to patient comfort and management must be considered when laser photocoagulation is compared with TUR of a bladder tumor. Although a patient undergoing Nd:YAG treatment may experience a minimal perception of heat, the majority of patients do not require general or regional anesthesia. The structural integrity of the bladder is maintained, and therefore a Foley catheter is not required. In addition, bleeding is not encountered (early or late) and the Nd:YAG laser can be used to treat patients receiving anticoagulants without discontinuing their medication. Because anesthesia is not usually necessary, the procedure can be performed on an outpatient basis. In contrast, many patients undergoing TUR of a bladder tumor are hospitalized, require a catheter, and may experience early or late bleeding. A further consideration is cost to the patient. The cost of treating a patient with a bladder tumor in the office or as an outpatient with the Nd:YAG laser is approximately one-third that of hospitalization for 1 day for TUR. The patient who has had laser therapy for transitional cell carcinoma can return to work immediately. Activity is not limited, and therefore productivity and life-style are not altered. Although certain biologic issues such as tumor recurrence remain to be settled, the advantages in patient comfort, management, and cost indicate that Nd:YAG laser treatment of bladder tumors is a useful therapeutic modality.

The technique of tumor treatment depends on the stage of tumor to be treated. The majority of bladder tumors that have been treated with the Nd:YAG laser in the United States and abroad have had a previous histologic diagnosis of transitional cell carcinoma and a visible tumor suggesting a papillary, low-stage lesion. The lesion may be confirmed histologically by any of the methods previously discussed. Exophytic tumors larger than 2.5 cm are difficult and time consuming to treat with the Nd:YAG laser. Larger tumors can be debulked with a resectoscope, although this approach would obviate many of the potential advantages of laser use. If a tumor is larger than 2.5 cm, I use the resectoscope for tissue removal and lase the base of the tumor only if frozen section pathologic analysis reveals invasion of the submucosa. Endoscopic laser treatment of bladder tumors can be performed anywhere an adequate cytoscopic examination can be carried out. Nd:YAG laser energy is easily transmitted by a flexible fiber (400 to 600 μm diameter) that can be inserted through the working channel of the cystoscope and directed by means of a modified Albarran apparatus. Most areas of the bladder are easily accessible for laser treatment, but lesions at the bladder neck may require the use of a flexible cystoscope for adequate direction of the laser energy.

Because full-thickness bladder penetration is unnecessary when superficial tumors are treated, laser specifications that safely allow penetration only to the superficial detrusor muscle should be used. The fiber is usually maintained 2 to 5 mm from the surface of the tumor, and 2 to 3 seconds of application of 20 to 40 W of energy results in the desired visible white discoloration of tumor tissue, which indicates adequate thermal destruction. Most experienced laser surgeons use the laser in a continuous mode to "paint" the tumor rather than in 2- to 3-second pulses. When possible, treatment begins with photocoagulation of approximately 0.5 cm of urothelium around the visible neoplasm and subsequent treatment of all of the malignant tissue (Figure 3–11). This technique is not always possible for larger tumors or those on the sidewalls of

A

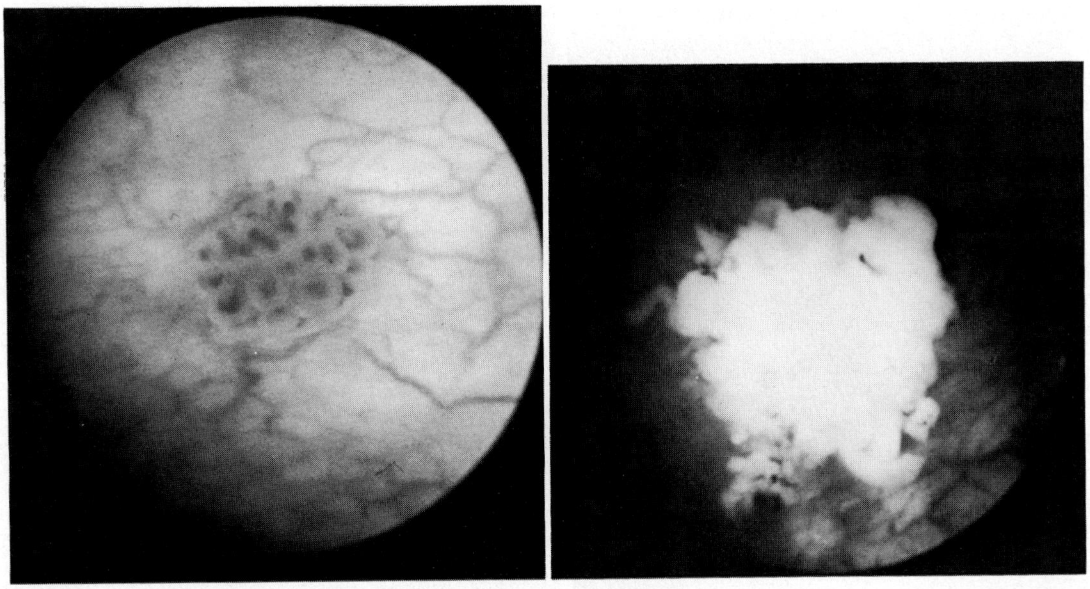

B

FIGURE 3–11. **A,** Papillary low-grade transitional cell carcinoma of the bladder. **B,** Same lesion after laser therapy (note whitish discolorations caused by protein denaturation).

the bladder or at the bladder neck; dislodging the superficial coagulated tissue may be necessary to visualize the remainder of the viable neoplasm.

Thousands of patients with noninvasive transitional cell carcinoma of the bladder have been treated with the Nd:YAG laser. Although results cannot be compared from one institution to another because of the differences in patient populations, grade of tumor, rate of previous recurrence, and length of follow-up, persistence of tumor in the treatment area has been reported to vary from 2% to 8% and tumor recurrences in remote areas from 16% to 58%.[20,26-31] These statistics compare favorably with electrocautery treatment of superficial bladder tumors. In addition, the low complication rate, lack of side effects, and ability to perform the procedure without anesthesia on an outpatient basis represent significant advantages to the patient.

The possibility of transmural photocoagulation of the bladder wall, the fact that the bladder wall will maintain its architectural integrity after a transmural injury, and the ability of the Nd:YAG laser to coagulate and seal lymphatic vessels led naturally to the consideration of laser treatment of muscle-invading bladder tumors. Application of 45 W of Nd:YAG laser energy for 3 seconds raises the temperature of the outer bladder wall to 65° C, enough to produce a full-thickness thermal necrosis, but adjacent loops of small bowel are not heated beyond 45° C. For these reasons laser treatment might offer an alternative means for local control of the tumor.

In reported series selection of patients for therapy has been based on patient preference or the surgeon's judgment that the patient was not a candidate for more conventional surgical approaches. Clinical staging is notoriously inaccurate and therefore interjects considerable bias into an examination of published series. In addition, all reported series recommend a vigorous TUR before laser therapy, and it is known that TUR of invasive bladder cancer can be curative. Nonetheless, laser treatment is capable of extending the margin of the electrocautery resection by approximately 4 to 5 mm, and therefore this approach may prove useful.

Most authors report treatment with a power of 45 to 50 W, a pulse duration of 3 to 4 seconds, and the tip held 2 to 3 mm from the tumor surface. It must be stressed that these parameters are generalizations and that treatment is dynamic. Unfortunately, because of previous TUR, color changes are less dramatic than with the treatment of noninvasive lesions, rendering the endpoint a more difficult judgment (Figure 3–12). In my experience patients are best served by Foley catheter drainage for 24 hours. Bleeding is rare, complications are minimal, and patients can generally be discharged from the hospital in 24 hours.

Results of laser treatment of invasive bladder tumors in what are admittedly carefully selected patients have been surprisingly good. Although survival is the preferable endpoint, studies have focused on reporting the rate of local tumor recurrence. Published results are shown in Table 3–2.[30,32-35]

Laser treatment seems reasonable for certain patients with stage T2 tumors, since it results in low morbidity and does not preclude or exclude other treatment options.

Lasers may also be used endoscopically in urology to produce reactions related not to the hyperthermic effect of the laser, but rather to the spectral output of the light the laser produces. Absorption of light by one molecule leading to the chemical alteration of another molecule is termed a photosensitizer, and the other molecule is termed the

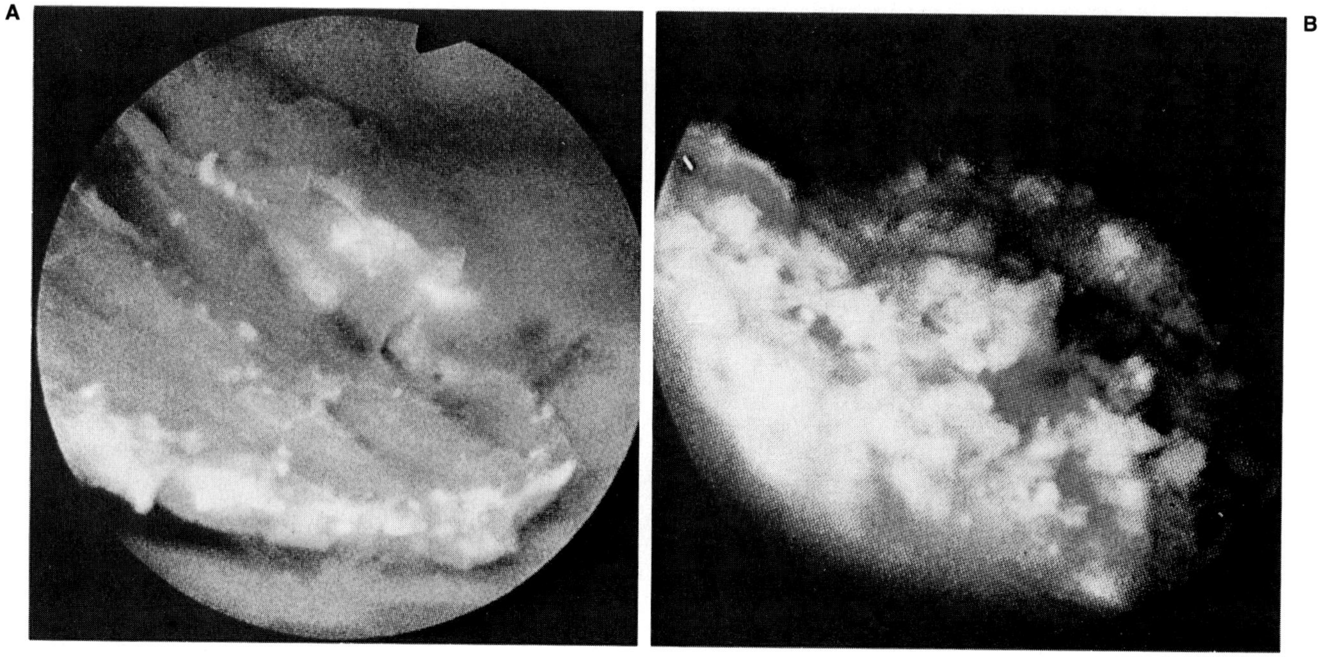

FIGURE 3–12. **A,** Stage T3a transitional cell carcinoma of the bladder after deep electrocautery resection. **B,** Same area after Nd:YAG laser treatment. (From Smith JA: Invasive bladder cancer. In Smith JA, Stein BS, Benson RC Jr [eds]: Lasers in urologic surgery, ed 2. Chicago: Year Book, 1989, pp 73-80. Used by permission.)

substrate of the reaction. Photosensitizers, light and oxygen, have been known for years to be toxic to cells.[36] This principle has led to a new approach to the treatment of various malignant lesions. It has been variously termed phototherapy, photoradiation therapy, photodynamic therapy, and photochemotherapy.

Although currently no photosensitizing drug is taken up or retained selectively by malignant tissue, several potentially useful photosensitizers are available for which such a tumor-specific characteristic has been claimed. These include berberine sulfate, fluorescein, eosin, tetracycline, acridine orange, and several porphyrins.[37-43] The porphyrins have been the drugs most completely investigated and at present they appear to be the most useful.

Hematoporphyrin, a product extracted by alcohol and sulfuric acid from hemoglobin, was discovered in the second half of the nineteenth century. Early investigators noted that hematoporphyrin localized in malignant tissues and caused tumor cells to fluoresce a salmon-red color when exposed to ultraviolet light. However, observed tumor fluorescence was inconsistent, making results unreliable. Investigators then ascertained that the commercially available hematoporphyrin product contained a mixture of porphyrins with varying localizing properties that in some cases exceeded those of pure hematoporphyrin. This prompted Lipson and colleagues to report on a method of preparing "hematoporphyrin derivative" (HpD), an acetic and sulfuric acid derivative of naturally occurring hematoporphyrin that showed greater effect for malignant tissue than hematoporphyrin.[39] HpD was subsequently found to be not only a tumor localizing agent, but also an active photosensitizing agent: cytotoxicity occurred in cells that had taken up HpD if they were exposed to wavelengths of light corresponding to the absorption spectrum of HpD.

The early observations prompted us to explore the use of HpD as a tumor localization agent for transitional cell carcinoma of the bladder. Our subsequent fluorescence bladder-mapping studies established that HpD does indeed localize preferentially in malignant and severely dysplastic transitional cells.[44] This fact, plus the knowledge that activation of intracellular HpD with light of appropriate wavelength results in cytotoxicity,

TABLE 3–2. Summary of Local Recurrence Rates for Patients Undergoing Nd-YAG Therapy for Invasive Transitional Cell Carcinoma of the Bladder

Reference	*Stage*				
	T1	*T2*	*T3a*	*T3b*	*T4*
Beisland[30]	0/47*	3/15†	—	—	—
Smith[32]	2/51	1/5	3/6	3/4	6/6
Hofstetter et al[33]	? < 2% (T1-T3)	—	—	—	—
Staehler et al[34]	3/60 (T0-T3a)	—	—	—	—
McPhee[35]	—	0/12	4/7	6/7	6/6

Local recurrence is defined as recurrence at the site of the original tumor.
*Cautery transurethral resection in 19 of 60 patients.
†Cautery transurethral resection in 6 of 10 patients.

prompted a trial of HpD photodynamic therapy in patients with focal and diffuse resistant carcinoma in situ (Tis) of the bladder. Production of the desired photochemical cytotoxic effect requires that the spectral output of the delivered light be matched closely with the absorption levels of HpD and that the total energy density irradiation of the cells be sufficient. (Energy density in joules per square centimeter [J/cm^2] is the product of the power intensity in watts per square centimeter and the irradiation time in seconds.) Red light (630 nm) has been most often used in the clinical setting because it penetrates tissue for approximately 1 cm. A suitable optical fiber is inserted through an open channel of the endoscope, and light of sufficient power is delivered into the bladder. The major problem is the focusing of light of high-power density into the proximal end of this fiber. Focusing enough power from external light sources, such as incandescent lamps and mercury arcs, into this filter is not technically possible. Most clinical studies use lasers for this purpose because their high-power density, small-diameter beam, and high coupling efficiency to optical fibers allow convenient delivery of light to many areas (Figure 3–13).

An argon ion laser pumped-dye laser system is the instrument most often used in the clinical setting. These systems are all similar and use a 5 to 20 W argon ion laser to pump a dye laser operating with a dye (rhodamine B or DCM) to produce light near 630 nm. The distal end of the fiber can be varied to accommodate the particular therapeutic situation: an optically flat end to produce an expanding cone of light, a rounded tip to further expand the spot, a cylindrical tip to diffuse the light within a narrow beam, or a "light bulb" tip for use in large, hollow organs such as the bladder.

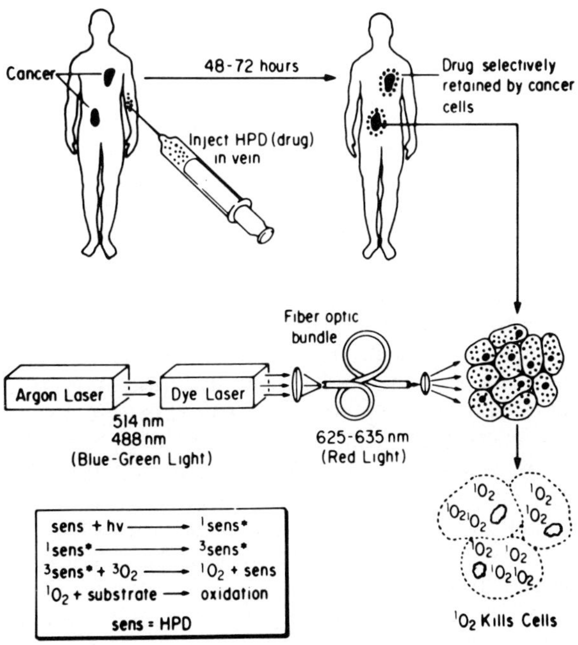

FIGURE 3–13. Schema illustrating hematoporphyrin derivative photodynamic therapy for cancer. (From Berns MW, Wilson M, Rentzepis P, et al: Cell biology of hematoporphyrin derivative [HPD]. Lasers Surg Med 2:261, 1983. Used by permission.)

The time between HpD administration and light delivery has varied from 48 to 22 hours. The proper light dose for maximal effect in the bladder is unknown, but doses should approximate 100 to 200 J/cm^2 for focal tumor therapy and 15 to 20 J/cm^2 for whole bladder therapy.

In 1976 Kelly and Snell reported on the first treatment of a human bladder carcinoma by transmission of white light (mercury vapor lamp) transurethrally through a quartz rod after intravenous administration of HpD.[45] The patient had multicentric noninvasive tumors, but only a small area was illuminated. Two days after treatment, histologic examination showed tumor necrosis in the treated area and unaltered tumor in the untreated areas. In 1983 our group and two groups in Japan published results of HpD phototherapy in which an argon ion pumped-dye laser was the source of red light.

Tsuchiya and associates treated six patients with Ta and T1 disease and two patients with T2 tumors.[46] Patients were given HpD intravenously at a dose of 2.5 mg/kg of body weight, and light (630 nm) was delivered 48 to 72 hours thereafter. The dose rate for Ta and T1 lesions was 120 to 360 J/cm^2 and for T2 lesions was 240 to 360 J/cm^2. Follow-up ranged from 6 to 18 months. All patients with Ta and T1 disease remained tumor free. One T2 tumor persisted, and one tumor recurred at 6 months.

Hisazumi and co-workers[47] administered HpD, 2 to 3.2 mg/kg body weight, to nine patients with Ta and T1 lesions. Between 48 and 72 hours later, red light was administered in a dose of 100 to 250 J/cm^2. These authors claimed complete tumor remission in five of six patients with tumors 1 cm or smaller in diameter but had less success with tumors greater than 1 cm in diameter.

Our group has directed treatment attempts primarily at patients with recurrent resistant Tis in whom all conservative treatment measures, including electrofulguration and various intravesical chemotherapautic agents, have failed.[48,49] Fifteen patients with focal resistant Tis have been treated and followed up for at least 6 months. All treated patients had biopsy and cytologic evidence of disappearance of the lesion in the treated area at the 3-month follow-up cytoscopic examination (Figure 3–14). Eight patients had one or more recurrent lesions, either in the treated area or at a remote site, in follow-up that ranged from 6 to 38 months. One patient underwent cystectomy and urinary diversion because of progression to T1 disease after multiple recurrences. Metastatic disease had not developed in any patient.

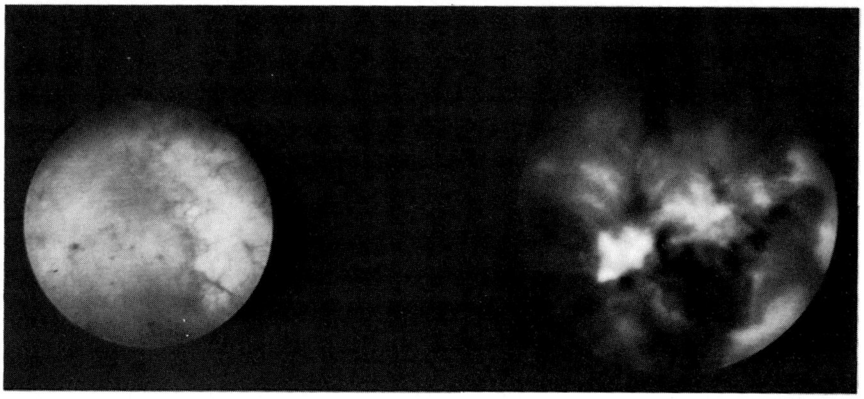

FIGURE 3–14. **A,** In situ transitional cell carcinoma of the bladder untreated (day 1). **B,** Same lesion 3 days after hematoporphyrin derivative photodynamic therapy shows marked hemorrhage, edema, and tissue necrosis.

The published recurrence rates for focal treatment of transitional cell carcinoma of the bladder with HpD phototherapy clearly show that they are not significantly different from those with conventional electrofulguration. For this reason several groups have investigated ways to deliver light of the appropriate dosage to the entire bladder in hopes of reducing recurrences. Jocham and coworkers and Baghdassarian and associates introduced the possibility of using a lipid-diffusing medium.[50,51] Hisazumi and colleagues devised a laser light–scattering optic coupled with a driving instrument that irradiates the entire bladder in sequential segmental strips.[47] Two patients had been treated with an argon ion pumped-dye laser as a light source; a dose of approximately 10 J/cm^2 was delivered to the entire bladder. Early results in two patients appeared encouraging because urinary cytologic findings returned to normal after treatment.

We have approached the problem of light delivery to the entire bladder by modifying the distal end of the delivery fiber. Our early attempts at forming a bulbous tip at this fiber end resulted in inadequate illumination at the bladder neck, but more recently we have used a fiber with a light bulb tip that delivers fairly uniform light to the entire bladder. Twelve patients with diffuse resistant Tis and an area of T1 have been treated with this fiber.[52]

In the eight patients with Tis alone, biopsy and urinary cytologic examination at the 3-month follow-up cystoscopic examination showed complete disappearance of tumor. Two patients who had both Tis and Ta lesions were noted to have disappearance of Tis but persistence of the Ta lesions, which in retrospect should have been treated with focal therapy before whole bladder therapy. The two patients who had diffuse Tis and also focal invasive disease were noted to have persistence of invasive disease and disappearance of Tis.[53,54]

Adverse effects of treatment have been minimal. Cutaneous photosensitivity (sunburn) is a risk, and patients must remain out of direct and indirect sunlight for 4 to 6 weeks. Irritative bladder symptoms and reduced bladder capacity have been noted in patients who have had whole bladder treatments, but those adverse effects have not lasted more than 2 months.

Relatively few patients with transitional cell carcinoma of the bladder have been treated with HpD phototherapy, and it remains an experimental technique. Several practical problems, such as optimal drug dosage, light wavelength, timing of light delivery, and light dose for the various stages of carcinoma to be treated, are yet to be resolved. Once these questions are answered, HpD and light may offer the urologist an additional means of diagnosing and treating transitional cell carcinoma of the bladder.

Benign Lesions

Benign tumors of the bladder are unusual, but hemangiomas are occasionally encountered and are extremely difficult to treat endoscopically because hemorrhagic complications may occur. Segmental resection remains the treatment of choice, but laser irradiation appears promising for patients whose lesions might not be amenable to surgical resection. Argon laser energy, which is readily absorbed by erythematous lesions, might seem ideal for treatment of bladder hemangiomas, but its limited penetration (approximately 1 mm) restricts its effectiveness to the smallest lesions. The Nd:YAG laser is usually more effective in treating larger lesions because of its greater depth of penetration.[55]

Interstitial cystitis has been a vexing chronic disease that responds quickly to numerous therapies but, unfortunately, recurs in most patients with advanced disease. Shanberg, Baghdassarian, and Tansey have described Nd:YAG therapy (25 to 30 W of energy for a pulse duration of 3 seconds) in five patients with interstitial cystitis.[56] Their technique involves laser treatment of all ulcerated and erythematous areas in the bladder, as well as laser photocoagulation of the entire trigone except the ureteral orifices. Objective measurements of bladder volumes before and after laser treatment showed improvement in all patients, and four of five patients had marked improvement in their nocturia pattern. A later expanded series of patients yielded similar results.[57] Shanberg's group believes that patients with frank ulcers have the best results. The mechanisms whereby bladder capacity increases in these patients are not clear but could result from partial denervation of the trigone in response to deep laser penetration. This question will be answered only by a randomized clinical trial, but the laser technique is a useful addition to the urologist's surgical armamentarium in the treatment of this difficult lesion. The incidence of bowel perforation with laser treatment is higher for interstitial cystitis than for bladder lesions. This may be because patients with interstitial cystitis could have undergone several previous surgical procedures with resultant adhesion of the small bowel to the bladder, because most ulcers are located in the dome of the bladder, or because the disease occurs most often in women, who probably have thinner bladders than men. For whatever reason, the laser surgeon must exercise caution when treating patients with interstitial cystitis.

Nd:YAG treatment of radiation-induced cystitis and drug-induced cystitis (cyclophosphamide) has been less promising. Published reports of significant series of patients are not available, but I have found that laser therapy only temporarily controls bleeding in these patients. We have treated three patients with significant hematuria secondary to radiation cystitis and two with cyclophosphamide cystitis with temporary but not lasting result. This outcome might be expected from a problem that causes a global pathologic condition of the bladder. Cystitis glandularis and eosinophilic cystitis, although rare conditions, have responded well to Nd:YAG treatment.

Prostate Gland

Malignancies

Use of the Nd:YAG laser for the treatment of localized (B1, B2) prostate cancer has been reported.[58] This novel approach involves preliminary extensive TUR (down to the capsule), followed in 3 to 6 weeks by laser photocoagulation of the prostatic fossa by a combined closed suprapubic and transurethral approach. The fossa is lased with 45 to 50 W of power at 4-second pulses. When a temperature-sensitive probe connected to a palpating finger was introduced rectally and pressed against the anterior wall of the rectum at the prostatic level, the maximal temperature recorded in seven patients during laser treatment was a safe 52° C.[59] Among 63 patients treated with the combined approach and followed up for longer than 6 months, 7 failures (biopsy-proven malignancies) were noted. Although follow-up times are short, this technique warrants further investigation, especially for patients who refuse surgery or radiation therapy for intracapsular prostate cancer.

Benign Lesions

The tissue vaporization ability of the CO_2 laser makes it theoretically attractive for the removal of obstructive prostatic tissue. However, its inability to be employed in a liquid medium, to be effectively passed down in a filter, or to control bleeding from vessels much larger than 1 mm precludes its transurethral use for the treatment of prostatic disease.

Nd:YAG laser treatment of prostatic tissue does not result in tissue vaporization but only protein coagulation and later tissue slough. It cannot be used to treat benign prostatic hyperplasia because sufficient tissue cannot be treated and tissue slough could cause obstruction. McPhee and colleagues have modified a standard resectoscope to enable positioning of a laser filter a fixed distance proximal to the cautery loop.[60] Using this instrument, they have been able to resect tissue with the loop and coagulate bleeding vessels with the Nd:YAG laser (40 W) in 11 patients with benign prostatic hyperplasia. TUR of the prostate can be performed in this manner, but the procedure is more tedious than using the resectoscope alone. Tissue can become entrapped between the loop and the laser fiber, obscuring the resectionist's view, and the laser cannot control bleeding from large vessels. This technique offers no improvement over standard TUR for benign prostatic hyperplasia.

Recently a novel approach to the application of Nd:YAG energy to benign prostatic hyperplasia was introduced. This system is called transurethral ultrasound-guided laser-induced prostatectomy (TULIP). The system employs a 20F transurethral probe with a miniature ultrasound transducer and a side-firing laser prism. The ultrasound image produced apparently allows adequate localization for safe laser energy application. It does not, however, allow exact visual appreciation of the depth of penetration of laser energy. A balloon is inflated in the prostatic urethra with the probe centered inside the balloon. The purposes of the balloon are to allow the ultrasound transducer to function, to distance the prostatic tissue from the laser energy source, and to compress the prostatic tissue and probably diminish its blood flow and reduce its heat sink effect. Apparently lased tissue does not slough off and cause significant problems with urethral obstruction, although edema is created, which often necessitates urethral catheterization for a period. The tissue effects known to result from the use of Nd:YAG laser in the bladder suggest that the zone of coagulative necrosis would not much exceed approximately 5 mm. Clinical trials with this new system are under way, and information regarding safety and efficacy may be forthcoming soon.

Shanberg, Tansey, and Baghdassarian have used the Nd:YAG laser to perform prostatotomy in 10 patients with obstructive voiding symptoms caused by benign prostatic hyperplasia.[61] The procedure involves direct contact of the laser fiber tip with prostatic tissue in the 5 and 7 o'clock positions, resulting in tissue vaporization. Incisions are carried out from the region of the trigone to the verumontanum. Because tissue contact overheats and carbonizes fiber tips, numerous fibers must be used to make a simple incision.

Shanberg and associates stated that all patients had marked improvement in voiding symptoms but that postoperative bleeding was significant in four of ten patients and that one patient had to be returned to the operating room for a standard TUR of the prostate for control of bleeding. No instance of retrograde ejaculation has been noted.

The availability of contact tips made from a synthetic sapphire crystal for Nd:YAG fibers might facilitate this procedure.[62] Such tips were designed to allow tissue contact and improve cutting ability. Nevertheless, this technique appears to have no advantage over standard transurethral incision or TUR of the prostate.

Laser prostatotomy can also be easily performed with the KTP laser. We have used this wavelength in several patients with small glands and have achieved gratifying results, although it affords no absolutely definable advantage over the other methods or wavelengths already mentioned.

Urethra

Malignancies

Urethral carcinomas are rare, and experience with laser treatment of these lesions is meager. Hofstetter and Frank have reported treating two patients, but both patients experienced recurrences.[17] Smith has successfully treated one elderly man with noninvasive transitional cell carcinoma of the proximal bulbar urethra with no recurrence noted in 18 months of follow-up.[63]

Benign Lesions

Techniques for the treatment of urethral strictures often fail. Urethral dilation is frequently followed by recurrence, and electrocautery resection with the resultant irregular urethral burns may actually accentuate recurrent scar tissue formation. Direct vision cold knife urethrotomy appears to have the best results, but recurrences remain common.

The use of lasers to treat urethral stricture disease is theoretically sound and based on the fact that lasers can produce either tissue vaporization (CO_2, KTP, and argon lasers) with little surrounding thermal effect or coagulation of tissues with subsequent tissue slough (Nd:YAG laser) and minimal scarring.

Bulow, Bulow, and Frohmuller were the first to report laser treatment of urethral stricture. Five patients were treated with an Nd:YAG laser with 40 W of power focused to a 1.5 mm spot.[64] The apparent success of the technique is somewhat surprising because the relatively deep penetration of this laser would be expected to produce further periurethral fibrosis and recurrent stenosis. The brevity of the follow-up period may be significant. Perez-Castro and Martinez-Pinero have described a technique of direct vision internal urethrotomy followed by Nd:YAG laser irradiation of the cut tissue edges, but only limited follow-up results are available.[66] Smith and Dixon have reported Nd:YAG laser treatment of benign strictures in 17 patients. All patients had had prior urethral dilations, and 13 had failed to improve with urethrotomy. The stricture was treated using a spot size of 0.2 cm at 1 cm from the fiber tip and a power setting of 40 to 50 W. A small urethral catheter was inserted through the lumen of the stricture before treatment, and the entire circumference of the strictured area underwent laser irradiation. After treatment was completed, the urethra was dilated to 24F because the edema caused by laser therapy created significant urethral obstruction. In 11 patients (63%) recurrent strictures developed within 6 months of treatment (Figure 3–15).

Shanberg, Chalfin, and Tansey initially reported on the treatment of six patients with benign stricture disease but have subsequently treated more than 30 patients.[67] Their techniques included the insertion of a guidewire through the stricture before circumferential destruction of scar tissue until healthy tissue was encountered. Although they reported excellent initial results, follow-up has demonstrated a recurrence of the stricture and a need for further treatment in 50% of the patients. One significant complication involved perforation of the urethra and subsequent urinary extravasation. This problem was controlled by cystotomy and local drainage.

Shanberg and his group at one time advocated internal urethrotomy at the 12 o'clock position using direct contact of the quartz tip of the laser fiber with the stricture.[68] However, careful follow-up showed failures in more than half of the patients who were followed for more than a year. Another way to increase the power density of an Nd:YAG laser (and decrease forward scatter) is to use sapphire contact tips, which are available in several configurations. These various tip shapes are made to enable, theoretically, the user to cut, cauterize, and perform other functions more effectively. Smith and his group attempted to treat 23 patients with benign urethral strictures using contact tips.[69] They were unable to complete the therapy in 10 patients because the cutting effect was inadequate. In the other 13 patients multiple urethrotomies were completed, but more than half of the patients have had recurrence over long-term follow-up. In general the treatment of urethral stricture with Nd:YAG lasers has been disappointing, and as Hofstetter and Frank concluded, at the present time

A B C

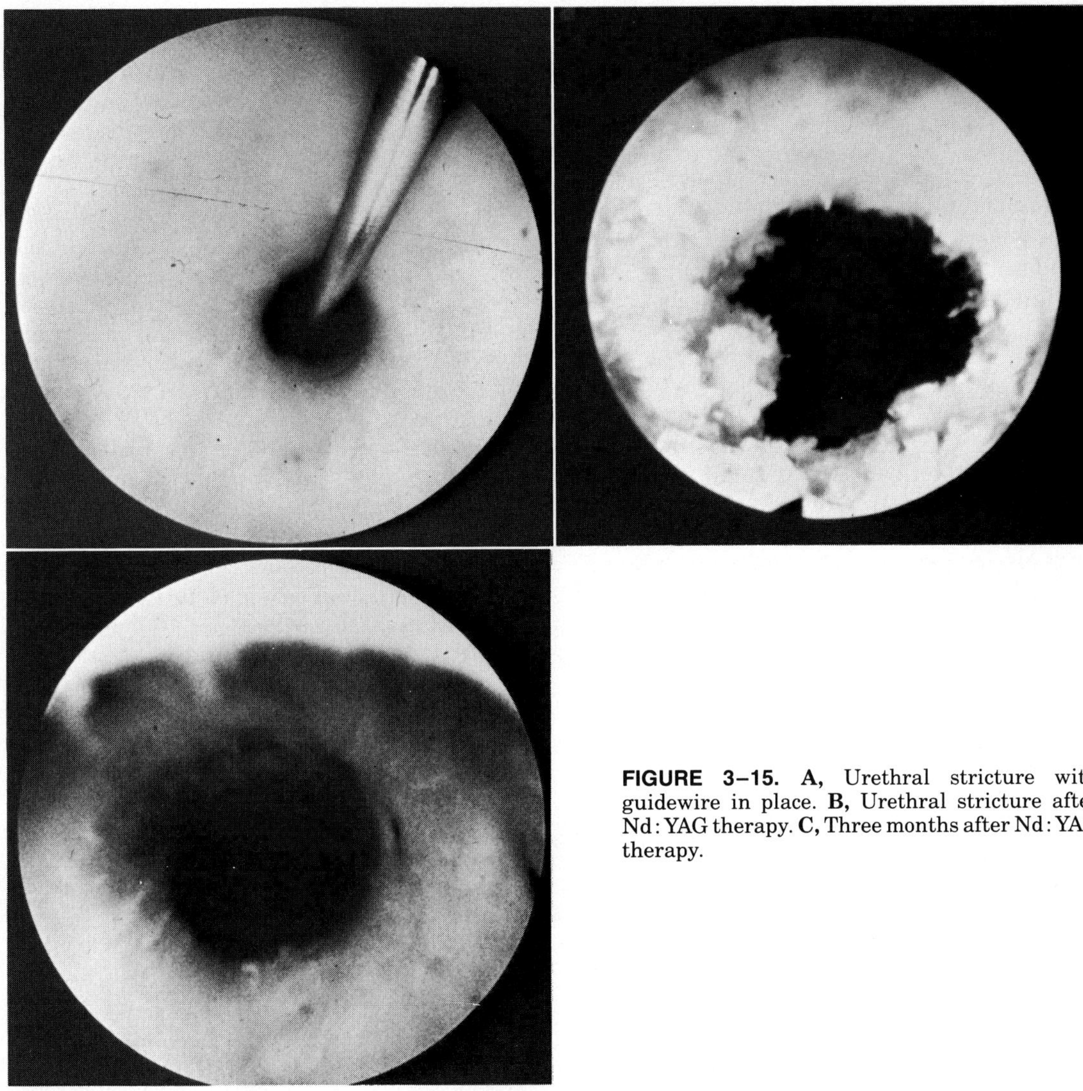

FIGURE 3–15. A, Urethral stricture with guidewire in place. **B,** Urethral stricture after Nd : YAG therapy. **C,** Three months after Nd : YAG therapy.

the Nd:YAG laser is unsuitable for the treatment of urethral strictures.[20]

Rothauge used the argon laser for the treatment of benign urethral strictures in 40 patients.[70] He stressed the necessity of removing the entire stricture down to the level of the corpus spongiosum. Although bleeding was negligible and urinary flow rates showed a statistically significant increase after laser urethrotomy, long-term follow-up is limited. Noske and co-workers later reported using the argon laser to treat 90 patients with urethral stricture. The recurrence rate was similar to that of conventional urethrotomy.[71]

The KTP-532 laser has properties similar to those of the argon laser and has recently been employed in and evaluated for treatment of urethral strictures. Shanberg and colleagues reported their results treating 22 recurrent strictures in 20 patients.[72] All strictures were vaporized in a circumferential manner. The laser was effective in 68% of the patients with relatively short follow-up periods, ranging from 6 to 14 months. A similar success rate has recently been cited by Turek and associates.[73] They treated 31 patients with a nonrecurrence rate of 59% (mean follow-up 9.7 months).

Among forms of laser radiation possibly available for stricture excision, the CO_2 laser seems the most promising. With this laser, precise removal can be accomplished with minimal bleeding. However, the strong absorption of CO_2 laser energy by water and the lack of a fiber to transmit the energy place significant practical limitations on the endoscopic use of this laser. Nevertheless, prototype CO_2 cystoscopes have had limited use in the treatment of urethral stricture disease. The high absorption of CO_2 laser energy by water and the accumulation of blood and urine on the lenses have necessitated infiltration of CO_2 gas during the procedure. Unfortunately, either because of the extent of the procedure and the proximity to the vascular corpus spongiosum or because of excessive gas pressures, fatal gas embolization has been noted in several patients.[11]

Lasers may offer an advantage in the treatment

of posterior urethral valves in children. Ehrlich, Shanberg, and Fine described a technique for destroying posterior urethral valves through a percutaneous cystotomy approach. A cystoscope is passed through the bladder neck, enabling a contact tip Nd:YAG fiber to destroy the valve.[74] More recently a KTP-532 laser has been used with the same technique. Adequate valve ablation has been uniformly achieved, and no urethral strictures have resulted.

Other benign lesions that have been effectively treated with the laser are urethral hemangiomas and condyloma acuminatum. Hemangiomas are unusual, and they are extremely difficult to treat because they are often extensive and electrofulguration might result in significant scarring of the urethra. Urethral hemangiomas or telangiectasis, particularly as may be seen in patients with Osler-Weber-Rendu syndrome or Klippel-Trenaunay-Weber syndrome, are especially amenable to laser therapy. If the lesion is small, the argon laser can be used. Larger lesions are best treated with the Nd:YAG laser.[55] Amagai and associates reported on the treatment of five patients with urethral hemangiomas: two with the CO_2, two with the argon, and one with the Nd:YAG laser.[75]

In 1980 Fuselier and co-workers reported using the CO_2 laser with a beam diameter of 1 mm and a power of 30 W to treat seven patients (six men, one woman) with a condyloma acuminatum of the urethral meatus.[76] Six of the seven had failed to improve with previous podophyllin or electrofulguration therapy. No recurrences were noted after laser treatment with follow-up periods ranging from 8 to 27 months. The application of the CO_2 laser to the treatment of accessible distal urethral lesions was later substantiated by Rosenberg and his group. They treated four men with condylomata of the urethra using a rapid superpulse carbon dioxide laser with a repetition rate of 100 pulses per second and a power ranging from 3 to 6.8 W.[77] The authors suggest that the superpulse mode is associated with less edema and tissue reaction because increased energy densities can be used. This same group later published the results of using a CO_2 laser coupled with an operating microscope to treat 22 patients with distal urethral meatal condylomata.[78] Lesions measuring 0.2 to 0.8 mm were treated with 2 to 6 W of energy and larger lesions with 10 to 15 W. Nineteen of the 22 patients were cured of their lesions after a single treatment, and more important no subsequent urethral strictures were noted. If lesions are extensive, the authors suggest treatment in two sessions 6 weeks apart.

Effective treatment of urethral condyloma acuminatum using the Nd:YAG laser has been reported by several groups.[79] Lesions in any portion of the urethra are easily accessible to treatment with the Nd:YAG laser (in contrast to the CO_2 laser) with power settings of approximately 35 W. As with the treatment of superficial bladder tumors, therapeutic effect is adequate when the lesions turn white because of protein denaturation. Most patients with extensive lesions require general or spinal anesthesia for treatment. Postoperative discomfort is minimal. No posttreatment urethral strictures have been noted. The apparent effectiveness of Nd:YAG laser treatment of intraurethral condyloma acuminatum and the lack of morbidity of this technique make it an attractive first-line therapy for this troublesome disease.

In women, intraurethral condylomata that frequently accompany extensive vaginal and meatal involvement are extremely difficult to treat with available methods. We treated two such patients, and all lesions were completely eradicated after three treatment sessions. No urethral strictures resulted from what was, in fact, laser treatment of 90% of the urethral mucosa (Fig. 3-16).

A

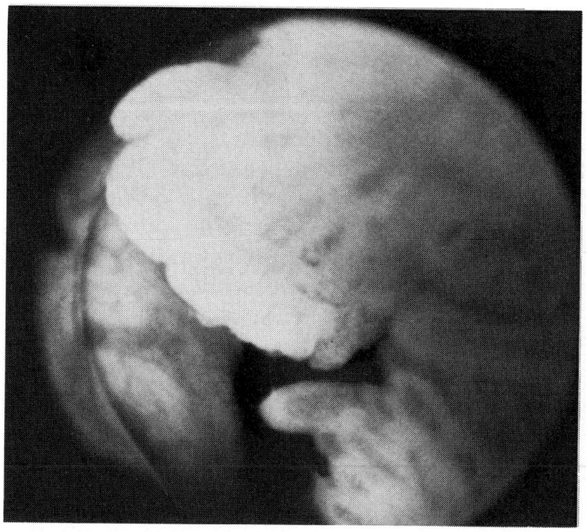

B

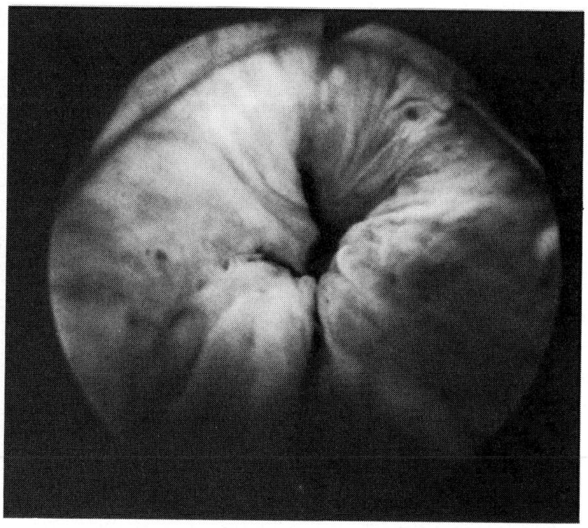

FIGURE 3–16. **A,** Extensive condylomata acuminata in the urethra of a female patient. **B,** Same area 3 months after Nd: YAG treatment.

Ureter and Renal Pelvis

Lasers can be used to treat transitional cell carcinomas of the ureter and renal pelvis in three ways: endoscopically, percutaneously, and through open surgical application. The first of these is clearly preferable and, with the availability of instruments that allow access to the ureter and renal collecting systems, has become a reality.

Although the indications for endoscopic laser treatment of ureteral and renal pelvic tumors continue to change with evolution of instrumentation and maturation of data, this treatment is new and the physician must adhere as strictly as possible to appropriate patient selection criteria. Although exceptions exist, a patient considered for this approach should either have a solitary kidney, significantly decreased renal function or bilateral synchronous tumors or be an unacceptable risk for open surgery. The tumor should be accessible, be smaller than 1.5 cm, and not be circumferential or occupy a long distance along the course of the ureter. Thorough endoscopic evaluation of the tumor and an adequate biopsy are essential, and at present only low-grade low-stage lesions should be treated.

From a technical standpoint either flexible or rigid ureteroscopes can be used, since a 400 laser fiber (either Nd:YAG or KTP-532) can be passed through either. The pressure of the irrigating fluid should not exceed 40 cm H_2O.

It is difficult to be dogmatic regarding power settings for use in the ureter or renal pelvis because assumptions must be based on animal studies.[80] It would appear that for the Nd:YAG laser powers should not exceed 20 W for 2 seconds and for the KTP-532 laser not more than 15 W for 2 seconds. Although these powers might be excessive, the fact that the operator can almost never achieve irradiation directly perpendicular to the lesion results in decreased power density and resultant decreased danger of overtreatment and damage to the ureteral wall or surrounding structures. In fact treating lesions in a "no touch" manner is often difficult because of the lack of room to maneuver the scope and fiber. Because of the inevitable edema after treatment, most authors recommend the placement of a double-J ureteral stent passed over the obligatory guidewire after completion of treatment.

Follow-up of patients treated with the laser is controversial. My practice has been to repeat ureteroscopy 4 to 6 weeks after treatment to assess treatment and healing. Thereafter patients are generally followed by urinary cytologic examinations, excretory urography, or retrograde pyelography (Figure 3-17).

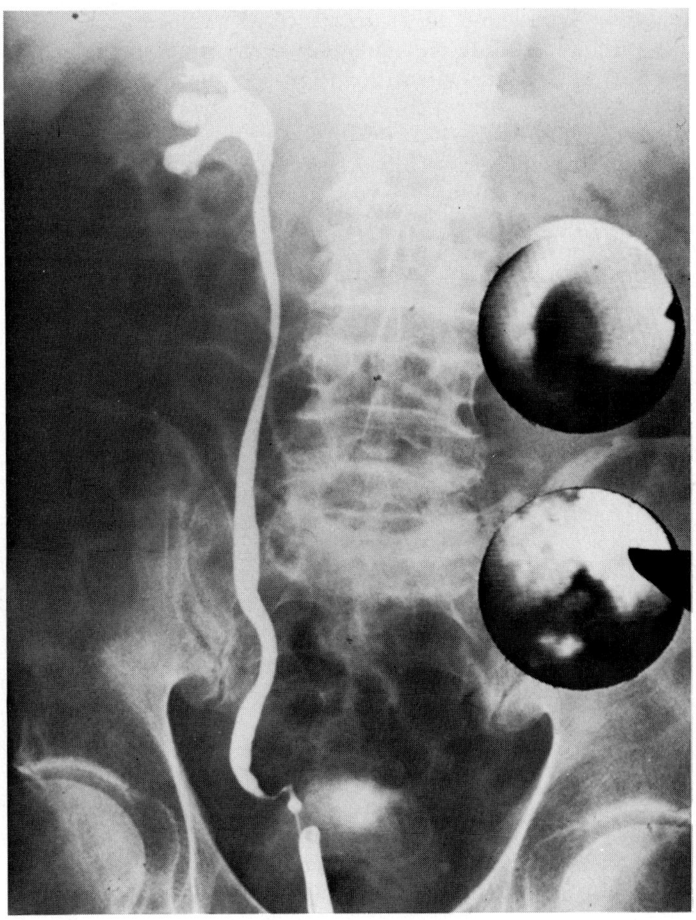

FIGURE 3–17. Pyelogram demonstrating filling defect in the upper pole calyx. Lower inset demonstrates endoscopic view of noninvasive transitional cell carcinoma. Upper inset is an endoscopic view of the same area 3 months after Nd:YAG therapy.

Hofstetter and Keiditsch were the first to report on the successful treatment of ureteral tumors with the Nd:YAG laser.[81] In the same year, Rothenberger and co-workers reported treating four patients with low-grade transitional cell carcinoma of the distal ureter with the Nd:YAG laser via the ureteroscope.[26] In all patients no evidence of recurrent disease was found 18 months after treatment. Following the success of this initial experience, 12 patients with a total of 16 biopsy-proven noninvasive tumors were treated with 40 W of power and 1- to 3-second pulses. During follow-up averaging 23 months, no local recurrences were noted.[82,83]

Hofstetter's group has expanded its experience to 20 patients with ureteral tumors treated by endoscopic means with either laser radiation or electroresection and laser radiation. With a median observation period of 13.8 months they noted three recurrences and four ureteral strictures. Three of the four strictures occurred in patients having TUR plus laser treatment.[80] This observation reinforces my opinion that lesions are best evulsed by using a biopsy forceps and treating the remaining tissue and base with the laser, or alternatively by cutting off the lesion using a contact laser (preferably the KTP-532) and subsequently lasing the base. Our experience with laser treatment of ureteral and renal pelvic lesions indicates that it is feasible and that recurrence rates approximate those noted with conservative open surgical approaches.[84]

Laser treatment of small ureteral tumors or accessible renal pelvic or calyceal tumors appears to be a promising alternative to open surgical techniques. However, many lesions in the renal pelvis or calyces (certainly the middle and lower pole calyces) are not accessible endoscopically. This fact leads many to consider a percutaneous approach to such lesions. Selection of patients for a percutaneous approach should be similar to that for an endoscopic approach: patients with a solitary kidney, renal insufficiency, or bilateral tumors in whom standard treatment would make the patient dependent on dialysis, patients who are too sick from other causes to undergo major abdominal surgery, and those who refuse operation.

The risks of a percutaneous approach are real. Seeding of tumor in the percutaneous tract is possible and has been reported in patients undergoing intraoperative rigid nephroscopy.[85] Long-term results are not yet available, and because of the difficulty of these procedures the physician must be a trained percutaneous surgeon in addition to having extensive laser experience. The popularity of this approach seems to be growing, however, and its use will probably increase as instrumentation improves.

Orihuela and Smith have used the Nd:YAG laser percutaneously as part of a second-look procedure.[86] During the initial operation they established and dilated a nephrostomy tract, obtained cold cup biopsy specimens, and resected the tumor and fulgurated the bed with a Bugbee electrode. In eight patients a second-look nephroscopy was performed several days later with Nd:YAG irradiation being delivered (15 to 20 W in 2-second pulses) to the tumor bed. During a follow-up of 1½ to 2 months, two recurrences necessitating nephroureterectomy were noted in these patients. Several authors[87,88] have reported similar success rates. My experience has been recurrence in two of seven patients treated percutaneously and followed up for more than 1 year (Figure 3–18).

Open Urologic Surgery

Kidney

Any discussion of the use of the CO_2 laser for renal surgery must be prefaced by the statement that this instrument cannot be used on renal parenchyma without first clamping the renal pedicle. Although the CO_2 laser is an effective cutting device, the relatively high pressure of flow through the arteries and larger caliber renal vessels exceeds the coagulative abilities of this laser, so that complete hemostasis within the renal parenchyma cannot be accomplished. In addition, once the renal collecting system is entered, extreme care must be taken to evacuate all urine because of the high absorption of CO_2 energy by water.

Mulvaney and Beck first reported an attempt at wedge resection of the canine kidney with a 50 W CO_2 laser; they found the incision to be slow and hemostasis unsatisfactory.[89] Hughes and Scott also examined the use of the CO_2 laser for partial nephrectomy in seven dogs in the hope that the procedure could be performed faster than conventional surgery and with less renal ischemia time and blood loss.[90] After transection of the parenchyma, the cut surface of the kidney was coagulated with the unfocused laser beam. The average time of ischemia was 15 minutes, and renal damage was limited to a 1 to 2 mm area of coagulation necrosis. No closure of the collecting system was performed other than laser coagulation, and subsequent x-ray evaluation indicated that urinary extravasation was not a problem. The authors were generally impressed by the ease with which the CO_2 laser could be used to perform partial nephrectomy in dogs. These observations were later confirmed in cats by Meiraz and associates,[91] who make the important point that although the CO_2 laser can seal vessels only up to a diameter of 0.5 mm, when blood flow is stopped temporarily while the tissue is divided, empty vessels up to 2 mm can be sealed. In 1982 Barzilay and associates reported on a careful comparative study in which the CO_2 laser was used in partial nephrectomies in dogs.[92] These authors claimed that the addition of the CO_2 laser shortened operating time, diminished blood loss, and did not interfere with final kidney function.

A

B

C

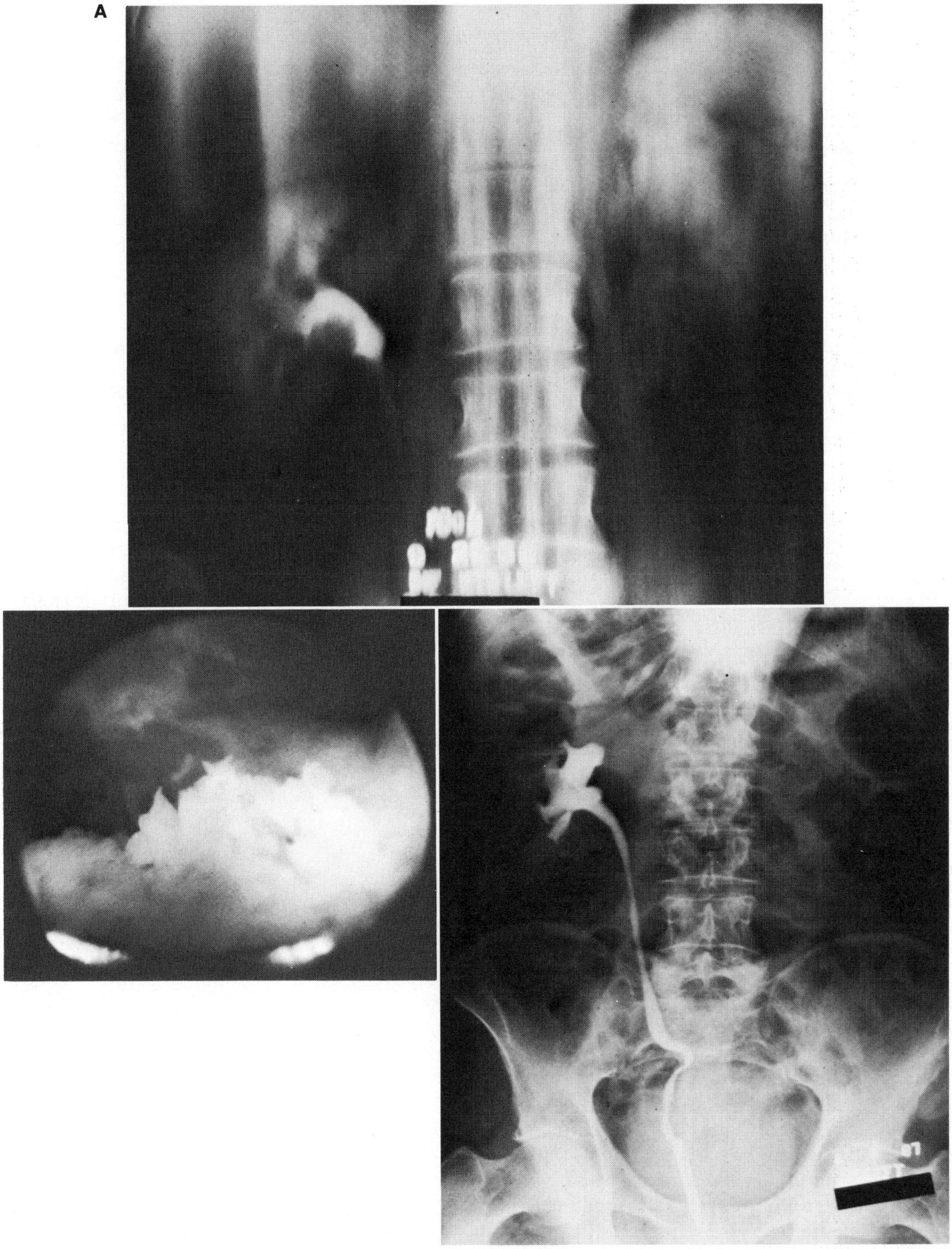

FIGURE 3–18. **A,** Excretory urogram demonstrating filling defect of the right renal pelvis and solitary right kidney. **B,** Percutaneous endoscopic view of papillary transitional cell carcinoma of the renal pelvis. **C,** Retrograde pyelogram 6 months after Nd:YAG therapy.

On the basis of these animal studies a number of investigators have used a CO_2 laser to perform partial nephrectomy and nephrolithotomy in humans. Pariente and d'Ovidio treated renal calculi with CO_2 laser nephrotomies and reported that "the incision of the renal parenchyma was always bloodless though we never practiced the clamping of the renal pedicle."[93] This observation is surprising and contrary to my experience. Barzilay and associates performed three partial nephrectomies (two patients with calculi, one with a calculus and xanthogranulomatous pyelonephritis) and one anatrophic nephrolithotomy using the CO_2 laser and were satisfied that the operation resulted in a minimum of blood loss and parenchymal damage.[94] Hall claimed that partial nephrectomy using the CO_2 laser in hemostasis was adequate but the incision was slow and prolonged renal ischemia times.[95]

Rosemberg and Lutz[96] and Rosemberg[97] reported on the successful performance of three anatrophic nephrolithotomies (for staghorn calculus) and three partial nephrectomies (for treatment of one congenital arteriovenous fistula, one segmental chronic atrophic pyelonephritis and calculus, and one bilateral renal mass). The surgical procedures were performed during regional hypothermia, but no mention of occlusion of the renal vessels was made. In the first three cases incision of the renal parenchyma with the CO_2 laser beam was slow, approximately 15 minutes. The average power used was 28 W and the optical spot size was 2 mm, corresponding to a power density of 700 W/cm^2. Because of the slowness the power densities were increased in the second three cases of 1000 to 1250 W/cm^2; this increase lowered the parenchymal incision time to 6 minutes. Total operation time ranged between 110 and 120 minutes, and the average estimated blood loss was 160 ml.

The cumulative experience with the CO_2 laser in renal surgery is contradictory, but theoretical considerations and practical experience seem to indicate that the instrument has little to offer over conventional surgery. With this laser, making the incision is slow, small vessels are well controlled but large vessels bleed readily, and the articulated arm of the instrument makes its use awkward. Unlike the CO_2 laser, the Nd:YAG laser has received relatively little use in renal surgery. Application of Nd:YAG energy causes protein denaturation, which results in deep thermal coagulation but no effective tissue vaporization. Therefore incision would be expected to be difficult and slow. We have found this laser, even with a focused beam, to be inefficient in the performance of partial nephrectomy and to cause tremendous tissue destruction. The Nd:YAG laser is effective in coagulating vessels up to 3 or 4 mm in diameter. Therefore, for hemostasis it may be preferable to use the Nd:YAG laser to coagulate a specific vessel on the cut surface of the kidney rather than to use cautery or a suture ligature. High power densities are required for this procedure, and use of 60 to 80 W for 1 to 3 seconds may be necessary. These energy levels may heat tissue too much and cause it to explode. Overheating can be prevented by irrigation of the cut surface of the kidney with saline. In addition, when cold knife incisions are made in the renal parencyhma, the brisk bleeding that occurs if the renal pedicle is not clamped may make effective application of the Nd:YAG laser to the bleeding site difficult. When the renal pedicle is clamped, the surface of the renal parenchyma can be coagulated; however, retraction of vessels may necessitate high powers to control bleeding, with resultant excessive tissue damage.

Benderev and Schaffer performed partial nephrectomy in six dogs using 100 W of focused Nd:YAG power to determine its hemostatic capabilities, safety, and effect on renal function and histologic pattern.[98] These studies were carried out with the renal pedicle clamped and with renal cooling. The renal collecting system was not closed. Hemostasis was reported to be excellent, but urinomas occurred in two dogs and the zone of necrosis produced by the laser energy penetrated as far as 7 mm. Because of this unacceptable amount of tissue necrosis, Melzer and associates combined the use of the Cooper Cavitron ultrasonic surgical aspirator for parenchymal dissection with the Nd:YAG laser for vessel coagulation.[99] They performed 20 partial nephrectomies in 10 dogs with the combination of these two instruments after the renal vessels had been isolated and temporarily occluded. Blood loss and total operating time were less than those in a control series of partial nephrectomies performed with a scalpel. The authors concluded that the combination of the Cavitron ultrasonic surgical aspirator and the Nd:YAG laser offers advantages over either method used alone and over standard techniques for partial nephrectomy. Since their original report, this combination of technologies has been used to perform three successful partial nephrectomies in humans.

Hofstetter and Frank have advocated Nd:YAG treatment of the renal parenchyma adjacent to an area where a small malignant renal lesion has been "shelled out" or removed by wedge resection.[20] This practice seems warranted, especially when the free tissue margin may be inadequate. Malloy has used a similar technique while performing partial nephrectomies for renal cell carcinoma in patients with one kidney or with bilateral renal cell carcinoma.[100] In this use of the Nd:YAG laser in combination with blunt dissection, the laser seals off the lymphatics and small vessels around the tumor before excision and limits the blood loss while the tumor is being surgically elevated and removed.

Miscellaneous Open Applications

The particular feature of the CO_2 laser that appealed to pioneers of laser surgery was the rapid and intensive localized heating it produced. This "laser scalpel" sealed blood vessels and lymphatics, facilitated incision of infected tissues, and sterilized the wound. The CO_2 laser has been used for skin incision, but in comparative trials it does not appear to be more rapid than the scalpel or electric knife.[92] In addition, the amount of necrosis at the margins of laser wounds, although small, is greater than that caused by scalpel incision. Hall, Hill, and Beach investigated whether this small amount of thermal necrosis would interfere with wound healing in rats.[101] They compared the laser with diathermy and scalpel incision, using the tensile strength of the wounds as a measure of healing. They found that laser and diathermy wounds of the skin healed more slowly than scalpel wounds and concluded that it was worse to use the CO_2 laser for incision of the skin. However, healing of abdominal muscle, fascia, and peritoneum was not delayed when the laser was used.

CO_2 laser incision of infected tissues and vaporization of abscess cavities have been performed in humans, but none of the wounds healed by primary intention despite the supposed sterilizing effect of the laser.[95] In addition, postoperative lymphatic drainage was not reduced in several patients undergoing pelvic or superficial inguinal lymphadenectomy with the aid of the CO_2 laser. Despite these observations, Lindstedt and Lundquist considered the CO_2 laser to be advantageous for minor procedures, such as circumcision and subcapsular orchiectomy, particularly in patients with bleeding disorders resulting from hemophilia, uremia, and anticoagulants.[102] d'Ovidio and Carmignani used the CO_2 laser in combination with microsurgical techniques and claimed several advantages: (1) with laser surgery, the target area is under continuous binocular vision, so that the progress of tissue destruction can be continuously monitored; (2) the hemostatic effect of the laser enables the surgeon to take full advantage of the excellent visualization provided by the microscope; and (3) operative and postoperative edema is limited.[103] They used this technique in testis autotransplantation, in vas deferens surgery, and in the repair of varicoceles.

Open cystotomy is rarely necessary in the treatment of transitional cell carcinoma, but several investigators have evaluated the use of the CO_2 laser in open ablation of these lesions.[93] In experiments on chemically induced bladder tumors in animals, hemostasis was satisfactory with the CO_2 laser, but the vessels encountered in rabbits, and even in dogs, do not compare in size to those of the human bladder. Hughes and Scott used the diffused laser beam through a large cystotomy in the dome of the bladder and coagulated 80% of the urothelium in seven dogs.[90] Histologic sections of tissue obtained immediately after coagulation revealed minimal damage to the underlying muscle, and examination of the bladders at 3 weeks showed reepithelialization. Hall, using the CO_2 laser in humans for open excision of multiple bladder tumors, indicated that "hemostasis was generally disappointing," particularly when he attempted to vaporize or excise tumors larger than 6 mm in diameter.[95]

Early attempts at the performance of open prostatic biopsies in dogs were disappointing because bleeding was difficult to control with the laser alone. Blood on the cut surface of the prostate absorbed the laser energy and effectively shielded the vessels from the cautery effect.[90] Transvesical prostatectomy in humans has been attempted with the CO_2 laser, but again, bleeding could not be adequately controlled with the use of the laser alone.[95]

Skin Lesions

For treatment of malignant and benign lesions of the external genitalia, lasers may prove to have a significant advantage over other methods of treatment. The Nd:YAG, CO_2, argon, and KTP-532 lasers have all been used for the treatment of skin lesions; the characteristics of each wavelength dictate the choice of instrument.

Premalignant and Malignant Lesions

Early experience with laser surgery for premalignant and malignant penile lesions has yielded promising results, although the number of cases reported is small. If long-term results substantiate the low recurrence rates observed thus far, the laser will be an important addition to the urologist's armamentarium for the treatment of these difficult problems. Laser therapy of penile lesions obviates mutilative surgery and results in less scarring and better cosmetic appearance than do current alternatives. To date, the premalignant lesions reported to have been treated with the CO_2 or Nd:YAG laser are Bowen's disease and erythroplasia of Queyrat. Rosemberg and Fuller used a rapid superpulsed CO_2 laser to treat erythroplasia of Queyrat involving the glans penis and coronal sulcus in one patient.[104] The cosmetic result was excellent, but long-term follow-up was not reported. I have successfully treated two patients with Bowen's disease (Figure 3–19),[105] one with erythroplasia of Queyrat, and one with leukoplakia of the glans penis using the Nd:YAG laser at a power setting of 20 W; there was no recurrence of disease at 8, 12, and 14 months after treatment.

In situ and invasive squamous cell carcinomas and malignant melanomas of the penis have been treated with the Nd:YAG laser. The one reported patient with malignant melanoma died of metastatic disease but pathologically proved local control was successfully achieved.[20]

Parsons, Campbell, and Thomley in 1968 were the first to report on laser therapy of squamous cell carcinoma of the penis.[106] They used a ruby laser to treat a patient who had invasive squamous cell carcinoma and refused partial penectomy. The treatment was performed under local anesthesia after the lesion was darkened with black shoe polish to enhance local energy absorption. At 3 months the cosmetic result apparently was excellent but a biopsy revealed persistent malignant disease. Repeat laser treatment was followed by partial penectomy. No tumor was found in the pathologic specimen.

B

A

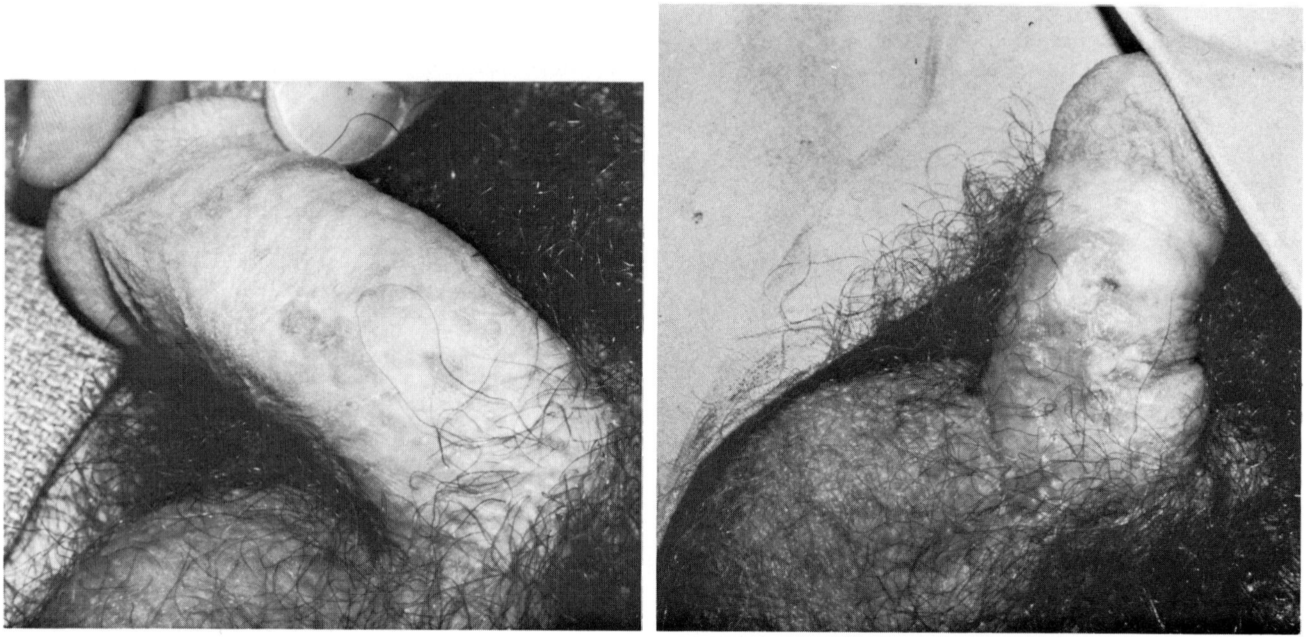

FIGURE 3–19. A, Bowenoid papules on the penile shaft before treatment. **B,** Penile shaft immediately after Nd:YAG laser treatment of bowenoid papules.

Squamous cell carcinoma of the penis is a lesion that might be ideally treated with the Nd:YAG laser because of the depth of energy penetration of this laser. I have treated four cases of in situ squamous cell carcinoma of the glans penis with the Nd:YAG laser; the cosmetic result was excellent and disease had not recurred in more than 1 year of follow-up. The advisability of laser treatment of invasive lesions remains conjectural, but the body of evidence for the efficacy of this therapy is increasing (Figure 3–20). In 1981 Numata and coworkers presented the "successful" treatment of three patients with squamous cell carcinoma of the penis treated by the Nd:YAG laser.[107] Treatment power ranged from 30 to 80 W, and a black cream was used to increase tissue absorption. In all patients large areas of the glans and foreskin were treated, and in one patient complete slough of the glans penis was noted.

Hofstetter and Frank have the largest experience with the use of the Nd:YAG laser to treat penile cancer.[20] They treated 17 patients who refused standard surgical therapy. The tumor and a 0.5 cm margin were treated with the Nd:YAG laser at a power setting of 40 W. Tissue slough, healing, and reepithelialization were complete by eight weeks, and cosmetic results were excellent. Eleven patients had follow-up of 11 to 39 months; only one patient had local recurrence. My experience has been that Nd:YAG therapy for local lesions in patients with demonstrated metastatic disease often provides excellent palliation and eliminates the

B

A

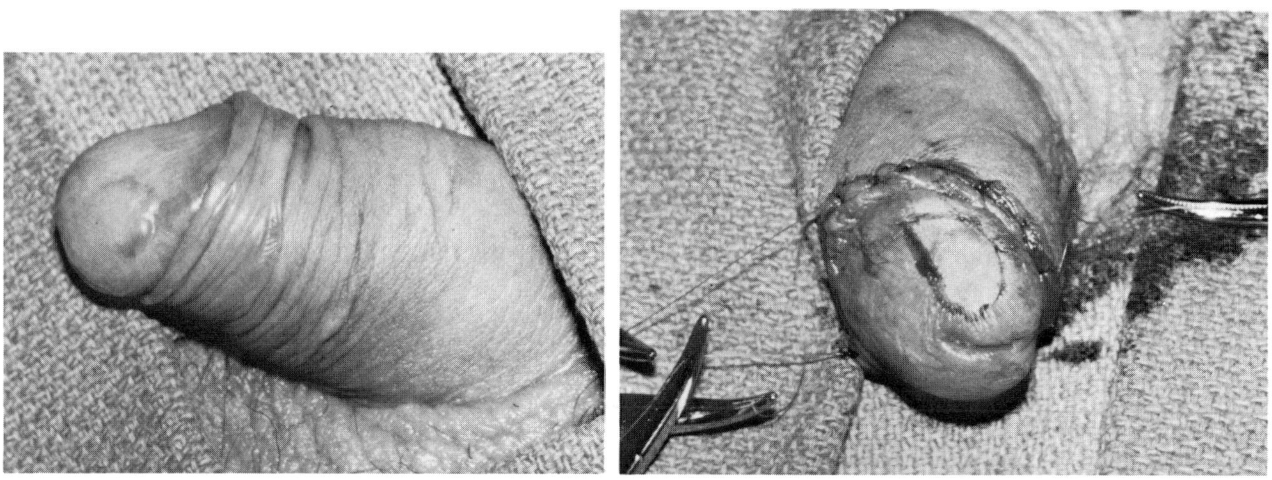

FIGURE 3–20. A, Area of noninvasive squamous cell carcinoma in the glans penis. **B,** Same area after Nd:YAG laser therapy and circumcision.

usual problems of secondary infection and urethral compression without the need for partial or total penectomy.

Malloy, Wein, and Carpiniello have published a similar report of experience with 16 men with squamous cell cancer of the penis who were treated primarily with the Nd:YAG laser.[108] Five patients had Tis, nine had T1 tumors, and two had T2 carcinomas. The patients were followed up from 12 to 36 months. At follow-up, five patients with Tis had no evidence of recurrent cancer. Of the nine patients with T1 disease, six (67%) were tumor free. The two with T2 cancer were not cured.

Evidence indicates that laser therapy may one day prove to be the preferred method of treatment for carefully selected patients with premalignant diseases of the penis.

Benign Lesions

Condyloma Acuminatum. The treatment of condyloma acuminatum with existing methods, for example, electrodesiccation, surgical excision, or topical application of a cytotoxic agent such as podophyllin or 5% fluorouracil cream, frequently results in recalcitrant lesions that are extremely difficult to eradicate. Recurrence often is due not only to treatment failure but also to the overlooking of extremely small early lesions. Examination should be performed after application of 3% to 5% acetic acid, and observation must be made under magnification. At present, accumulated clinical experience with all types of lasers indicates that laser therapy is effective for condylomata that are refractive to other treatments.

The CO_2 laser has been used most frequently for the treatment of genital condylomata. Local infiltration with 1% lidocaine (Xylocaine) or 0.25% bupivacaine (Marcaine) provides sufficient anesthesia for the treatment of small penile or vulvar condylomata, but extensive lesions or perianal lesions require regional or general anesthesia. For the treatment of small lesions, a setting of 2 to 20 W on a continuous wave or rapid superpulse mode is sufficient because vaporization proceeds rapidly and overtreatment can lead to a significant skin defect. Precise control of the incident beam confines injury of adjacent tissue to an area not exceeding 2 mm, facilitates healing, and minimizes fibrosis. In addition, the use of a rapid superpulse laser (100 pulses per second) creates a lesion to a predetermined depth with a lower average power density than that of the continuous wave mode.[109] When comparable power densities are used in both modes, the rapid superpulse laser results in less edema and tissue necrosis, so that healing is faster and is accompanied by less scarring. Each pass of the laser beam creates a U-shaped crater of vaporized tissue whose diameter is about that of the focused laser beam. If the beam were moved randomly, skip areas of untreated diseased tissue would result. An organized pattern of transverse movement of the beam across the tissue results in a uniform ablation of tissue. When the laser is operated in this fashion, the heat conducted to the underlying tissue is distributed evenly along the surface of the lesion. The cross-hatched matrix produced by directing the laser beam vertically, horizontally, and obliquely ensures that all ridges and islands of tissue left behind will be vaporized. A moistened sponge should be used to wipe the surface clear of carbonized tissue to expose deeper layers for treatment. Large, bulky lesions may require high power outputs (20 to 30 W). Treatment of small or subclinical lesions is often facilitated by the use of the operating microscope.

The safety and efficacy of CO_2 laser treatment of condyloma acuminatum have been demonstrated by many authors. In 1980, Baggish, in a report on the treatment of 110 female patients with condyloma of the vagina, cervix, and urethral meatus, cited a 5.5% recurrence rate without associated morbidity and indicated the necessity for staging procedures when a large area of condylomatous involvement was present.[110] Fuselier and associates reported on their experience with 10 patients who had condylomatous involvement of the penile shaft, vaginal introitus, and urethral meatus treated with CO_2 laser energy.[76] In eight of these patients, various previous therapies had failed and the authors noted no recurrence and no morbidity after 10 to 34 months of follow-up. Similar results were achieved by Rosemberg in 61 patients treated for penile condylomata; the cure rate from a single treatment was 88%.[111] Lundquist and Lindstedt treated 150 male patients for podophyllin-resistant genital warts.[112] In this group of patients the authors achieved a cumulative success rate of 95% with one to three treatments and a follow-up duration of 6 months. More recently Carpniello and associates reported on the results of CO_2 laser treatment of 127 high-risk males with biopsy-proven subclinical human papillomavirus (HPV) infection found by magnified penile surface scanning.[113] At a mean follow-up of four months a 66% recurrence rate of microscopic condyloma was encountered. This study underscores the fact that previously reported high cure rates were for grossly visible lesions, which are generally viral subtypes 6 and 11, and that cure of the possibly carcinogenic subtypes 16, 18, and 31 is problematic with any type of focal therapy. Giant condyloma (Buschke-Lowenstein tumor) has also been successfully treated with the CO_2 laser, the sheer size of the lesion often necessitating more than one treatment session.[114]

The argon laser has rarely been used to treat condyloma acuminatum. Aledia reported the successful treatment of three patients with penile condylomata without subsequent recurrence, and Amagai and associates treated six patients but did not give follow-up results.[75,115] The KTP-532 laser can also be used to treat condyloma effectively at power settings of 7 to 9 W (Figure 3–21). As is true with the argon laser, KTP laser energy is absorbed by melanin, and therefore the KTP laser is useful in treating condyloma in black patients.

Effective Nd:YAG laser treatment of genital warts has been reported by several authors.[116] Therapy can usually be delivered with use of local anesthesia in the outpatient setting; only extremely large or perianal lesions require hospitalization and general anesthesia (Figure 3–22). Because penetration of Nd:YAG energy is significantly deeper than that of the CO_2 laser, care must be taken not to overtreat lesions. Large lesions can be treated with power outputs of 35 to 40 W, but my preference is to treat smaller lesions with 11 to 15 W to prevent significant scar formation. Stein treated 12 patients with condylomata, including one with meatal involvement and one with extensive perianal involvement. In all cases excellent cosmetic results with no recurrences were noted in follow-up of more than six months.[117] Hofstetter and Frank used the Nd:YAG laser to treat 30 patients with condylomata, and recurrent lesions developed in only two.[20] The epithelium for up to 6 mm around the lesion should be treated because it has been shown that HPV can extend this distance from the base of the lesion.[118]

Miscellaneous Benign Lesions. Baggish reported on CO_2 laser treatment of 78 women with herpes simplex virus type 2 (HSV-2) infections of the vulva, vagina, or cervix, separately or in combination.[119] Since the viral organisms replicate in the basal or prickle cell layers of the epithelium, deep laser treatment is not necessary. After laser vaporization even women with extensive herpes had relief of pain. Four patients who had been receiving systemic analgesics and who had urinary catheters to prevent retention were able to void and to leave the hospital. Of the 30 patients who had

A

B

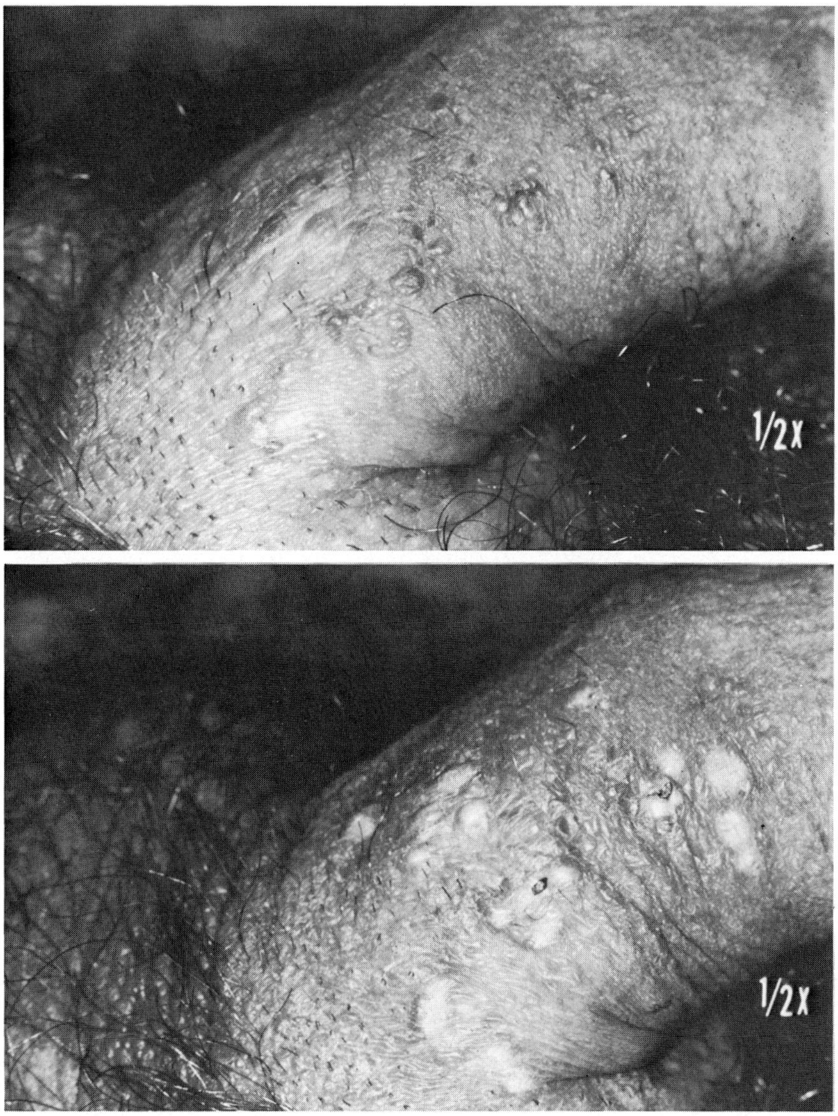

FIGURE 3–21. **A,** Same condylomata acuminata of the penile shaft. **B,** Same lesions immediately after KTP laser treatment.

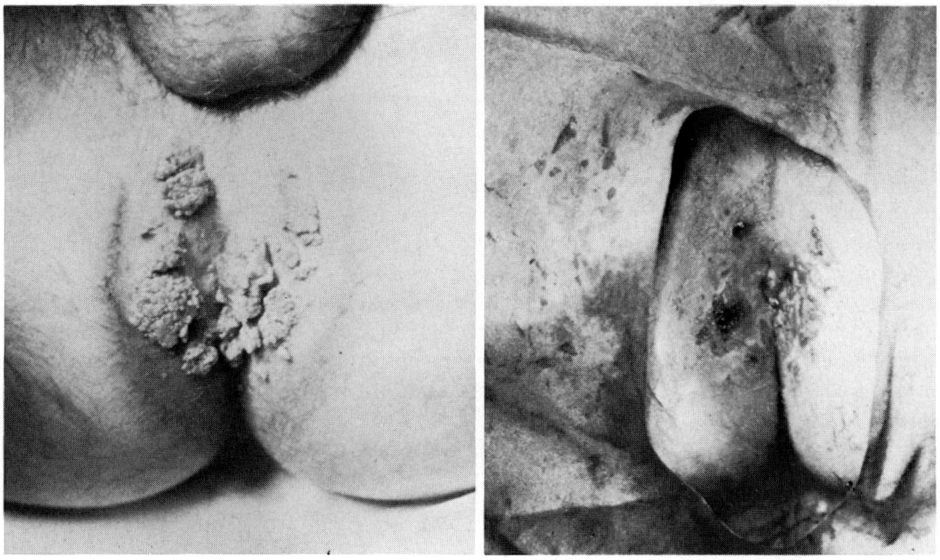

FIGURE 3–22. A, Extensive perianal condylomata acuminata. **B,** Same lesions after Nd:YAG treatment.

primary HSV-2, 84% had complete remission with no further recurrences. Of the 48 women with recurrent HSV-2, 33% had no further infections after laser treatment.

Successful laser treatment of urethral caruncles has been reported by several groups. Amagai and associates treated nine patients with the CO_2 laser and three with the Nd:YAG laser without reported morbidity.[75] Kleinman and Russin treated four patients and emphasized that the procedure took less time than standard surgical techniques and hospitalization was shorter.[120] In addition, they claimed that postoperative pain, bleeding, and use of a catheter were eliminated. A 1-year follow-up study revealed complete resolution of the lesion without stricture formation.

Penile or urethral hemangioma or telangiectasis is amenable to laser therapy. If the lesion is small, the argon laser can be used because of its selective absorption by hemoglobin. Larger lesions are best treated with the Nd:YAG laser because of the need for deeper penetration. Amagai and colleagues treated five urethral hemangiomas: two with the CO_2, two with the argon, and one with the Nd:YAG laser.[75] Smith and Dixon treated four such patients.[55] Three men who had multiple small lesions were treated with the argon laser, and the fourth patient had both argon and Nd:YAG therapy. Stein also recently reported successful Nd:YAG treatment of a large periurethral hemangioma in a woman with Osler-Weber-Rendu disease.

Rosemberg and Jacobs used the CO_2 laser to treat three patients with balanitis xerotica obliterans.[121] Short-term results were excellent; functional morbidity was less and cosmetic appearance was better than with other methods of treatment.

Calculi

Tanahashi and associates first reported using 50 to 70 W of Nd:YAG power to disintegrate known urinary calculi transplanted into the canine bladder.[122] However, Pensel and colleagues were less successful in destroying bladder calculi with the laser.[123] It has recently demonstrated that it is possible to fragment ureteral calculi via a ureteroscope using either Q-switched Nd:YAG laser or tunable pulsed-dye laser energy passed down a fiber.

The ability to create a shock wave strong enough to break stones without producing enough heat to damage tissue is the major advantage of using a laser to fragment stones. Three characteristics of a laser allow it to do this. First, wavelength can be made specific to the task—that is, a wavelength that is well absorbed by the calculus but poorly absorbed by tissue. Second, laser energy can be delivered in short bursts to prevent heat buildup. Investigators have shown that continuous wave lasers produce too much thermal effect with subsequent damage to surrounding tissue to be used for fragmentation of urinary stones. Therefore only pulsed dye or Q-switched lasers can produce the power density necessary for stone fragmentation without heat buildup. Third, laser energy can be transmitted by optical fibers that can be passed through small-diameter semirigid or flexible ureteroscopes.

The development of the flashlamp-excited pulsed dye laser has opened new possibilities for the fragmentation of calculi.[124] This laser is used with pulse durations in the microsecond range, and a large amount of energy can be released in a short time, resulting in a pulse of high energy with very little heat. The uniqueness of the dye laser is that the wavelength of the laser light is determined by the color of the dye in the laser reservoir. The laser medium is a coumarin green dye that is externally excited by means of a high-intensity flashlamp. The excited dye fluoresces, and the light generated is raised to laser threshold by the presence of resonator mirrors. The laser light is focused through the partially reflective mirror into a 250 μm (200 μm core) quartz fiber that forms the delivery system. Basic laboratory studies have shown a wavelength of 504 nm to be optimal for laser fragmentation because of its absorption selectivity: it is well absorbed by stone material but not by the ureter or the kidney. The controlled fragmentation of urinary calculi can occur with no risk of laser-induced trauma to the ureter.

By the following equation the power density is related to energy of the laser, pulse duration, and size of the fiber diameter:

$$\text{Power density (watts/cm}^2\text{)} = \frac{\text{Energy (mJ/pulse)}}{\text{Pulse duration } (\mu \text{ sec}) \times \text{Fiber area } (\mu\text{m})}$$

It can be seen that the size of the fiber in addition to pulse duration can significantly affect the power density at the point of exit energy. Laboratory data have demonstrated that the smaller the fiber, the more effective the fragmentation for relatively fragile calculi. A 50 to 100 μm fiber burns out at the needed energy; however, the 250 μm silica-coated quartz fiber is suitable for generation of power density that will both fracture calculi and prevent fiber burnout. Laboratory studies have also shown that the shorter the pulsation, the less energy required per pulse for irradiation of stone fragmentation. One microsecond was found to be optimal for stone fragmentation when the pulsed dye laser is used. Most stones can be fragmented by a series of pulses from 30 to 60 mJ.

The Q-switched Nd:YAG laser is also being used for stone fragmentation. This laser is used at 35 to 80 mJ per pulse at pulse rates of 10 to 50 Hz with pulse durations of 8012 nsec. Like the dye laser, it causes no significant damage to adjacent tissue. This laser generally requires a larger fiber size (600 nm) and has also been used with an optomechanical coupler at the filter tip.[125,126] However, use of this laser with spherically polished fibers as small as 200 nm has been reported. The extent of fiber damage with smaller fibers remains controversial.

Several other lasers are being evaluated for their efficacy in lithotripsy. The solid state alexandrite laser[127] and the holmium laser are being investigated, and efficacy data may emerge soon.

Depending on the laser type, three mechanisms for stone disintegration are possible. Continuous wave lasers induce a thermal stress on the stone by heating the surface. Flashlamp-pulsed lasers (e.g., dye lasers) act by optoacoustic-released mechanical stress. Absorption at the stone creates a "plasma" with optoacoustic effects. Q-switched lasers (e.g., Nd:YAG) set off a laser-induced breakdown in the liquid around the stone. The stone composition is no longer decisive, unlike the situation with the dye laser, in which a certain wavelength is selected for absorption of the stone. With the Nd:YAG laser the liquid around the calculus acts as an energy converter, propagating the laser-induced shock wave to the stone, whereas the stone itself is used for energy transformation in the dye laser application. Peak pressures of 1000 bar have been generated at the cone tip of a 600 nm quartz fiber. Since the absorption of the Nd:YAG wavelength by the stone is not sufficient for stone fragmentation, focusing of the laser energy at the tip of the fiber is required. One method used has been the fabrication of a polished cone tip on the fiber. A second method is the use of an optomechanical coupler. This is a 0.5 mm bar of tungsten or titanium at the tip of a metal tube containing the laser-carrying fiber. The laser pulse is directed at the bar, causing vaporization and ionization of the material of the bar, which is the source of the shock wave. The tube containing the laser and the bar is 2.9 nm (8.7F).

When a 200 nm core fiber with a rigid ureteroscope is used, it is generally passed through a 4F ureteral catheter for stability. With the dye laser the fiber must be placed directly on the stone rather than being focused as with the Nd:YAG laser.

Stones of differing composition respond differently to laser lithotripsy. Twice as many pulses per square millimeter of stone are needed to break monohydrate as to break calcium oxalate dihydrate. Calcium oxalate dihydrate stones can be broken in moments to particles less than 2 mm in diameter, whereas the monohydrate takes a longer time and fragments are larger, often requiring basket extraction.

Dretler has recently reported successful stone fragmentation in approximately 80% of 225 patients with the pulsed dye laser.[128] All patients had calculi too large to pass spontaneously or to be basket extracted. Ureteral damage was not observed, and no ureteral strictures were reported. Bagley and associates reported a 100% success rate in 70 stones, 65% of which were calcium oxalate monohydrate.[129] When the Q-switched Nd:YAG laser was used without a coupler, fragmentation was reported in 14 of 120 calculi.[125] With an optomechanical coupler 11 of 15 stones were completely fragmented and 3 stones showed partial fragmentation.[126]

The clear advantages of laser and fiber lithotripsy are the ability to use them with small-diameter endoscopes, obviating the need for ureteral orifice dilation, and the low risk of thermal injury. Stones at the ureteral orifice, steinstrasse, and impacted calculi that have been difficult problems in the past are resolved more easily with this technology (Figure 3–23).

A

B

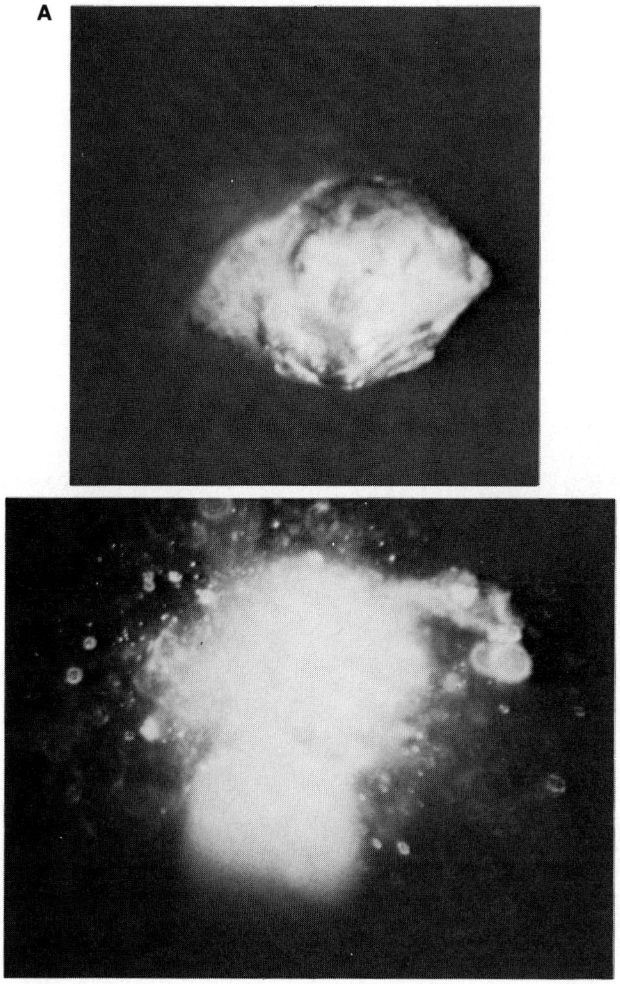

FIGURE 3–23. **A,** Stone impacted in ureteral orifice. **B,** Laser fragmentation of impacted stone.

Tissue Welding

"Tissue welding" is a promising future use of laser technology in urology. The Nd:YAG laser, CO_2 laser, and argon laser have all been successfully used in the animal laboratory to weld small blood vessels (arteries and veins), peripheral nerves, skin, urethra, and the vas deferens. Although reports are encouraging, few comparative studies have been performed. These techniques await refinement and judicious scrutiny before they can be considered superior to current microvascular techniques. Laser welding may prove superior to microsurgery because anastomosis would theoretically be less time consuming, require less surgical dexterity, and result in a stronger tissue bond. Although no vascular welding studies strictly pertaining to urology have been performed, a number of reports indicate that laser welding of vessels is feasible.

Jain and Gorisch[130] and Jain[131] were the first to report on microvascular repair of arteries and veins with the Nd:YAG laser. They compared its efficacy with that of bipolar coagulation and microsuture technique. When rat vessels ranging in diameter from 0.3 to 1.1 mm were treated, no vessels between 0.7 to 1.1 mm became occluded after laser repair. In addition, for vessels as small as 0.3 mm in diameter, laser welding was the only technique that significantly preserved vessel patency. If the vessel edges tended to gape, a small piece of vein or muscle was placed over the area to be welded and was fused to the vessel wall. Tensile strength measurements of the laser-repaired veins and arteries showed no disruption with intraluminal pressures as high as 300 mm Hg.

Gomes and colleagues used the argon laser to perform vascular anastomosis in dogs.[132] Three types of vascular anastomosis were accomplished: saphenous vein–intercarotid artery bypass; left mammary artery–left anterior descending coronary artery bypass; and venovenous anastomosis. In all groups 0.8 to 1.5 W of argon laser power was applied for 90 to 300 seconds. The lower power was for venovenous anastomoses and the greater for arterial anastomoses. The mean values of resistance of the laser anastomoses to pressure-induced rupture were greater than 30 mm Hg in the immediate postoperative period but increased to 2000 mm Hg 30 days after surgery. No signs of occlusion were demonstrated at the anastomotic sites by angiographic and anatomopathologic studies. The exact mechanism of action of laser welding is not clear. Heat produced at the site of input is high enough to discolor the vessel surface, and heat can cause fusion of collagen in the media of blood vessels.

Vasectomy in dogs was performed with the CO_2 laser as early as 1972, but a significant number of vasa were noted to recanalize by 6 weeks. Of particular interest to the urologist is the possibility of using the laser in vasovasostomy. Lynne and coworkers used a specially constructed optical bench and a continuous wave, RF-excited CO_2 laser delivering 100 to 200 mW of energy with a beam spot size of 0.2 to 0.5 mm to weld the edges of rat vasa held in approximation with three sutures (Figure 3–24).[133] The wall of the healed vas was thin in the region of anastomosis, but no sperm granulomas and very little inflammatory response were noted in the surrounding scar tissue. Rosemberg, Elson, and Nathan, using 1.8 W of power from a continuous wave mode CO_2 laser with a spot size of 2 mm and a pulse duration of 0.2 second, performed similar experiments in dogs.[134] They concluded that speed of performance, patent vas lumen, and lack of sperm granuloma formation supported the CO_2 laser's ability to simplify the technique of vasovasostomy. Rosemberg was the first to describe laser-assisted vasovasostomy in patients.[135] In four patients a 100% patency rate with a 50% pregnancy rate was reported. The follow-up period was 3 to 9 months with no evidence of sperm granuloma re-

A

B

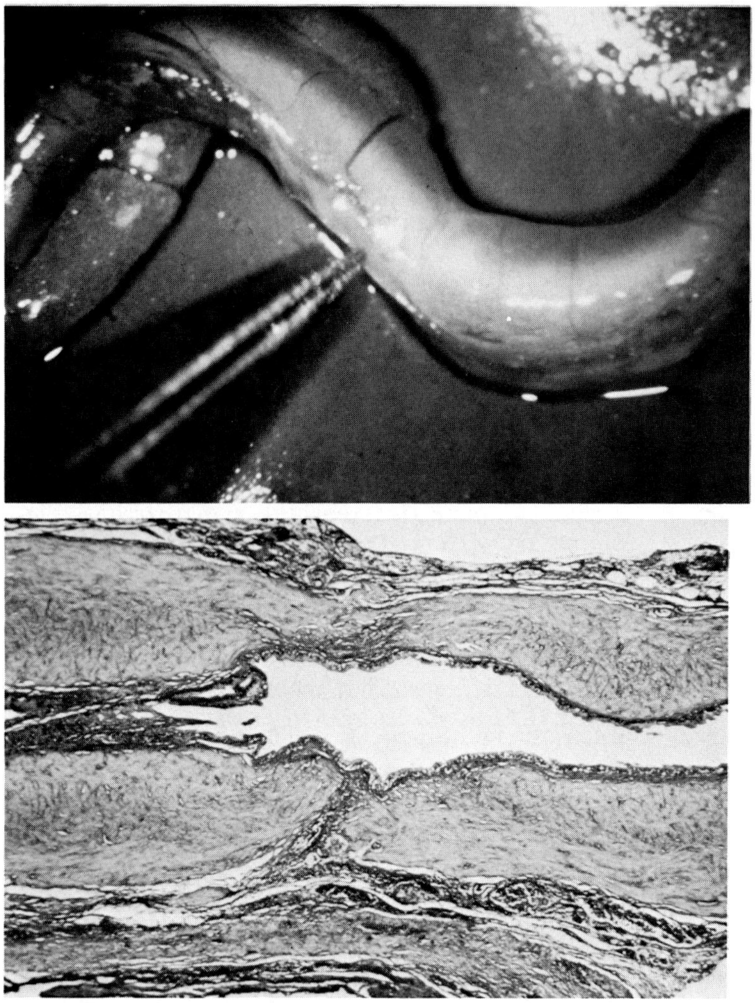

FIGURE 3–24. **A,** Rat vas deferens 3 months after laser-assisted vasovasostomy. Forceps indicates area of laser weld. **B,** Rat vas deferens 3 weeks after laser-assisted vasovasostomy. Connective tissue in the midportion of the muscularis indicates area of weld.

ported. Recently Shanberg and associates reported laser-assisted vasectomy reversal in 32 patients.[136] They employed three 9-0 sutures for approximation. The vasa were then welded with a CO_2 laser with average settings of 90 to 120 mW, a spot size of 100 nm, and a pulse duration of 0.1 second. Success rates for sperm in the ejaculate of patients who underwent vasectomy less than 10 years previously approached 95%. The pregnancy rate in this group was 35%. In patients whose vasectomy was performed more than 10 years before reversal, the success rate for sperm in ejaculate was only 36% and the pregnancy rate 9%.

CO_2 laser welding has been used successfully in the ureter, bladder, and urethra of animals. In rabbits an end-to-end ureteral anastomosis has been created by using an average power of 300 mW and a spot size of 1 mm.[137] Results of laser repair were similar to those of standard suture repair. Similar results have been reported in dog ureters. Poppas and co-workers recently reported a study in which partial urethral transection in rats was reconstructed using microsuture, laser, or laser plus solder (egg albumin).[138] Suture repair and repair with the laser produced similar results. This group later examined free preputial skin patch grafts in the ventral urethra of rats using the same methods. Comparable results were seen with conventional repair and laser plus solder repair.[139]

Although many questions await resolution, laser welding appears to be a valuable new technology, especially in dealing with very small, sometimes inaccessible tubular strictures that require a fluid-impermeable anastomosis.

REFERENCES

1. Einstein A: Zur Quantentheorie der Strahlung, Physiol Z 18:121-128, 1917.
2. Maiman TH: Stimulated optical radiation in ruby. Nature 178:493-494, 1960.
3. Javan A, Bennett WR Jr, Herriott DR: Population inversion and continuous optical maser oscillation in a gas discharge containing an HeNe mixture [Letter]. Physiol Rev 6:106-110,1961.
4. Johnson LF: Optical maser characteristics of rare-earth ions in crystals. J Appl Physiol 34:897-909, 1961.
5. Patel CKN, McFarlane RA, Faust WL: Selective excitation through vibrational energy transfer and optical maser action in N_2-CO_2. Physiol Rev 13:617-619, 1964.
6. Fuller TA: Fundamentals of lasers in surgery and medi-

cine. In Dixon JA (ed): Surgical application of lasers. Chicago: Year Book, 1983, pp 11-28.
7. Stein BS, Kendall AR: Lasers in urology. I. Laser physics and safety. Urology 23:405, 1984.
8. Bellina JH: Lasers in gynecology. World J Surg 7:692, 1983.
9. Rosemberg SK, Fuller TSA: Carbon dioxide rapid superpulsed laser treatment of erythroplasia of Queyrat. Urology 16:181, 1980.
10. Willscher MK, Filoso Am, Jako GJ, et al: Development of a carbon dioxide laser cystoscope. J Urol 119:202, 1978.
11. Voure'h, Bereti E, Trichet B, et al: Two unusual cases of gas embolism following urethral surgery under laser. Intensive Care Med 8:239, 1982.
12. Bulow H, Lavene S: Development of a carbon dioxide laser endoscope without a mobile arm system. Urol Res 7:31, 1979.
13. Rothauge CF: Transurethrale Behandlung vos Blasentumoren mit Laser. Helv Chir Acta 45:233, 1978.
14. Smith JA Jr, Dixon JA: Argon laser phototherapy of superifical transitional cell carcinoma of the bladder. J Urol 131:655, 1984.
15. Hofstetter A, Staehler G, Keiditsch E: Experimentelle Erzeugung von malignee tumoren au der Kaninchen. Harnblase Fortschr Med 95:346, 1977.
16. Staehler GN, Hofstetter A: Transurethral laser irradiation of urinary bladder tumors. Eur Urol 5:64, 1979.
17. Hofstetter A, Frank F: The neodymium-YAG laser in urology. Basel: Hoffman-LaRoche, 1980.
18. Frank F, Hofstetter A, Keiditsch E: Experimental investigation and new instrumentation for Nd:YAG laser treatment in urology. In Bellina JH (ed): Gynecologic laser surgery. New York: Plenum Press, 1981, p 345.
19. Keiditsch E, Hofstetter A, Rothenberger K, et al: Comparative morphological investigation of the effects of the neodymium-YAG laser and electrocoagulation in experimental animal research. In Bellina JH (ed): Gynecologic laser surgery. New York: Plenum Press, 1981, p 327.
20. Hofstetter A, Frank F: Laser use in urology. In Dixon JA (ed): Surgical application of lasers. Chicago: Year Book, 1983, pp 146-162.
21. Soloway MS, Masters S: Implantation of transitional tumor cells on the cauterized murine urothelial surface. Proc Am Assoc Cancer Res 20:256, 1979.
22. See WA, Chapman WH: Tumor cell implantation following neodymium-YAG bladder injury: a comparison to electrocautery injury. J Urol 137:1266-1289, 1987.
23. Hofstetter A, Frank F, Keiditsch E: Laser treatment of the bladder: experimental and clinical results. In Smith JA (ed): Lasers in urologic surgery. Chicago: Year Book, 1985, p 63.
24. Beisland HO, Seland P: A prospective randomized study on neodymium-YAG laser irradiation versus TUR in the treatment of urinary bladder cancer. Scand J Urol Nephrol 20:209-212, 1986.
25. Zimmermann I, Stern J, Frank F, et al: Interception of lymphatic drainage of Nd:YAG laser irradiation in rat urinary bladder. Laser Surg Med 4:167, 1984.
26. Rothenberger K, Pensel J, Hofstetter A, et al: Transurethral laser coagulation for treatment of urinary bladder tumors. Laser Surg Med 2:255, 1983.
27. Smith JA, Middleton RG: Bladder cancer. In Smith JA (ed): Lasers in urologic surgery. Chicago: Year Book, 1985, pp 52-62.
28. Stein BS, Kendall AR: Lasers in urology. II. Laser therapy. Urology 23(5):411, 1984.
29. Okada K, Asaoka H, Amagai T, et al: Transurethral neodymium-YAG laser surgery for bladder tumors. Urology 20(4):404, 1982.
30. Beisland HO, Sander S, Fossberg E: Neodymium-YAG laser irradiation of urinary bladder tumors: follow-up study of 100 consecutively treated patients. Urology 25(6):559, 1985.
31. von Eschenbach AC, Anderson Hospital and Tumor Institute, Houston: Personal communication, 1991.
32. Smith JA: Treatment of invasive bladder cancer with a neodymium-YAG laser. J Urol 135:55, 1986.
33. Hofstetter A: Treatment of urological tumors by neodymium-YAG laser. Eur Urol 12(suppl 1):21, 1986.
34. Staehler G, Chaussy C, Jocham D, Schmiedt E: The use of neodymium-YAG lasers in urology: indications, technique and critical assessment. J Urol 134:1155, 1985.
35. McPhee MS, Arnfield MR, Tulip J, Lakey WH: Neodymium-YAG laser therapy for infiltrating bladder cancer. J Urol 140:44-46, 1988.
36. Blum HF: Photodynamic action and diseases caused by light. New York: Reinhold, 1941.
37. Auler H, Banzer G: Untersuchungen uber die Rolle der Prophyrine bei geschwulstrkranken Menschen und Tieren, Z Krebsforsch 53:65, 1942.
38. Figge FHJ, Weiland GS, Manganiello LOJ: Cancer detection and therapy: affinity of neoplastic embryonic and traumatized tissues for porphyrins and metalloporphyrins. Proc Soc Exp Biol Med 68:640, 1948.
39. Lipson RL: The photodynamic and fluorescent properties of a particular hematoporphyrin derivative and its use in tumor detection. Thesis, Mayo Graduate School of Medicine, Rochester, Minn, 1959.
40. Mellors RC, Glassman A, Papanicolaou GN: A microfluorometric scanning method for the detection of cancer cells in smears of exfoliated cells. Cancer 5:458, 1952.
41. Moore GE: Diagnosis and localization of brain tumors: a clinical and experimental study employing fluorescent and radioactive tracer methods. Springfield, Ill: Thomas, 1953.
42. Policard A: Etude sur les aspects offerts per des tumeurs experimentales examinees a la lumiere de Wood, Compt Rend Soc Biol 91:1423, 1924.
43. Tomson SH, Emmett EA, Fox SH: Photodestruction of mouse epithelial tumors after oral acridine orange and argon laser. Cancer Res 34:3124, 1974.
44. Benson RC Jr, Farrow GM, Kinsey JH, et al: Detection and localization of in situ carcinoma of the bladder with hematoporphyrin derivative. Mayo Clin Proc 57:548, 1982.
45. Kelly JF, Snell MD: Hematoprophyrin derivative: a possible aid in the diagnosis and therapy of carcinoma of the bladder. J Urol 115:150, 1976.
46. Tsuchiya A, Obara N, Miwa M, et al: Hematoporphyrin derivative and laser photoradiation in the diagnosis and treatment of bladder cancer. J Urol 130:79, 1983.
47. Hisazumi H, Misaki T, Miyoshi N: Photoradiation therapy of bladder tumors. J Urol 130:685, 1983.
48. Benson RC Jr: Photochemotherapy of bladder cancer. In Spitzy KH, Karrer K (eds): Proceedings of the 13th International Congress on Chemotherapy, Vienna, Aug 28–Sept 2, 1983, pp 31-35.
49. Benson RC Jr, Kinsey JH, Cortese DA, et al: Treatment of transitional cell carcinoma of the bladder with hematoporphyrin derivative phototherapy. J Urol 130:1090, 1983.
50. Jocham D, Staehler G, Chausz C, et al: Integral dye-laser irradiation of photosensitized bladder tumors with the aid of a light-scattering medium. In Doran DR, Gomer CJ (eds): Porphyrin localization and treatment of tumors. New York: Liss, 1984, pp 249-256.
51. Baghdassarian R, Wright MW, Vaughn SA, et al: The use of lipid emulsion as an intravesical medium to disperse light in the potential treatment of bladder tumors. J Urol 133:126, 1985.
52. Benson RC Jr: Treatment of diffuse transitional cell carcinoma in situ by whole bladder hematoporphyrin derivative photodynamic therapy. J Urol 134:675, 1985.
53. Benson RC Jr: Endoscopic management of bladder cancer with hematoporphyrin derivative phototherapy. Urol Clin North Am 2:637, 1984.
54. Benson RC Jr: Hematoporphyrin in photodynamic ther-

apy for transitional cell carcinoma of the bladder: an update. In Kessel D (ed): Methods in porphyrin photosensitization. New York: Plenum Press, 1985, pp 1-13.
55. Smith, JA, Dixon JA: Laser treatment of bladder hemangioma. Urology 24:134, 1984.
56. Shanberg AM, Baghdassarian R, Tansey LA: Treatment of intersitial cystitis with the neodymium-YAG laser. J Urol 134:885, 1985.
57. Shanberg AM, Malloy T: Treatment of intersitial cystitis with neodymium-YAG laser. Urology 29(suppl 4):31-33, 1987.
58. Sander S, Beisland HO: Lasers in the treatment of localized prostatic carcinoma. J Urol 132:280, 1984.
59. Beisland HO, Stranden E: Rectal temperature monitoring during neodymium-YAG laser irradiation for prostatic carcinoma. Urol Res 12:257, 1984.
60. McPhee MS: Edmonton, Alberta, Canada: Personal communication, 1991.
61. Shanberg AM, Tansey LA, Baghdassarian R: The use of the neodymium-YAG laser in prostatomy. J Urol 133(4), part 2:196A, 1985.
62. Daikuzono N, Joffe SN: Artificial sapphire probe for contact photocoagulation and tissue vaporization with the Nd:YAG laser. Med Instrum 19:173, 1985.
63. Smith JA Jr: University of Utah, Salt Lake City: Personal communication, 1991.
64. Bulow H, Bulow U, Frohmuller HG: Laser investigations of the strictured dog urethra. Invest Urol 16:403, 1979.
65. Perez-Castro E, Martinez-Pinero JA: Endoscopic urethrotomy plus laser photocoagulation in urethral strictures. In Proceedings of the 19th International Congress of the Societe Internationale d'Urologie, abstract 473, San Francisco, 1982.
66. Smith JA, Dixon JA: Neodymium:YAG laser treatment of benign urethral strictures. J Urol 131:1080, 1984.
67. Shanberg, AM, Chalfin SA, Tansey LA: Neodymium:YAG laser: new treatment for urethral stricture disease. Urology 24:15, 1984.
68. Shanberg AM, Tansey LA: Laser treatment of urethral strictures. In Smith JA (ed): Lasers in urologic surgery. Chicago: Year Book, 1985, pp 43-51.
69. Smith JA Jr: University of Utah, Salt Lake City: Personal communication, 1991.
70. Rothauge CF: Urethroscopic recanalization of urethral stenosis using an argon laser, Urology 16:158, 1980.
71. Noske HD, Krashan J, Wentzal H, Rothauge CF: Argon laser therapy on bladder tumor and urethral stricture, 1981. In Proceedings of the 4th International Symposium on Laser Surgery. Cited in Hall RR: Report to the standing committee on urological instruments: lasers in urology. Br J Urol 54:421, 1982.
72. Shanberg A, Baghdassarian R, Tansey L, Sawyer D: KTP 532 laser in treatment of urethral strictures. Urology 32(6):517-520, 1988.
73. Turek PJ, Malloy TR, Cendron M, et al: KTP-532 laser ablation of urethral strictures. Accepted for publication in Urology.
74. Ehrlich RM, Shanberg A, Fine RN: Neodymium:YAG laser ablation of posterior urethral valves. J Urol 138:959-961, 1987.
75. Amagai T, Onoe Y, Okada K, et al: Laser application for urological disease. In Proceedings of the 4th International Congress of Laser Medicine and Surgery, Tokyo, 1981.
76. Fuselier HA, McBurney EI, Brannan W, Randrup E: Treatment of condylomata acuminata with carbon dioxide laser. Urology 15(3):265, 1980.
77. Rosemberg SK, Fuller T, Jacobs H: Rapid super-pulse carbon dioxide laser treatment of urethral condylomata. Urology 17(2):149, 1981.
78. Rosemberg SK, Jacobs H, Fuller T: Some guidelines in the treatment of urethral condylomata with carbon dioxide laser. J Urol 127:906, 1982.
79. Knoll LD, Benson RC, Furlow WL: Condyloma acuminata in males: the urologist's role. J Tenn Med Assoc 83(5):230, 1990.
80. Schmeller NT, Pensel J: Ureteral tumors. In Smith JA, Stein BS, Benson RC (eds): Lasers in urologic surgery. Chicago: Year Book, 1989, pp 81-91.
81. Hofstetter AG, Keiditsch E: Lasers for renal pelvis and ureteral tumors. Laser 1:75, 1985.
82. Hofstetter A: Laser application for destroying ureter tumors [Abstract]. Laser Surg Med 2:255, 1983.
83. Bowering R, Hofstetter A, Keiditsch E, Frank F: Treatment of ureteral tumors by endoscopic neodymium:YAG laser irradiation [Abstract]. J Urol 133(4), Part 2:236A, 1985.
84. Blute M, Segura JW, Patterson D, et al: Impact of endourology on diagnosis and management of upper urinary tract urothelial cancer. J Urol 139(2):169A, 1987.
85. Tomera KT, Leary FJ, Zincke H: Pyeloscopy of urothelial tumors, J Urol 127:1088, 1982.
86. Orihuela E, Smith AD: Percutaneous treatment of transitional cell carcinoma of the upper urinary tract. Urol Clin North Am 15:424-431, 1988.
87. Streem SB, Pontes EJ: Percutaneous management of upper tract transitional cell carcinoma. J Urol 135:773-775, 1986.
88. Woodhouse CRJ, Kellett MJ, Bloom HJG: Percutaneous renal surgery and local radiotherapy in the management of renal pelvic transitional cell carcinoma. Br J Urol 58:245-249, 1986.
89. Mulvaney WP, Beck CW: The laser beam in urology, J Urol 99:112, 1968.
90. Hughes BF, Scott WW: Preliminary report on the use of a CO_2 laser surgical unit in animals. Invest Urol 9:353, 1972.
91. Meiraz D, Peled I, Gassner S, et al: The use of the CO_2 laser for partial nephrectomy: an experimental study. Invest Urol 15:262, 1977.
92. Barzilay B, Lijovetzky G, Perlberg S, et al: Comparative experimental study on the use of the carbon dioxide laser beam in partial nephrectomy. Laser Surg Med 2:73, 1982.
93. Pariente R, d'Ovidio M: Cited by Willscher MK: Endoscopic delivery of CO_2 laser energy. In Smith JA (ed): Lasers in urologic surgery. Chicago: Year Book, 1985, pp 138-150.
94. Barzilay B, Lijovetzky G, Shapiro A, et al: The clinical use of CO_2 laser beam in the surgery of kidney parenchyma. Laser Surg Med 2:81, 1982.
95. Hall RR: Report to the Standing Committee on Urological Instruments: lasers in urology. Br J Urol 54:421, 1982.
96. Rosemberg SK, Lutz SJ: Some clinical applications of carbon dioxide laser in urologic surgery. Urology 23:240, 1984.
97. Rosemberg SK: Clinical experience with carbon dioxide laser in renal surgery. Urology 25:115, 1985.
98. Benderev TV, Schaeffer AJ: Efficacy and safety of the Nd:YAG laser in canine partial nephrectomy. J Urol 133:1108, 1985.
99. Melzer RB, Wood TW, Landau ST, et al: Combination of CUSA and neodymium:YAG laser for canine partial nephrectomy. J Urol 134:620, 1985.
100. Malloy TR: Laser treatment of ureter and upper collecting system. In Smith JA (ed): Lasers in urologic surgery. Chicago: Year Book, 1985, pp 82-93.
101. Hall RR, Hill DW, Beach AD: A carbon dioxide surgical laser. Ann R Coll Surg Engl 48:181, 1971.
102. Lindstedt EM, Lundquist SB: Cited by McPhee MS: Application of laser energy in open urologic and renal surgery. In Smith JA (ed): Lasers in urologic surgery. Chicago: Year Book, 1985, pp 94-102.
103. d'Ovidio M, Carmignani G: Laser-micro-surgery in urology [Abstract]. Laser Surg Med 3:114, 1983.
104. Rosemberg SK, Fuller TA: Carbon dioxide rapid superpulsed laser treatment of erythroplasia of Queyrat. Urology 16(2):181, 1980.

105. Knoll LD, Segura JW, Benson RC Jr, Goellner JR: Bowenoid papulosis of the penis: successful management with neodymium:YAg laser. J Urol 139:1307, 1988.
106. Parsons RL, Campbell JL, Thomley MW: Carcinoma of the penis treated by the ruby laser. J Urol 100:38, 1968.
107. Numata I, Tanahashi R, Harada K, et al: Cited by Stein BS: Laser therapy for carcinoma of the penis. In Smith JA (ed): Lasers in urologic surgery. Chicago: Year Book, 1985, pp 32-42.
108. Malloy TR, Wein AJ, Carpiniello VL: Carcinoma of the penis treated with neodymium:YAG laser. Urology 3(1):26-29, 1988.
109. Rattner WH, Rosemberg SK, Fuller T: Difference between continous wave and superpulse carbon dioxide laser in bladder surgery. Urology 13:264, 1979.
110. Baggish MS: Carbon dioxide laser treatment for condylomata acuminata venereal infections. Obstet Gynecol 55:711, 1980.
111. Rosemberg SD: The use of CO_2 laser in urology [Abstract]. Laser Surg Med 3:114, 1983.
112. Lundquist SB, Lindstedt EM: Laser treatment of condylomata acuminata [Abstract]. Laser Surg Med 3:152, 1983.
113. Carpiniello V, Sedlacek TV, Cunnane M, et al: Magnified penile surface scanning in the diagnosis of penile condyloma. Urology 28:190, 1986.
114. Rosemberg SK, Fuller T, Jacobs H: Continuous wave carbon dioxide laser treatment of giant condylomata acuminata of the distal urethral and perineum: technique. J Urol 126:827, 1981.
115. Aledia FT: Clinical experience with laser in urologic surgery [Abstract]. Laser Surg Med 3:115, 1983.
116. Malloy TR, Wein AJ: Laser treatment of bladder carcinoma and genital condylomata. Urol Clin North Am 14(1):121-126, 1987.
117. Stein BS: Treatment of lesions of the external genitalia. In Smith JA (ed): Lasers in urologic surgery. Chicago: Year Book, 1985, pp 32-42.
118. Ferenezy A, Mitao M, Nagai N, et al: Latent papilloma virus and recurrent genital warts. N Engl J Med 313:784-788, 1985.
119. Baggish MS: Laser surgery in gynecology. In Dixon JA (ed): Surgical application of lasers. Chicago: Year Book, 1983, pp 102-145.
120. Kleinman SZ, Russin D: The use of the carbon dioxide laser in the treatment of urethral caruncles: a preliminary report [Abstract]. Laser Surg Med 3:152, 1983.
121. Rosemberg SK, Jacobs H: Continuous wave carbon dioxide treatment of balanitis xerotica obliterans. Urology 19:539, 1982.
122. Tanahashi Y, Numata Kambe K, Harada K, et al: Transurethral disintegration of urinary calculi by the use of laser beams. In Proceedings of the 4th International Symposium on Laser Surgery. Cited in Hall RR: Report to the Standing Committee on Urological Instruments: lasers in urology. Br J Urol 54:421, 1982.
123. Pensel J, Frank F, Rothenberger KH, Unsold E: Destruction of urinary calculi by neodymium laser irradiation. In Proceedings of: the 4th International Symposium on Laser Surgery. Cited in Hall RR: Report to the Standing Committee on Urological Instruments: lasers in urology. Br J Urol 54:421, 1982.
124. Watson GM, Murray S, Dretler SP, et al: Pulsed dye laser for fragmenting urinary calculi. J Urol 138:195-199, 1987.
125. Hoffman R, Hartuug R, Schmidt-Kloiber, Reichel E: Laser-induced shock wave ureteral lithotripsy using Q-switched Nd:YAG laser. J Endourol 4(2):169-174, 1990.
126. Maghraby H, Knipper A, Muschter R, Hofstetter AG: Laser lithotripsy: further experience with Nd:YAG laser. J Endourol 4(2):161-167, 1990.
127. Weber HM, Miller K, Ruschoff J, et al: Alexandrite laser lithotripter in experimental and first clinical application. J Endourol 5(1):51-55, 1991.
128. Dretler SP: An evaluation of ureteral laser lithotripsy: 225 consecutive patients. J Urol 143:267-272, 1990.
129. Bagley DH, Grasso M, Shalaby M, El-Akkad MA: Ureteral laser lithotripsy using the pulsolith. J Endourol 3(1):91-97, 1990.
130. Jain KK , Gorisch W: Microvascular repair with neodymium:YAG laser. Acta Neurochir (Wien) 28(suppl):260, 1979.
131. Jain KK: Sutureless microvascular anastomosis using a neodymium:YAG laser. J Microsurg 1:436, 1980.
132. Gomes OM, Macruz R, Armelin E, et al: Vascular anastomosis by argon laser beam. Tex Heart Inst J 10:145, 1983.
133. Lynne CM, Carter M, Morris J, et al: Laser-assisted vas anastomosis: a preliminary report. Laser Surg Med 3:261, 1983.
134. Rosemberg SK, Elson L, Nathan LE Jr: Carbon dioxide laser microsurgical vasovasostomy. Urology 25(1):53, 1985.
135. Rosemberg SK: Clinical use of carbon dioxide (CO_2) laser in microsurgical vasovasostomy. Urology 29:372-374, 1987.
136. Shanberg A, Tansey L, Baghdassarian R, et al: Laser assisted vasectomy reversal: experience in 32 patients. J Urol 143:528-530, 1990.
137. Merguerian PA, Rabinowitz R: Dismembered nonstented ureteroureterostomy using the carbon dioxide laser in the rabbit: comparison with suture anastomosis. J Urol 136:229-231, 1986.
138. Poppas DP, Schlossberg SM, Richmond IL, et al: Laser welding in urethral surgery: improved results with protein solder. J Urol 139:415-417, 1988.
139. Ganesan G, Poppas DP, Devine CJ, Schlossberg SM: Urethral reconstruction using the carbon dioxide laser: an experimental evaluation. J Urol 142:1139-1141, 1989.

CHAPTER 4

PROSTHETICS

TERRENCE R. MALLOY and PAUL TUREK

Functional prosthetics in urology are a recent addition to the urologic surgeon's armamentarium. Before 1970 no truly effective mechanical prostheses were available to correct problems with organic erectile impotence and urinary incontinence.

F. Brantley Scott pioneered development of an inflatable penile prosthesis[1] and implantable urinary prosthetic sphincter.[2] Since the early 1970s considerable improvement has been made in the construction, function, and number of urologic prostheses.

PENILE PROSTHESES

History

In 1936 Bogoras described the use of rib cartilage implanted into a tube skin graft to reconstruct the penis for sexual function.[3] In 1944 Frumpkin reported on further efforts at penile reconstruction using bone graft.[4]

Goodwin and Scott were the first to report on their experience with inert penile implants using acrylic splints for erectile impotence.[5] In 1958 Behari first described intrapenile stents using polyethylene rods.[6] Pearman first used silicone rubber to treat impotence, but the stents were often extruded from their position between Buck's fascia and the tunica albuginea.[7] It was not until 1973 that Small and his co-workers developed a paired intracavernosal silicone rubber penile prosthesis.[8] At approximately the same time Scott introduced an inflatable four-piece silicone rubber prosthesis with inflatable cylinders in each corpus, a reservoir, and a pump located in the scrotum.

Various modified semirigid prostheses were introduced later by Finney[9] and Jonas.[10] Dacomed Incorporated introduced the OmniPhase prosthesis in 1986 and subsequently the DuraPhase implant.[11]

In 1981 Mentor Incorporated introduced a modified version of an inflatable penile prosthesis constructed of polyurethane.[12] American Medical Systems Incorporated introduced a fluid self-contained prosthesis (Hydroflex), and Surgitek Incorporated developed a similar product (Flexi-flate).

In the 1990s with newer and more varied prostheses, the surgeon has numerous options from which to choose the best prosthesis for the impotent patient who requires surgery.

Presurgical Evaluation of Impotent Patients

Every patient with erectile impotence being considered for penile prosthesis surgery should have a complete evaluation to determine the cause of his sexual dysfunction. The cause of the problem must be determined so that the patient can be informed of alternative therapies that might be of benefit before surgery is tried. The most common medical malpractice claim against urologists involving prosthesis surgery has been the failure to pursue conservative alternative therapies before prosthetic surgery. In evaluating patients the urologist cannot fixate on surgery but must look at the problem as part of the patient's overall psychologic and physiologic condition.

In the 1980s the diagnosis, testing, and medical treatment of erectile impotence have improved rapidly. Therapies abound for diseases that cause sexual dysfunction. With this new medical therapeutic regimen, irreversible surgery such as the implantation of prostheses must be considered only if no other medical treatment can be used.

Despite the claims of success for intracavernosal pharmacotherapy,[14,15] penile revascularization, venous ligation, and penile suction devices, penile prosthesis surgery has the highest rate of success in the largest proportion of patients.

Patient's History

A complete history of the patient's sexual dysfunction is essential for optimum results of therapy. A previsit questionnaire helps to establish what the patient perceives as his sexual dysfunction and what he expects treatment to do. On this form the patient is asked to list his medical history, the drugs he uses, and other factors that can affect his sexual function. He is asked to describe his sexual function before the onset of the problem to determine what he expects from treatment.

With this information the initial history can be taken from the patient more efficiently. On first meeting the urologist the patient may be reluctant to provide intimate details of his medical and sexual history. However, after completing a questionnaire he is likely to be more candid about his problems and history. Urologists should carefully question the use of medications that are not prescribed but are bought over the counter. These drugs can often affect the ability to obtain and maintain an erection. Patients often are reluctant to admit to the use of illegal drugs, such as marijuana, that can affect sexual performance. Furthermore, patients generally do not acknowledge the full amount of alcohol consumption, and careful questioning is needed to elicit their true drinking history. With a complete history the surgeon gains considerable insight into what the patient wants and expects from therapy and how far he is willing to proceed with testing.

Physical Examination

The physical examination is important to determine the general medical health of the patient. A complete urologic, vascular, and neurologic evaluation should be performed. Medical conditions that might influence surgery or the patient's ability to use a prosthesis must be determined. Patients with impaired vision or decreased manual dexterity would have problems using an inflatable prosthesis. Mental deficiencies or confusion would also prohibit the use of more complicated prostheses. The general examination should determine not only the mental status of the patient but also the overall condition, including blood pressure and cardiovascular and pulmonary status. The urologic examination should determine that no urinary infections or urinary obstruction needs to be corrected before insertion of a penile prosthesis. Peyronie's disease is often undiagnosed until a careful physical examination of the penis has been done. This may be the primary cause of the impotence. Corrective surgery to straighten the penis and to improve rigidity might be necessary. Vascular assessment of the penile blood pressure should be accomplished with the Doppler stethoscope. Vasculogenic components and the cause of sexual dysfunction can be determined by more complete vascular evaluation if appropriate. Careful rectal examinations should be performed to determine the status of the prostate gland and to rule out carcinoma or obstruction as the cause of sexual dysfunction.

A complete neurologic examination should be performed to determine the sensation and the competency of the sacral nerves, as well as the various sphincter tones. Prediabetics often have neurologic impairment that is not appreciated as a cause of their erectile dysfunction. After the complete physical examination the urologist can best determine what laboratory tests and additional studies are required.

Laboratory Testing

The patient should have a full assessment including a complete blood count, sequential multiple analysis (SMA-12 or SMA-23), and measurement of serum testosterone, prolactin, prostatic specific antigen, and acid phosphatase levels. These tests will illuminate medical conditions that might affect erectile function. Psychologic tests such as the Minnesota Multiphasic Personality Inventory may be indicated to give the urologist a better picture of the patient's emotional and psychologic state. In patients with vasculogenic impotence, duplex ultrasonography studies may be indicated to determine the cause of the vascular deficiencies. The patient can be tested in the office with intracavernosal administration of prostaglandin E_1 or papaverine with phentolamine (Regitine) to see whether an erection can be induced. If an erection is produced with these medications, it usually indicates a competent arterial inflow and a functioning venoocclusive mechanism.

In a second visit the patient will receive a general diagnosis based on the history and physical and laboratory assessments. In some cases a clear-cut cause of organic impotence can be determined, and in others psychogenic impotence can be established. When there is doubt or a need for more precise diagnoses, special studies can be undertaken.

If the patient appears to be an appropriate candidate for vascular corrective surgery, dynamic corpora cavernosography should be undertaken and sometimes penile arteriography. If venous leaks are found on corpora cavernosography, the patient might benefit from venoocclusive surgery. When arterial deficiencies are determined, revascularization may seem appropriate. Before proceeding with these more complicated tests, however, the urologist should determine whether the patient has a reasonable chance for success based on his other medical conditions and age. If the patient is elderly or diabetic, the results of revascularization procedures are usually poor and the testing could be nonproductive.

If the patient obtained satisfactory erection with intracavernosal injection of papaverine or prostaglandin, a program of pharmacologic intracavernosal therapy may alleviate his impotence. None of these drugs has approval from the Food and Drug Administration (FDA) at present, so the urologist has to caution the patient and obtain an informed consent. The patient should be closely monitored.

Before any surgical procedure is considered, the

patient should undergo nocturnal penile tumescence studies. This testing is the standard required by third-party insurance carriers in cases of impotence arising from accident or trauma. The lack of a nocturnal penile tumescence study places the patient and the surgeon at risk that third-party insurance carriers will register claims of an incomplete workup. If the patient is dissatisfied with a subsequent surgical procedure, the nocturnal penile tumescence study will have clearly established that the impotence was organic and the urologists did not proceed without a firm diagnosis.

Decision to Proceed with Penile Prosthesis

When the diagnostic evaluation of the impotent patient has been completed, the patient should be apprised of all the results and the diagnosis. The surgeon can then detail the possibilities of therapy.

No Active Therapy

After a complete evaluation certain patients, particularly the elderly, wish to determine whether anything conservative could be done to correct their sexual dysfunction. They have no interest in surgery or complicated tests. They may decide to accept their condition or to try alternative sexual patterns. In these cases a referral to a sex therapist can sometimes alleviate some of their concerns and help them deal with their problems.

Sexual Therapy

Patients, including those with organic impotence, often benefit from sexual therapy either before surgery or concurrent with prosthetic implantation.[16,17] If a patient hesitates to proceed with surgery, a conservative course of sexual therapy may improve his self-image and alleviate anxieties.

Conservative Medical Therapy

In appropriate men, yohimbine or isoxuprine may be beneficial to improve erectile function. If the patient has a low serum testosterone level, a course of biweekly intramuscular testosterone injections may improve libido and sexual erectile function. Certainly, conservative medical therapy can be used while the patient is trying to determine what further therapy he wishes to pursue.

Intracavernosal Drug Therapy

Intracavernosal testing with papaverine or phentolamine and more recently with prostaglandin E_1 has become part of the standard diagnostic regimen for most urologists. If the patient obtains a satisfactory erection with these drugs, he should be told of the availability of this therapy and of the risks and long-term results. The patient should be told that this is not an FDA-approved drug. He will need close follow-up. The patient should sign an informed consent to eliminate misunderstanding about the nature of the medication and potential problems such as priapism or prolonged erections. Cardiovascular complications and long-term scarring in the corpora cavernosa have been reported with the use of papaverine. All these potential complications should be described to the patient.

If the patient decides to proceed with intracavernosal therapy, he should be given a 1-month supply of the medicine. He should be carefully trained in the use of the medication, particularly where to insert it. The patient should be followed at least every month for several months to ensure that he is taking the drugs properly and is not obtaining prolonged erections. If papaverine or phentolamine is used, the penis should be carefully inspected for signs of scarring in the corpora cavernosa.[18]

External Penile Vacuum Devices

Although vacuum "suction" devices that produce erection have proponents, many long-term studies have shown limited results.[19] However, the patient should be given literature about the device and information on the long-term results. If used properly the device causes no long-term problems, and it can be used while the patient is deciding whether he wants a more permanent surgical correction for his impotence. In our experience the dissatisfaction rate with these devices has been high.

Revascularization Surgery

In certain patients after complete evaluation, vascular surgery may be a viable alternative. If dynamic corpora cavernosography shows considerable venous leaks, ablation of the penile veins and dorsal veins may help restore erectile function. In patients with arterial insufficiency, especially younger men with a history of trauma, revascularization may reestablish potency. Patients considering this surgery should consider the long-term success rates of both types of surgery. The urologist should emphasize that if the surgery is not successful, penile prostheses can be inserted as a second surgical procedure. With an informed consent the patient certainly can try vascular surgery to alleviate his condition. Recent detailed anatomic dissections of the penis by Lue and associates have furthered the understanding of the vascular function of the penis and have improved methods for correcting inadequacies.[20]

Penile Prosthesis Selection

When the patient has decided that he wants a penile prosthesis, the type of prosthesis to implant

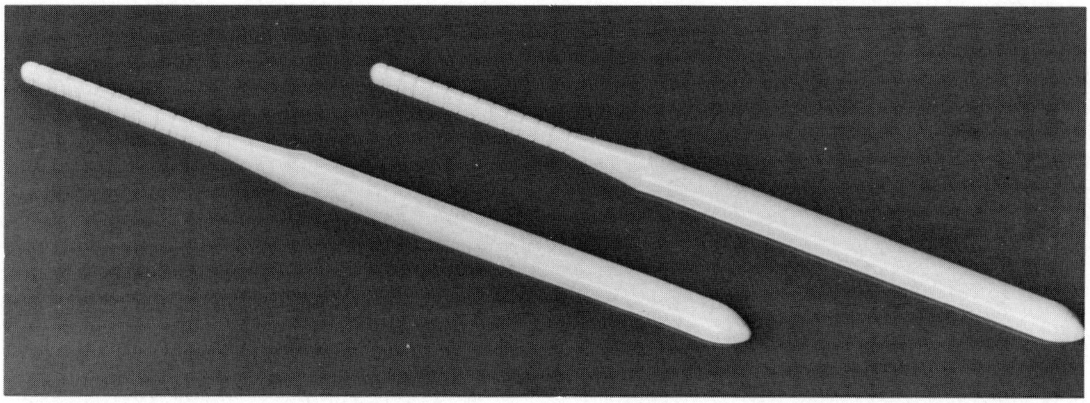

FIGURE 4–1. Flexi-Rod II penile prosthesis. (Courtesy of Surgitek Corporation, Racine, Wisconsin.)

should be determined by the patient in consultation with the urologist. The device chosen should be ideal for the patient's circumstances. All the prostatic types should be discussed in detail and their advantages and disadvantages explained.[21] Long-term success rates must be discussed. Manufacturers' literature and videotapes can be used to educate the patient. Patients who have had prosthetic surgery make excellent references. The patient should have enough time and information to discuss and select a prosthesis that meets his requirements. It is essential that the patient receive the prosthesis that he wishes and not the one that is easiest for the urologist to implant.

Semirigid and Malleable Rod Prostheses

The malleable rod prostheses have the advantage of simplicity of surgical insertion, long-term mechanical stability, and low malfunction rates. These devices have been used since the early 1970s and have generally had a satisfactory success rate. The devices, however, all have the same basic disadvantage: they provide no increase in girth or length of the penis with intercourse. Although the device can be positioned for intercourse and then repositioned for concealment, the penis obviously does not have a normal appearance. Concealment in public places is difficult. The device is easily palpable by patient and partner, resulting in complaints of artificial sensation. The device can migrate proximally, producing a deformity in the penis that resembles an SST airliner. This "SST" problem leaves the glans penis sloping over the tips of the rods. The rod produces constant pressure on the glans, which may lead to erosion.

The Small-Carrion device produced by the Metro Corporation has a long implant history.[22] Success rates have been satisfactory. The device is not malleable, so positioning for concealment can be a problem. Mechanical failure rates have been low. Comparison studies with inflatable prostheses have shown that the device can be satisfactorily used if patients are carefully selected.[23]

The Flexi-rod II by Surgitek Corporation is a silicone rod with a softer zone at the flex point to facilitate concealment (Figure 4–1). The proximal tail is cut to adjust for the appropriate size. At times, however, because of the narrow tail the proximal stability has not been ideal. Good results have been reported by Finney, Sharpe, and Sadlowski.[24]

Malleable rod prostheses such as the AMS 600 (Figure 4–2), the Bard Corporation's Jonas pros-

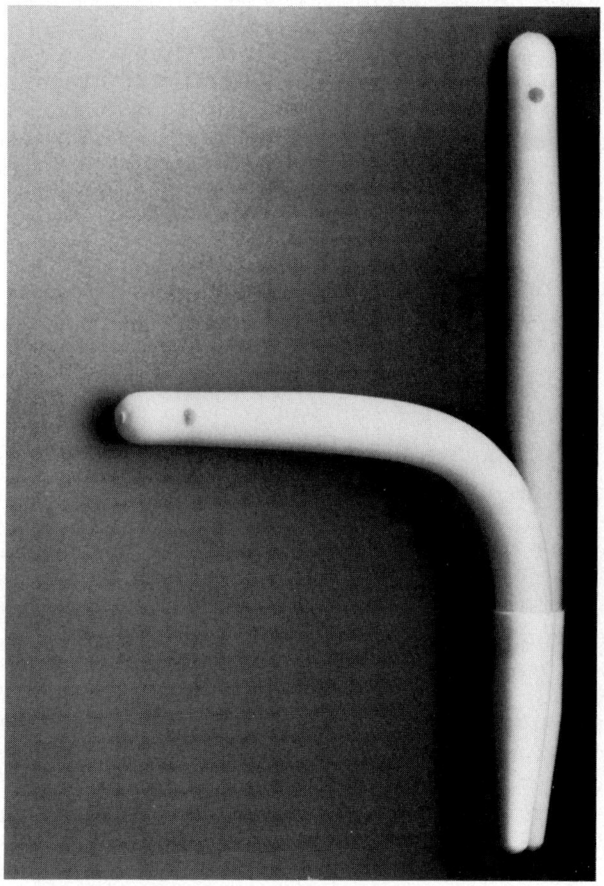

FIGURE 4–2. AMS 600 penile prosthesis. (Courtesy of American Medical Systems, Minnetonka, Minnesota.)

thesis, and the Metro Corporation's malleable prosthesis rely on an inner core that bends to allow the prosthesis to be positioned for intercourse in an upright direction and then flexed down for concealment. The inner core consists of stainless steel wires or silver alloy wires that allow proper positioning. Sizes are adjusted with rear tip extenders or ends that are trimmed and capped.[25,26] Dacomed Corporation has added devices to the rod prosthesis category. DuraPhase (Figure 4–3) has a central stainless steel cable passing through ball-in-socket disks. Tension by springs allows positioning. The device exhibits good rigidity upward and mobility downward. Positional integrity with intercourse has been adequate. Long-term mechanical stability is not yet known.[11]

The OmniPhase prosthesis (Figure 4–4) is relatively easy to operate and does not require fine motor coordination of the fingers. The prosthesis consists of paired cylinders, each composed of three parts: a central body, a proximal tip, and a distal tip. The body contains a series of polysulfone plastic balls and sockets that articulate one with the other. The stainless steel cable runs through the center of the balls and sockets and is fixed at one end. The other end of the cable is attached to the activator mechanism, and the entire body is covered by polytetrafluoroethyelene and sleeved in an outer layer of silicone to prevent adherence. The activator mechanism is a series of springs and levers that shortens and lengthens the cable. When the cable is shortened, it becomes taut and pulls the balls and sockets together. When the joints articulate, the device becomes firm and can be bent with good range of motion. When the cable lengthens, the balls and sockets separate and the device becomes relatively loose. The patient activates the device by bending the penis under the scrotum and then releasing it. Again, long-term results on satisfaction with this prosthesis are not available.[27]

Fluid Malleable Prostheses

Fluid malleable prostheses have better concealment and more normal appearance and sensation on palpation than rod prostheses. However, no increase in girth or length occurs with activation of the device and there is a chance of mechanical failure with fluid loss. The Dynaflex penile prosthesis (Figure 4–5) by American Medical Systems is the second-generation prosthesis after the Hydroflex prosthesis. It consists of paired cylinders filled with isotonic saline solution. The pump is in the most distal portion of the cylinder and when implanted fits beneath the glans penis. A release valve sits in a more proximal position and can be activated by bending the penis down. When the distal end is pumped, fluid is transferred from a proximal tip into an inflatable chamber, producing the desired erectile rigidity. The principal problem with this type of device has been difficulty in teaching patients how to activate and deactivate both cylinders. Disappointment with lack of increase in girth and length has also been expressed by patients who previously had an inflatable four-piece penile prosthesis.

The Surgitek Corporation produces Flexi-flate II (Figure 4–6), which has a distal pump mechanism with a proximal deflate valve that is activated by bending the penis. This device can be operated by the patient, but spontaneous deflation has occurred during intercourse.[30] Mechanical failure rates have been low with both Hydroflex and Flexi-flate. However, rigidity, appearance, and concealment certainly cannot compare to those of inflatable devices. The lack of increase in circumference and length has disappointed some patients.

Inflatable Penile Prostheses (Four-Piece)

The standard four-piece inflatable penile prosthesis still produces the erection with the best rigidity and most normal appearance. The device feels natural to palpation for the patient and partner alike. When deflated the penis appears normal and causes no embarrassment in public places. Endoscopic procedures through the penis present no problem. The erection that is produced increases the penis' circumference and, to some degree, length. The rigidity accomplished with this device is the best among penile prostheses.

The principal initial disadvantage of inflatable penile prostheses was its mechanical failure rate.[31-33] In the past decade manufacturers have refined the devices so that long-term reliability has improved dramatically.

The AMS 700 Ultrex penile prosthesis (Figure 4–7) features an abdominal reservoir, a scrotal pump, and paired cylinders in each corpus cavernosum. The Ultrex cylinder consists of the same molded front and rear tip as the original 700 CX cylinder. The input tube and sleeve on the Ultrex are identical to those on the 700 CX cylinder. The inner and outer silicone tubes of the Ultrex were modified to prevent any limitation of the functional length expansion of the fabric. The inner fabric layer is completely new. It is woven from a composite yarn of Lycra and Dacron. The diametric expansion occurs at a lower pressure, and a longitudinal expansion occurs at a slightly higher pressure. These pressure characteristics allow a girth expansion to occur first, and subsequent length expansion that the patient's anatomy will allow should not compromise rigidity. The flaccid diameter of the cylinder is 12 mm, and the fully erect diameter is 18 mm. The Ultrex fabric is designed to allow 15% to 25% lengthening measured from the resting state. This expansion may not result in penile lengthening, depending on the patient's anatomy. The lengthening occurs in most patients'

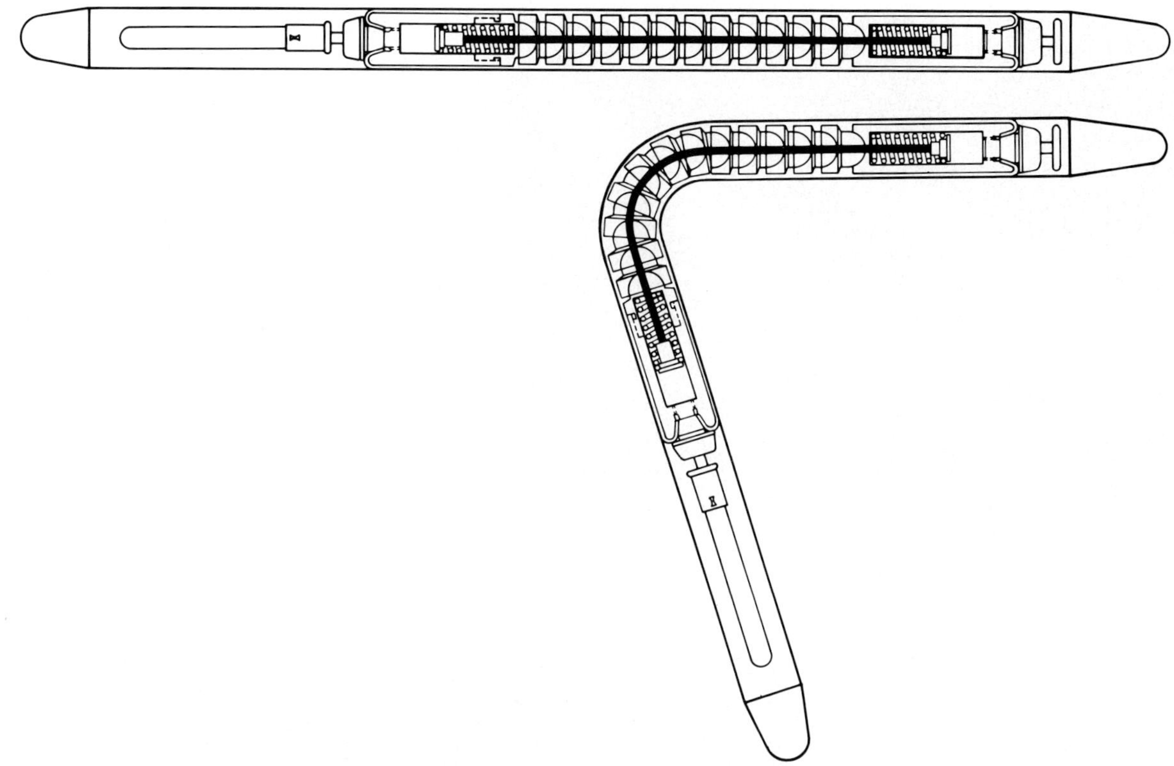

FIGURE 4–3. DuraPhase prosthesis. (Courtesy of Dacomed Corporation, Minneapolis, Minnesota.)

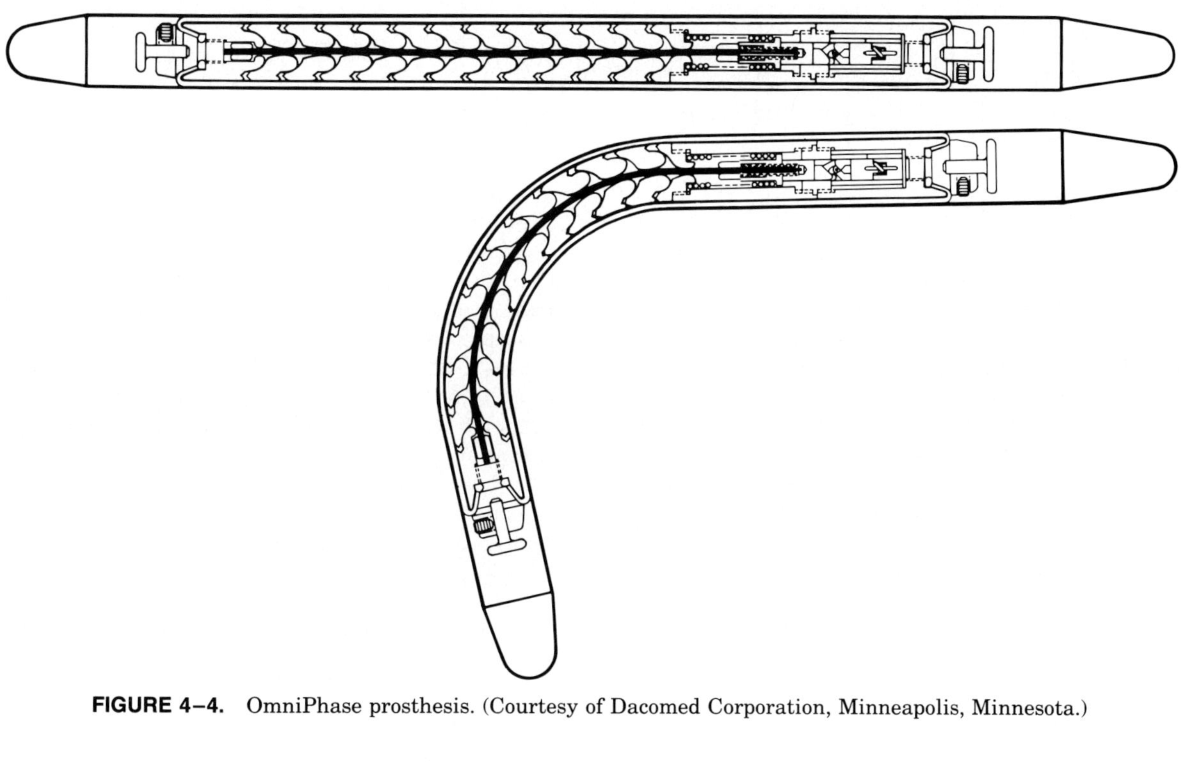

FIGURE 4–4. OmniPhase prosthesis. (Courtesy of Dacomed Corporation, Minneapolis, Minnesota.)

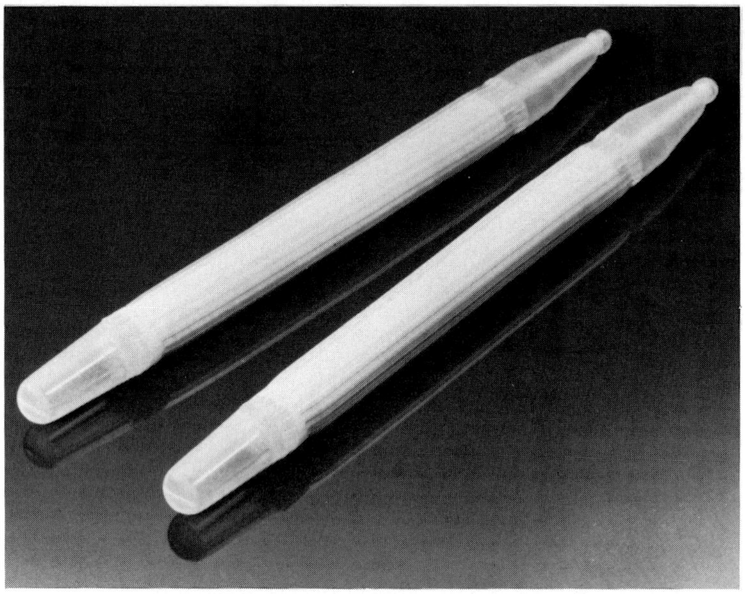

FIGURE 4–5. Dynaflex penile prosthesis. (Courtesy of American Medical Systems, Minnetonka, Minnesota.)

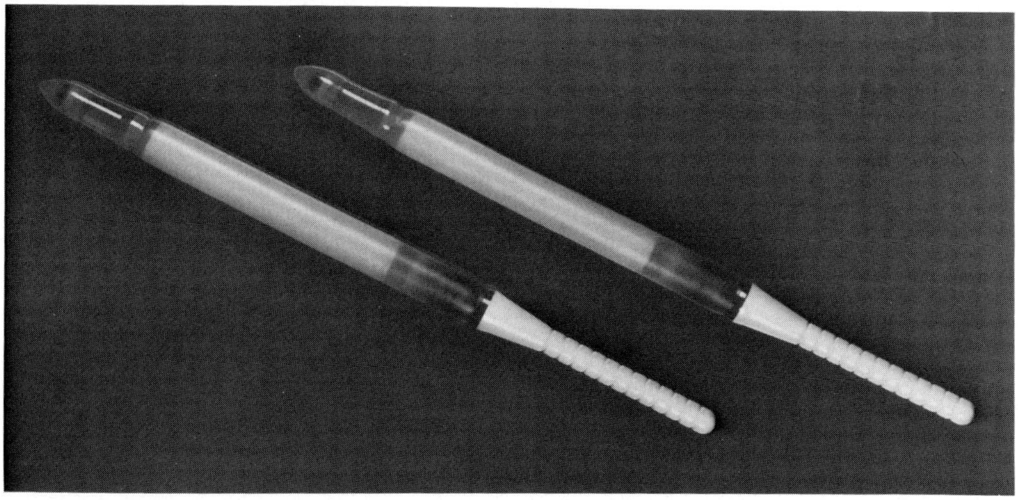

FIGURE 4–6. Flexi-flate II prosthesis. (Courtesy of Surgitek Medical Engineering Corporation, Racine, Wisconsin.)

penises and allows better anatomic fit over time. Any lengthening of the corpora depends on the patient's anatomy and ability to inflate the device. The device comes in various sizes and is fitted with rear tip extenders. The 18 and 21 cm Ultrex cylinders require a 100 ml reservoir. Excellent mechanical stability has been reported from several medical centers.[34-36]

The Mentor Corporation's Alpha I inflatable penile prosthesis (Figure 4–8) has also produced excellent long-term results.[37,38] The cylinders are constructed of a silicone-polyurethane blend that produces excellent durability. The Mentor Corporation believes that their polyurethane material is stronger and more abrasion resistant than silicone. These properties have reduced failures and eliminated aneurysms. The diameter of expansion of the cylinders depends on the cylinder's length. A 12 cm cylinder will reach a diameter of 17 cm. A 22 cm cylinder will expand to a diameter of 20.8 cm. Early problems with the pump release mechanism of this device have been corrected. In its deflated state the cylinders do not deflate as naturally as silicone cylinders, but concealment is not a major problem.

The four-piece inflatable prosthesis remains the state-of-the-art penile prosthesis for the most nearly natural and functional erections and the most natural concealment pattern when the prosthesis is flaccid.

Inflatable Penile Prostheses (Three-Piece)

Recent additions to the inflatable prosthesis field include three-piece inflatable prostheses. These devices consist of paired cylinders implanted within the corpora cavernosa and connected to

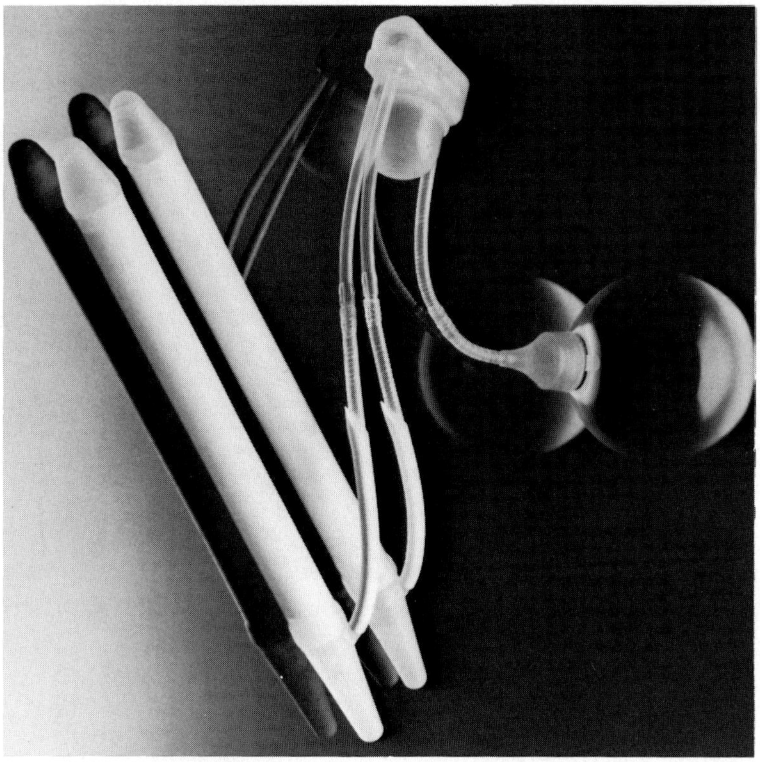

FIGURE 4–7. AMS 700 Ultrex penile prosthesis. (Courtesy of American Medical Systems, Minnetonka, Minnesota.)

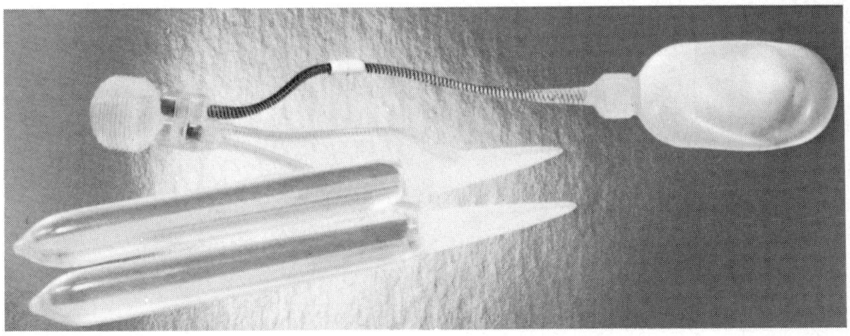

FIGURE 4–8. Alpha I inflatable penile prosthesis. (Courtesy of Mentor Corporation, Goleta, California.)

a combined pump reservoir in a subcutaneous pouch in the scrotum.

The Surgitek Corporation has produced the Uniflate 1000 (Figure 4–9) with proximal trimmable tips for positioning of the cylinders within the corpora cavernosa. The Mentor Corporation has produced the Mark II inflatable penile prosthesis (Figure 4–10), which features the two cylinders connected to a pump-reservoir combination in the scrotum. The advantage of both of these inflatable prostheses is simplicity of surgery and elimination of the need to implant an abdominal reservoir. This is beneficial in patients with previous abdominal surgery such as cystectomy and radical prostatectomy, in which the space of Retzius may be obliterated. The disadvantage of these devices is the size of the pump-reservoir, which may be cumbersome in the scrotum. More important, there may be too little fluid in the pump-reservoir to give complete expansion and rigidity to the cylinders. The long-term success rate will have to be evaluated to see whether patients' satisfaction is similar to their satisfaction with the standard four-piece inflatable penile prosthesis.

Prosthetic Surgery

The patient should be given adequate time to select a prosthesis. The urologist should show the patient representative samples of each type of device: malleable rod, fluid malleable, and inflatable. Videotapes provided by manufacturers should also be used if the patient has questions about how the prosthesis works. The patient should be allowed to talk with men who have received prostheses so all his questions can be addressed. If a surgeon is inexperienced or uncomfortable with a certain type of prosthesis, he should refer the patient to a urologist with experience in that type of prostatic surgery.

Informed consent is essential and should be ob-

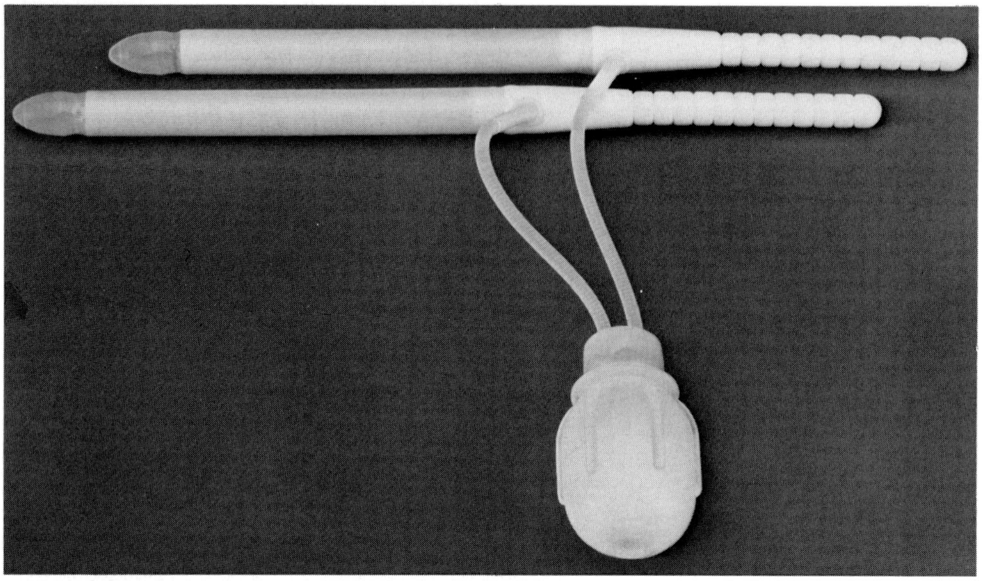

FIGURE 4–9. Uni-flate 1000. (Courtesy of Surgitek Corporation, Racine, Wisconsin.)

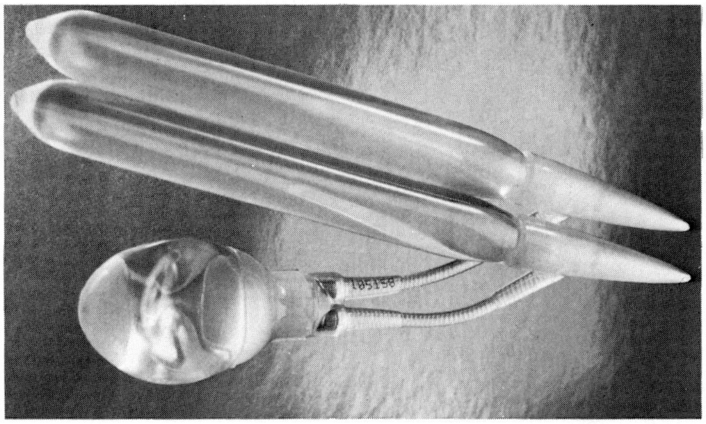

FIGURE 4–10. Mark II inflatable prosthesis. (Courtesy of Mentor Corporation, Goleta, California.)

tained before admission to the hospital. The informed consent should be of the urologist's own design and not a standard hospital form. A consent should include warnings about mechanical failure, infection, bleeding, and the need for prosthesis removal. The consent should state that no guarantee is made that the penis will be longer than before the premorbid condition. No guarantee should be given as to the performance of the device. The manufacturers do not guarantee the performance of their prostheses, nor should the urologist. The patient should read and sign this consent form before admission to the hospital so that no claim can be made that he did not have time to understand the surgery before being admitted. Nor can the patient claim that he was under pressure the night before surgery to sign the consent that he did not understand. The consent form should be sent to the patient weeks in advance and returned to his chart before any plans for admission are made.

Preoperative preparation consists of two Betadine scrub showers directed to the surgical area the night before surgery. Infection in urine and skin areas should be eliminated before surgery is considered. Preoperative antibiotics are beneficial and administered just before the patient is taken to the operating room. A surgical shave and preparation should be done in the operating room immediately before surgery. The type of intravenous (IV) antibiotic to be used preoperatively depends on the patient's tolerance to antibiotics. In our practice one dose of an aminoglycoside type of antibiotic and a cephalosporin antibiotic has been used.

The surgical approach should be one that is familiar to the surgeon to maximize results and minimize complications. Penile incisions should be avoided in most patients. Such incisions may damage the neurovascular bundle or cause pain or deformity in the penile skin. Infection or scarring also may harm penile appearance. All types of prostheses can be inserted via the suprapubic or the penoscrotal approach. With these excellent approaches there is no need for penile incisions that may result in medicolegal complications or complaints.

Before surgery commences, an artificial erection

should be produced to ascertain that no angulation or Peyronie's plaques are present within the penis. Corrective corporaplasties may have to be performed after the prosthesis is inserted if the penis is not straight. The use of intraoperative antibiotic irrigation has helped to prevent infection. Dissection should be carried out to the glans penis and proximally to the crus. Careful dilations should be accomplished so that the proximal crura are not perforated with the rear tip of the prosthesis migrating into the perineal area. Measurements should be carefully made. If one corporal tunnel appears much greater than the other, the possibility of a crural perforation should be established.

The cylinders chosen for implantation should be basically the same size. A slight difference in length can be adjusted by trimming the proximal portion of the prosthesis, as in the Flexi-flate type, or by adding rear tip extenders.

The tunica albuginea should be closed with care. Preplacement of sutures helps prevent trauma to the silicone rubber or the lining of the cylinder walls.

With inflatable prostheses the tubing should be measured for a comfortable fit of the prosthesis pump in the most dependent portion of the scrotum. If the tubes are too short, the pump will rise into the region of the external inguinal ring and cause discomfort and pain when the prosthesis is operated. The appropriate connectors should be used and tested several times before the wound is closed. Bleeding points should be inspected and coagulated before closure is attempted. With the inflatable prostheses the rectus fascia should be carefully closed to prevent incisional hernias. The reservoir should be placed in the space of Retzius to prevent migration.

A Jackson-Pratt-type suction drain should be inserted before closure, especially with inflatable prostheses. The drain prevents accumulation of a hematoma or fluid in the postoperative period. This allows early healing of the pump in a comfortable position so the pump can be activated. The drain is generally left in place for 18 hours.

In the immediate postoperative period the patient is treated with IV antibiotics. We have used IV cephalosporin with excellent results. The patient is kept in a Trendelenburg position with an ice pack in the scrotum for the first 18 hours. This prevents swelling and minimizes discomfort. Foley catheter drainage is maintained for 6 hours until the patient can urinate comfortably. The incision should be closed with a subcuticular suture to ensure early adherence of the wound and to prevent sepsis. Patients receiving an inflatable prosthesis generally require a 1- or 2-day hospital stay. After discharge the antibiotics should be continued for 10 to 14 days.

When the swelling and pain have subsided, the patient will require careful instruction in the operation of the device. The patient must be given instruction materials. Ample opportunity should be provided for the patient to learn how the prosthesis works. Follow-up studies have often indicated that patients are confused about the use of their prostheses.

Periodic follow-up examinations by the urologist are recommended to determine that the prosthesis is working properly and that no complications, such as proximal migration of rods or cylinders have arisen.[39]

Results with Penile Prostheses

The results of penile prosthesis surgery in a large series reveal overall excellent results. Depending on the type of prosthesis installed and the patients' expectations, the satisfaction rate varies. If patients are carefully screened and informed about the prosthesis they choose, the satisfaction rate is usually above 85%.

Malleable rod prostheses have shown a 90% to 95% reliability rate within the first 3 years with no problems in mechanical function or removal for pain, edema, or infection. Again, the satisfaction rate with this type of prosthesis depends on the information the patients receive before surgery and their acceptance of the limitations of the device.[40]

Patients in whom the Dynaflex- and Hydroflex-type prostheses were inserted have had good mechanical stability postoperatively. However, satisfaction rates have varied depending on the patients' ability to activate and deactivate the device. Patients considering this device should be informed that the firmness is not as great as that achieved with the traditional four-piece inflatable penile prosthesis.[13]

Results with the Flexi-flate II fluid malleable prothesis are similar except that in the initial series patients had up to a 30% rate of spontaneous deflation of the device during intercourse.[30]

Results with the standard four-piece inflatable penile prosthesis have improved dramatically over the years. The initial inflatable prostheses were troubled by leaks from the cylinder wall and problems with inflate tubing erosion of the cylinder wall. In some cases the cylinders formed aneurysmal bulges. With the development of the AMS M700 series of prostheses and the Mentor Alpha I inflatable protheses, most of these mechanical problems have been addressed. At present the patient can be assured that the mechanical stability of these devices will exceed 5 years and may last as long as 8 to 10 years.[34-40] However, the patient should be told that no device will last forever. Whatever type of device is chosen, the patient will probably need revision surgery at least once in his lifetime. Patients who are aware of this potential problem are much less likely to be dissatisfied with the device.

VACUUM PENILE ERECTILE DEVICES

The concept of a vacuum external device placed around the penis has been discussed for many years in the nonmedical literature. Men with impotence problems often place rubber bands at the base of the penis in an attempt to produce or prolong erections. In 1974 Witherington introduced a vacuum constriction device consisting of a plastic cylinder, vacuum pump with tube, and elastic constriction bands (Figure 4–11).[41] The cylinder is placed on the penis with the base open. A constriction band is placed around the base of the cylinder. Suction on the cylinder is created with a pump that augments a semierection that is already present or produces an erection-like state. When maximum penile engorgement is obtained, the band is guided over the base of the penis, the cylinder is removed, and sexual activity is initiated. The band at the base of the penis must not be left for a long time or it will cause penile blood flow constriction.

The major concern with the external vacuum device systems is diminished penile blood flow. The possibility of ischemic penile injury, especially with prolonged use, is worrisome. Katz and associates found that the xenon washout rate did not change with the Synergist erection system but was significantly reduced with the Osbon ErecAid System.[42] The degree and duration of decrease in penile blood flow that may result in ischemic changes are unknown.

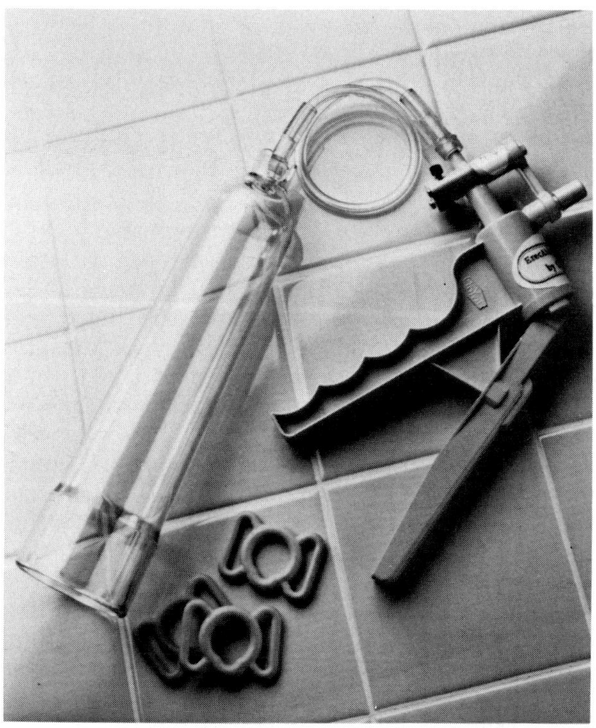

FIGURE 4–11. External vacuum erectile device, the ErecAid System. (Courtesy of Osbon Medical Systems, Augusta, Georgia.)

Nadig, Ware, and Blumoff reported satisfactory results with their vacuum device,[43] as did Witherington with his model.[44] However, true satisfaction rates are hard to determine from these studies. Trapping blood in the penis while the proximal corpora remains flaccid is not a physiologic erection. The urethra is compressed, obviously altering the sensation and force of ejaculation. Sensation to the more sensitive glans penis is also altered. Vacuum devices must be used with caution. Thirty-seven percent of patients initially described penile pain and ecchymosis in Witherington's report on 1517 patients.[41]

PROSTHETIC TREATMENT OF URINARY INCONTINENCE

History of Incontinence Therapy

Efforts to attain continence in incontinent patients have generated numerous drugs, devices, and operations over many years. The sheer number of reported techniques reflects the difficulty of producing consistent results.

Since 1960 prosthetic treatment for severe urinary incontinence has been attempted.[45] The first prostheses were compressive devices that maintained continence by obstructing the urethra while allowing voiding by sufficient elevation of the intraabdominal and intravesical pressure. In 1961 Berry described an acrylic prosthesis that was implanted between the bulbous urethra and bulbocavernosus muscle.[46] Failures resulted from dislocation of the device.

In 1973 Kauffman reported on a silicone gel prosthesis that was placed against the bulbous urethra and maintained in position by straps around the crura and the pubic rami.[47] Like Berry's device, it could be used only in males. It was an unphysiologic approach to continence because only urethral obstruction was used to maintain continence.

Urologists considered the ideal continence device to be one that could produce urethral compression while maintaining periurethral tissue viability, was reliable, and was reversible so that a normal voiding pattern could be established. The first successful device with these characteristics was reported by Scott and co-workers in 1973.[2]

The original Scott sphincter, designated AS721, was composed of medical-grade silicone elastomer and stainless steel. It had four components: a fluid reservoir, an inflatable cuff, and two pumps. The cuff could be implanted around the bulbous urethra of the bladder neck. The fluid reservoir was implanted intraabdominally underneath the rectus muscles. The inflation and deflation pumps were placed on opposite sides of the scrotum or labia majora. The device was filled with isotonic saline solution or contrast material so that it could be followed by radiologic study. To urinate, the patient pressed the deflation bulb located on the left scrotum or labium. This removed fluid from the cuff into the reservoir. To regain continence, the patient squeezed inflation bulb on the opposite labium or scrotum to pump fluid from the reservoir back to the cuff. The pressure in the cuff was regulated by a V-4 valve that was set below tissue perfusion pressure to prevent tissue necrosis.

A disadvantage of the Scott device was the large number of components, which made the device more difficult to implant and more prone to mechanical failure. Loss of pressure of the V-4 valve was a constant problem. Various revisions were made until an AS742 sphincter was devised. In this device the components were consolidated, with a pressure-regulating balloon serving as a reservoir for the cuff fluid during voiding. This device also eliminated the inflation pump because the balloon reservoir automatically refilled the cuff after urination. The addition of a delay-fill resistor between the balloon and the cuff slowed the return of the fluid to the cuff, allowing the patient sufficient time to empty the bladder. Success rates with the 742 model were significantly better than with the 721 model.

The next revision was the AS791-792, in which the valves and resistor of the 742 model were miniaturized and placed in a single unit or control assembly. The difference was the location of the control assembly on the cuff at either the bulbous urethra or the bladder neck.

The problem with the AS791-792 was that 6 weeks after the device had been implanted, a second operation was necessary to activate it. The cuff would not cause constant pressure on the bulbous urethra for the initial 6 weeks. However, the results were superior to those with the other earlier sphincters.[48]

AMS Sphincter 800 Urinary Prosthesis

The AMS sphincter 800 urinary prosthesis (Figure 4–12) is the culmination of the research and work done on the earlier genitourinary sphincters. The device consists of an inflatable cuff, a pressure-regulating balloon, and a pump. A valve, a refill-delay resistor, and a deactivation pump are incorporated into the one-unit pump mechanism. The deactivation mechanism provides a means of deactivating the prosthesis by external manipulation. This allows the cuff time to heal postoperatively around the bladder neck or bulbous urethra without undue pressure. Pressing the deactivation button on the side of the pump locks the position so that no fluid is transferred into the cuff. A forceful pump on the pumping mechanism releases the deactivation valve and activates the device.

The device functions in the following manner.

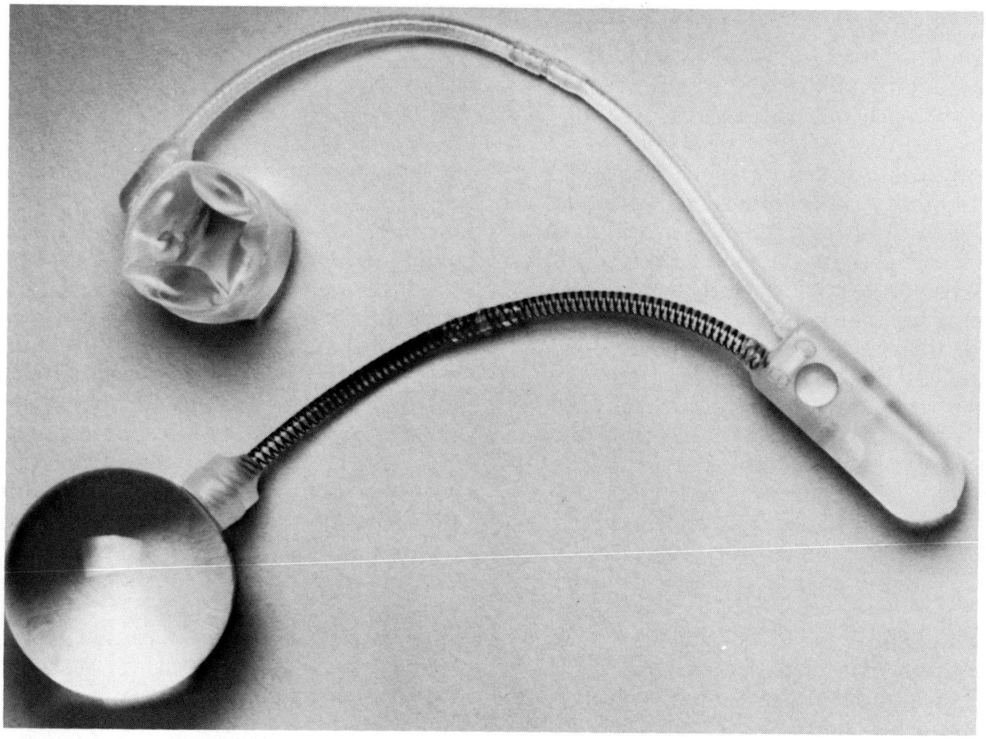

FIGURE 4–12. AMS sphincter 800 urinary prosthesis. (Courtesy of American Medical Systems, Minnetonka, Minnesota.)

The pump is squeezed three or four times, which transfers fluid from the cuff into the pressure-regulating balloon in the perivesical space. The pressure-regulating balloon begins automatic repressurization of the cuff, but the resistor delays refill of the cuff. The delay lasts 90 to 120 seconds, which allows time for complete urination. When the cuff refills, pressure is maintained around the urethra to provide continence.

The pressure-regulating balloon is constructed of a silicone rubber polymer with a dip coating process so that it provides pressure over a certain range. The thickness of the wall of the balloon determines the pressure characteristic. The reservoir can maintain pressure from 51 to 100 mm H_2O, depending on the balloon chosen. The cuff surrounding the urethra or bladder neck is also produced by a dip coating method to prevent sharp seams that might lead to erosion.

A major advantage of the AMS 800 device is the one-operation installation.

Patient Selection

The patients selected for treatment with the M800 genitourinary sphincter should have sphincteric incompetence as the sole cause of their urinary incontinence. The ideal candidate has a normal bladder that has become incontinent after a surgical procedure such as a radical prostatectomy or a transurethral resection of the prostate.

In evaluating patients an intravenous urogram is necessary to exclude structural abnormalities or problems that might be adding to the incontinence. A voiding cystourethrogram is also obtained to evaluate the bladder capacity and to rule out urethral stricture. Vesicoureteral reflux should be evaluated if present.

Urodynamic studies are critical, since the patient must be able to empty the bladder. A patient who has uninhibited contractions but still has a strong detrusor force can be treated with a sphincter and medication. However, a patient with a motor paralytic neurogenic bladder will not be able to empty the bladder with a sphincter in place. Such a patient is not good candidates for the sphincter. Low-compliance small bladders may require augmentation before use of the sphincter to restore continence is considered. Cystoscopy should be performed to delineate any strictures or bladder neck contractures. Stones or infection in the bladder should be eliminated. Urine cultures should be obtained to ensure urine sterility before sphincter surgery.

The patient's general medical health should be assessed before surgery to ascertain that the patient has the intelligence and manual ability to operate the pump. A quadriplegic with poor eye-hand coordination would probably not benefit from a urinary sphincter. The physician should obtain informed consent after explaining to the patient that additional surgery may be necessary or that erosion or infection that necessitate removal of portions of the device.

Genitourinary Sphincter Implantation

The patient should be given prophylactic antibiotics before surgery. A surgical "prep" should be done in the operating room, and the operative area should have a surgical scrub for at least 15 minutes prior to surgery. The patient should have scrubbed the area with Betadine showers on least two occasions the night before surgery.

The incision used depends on the area in which the cuff will be placed. If the cuff is being placed at the bladder neck in either a male or a female patient, a low transverse or midline abdominal incision may be used. The surgeon must have adequate exposure to view the bladder neck and to obtain space to dissect between the urethra and rectum or the urethra and vagina. The endopelvic fascia is incised adjacent to the bladder neck bilaterally. An indwelling Foley catheter is palpated to locate the bladder neck. If the dissection proves difficult, the bladder should be opened so the bladder neck can easily be visualized. Right-angle dissecting scissors and right-angle clamps of various sizes are useful in making the passage around the urethra at the bladder neck. After the passage is made, a measuring cuff is placed in this area to determine the proper circumference for the cuff. The cuff inserted should be snug but not obstructive. The urethra and bladder should be carefully inspected for injury or perforation. Irrigation of the Foley catheter allows the surgeon to observe any leaks.

If the cuff is being placed in the vicinity of the bulbous urethra, a perineal incision is made in the midline. The bulbourethralis and rectourethralis muscles are dissected until the bulbous urethra is exposed. Careful dissection is done to circumscribe the bulbous urethra. Care is taken at the 12 o'clock position to avoid injuring the most superior portion of the bulbous urethra. Simultaneous urethroscopy ensures that no damage is done to the urethra. A measuring tape is passed around the bulbous urethra to determine the proper circumference for the cuff. Generally the cuff should be 4.5 to 5 cm. If the measurement is larger, careful attention should be made to the dissection so that the passage is only around the bulbous urethra. In patients having a bulbous urethral placement, an inguinal incision approximately 6 cm in length is made. The dissection is deepened to the region of the external inguinal ring. The spermatic cord structures are carefully retracted, and the transversalis fascia at the floor of the inguinal canal is opened. The space over Cooper's ligament is carefully dissected, and a pressure-regulating balloon is placed in this area. The amount of pressure for a bulbous urethral placement varies from 51 to 80 cm H_2O. Pressures greater than this range may cause erosion of the cuff through the bulbous urethra. The transversalis fascia is closed after the pressure-regulating balloon has been inflated. The pump mechanism is placed in a subcutaneous pouch on the ipsilateral scrotum. The appropriate tubing from the pump is connected to the pressure-regulating balloon with a quick connector or a tie connector. The tubing from the cuff around the bulbous urethra is passed via a needle through the perineum into the inguinal area and is similarly attached to the pump. The device is activated several times to prove the competence of the pressure around the bulbous urethra. Urethroscopy is repeated to ascertain that the bulbous urethra is not damaged or eroded. The pump should be left in a deactivated position for 6 to 8 weeks to prevent undue pressure on the bulbous urethra. The perineal incision is closed carefully, reapproximating the bulbourethralis and rectourethralis muscles in the subcutaneous tissue. The perineal incision is closed with a subcuticular suture to prevent infection. The inguinal incision is similarly closed.

When cuff placement is at the bladder neck, no additional incisions are needed. The pressure-regulating balloon is placed in a space lateral to the bladder wall, and the tubes from both the cuff and pressure-regulating balloon are brought up into the inguinal area. A pump is similarly placed in a subcutaneous pouch within the scrotum or labia, and the tubes are connected to their appropriate components. The device should be activated and deactivated several times. Cystoscopy should be performed to determine that no damage or erosion has occurred at the bladder neck. The pump should be placed in the most dependent portion of the scrotum or labia and should be easily palpable. The bladder, if open, should be closed in a watertight fashion using two layers. The device is left in a deactivated position. A Foley catheter is left in place for 24 to 72 hours. The patient is treated postoperatively with IV antibiotics. The patient can be discharged from the hospital on the second to fourth postoperative day, depending on the postoperative course. The cuff should not be activated until the wound is well healed and no edema or pain is detected when the pump is palpated in the scrotum or labia.

Results with Artificial Genitourinary Sphincters

Although the genitourinary sphincter was designed primarily for patients with neurogenic bladder, it has found wider application and success. It has been used in a number of postoperative conditions in which urinary incontinence results.

Success rates after genitourinary sphincter placement vary widely among reported series. Length of follow-up also varies in the published series, and results are often difficult to evaluate because various definitions of continence and success were used.[45-51]

Generalizations from the various series can be made, however. Implantation of the artificial sphincter has been very successful in patients incontinent from prostatic surgery, including radical retropubic prostatectomy, suprapubic prostatectomy, and transurethral resections of the prostate. Continence rates have ranged from 74% to 93%. Series of reimplantation of artificial sphincters after malfunction or erosion have produced success rates approaching 80%.[47] Patients with neuropathic bladder generally have a lower success rate.[53] Sphincter implantation for urinary stress incontinence has had excellent results, with continence rates of 90%.[54,55] In summary, patients with pure sphincter incompetence and minimal complicating factors seem to have the best chance for success with urinary sphincters.

Complications after artificial sphincter surgery have included urethral erosions, bladder neck erosions, and infections. If hematoma formation is a possibility, drains should be left in the postoperative period. The device should be activated and deactivated several times at the operating table before closure of the wound to guarantee proper function. Urethroscopy and cystoscopy should be performed after the cuff is implanted to ensure that urethral erosion and trauma are absent. The bladder should be drained postoperatively with a small catheter.

Cuff erosion is still the primary problem when the cuff is placed at the bulbous urethra in males and at the bladder neck in females. Careful measurement of the urethral circumference should allow selection of a cuff that is not too tight. Appropriate selection of the pressure-regulating balloon prevents undue pressure on the urethra. Deactivation of the cuff for 6 to 12 weeks allows proper healing before pressure is placed on the urethra or bladder neck. Meticulous care in the surgical approach to the urethra or bladder neck should minimize the chances of trauma to the urethra.

Despite complications, the genitourinary sphincter has proved valuable in correcting incontinence. It has restored continence to patients whose sphincter competence had not returned after surgery. It has also led to urinary continence in children and young adults with congenital conditions that would not have allowed them to become continent.

INJECTION THERAPY FOR INCONTINENCE

The injection of synthetic substances into the body to effect anatomic changes is not a new concept. Otolaryngologists and plastic surgeons routinely perform injection therapy of the vocal cord.

Arnold first used polytetrafluoroethylene (Teflon) to improve vocal cord closure in cases of congenital deficiency.[61] Teflon's application to urology, specifically for urinary incontinence, was initiated by Berg[62] and subsequently Politano and associates[63] in 1973. Berg presented three patients in whom 5 to 10 ml of Teflon had been injected submucosally into the periurethral tissues. Although all three patients required repeat injections, they were continent after relatively short follow-up.[62] Politano in a series of 32 selected patients, both male and female, treated various cases of incontinence including cases of failed prior surgical attempts to obtain continence. His success rate was 60%.[63] Teflon injections work because they produce a periurethral mass that anatomically alters urethral resistance. Teflon appears to maintain its anatomic position through fibrous encapsulation by tissue and secondarily may cause a continuous low-grade inflammatory response with giant cell reaction.[63-65] This systemic reaction has created concern about the safety of Teflon injection.[65]

Patient selection depends on a thorough preoperative workup. Previous therapy and surgery should be investigated, and complete evaluation, including urodynamics, voiding cystourethrography, and cystoscopy, should be performed. Vaginal fistulas and urethral diverticula should be ruled out. External genitalia must be carefully examined. Urine cultures should be obtained and any infection treated before injection therapy. The upper urinary tract should be assessed with intravenous pyelography or renal ultrasound before therapy. A voiding cystourethrogram delineates the urethral anatomy and is valuable in comparing the preoperative condition with the postoperative effect. The best candidates for injection therapy are incontinent patients who have the ability to empty their bladders and do not have motor neurogenic bladders.

The surgery can be performed by various methods, depending on the type of syringe used to inject the Teflon paste. The patient is positioned in the dorsal lithotomy position, and endoscopy is concomitantly performed. Under direct vision 4 to 5 ml of paste is injected in the 3, 6, and nine o'clock positions around the urethra in the bladder neck area in a female patient. In a male patient the same areas are infiltrated through a perineal injection that places the Teflon around the membranous urethra. The Teflon can be injected endoscopically through a needle placed suburethrally under direct vision. The mass produced by the paste can be judged endoscopically and repeat injections given if necessary. A Foley catheter is usually left in place for 24 hours after the procedure. Some patients have postoperative urinary retention and require intermittent catheterization. Antibiotic prophylaxis should be given for at least 1 week after injection therapy.

Follow-up therapy should ensure that the patient is evacuating the bladder satisfactorily and is not carrying large volumes of residual urine. If the completeness of evacuation is in doubt, the upper urinary tract should be evaluated to rule out hydronephrosis.

Reports on the use of Teflon injection for urinary incontinence reveal improvement in various clinical situations. Politano reported on Teflon injection for 69 postprostatectomy patients.[66] The improvement rate was 85% in the patients incontinent after transurethral resection of the prostate and 48% in patients incontinent after radical prostatectomy. Corrie, Rodriguez, and Thompson found a 60% improvement in 10 patients with postprostatectomy incontinence.[67] Osther, however, reported a disappointing 24% improvement rate and concluded that other forms of continence therapy were preferable.[68]

Teflon injections have been more successful in women with stress incontinence. Vesey, Rivett, and Boyle reported a 78% success rate in 36 patients with urinary stress incontinence.[69] Lockhart and co-workers in a series of 20 patients with Teflon injection found 85% cured or improved after limited follow-up.[70] Schulman and associates reported an 86% rate of improvement or cure in 56 patients with urinary incontinence.[71]

Complications after periurethral Teflon injection have been few. Intraoperative extrusion of paste into the urethra appears not to have a serious effect on bladder or urethal function if the area is well irrigated. Perineal abscesses have been reported infrequently, and only occasional cases of postoperative urinary retention have been reported.[72] A more profound concern with Teflon injection therapy is the possibility of particle migration, embolization, and neoplastic transformation. In short- and long-term histologic studies of dogs and monkeys, Malizia found migration of small Teflon particles to pelvic lymph nodes, brain, lung, kidney, and spleen.[65] Most particles were smaller than 100 μm, but particles of 80 μm were found outside the injection site. Pulmonary migration of Teflon particles and pulmonary granulomas, neither of which were fatal, have been reported.[73,74] The degree of foreign body reaction seen in histologic studies of animals given Teflon injection produces the troublesome question of possible carcinogenic effects of the Teflon paste in embolized sites. Although the use of Teflon in the vocal cords has been safe and successful, other areas of the body may not be as immune to the foreign body reaction. Teflon therapy for urologic incontinence has not been approved by the FDA. Treatment therefore should be done with care, and informed consent should be obtained. Teflon should be used with caution in young adults and children because the long-term effects of the substance on soft tissue are unknown.

Collagen Injection Therapy

Since the introduction of Teflon injection for treatment of urinary incontinence, other substances have been investigated. Glutaraldehyde cross-linked collagen, composed of purified bovine dermal collagen suspended in lidocaine, was recently used in 17 female patients with urinary incontinence.[75] The collagen preparation is identical in composition to a commercially available collagen implant (Zydem), which has FDA approval for use in the correction of dermal contour defects. Cross-linking is absent in the Zydem product. Cross-linking is assumed to decrease autogenicity and stabilize the collagen. Patients were preoperatively tested for localized hypersensitivity to subdermally placed collagen. No patient had a serious reaction. With an endoscopic needle, perisphincteric injections were placed circumferentially at the bladder neck. Suprapubic tubes were placed during surgery and removed after satisfactory urethral voiding was established. Of 17 patients followed up for 9 to 23 months, 9 (39%) were cured or improved. Urethal pressure profiles did not change significantly in this group of patients, and other urodynamic parameters were not affected. McGuire and associates recently presented 1-year follow-up results of collagen injections for urinary incontinence in 30 males and 35 females and reported 83% and 94% improvement or cure rates, respectively.[76] Peak urethral profile values did not reflect continence function. However, increased leak point pressures were found in successfully treated patients.

Clinical trials are evaluating the efficacy of percutaneously placed inflatable silicone spheres (Genisphere) in the treatment of incontinent female patients.[77] With the patient under local anesthesia, the spheres are introduced via a trocar delivery system and are placed in the periurethral tissue under fluoroscopic guidance. The spheres are subsequently inflated to effect coaptation of the urethral walls. Of 39 patients injected, 76% were improved or cured at a mean of 6 months' follow-up. In four patients the spheres were extruded, but no lasting adverse urethral effects were noted.

Periurethral autologous subcutaneous fat tissue was recently substituted for Teflon in an injection study reported by Palma and associates.[78] Ten patients were endoscopically injected with fat obtained by simultaneous suprapubic liposuction. A 90% cure rate was seen with mean follow-up of 9 months. Long-term continence rates and incidents of fat emboli are not yet reported.

Injection therapy by whatever means has the appeal of ease of placement and reliance on compression to obtain urinary continence. Long-term results will have to be evaluated to ascertain continence rates and any long-term adverse effects.

REFERENCES

1. Scott FB, Bradley WE, Timm GW: Management of erectile impotence: use of implantable inflatable prosthesis. Urology 2:80, 1973.
2. Scott FB, Bradley WE, Timm GW: Treatment of urinary incontinence by an implantable prosthetic sphincter. Urology 1:252, 1973.
3. Bogoras NA: Ubeir die volle plastiche Wiederherstellung eines rum Koitus Fahigen Penis (Peniplastica Totalis). Zentrabl Chir 63:1271, 1937.
4. Frumpkin AP: Reconstruction of the male genitalia. Am Rev Soviet Med 2:14, 1944.
5. Goodwin WE, Scott WW: Phalloplasty. J Urol 68:903, 1952.
6. Behari GE: Surgical treatment of impotence. Plast Reconstr Surg 38:92, 1966.
7. Pearman RO: Treatment of organic impotence by implantation of a penile prosthesis. J Urol 97:716, 1967.
8. Small MP, Carrion HM, Gordon JA: Small-Carrion penile prosthesis: new implant for management of impotence. Urology 5:479, 1975.
9. Finney RP: New hinged silicone penile implant. J Urol 118:585, 1977.
10. Jonas U, Jacob GH: Silver-Silicone penile prosthesis. J Urol 123:865, 1970.
11. Mulcahy JJ: The OmniPhase and Duraphase penile prosthesis. Urol Clin North Am 6:25, 1989.
12. Merrill DC: Mentor inflatable penile prosthesis. Urology 22:504, 1983.
13. Mulcahy JJ: The self-contained inflatable and mechanical prosthesis. AUA Update Series 6:20, 1987.
14. Malloy TR, Malkowicz B: Pharmacologic treatment of impotence. Urol Clin North Am 14:297, 1987.
15. Puppo P, DeRose AF, Pittaluga P, et al: Diagnosis of male impotence after intracavernosa papaverine test. Eur Urol 15:213, 1988.
16. Stewart TD: Penile prostheses: potential value of medical psychiatric assessment and psychotherapy. Psychother Psychosom 44:18, 1985.
17. Schover LR: Sex therapy for the penile prosthesis recipient. Urol Clin North Am 16:91, 1989.
18. Krane RJ, Goldstein I, Tejada IS: Medical progress: impotence. N Engl J Med 321:1648, 1989.
19. Asopa R, Williams G: Use of the "Correctaid" device in the management of impotence. Br J Urol 63:546, 1989.
20. Breza J, Aboseif SH, Orvis R, et al: Detailed anatomy of penile neurovascular strictures: surgical significance. J Urol 141:437, 1989.
21. Montague DK: Penile prosthesis: an overview. Urol Clin North Am 16:7, 1989.
22. Small M: Small-Carrion penile prosthesis: a report on 160 cases and review of the literature. J Urol 119:365, 1978.
23. Malloy TR, Wein AJ, Carpiniello VL: Comparison of the inflatable penile and the Small-Carrion prostheses in the surgical treatment of erectile impotence. J Urol 123:678, 1980.
24. Finney RP, Sharpe JR, Sadlowski RW: Finney hinged penile implant: experience with 100 cases. J Urol 124:480, 1980.
25. Benson RC, Patterson DE, Barrett DM: Long term results with the Jonas malleable penile prosthesis. J Urol 134:899, 1985.
26. Moul JW, McLeod DG: Experience with the AMS 600 malleable penile prosthesis. J Urol 135:929, 1986.
27. Krane RJ: Omniphase penile prosthesis. Semin Urol 4:247, 1986.
28. Mulcahy JJ: The Hydroflex self-contained inflatable prosthesis: experience with 100 patients. J Urol 140:1422, 1988.
29. Fishman IJ: Experience with the Hydroflex penile prosthesis. Semin Urol 4:239, 1986.
30. Stanisic TH, Dean JC, Donovan JM, et al: Clinical experience with a self-contained inflatable penile implant: the Flexi-flate. J Urol 139:947, 1988.

31. Malloy TR, Wein AJ, Carpiniello VL: Improved mechanical survival with revised model inflatable penile prosthesis using rear-tip extenders. J Urol 128:489, 1982.
32. Scott FB, Byrd GJ, Karacan I, et al: Erectile impotence treated with an implantable penile prosthesis. J Urol 124:611, 1980.
33. Furlow WL: Surgical management of impotence using the inflatable penile prosthesis: experience with 103 patients. Br J Urol 18:49, 1977.
34. Malloy TR, Wein AJ, Carpiniello VL: Reliability of AMS M700 inflatable penile prosthesis. Urology 28:385, 1986.
35. Mulcahy JJ: Use of CX cylinders in association with AMS 700 inflatable penile prosthesis. J Urol 140:1420, 1988.
36. Furlow WL, Motley RC: The inflatable penile prosthesis: clinical experience with a new controlled expansion cylinder. J Urol 139:945, 1988.
37. Engle RM, Smolev JK, Hackler R: Mentor inflatable penile prosthesis. Urology 29:498, 1987.
38. Merrill DC: Clinical experience with the Mentor inflatable penile prosthesis in 301 patients. J Urol 140:1424, 1988.
39. Pedersen B, Tiefer L, Ruiz M, et al: Evaluation of patients and partners 1 to 4 years after penile prosthesis surgery. J Urol 139:956, 1988.
40. Nielsen KT, Bruskewitz RC: Semirigid and malleable rod penile prosthesis. Urol Clin North Am 16:13, 1989.
41. Witherington R: Vacuum constriction device for management of erectile impotence. J Urol 141:320, 1989.
42. Katz PG, Haden HT, Mulligan T, Zasler ND: The effect of vacuum devices on penile hemodynamics. J Urol 143:55, 1990.
43. Nadig PW, Ware JC, Blumoff R: Noninvasive device to produce and maintain an erection-like state. Urology 27:126, 1986.
44. Witherington R: Suction device therapy in the management of erectile impotence. Urol Clin North Am 15:123, 1988.
45. Montague DK: Evolution of implanted devices for urinary incontinence. Cleve Clin Q 51:405, 1984.
46. Berry JL: A new procedure for correction of urinary incontinence: preliminary report. J Urol 85:771, 1961.
47. Kauffman JJ: Treatment of post-prostatectomy urinary incontinence using a silicone gel prosthesis. Br J Urol 45:646, 1973.
48. Montague DK: The Scott-Bradley-Timm artificial urinary sphincters. J Urol 125:796, 1982.
49. Scott FB, Bradley WE, Timm GW, et al: Treatment of incontinence secondary to myelodysplasia by an implantable prosthetic urinary sphincter. South Med J 66:987, 1973.
50. Scott FB: The artificial sphincter in the management of incontinence in the male. Urol Clin North Am 5:375, 1978.
51. Barrett DM, Motley RC: Artificial urinary sphincter cuff erosion: experience with reimplantation in 38 patients. Urology 35:215, 199.
52. Hold T: The artificial sphincter in the treatment of congenital incontinence. Acta Urol Belg 57:545, 1989.
53. Gonzalez R, Koleilat N, Austin C, Ami Sidi A: The artificial sphincter AS800 in congenital urinary incontinence. J Urol 142:512, 1989.
54. Boyd SD: The role of the urethral reconstruction in artificial sphincters in complicated salvage radical prostatectomy. Urology 32:304, 1988.
55. Fishman IJ, Shabsigh R, Scott FB: Experience with the artificial urinary sphincter Model AS800 in 148 patients. J Urol 141:307, 1989.
56. Malloy TR, Wein AJ, Carpiniello VL: Surgical results with the artificial urinary sphincter. Urology 19:602, 1982.
57. Malloy TR, Wein AJ, Carpiniello VL: Surgical success with AMS M800 GU sphincter for male incontinence. Urology 33:274, 1989.
58. Light JK, Scott FB: Use of the artificial urinary sphincter in spinal cord injury patients. J Urol 130:1127, 1983.
59. Light KJ, Scott FB: Management of urinary incontinence in women with the artificial urinary sphincter. J Urol 134:476, 1985.
60. Scott FB: Use of the artificial sphincter in the treatment of urinary incontinence. Clin Obstet Gynecol 12:415, 1985.
61. Arnold GE: Further experience with intrachordal Teflon injection. Laryngoscope 17:802, 1964.
62. Berg S: Polytef augmentation urethroplasty. Arch Surg 107:379, 1973.
63. Politano VA, Small MP, Harper JM, et al: Periurethral Teflon injection for urinary incontinence. J Urol 111:180, 1974.
64. Toomey JM, Brown BS: The histological response to intrachordal injection of Teflon paste. Laryngoscope 77:110, 1967.
65. Malizia AA, Reiman HM, Myers RP, et al: Migration and granulomatous reaction after periurethral injection of polytef (Teflon). JAMA 251:3277, 1984.
66. Politano VA: Periurethral polytetrafluoroethylene injection for urinary incontinence. J Urol 127:439, 1982.
67. Corrie D, Rodriquez FR, Thompson IM: Periurethral polytetrafluoroethylene injection for post-prostatectomy incontinence. Milit Med 154:442, 1989.
68. Osther PJ: Teflon injections in post-prostatectomy incontinence. Scand J Urol Nephrol 22:171, 1988.
69. Vesey SG, Rivett A, O'Boyle PT: Teflon injection in female stress incontinence: effect on urethral pressure profile and flow rate. Br J Urol 62:39, 1988.
70. Lockhart JL, Walker RD, Vorstman B, Politano VA: Periurethral polytetrafluoroethylene injections following urethral reconstruction in female patients with urinary incontinence. J Urol 140:51, 1988.
71. Schulman CC, Simon J, Wespes E, Germeau R: Eur. endoscopic injection of Teflon for female urinary incontinence. Urology 9:246, 1983.
72. Boykim W, Rodriquez FR, Brizzolara JP, et al: Complete urinary obstruction following periurethral polytetrafluoroethylene injection for urinary incontinence. J Urol 141:1199, 1989.
73. Claes H, Stroobants D, Van Meerbeck J, et al: Pulmonary migration following periurethral polytetrafluoroethylene injection for urinary incontinence. J Urol 142:821, 1989.
74. Mittleman RE, Marraccini JV: Pulmonary Teflon granulomas following periurethral Teflon injections for urinary incontinence. Arch Pathol Lab Med 107:611, 1983.
75. Daikiri-Shortliffe IM, Freiha FS, Kessler R, et al: Treatment of urinary incontinence by periurethral implantation of glutaraldehyde cross-linked collagen. J Urol 141:538, 1989.
76. McGuire EJ, Wang SC, Appel R, et al: Treatment of urethral incontinence by collagen injection: one year follow-up [Abstract 142]. J Urol 143:224A, 1990.
77. Barrett DM, Ghoniem G, Bruskewitz R, et al: The Genisphere: a new percutaneously placed anti-incontinence device [Abstract 141]. J Urol 143:224A, 1990.
78. Palma PR, Netto NR, Ikari O, D'Ancora CA: Paraurethral autologous subcutaneous fatty tissue injection for female urinary stress incontinence [Abstract 140]. J Urol 223A, 1990.

CHAPTER 5

ULTRASOUND IN UROLOGY

ALBERTO D. HERNANDEZ and JOSEPH A. SMITH, JR.

HISTORICAL PERSPECTIVE

The use of ultrasound for medical diagnosis began in the late 1940s and early 1950s with application of the piezoelectric phenomenon described at the beginning of the twentieth century. The development of equipment with the sensitivity to detect tissue interfaces allowed Howry, Bliss, and Holmes to produce the first cross-sectional ultrasound image scanner.[1] The clinical application of this prototype scanner had obvious limitations but encouraged other researchers to investigate this new noninvasive diagnostic modality. By the late 1950s, sonographic visualization of brain, intraocular, and cardiac structures, as well as obstetric and gynecologic applications, were described. The development of gray scale ultrasound provided increased parenchymal visualization from tissue interfaces. Other innovations allowed dynamic visualization of structures by real-time scanners, as well as more precise focusing and transducer resolution, which ultimately improved the diagnostic capabilities of ultrasonography.

The detection and staging of prostatic cancer by transrectal ultrasonography fostered enthusiasm and interest among urologists and led to the incorporation of ultrasonography into routine clinical urology. In 1971 Watanabe published the results of size and volume measurements of the prostate gland determined by transrectal ultrasonography, and in 1975 he suggested its utility in staging and monitoring prostate cancer.[2] Harada and co-workers originated the gray scale transrectal sonographer in 1980, making possible visualization of the internal architecture of the prostate gland and the identification of two distinct zones.[3] By 1985 the introduction of 5 mHz scanners improved visualization of prostate tumors and allowed better definition of their echo characteristics.[4] The availability of high-resolution, real-time ultrasound scanners, together with increasing development in bioengineering, has provided the equipment that has become an essential diagnostic and interventional modality in urologic surgery.

FUNDAMENTALS AND PHYSICAL PRINCIPLES

Transducer

The transducer is the source of ultrasonic energy. A transducer is a device that converts one form of energy into another, such as electrical energy into mechanical sonic energy and vice versa. Transducer physics are based on the piezoelectric effect, described by Pierre Curie in 1880. Certain crystals have the inherent quality of vibrating in response to an electric stimulus. When the crystals are deformed, the alignment of charged molecules is altered, generating an electric signal. The crystals, such as lead zirconate and lead titanate (synthetic ceramics), vibrate at any frequency, depending on the voltage of the electric stimulus. The transducer is also the receiver of the transmitted sound that is reflected when it passes through different tissues. This reflected wave hits the crystal and distorts its shape, causing a small electric signal to be generated. The crystal, acting as both a transmitter and a receiver of ultrasound, forms the basis of the pulsed mode ultrasound (Figure 5–1).

A pulsed wave is commonly used in diagnostic ultrasonography. It can be pulse excited by discharging a capacitor through the transducer crystal or by gating a continuous alternating voltage. The other type of transducer excitation is the continuous wave in which the transducer is constantly supplied with an appropriate alternating voltage. This is the mode of operation used in most diagnostic Doppler instruments.

Ultrasound images are cross-sectional representations of the tissues (tomograms) that, in contrast to electromagnetic waves (x rays), require a medium for propagation. The interaction of the medium (tissue) with the ultrasound beam generates particle vibration. This process of transmitted vibrations from particle to particle leads to the propagation of the ultrasound wave (Figure 5–2).

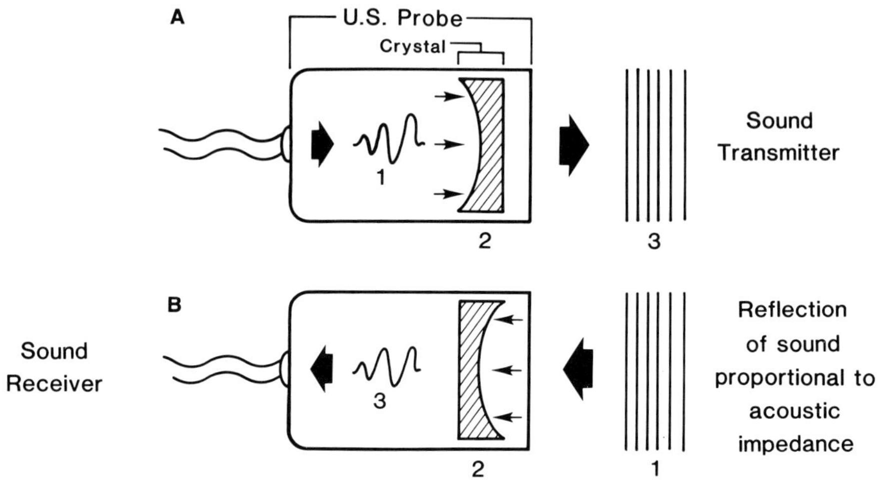

FIGURE 5–1. Physical principles behind an ultrasound transducer. **A,** Electrical voltage *(1)* deforms the crystal *(2)* and vibrates, generating an ultrasound pulse *(3)*. **B,** The reflected sound *(1)* deforms the crystal, vibrates *(2)*, and generates an electrical signal *(3)*, which is eventually transformed into an image.

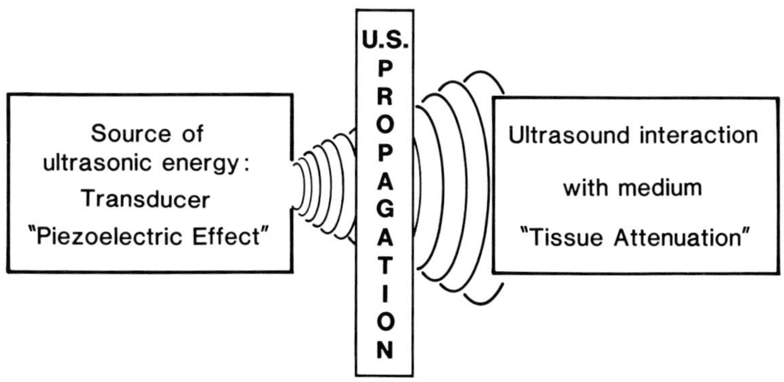

FIGURE 5–2. The piezoelectric effect generates a wave phenomenon that propagates and interacts with the medium.

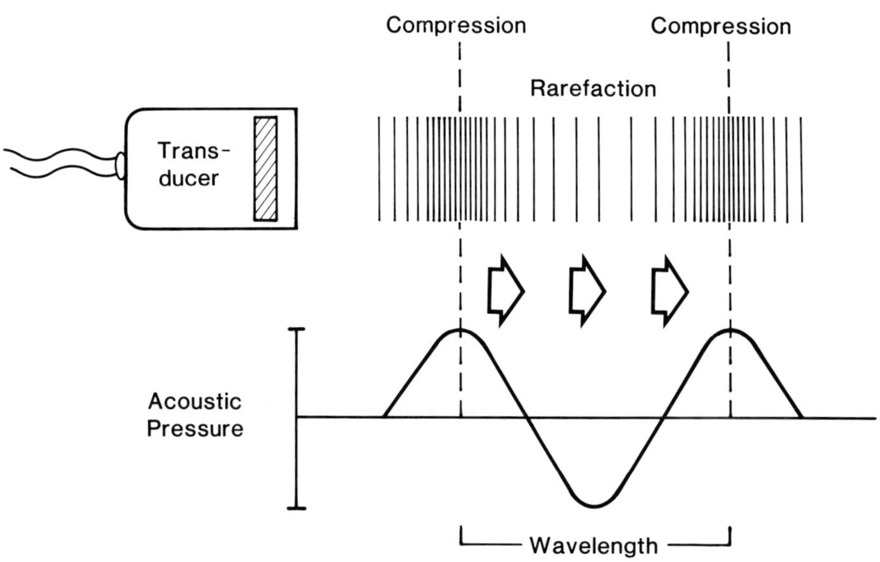

FIGURE 5–3. Ultrasound propagation. The arrow indicates the propagation of the longitudinal wave emitted by the transducer.

Ultrasound Propagation

Sound initiates a local vibratory disturbance in the medium between the source and the receiver. This type of vibratory disturbance propagation is described as a wave. The particles vibrate back and forth along the line of travel of the sound wave. The particles do not move from the source to the receiver of the sound, but mechanical energy (ultrasound) is propagated and ceases whenever the vibratory stimulus stops (Figure 5–3).

The vibratory movement of the particles in the medium creates longitudinal waves. They contain areas of rarefaction where the particles are spread apart, reducing pressure. Regions of increased pressure in the wave increases are called areas of compression. These correspond to areas where the vibrating particles are close together. The elevation in acoustic pressure results in compression of the medium, whereas reduction in this pressure corresponds to rarefaction. The distance from one compression area to another with one rarefaction area in between (one complete sinusoidal cycle) is called a wavelength. Wavelength can also be measured from one rarefaction area to another. The number of such complete cycles occurring each second is called frequency and is measured in Hertz (Hz) or cycles per second (c/s). Sound consists of waves of frequency between 20 Hz and 20 kHz (audible sound). Frequencies lower than 20 Hz are called infrasound, and frequencies above 20 kHz are called ultrasound.

Sound or ultrasound travels at different speeds (velocity) determined by the density, compressibility, and elasticity of the medium. The speed in each medium is constant and is measured in meters per second (m/s) (Figure 5–4). Ultrasound always requires a mechanical medium for propagation (gas, liquid, or solid) and does not propagate through a vacuum because the particles are not allowed to vibrate. Most abdominal and pelvic ultrasound scanning is performed with transducers having a frequency between 3 and 7 mHz (3 to 7 million c/s) (Figure 5–5).

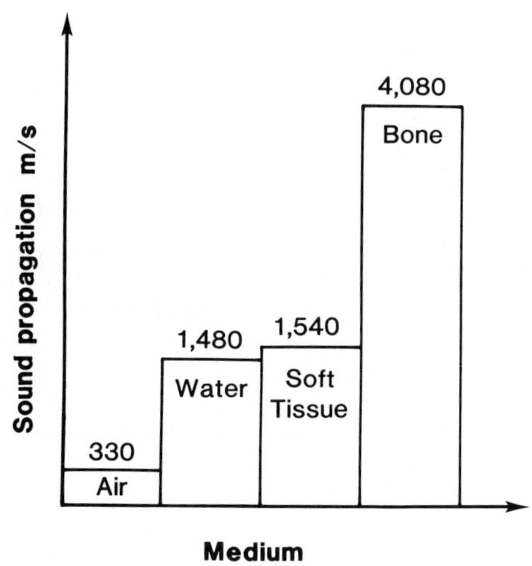

FIGURE 5–4. Sound propagation through different media.

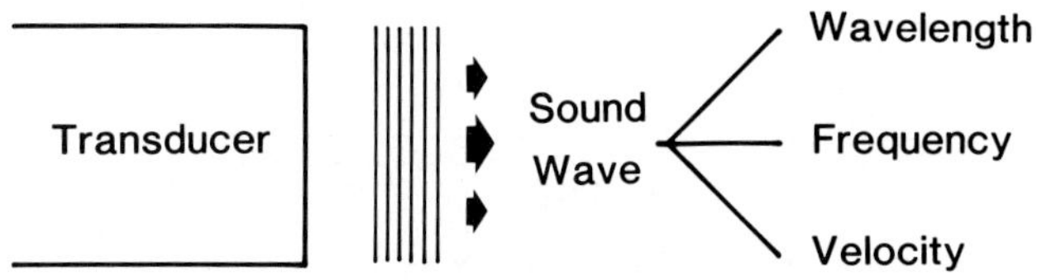

FIGURE 5–5. Sound wave characteristics.

Ultrasound Interaction with the Medium

The preceding description refers to ultrasound propagation as homogeneous, but body tissues actually behave as a complex inhomogeneous medium. When an ultrasound wave reaches a boundary between two media of different acoustic properties, part of the sound is transmitted through the boundary and part is reflected (echo). The amount of sound reflected depends on the acoustic properties (acoustic impedance) of the two adjacent media and on the angle at which the beam strikes the boundary (angle of incidence). Acoustic impedance is equal to the product of the density of the medium and the velocity of the sound in the medium. If two media have the same acoustic impedance, no sound is reflected. The greater the difference in acoustic impedance, the greater the sound reflected and the less the sound transmitted. All of the sound is reflected at a muscle-air interface, which explains the inability of ultrasound to penetrate air-filled structures (Figure 5–6).

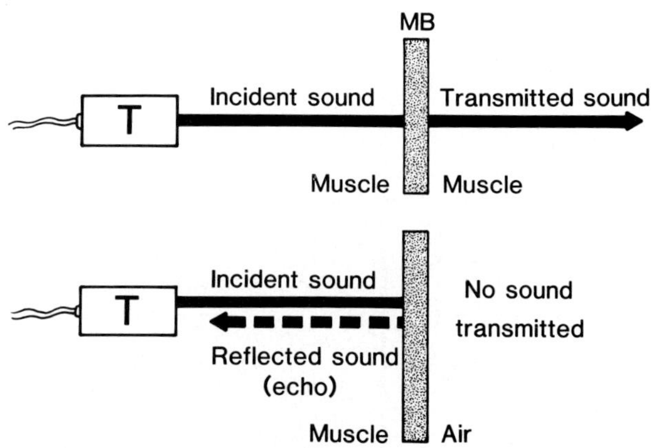

FIGURE 5–6. Ultrasound interaction with medium. The upper portion shows a schematic representation of an ultrasound wave reaching a boundary between two media with the same acoustic impedance. Since there is no sound reflection, the ultrasound wave is transmitted. The lower portion of the diagram shows the situation when the difference in acoustic impedance increases. More sound is reflected (echo), and less is transmitted. *T*, Transducer; *MB*, medium boundary.

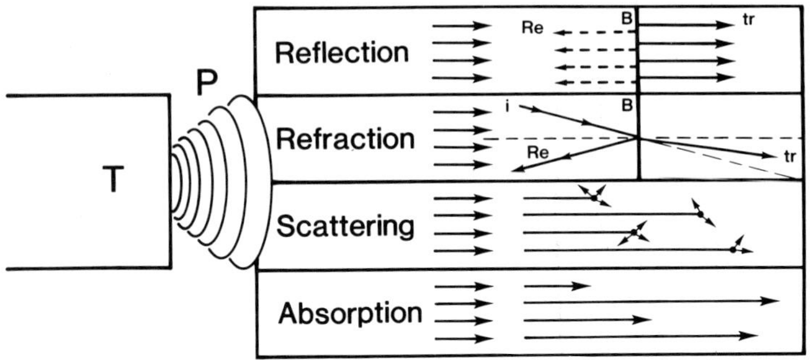

FIGURE 5–7. Schematic drawing of the process of attenuation. Sound waves emitted by a transducer *(T)* are propagated *(P)* and interact with the medium, creating reflection, refraction, scattering, and absorption. *B,* Medium boundary; *i,*incident sound; *Re,*reflected sound; *tr,*transmitted sound.

The intensity and amplitude of a sound wave decrease with increasing distance from the sound source (transducer). This phenomenon is called attenuation. Several mechanisms, including reflection, refraction, scattering, and absorption, may attenuate a sound wave (Figure 5–7).

As previously stated, the amount of sound reflected depends on the acoustic impedance of two adjacent media and on the angle of incidence of the propagated sound wave. If a sound wave strikes a boundary at a right angle, the reflected wave is specular and the transmitted sound does not deviate from its original course. If an incident sound wave strikes a boundary at an angle other than 90 degrees, the reflected wave travels back into the first medium with an angle of reflection and the transmitted sound is refracted (Figure 5–8).

Scattering occurs when the sound wave interacts with small reflectors, causing dispersion in all directions. The energy of each of the scattered echoes is small. The ones generated back in the direction of the sound source are termed back scatter. The intensity of the wave beyond the reflectors is reduced.

Some of the ultrasound mechanical energy is converted into heat by a process called absorption. Ultrasound originates the vibration of particles in the medium, creating friction. The particle vibration depends on the viscosity of the medium, defined as the property that tends to oppose the vibratory motion. This friction creates energy loss in the form of heat, decreasing the sound intensity as it propagates.

Both absorption and scattering depend strongly on frequency, and consequently the overall attenuation is also frequency dependent. The higher the frequency, the greater the attenuation. Attenuation is a measurable property that can be quantified with a decibel notation and has an exponential decrease (Figure 5–9).

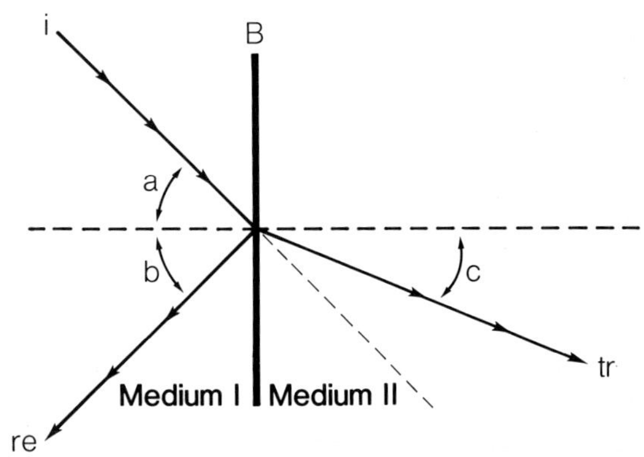

FIGURE 5–8. Process of reflection and refraction. In medium I the angle of reflection *(b)* is equal to the angle of incidence *(a)*. In medium II the angle of refraction *(c)* is different from the original angle of incidence. *i,* Incident sound; *re,* reflected sound; *tr,* transmitted wave.

Signal Processing

Gray Scale

The interaction of the ultrasound wave with the medium determines the intensity of sound reflected. The number of interfaces and the acoustic impedance depend on the tissue through which the sound is traveling. In brightness mode (B-mode) scanners, echoes with different intensity are displayed with varying shades of gray. This conveys an impression of tissue texture and is an important factor in the ability to differentiate between tissues of similar echogenicity. The echo signal is processed before it is displayed. A range of signal voltage levels is assigned to each available gray shade, creating a relationship between the voltage produced by the echo and the gray shade. Thus the stronger the echo signal amplitude, the brighter its appearance in the display. The gray scale may be modified to obtain an interpretable visual representation of the tissue being scanned, but care must be taken to ensure that small changes in the appearance of parenchymal echoes are not suppressed.

Time Gain Compensation

As mentioned previously, attenuation is the sum of acoustic energy losses resulting from reflection, refraction, absorption, and scattering of the ultrasound beam as it travels through tissue. Echoes near the transducer are relatively intense compared with those far from it, although both echoes

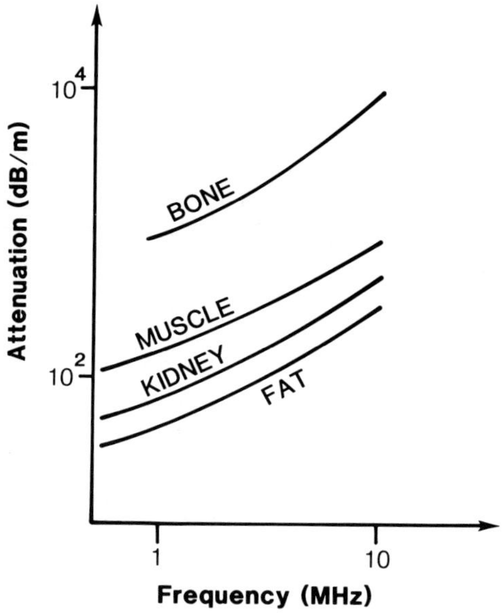

FIGURE 5–9. Attenuation is frequency dependent. The higher the sound frequency, the higher the medium attenuation and the poorer the penetration.

originate from similar reflected surfaces at different distances.

Electronic correction for the progressive decrease in echo intensity is necessary to obtain a more realistic impression of the reflectivity of structures scanned. This correction is obtained by "time gain compensation" in which the amplification (gain) applied to echo signals is progressively increased as the signals arrive from deeper structures. The greater the distance between the transducer and the echo's origin, the greater the amplification of that echo relative to echoes originating closer to the transducer.

Time gain compensation can be expressed in terms of a curve with three modifiable sections. The part closest to the transducer, the first portion of the curve, is called "near gain" and is used to adjust the amplitude of the proximal high-intensity echoes. The "slope" of the time gain compensation curve, the middle portion, varies the steepness of the slope reflecting the relative amplification over distance. The "far gain" is the last portion of the curve and indicates the distance from the transducer at which amplification is maximal.

The signal received by the transducer can be displayed on ultrasound instruments in a variety of ways. The information is usually displayed on a cathode-ray tube or a television monitor, and each mode has different appearances and clinical applications.

Scanning Mode

Amplitude mode (A-mode) scanning was the earliest ultrasound technique developed for medical diagnostic purposes. It consists of an oscilloscope mapping of the received voltage on the x-axis and time on the y-axis, which is linearly related to the distance (Figure 5–10). A-mode scanning obtains information only at a single line through the tissue at any particular position of the probe. The most common applications are to measure distances between various structures of the eye, to determine the antenatal biparietal diameter of the fetus, or as a echoencephalogram.

B-mode imaging yields a two-dimensional cross-sectional spatial representation of the examined tissue on the horizontal and vertical axes. A gray scale is assigned to each echo voltage received by the transducer, and the instrument can compute the distance from the time an echo takes to return (Figure 5–11). Instead of spikes representing the returning echoes (A-mode), a series of dots with different brightness is displayed along the longitudinal axis of propagation of the ultrasound beam. The computed integration of the sum of many B-mode lines through an object in one plane creates a B-scan image. This static B-mode scanner requires a memory system to store the different views and a probe-coordinating measuring device to detect the position and orientation of the probe at all times, making the machine nonportable. Another limitation of the static B-mode scan is that it requires a long time to generate the image, which can be blurred if the patient or the internal organs move during the image buildup.

Real-time B-mode scanning techniques have been developed to overcome the time limitation. Real-time or dynamic imaging instruments produce several cross-sectional images per second. Between 10 and 60 images are displayed per second (frame rate), yielding what appears to be a contin-

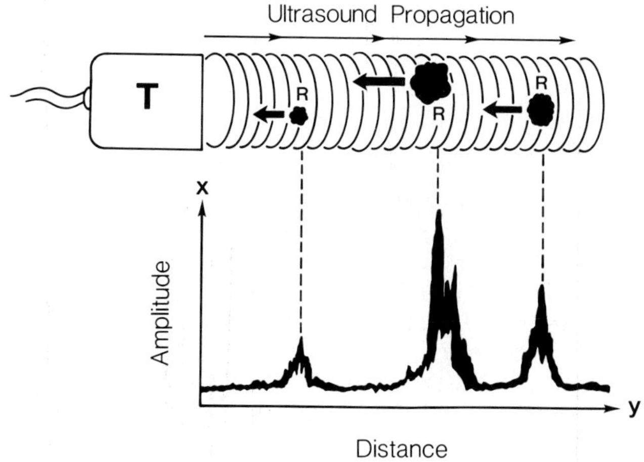

FIGURE 5–10. Schematic representation of an A-mode image. The transducer receives sound waves from the reflectors *(R)*. Interpretation of the image is based on the amplitude of the echo (x-axis). The y-axis plots the distance from the transducer.

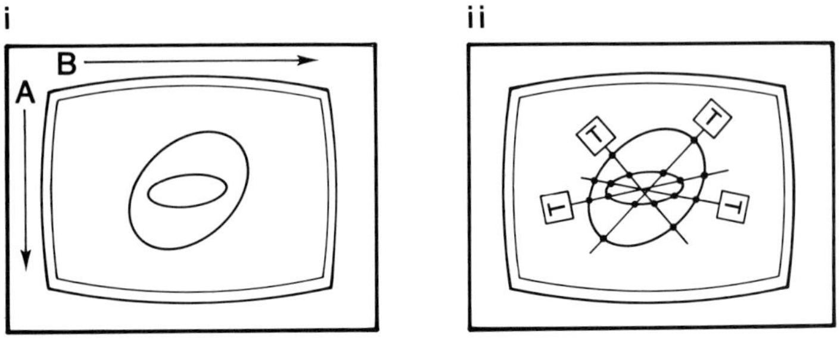

FIGURE 5–11. On the left *(i)* a B-mode display is shown on a television monitor. A two-dimensional cross-sectional representation of the object scanned is seen in depth *(A)* and width *(B)*. On the right *(ii)*, generation of the B-scan image occurs after the sum of several B-mode lines through the scanned object is stored and integrated by the instrument. The transducer *(T)* lines represent the interaction of the longitudinal ultrasound beam with the scanned object.

uously changing image. The images are produced rapidly in sequence, and memory is not required, although static image (freeze-frame) capability is available.

The basic concept of a real-time transducer requires a rapid and repetitive sweep of the sound beam through the tissues. Two methods are possible. The first, mechanical scanning (sector scan), is accomplished by oscillating a transducer at an angle. It is rocked back and forth by an appropriate device mechanism or by rotating a transducer or a group of transducers. The second mechanism is the use of electronic scanning or phased array, which is performed by using an array of identical small transducers arranged in a line (linear array) or ring shape (annular array).

Motion mode (M-mode) operation is a B-mode operation in which the motion of the reflector is detected by a strip chart recorder that moves across the face of the display and records its movement. During the generation of M-mode images the transducer is held immobile against a moving object. M-mode imaging is used primarily in echocardiology.

Artifacts

An artifact is anything not properly indicative of the structures imaged. It can be a structure that is not real, is missing, is improperly located, or has a different size or shape from the actual structure. Some artifacts are produced by inadequate equipment operation or settings, others result from improper scanning technique, and still others are inherent to the method and can occur even with proper equipment and technique. The identification and characterization of artifacts are among the most difficult areas of ultrasound interpretation and can lead to confusion and errors in diagnosis.

Reverberation. Reverberation may occur whenever an intense echo is generated, as when a transrectal ultrasound probe is used with a water-filled balloon. The echoes from the transducer travel through the medium (water) with minimal attenuation. When they strike the balloon compressed against the rectal wall, the acoustic impedance is of such magnitude that it creates an intense reflected echo. This echo is not entirely absorbed by the transducer material, and some of the energy is reflected back into the medium from the transducer face. This reflected energy acts as if it were a new pulse generated by the transducer and produces another echo, which strikes the reflector. The ultrasound machine interprets the signal and displays it at a distance twice as deep as the true echo. The intensity of the primary reflected echo determines the amount of reverberating echoes. Reverberations may be recognized because they are displayed parallel at regular intervals to the true image of the strongly reflecting surface and are separated from each other by the depth of that reflector. Another characteristic of reverberations is that their intensity decreases as they separate from the transducer (Figure 5–12).

Shadowing. An acoustic shadow occurs when there is absence of sound distal to a reflector. Again, the artifact depends on the acoustic properties of the tissue in which the ultrasound is traveling and creating attenuation (reflection, refraction, and absorption). The most common cause of shadowing is when the sound beam strikes a concretion (Figure 5–13).

Image Enhancement. Enhancement is essentially the reverse of shadowing. It occurs when some

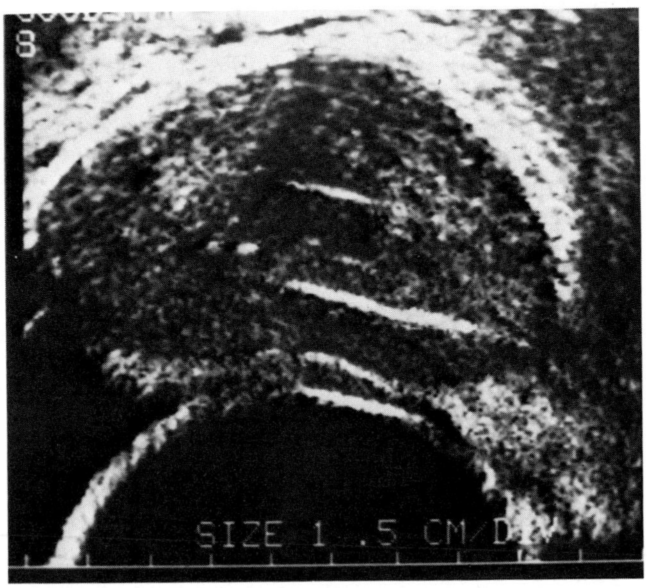

FIGURE 5–12. Reverberation artifact is seen displayed as parallel white lines at regular intervals. The intensity decreases as the distance from the transducer increases.

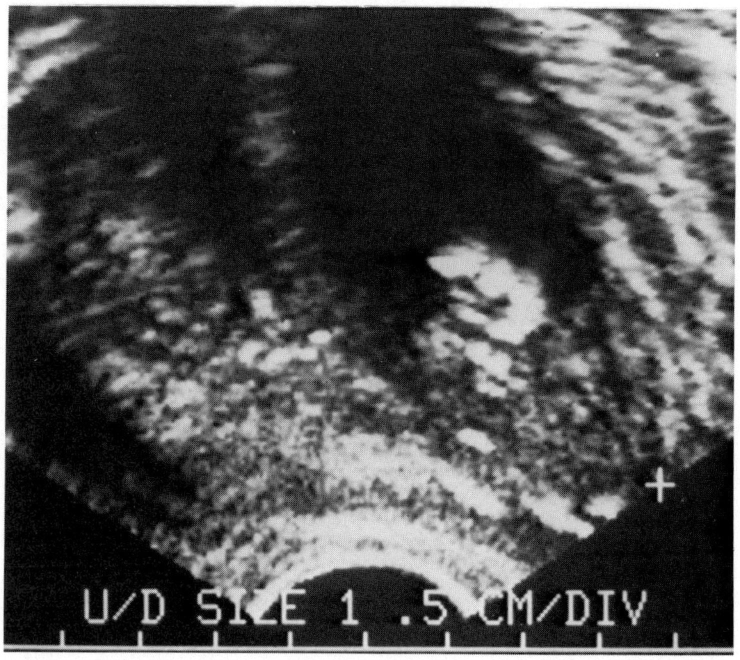

FIGURE 5–13. Shadowing from a concretion in the prostate gland. The white reflective surface of the stone can be seen with intense shadowing beyond the reflective surface.

of the superficial tissues have low attenuation and the echo signals from some of the deeper tissues are overcompensated by the time gain compensation. Thus distant structures appear to be echogenic when contrasted with similar structures at the same depth (Figure 5–14).

Edge Effect. Edge effect is an acoustic shadow in which the mechanisms of attenuation are primarily refraction and reflection. When an ultrasound beam strikes a cystic structure, the angle of incidence at the margin of a round structure with a smooth wall reflects the beam away from its original path. In addition, the sound is refracted when the ultrasound beam strikes the boundary between the fluid of the cystic structure and its wall at an angle other than 90 degrees. Both reflection and refraction create the acoustic shadow seen at the edge of a cyst when the beam is diverted from its axial course. Edge effect can also be identified at the margins of round, noncystic structures such as the lateral margin of the prostatic capsule (Figure 5–15).

Refraction. Refraction can cause a reflector to be improperly positioned on the display (Figure

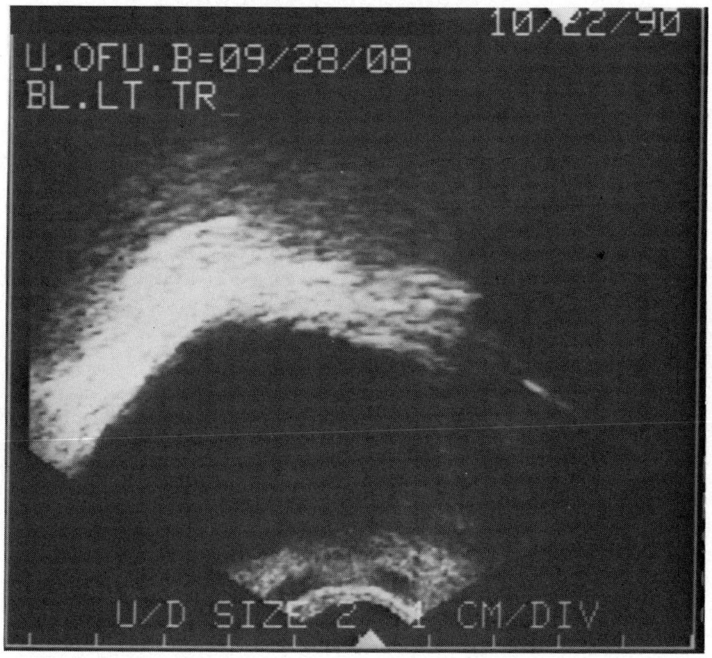

FIGURE 5–14. Image enhancement beyond a fluid-filled bladder. The distant structures appear to be highly echogenic because of overcompensation in signal reception.

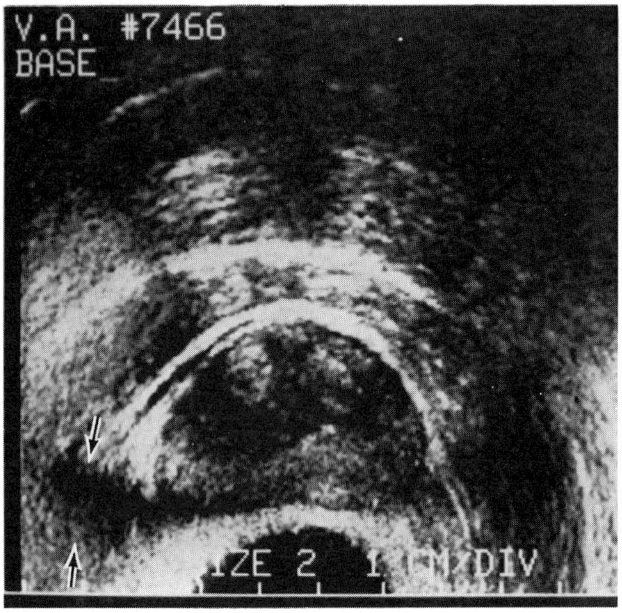

FIGURE 5–15. The edge effect appears as an acoustic shadow, primarily because of refraction and reflection of the sound wave. In this transrectal prostate image, the edge effect on the left side of the photograph *(arrow)* could be misinterpreted as a hypoechoic area.

5–16). This occurs with multielement arrays when secondary sound beams of less intensity are generated at angles from the main beam. They interact with the medium and create echoes that may be displayed at an incorrect position because the transducer interprets them as coming from a reflector along the axis of the main beam.

Multiple Path Artifact. The term "multiple path" describes the situation in which the paths to and from the reflector are different. This results in improper reflector image positioning.

Other Artifacts. Other artifacts depend on the characteristics of the transducer. For example, the material producing an acoustic shadow must be located within the focal zone of the transducer where the width of the beam is small relative to the size of the reflector. If the reflector lies proximal or distal to the focal zone of the transducer, the wide beam masks the acoustic shadow (Figure 5–17). The width of the beam can also create an artifact that simulates debris inside a cystic formation or a full bladder. This has been termed slice thickness artifact. It is caused by the increased width of the beam beyond the focal zone of the transducer (Figure 5–18). This meniscus-shaped artifact disappears when the area is scanned at different angles.

Artifacts produced by velocity variations cause incorrect computation of the position of the tissue resulting from a returned echo. For diagnostic instruments a speed of 1540 m/s is assumed. If the propagation of the medium is greater, the calculated distance to the reflector is too small and the display places the reflector too close to the transducer. The opposite happens if the ultrasound speed propagation is less than 1540 m/s.

Transducer Selection

To avoid some of the artifacts just described, the ultrasonographer must select an appropriate transducer frequency, focal zone, and face diameter. The anticipated depth and width of the structure to be scanned must be estimated. Structures close to the transducer head require little penetration. A high-frequency transducer results in better axial resolution. The axial resolution is the minimum reflec-

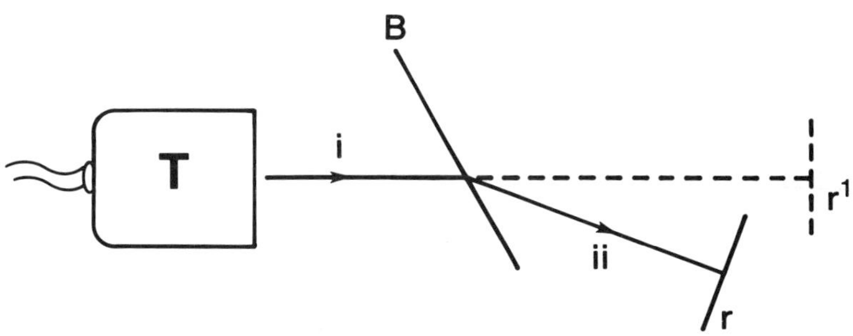

FIGURE 5–16. Refraction occurs when the ultrasound beam *(i)* from the transducer *(T)* interacts with the boundary *(B)* and is refracted *(ii)*. When the beam strikes a reflector (r^1), the ultrasound machine may display an incorrect position because of the refraction of the original ultrasound beam *(i)*.

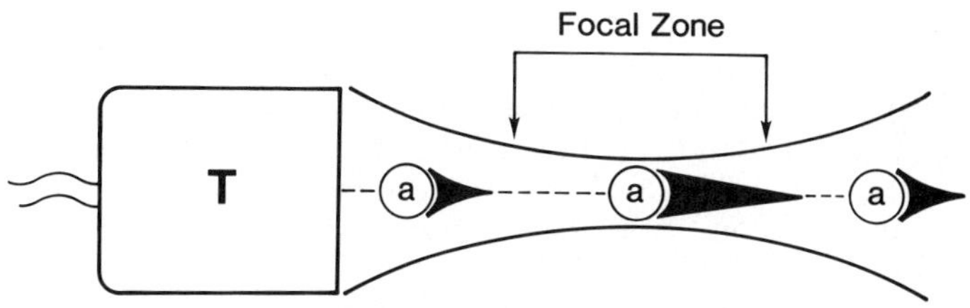

FIGURE 5–17. The focal zone of the transducer is important in interpreting the image. The same size reflector *(a)* generates a longer acoustic shadow when placed within the focal zone. *T*, Transducer.

tor separation required along the direction of the sound travel so that separate reflections will be produced. It depends on the spatial pulse length, which is the product of wavelength and the number of cycles in the pulse. The smaller the spatial pulse length, the better the axial resolution. This is a characteristic of a sound wave. The higher the frequency, the shorter the wavelength, resulting in less tissue penetration but better image quality. Conversely, visualizing deep structures requires more penetration and a lower frequency transducer. The operator should choose the highest frequency transducer that allows adequate penetration.

The focal zone is another aspect to consider. The distance from the surface to the scanned structure must be measured at the beginning of the scan and matched with the corresponding focal zone of the transducer. The focal zone of the transducer is expressed as a distance range at which the lateral resolution is optimal. Lateral resolution describes the minimal separation (in the direction perpendicular to the direction of the sound beam) between two reflectors. When the beam is scanned across the reflectors, two separate reflections are produced. Lateral resolution is equal to the beam diameter and varies with the distance from the transducer. The lateral separation between two reflectors must be greater than the beam diameter for them to be visualized as two separate structures. Accordingly, the optimal lateral resolution occurs within the focal zone.

The configuration of the transducer face is also an important factor. The transducer face should be small to allow scanning through the intercostal space. Linear arrays cannot be used to obtain transverse transrectal images. Finally, superficial structures are often not well seen with larger transducer faces because the sound beam is too wide near the transducer face.

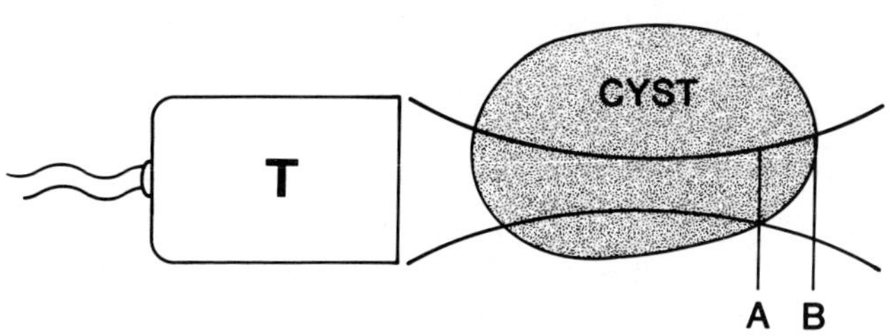

FIGURE 5–18. Slice thickness artifact occurs when the curved margin of the cyst makes the beam interact with both fluid and solid tissue at the same depth (between *A* and *B*) and the border is beyond the focal zone of the transducer *(T)*.

Imaging Conventions

Enough information regarding the plane of each scan must be provided by the ultrasound operator so that the image can be properly interpreted and reproduced. Certain conventions for image presentations have been established by the American Institute of Ultrasound in Medicine (AIUM). All transverse scans are oriented as if viewed from the patient's feet. With the patient supine, the patient's right side appears on the left of the image and the left side on the right. The anterior abdominal wall is at the upper portion of the image, and the posterior aspect of the patient is at the lower border of the image. Prone transverse images are oriented in the opposite manner, with the patient's left side on the left side of the image and the posterior portion in the upper part of the image. Longitudinal or sagittal scans are presented with the patient's head (cephalad) to the left of the image and the feet (caudal) to the right of the image in both the supine and the prone positions. Parasagittal views are labeled with an R (right) or L (left) followed by the number in centimeters from the midline.

Safety of Diagnostic Ultrasound

Vibratory motion of the particles of the medium and their interaction with the propagated ultrasound wave form the basis of diagnostic ultrasonography. A reversible rupture of the equilibrium of the medium originated by the ultrasound wave produces oscillatory changes in density and temperature of the medium. Generally, the tissue returns to its original equilibrium without suffering any damage when the sound stops. However, some irreversible absorption occurs. Absorption by the tissue results from the conversion of mechanical energy into heat. The amount of heat produced depends on the ultrasound intensity and the absorption coefficient of the medium. In living tissues, heat is dissipated by the effects of blood circulation. Within limits, this buffers any significant temperature increase.

Cavitation is another mechanism by which ultrasound can produce biologic effects in tissues. With higher intensity levels, drastic rupturing of the medium can occur. With large pressure fluctuations, bubbles are formed during rarefaction but decrease in size during the compression phase. If the intensity is not excessive, the bubbles grow and disappear during each cycle of the wave, resulting in a process of stable cavitation. If the intensity is very high, the bubbles accumulate and eventually implode with changes in temperature and pressure, causing damage to the tissue. In an aqueous medium, at the frequencies commonly used, cavitation occurs only at intensities greater than 10^6 W/m^2. The intensities needed to produce cavitation in more viscous media such as biologic tissue are greater than for aqueous media.

A nonthermal, noncavitational mechanism by which ultrasound can produce biologic effects exists. The intensity dependence and mechanism are not well defined. Nevertheless, information from in vitro and in vivo experimental studies and from epidemiology has yielded no known risk in the use of ultrasound in medical imaging.[5]

ULTRASONOGRAPHY IN ADULT UROLOGY

Renal Scanning Techniques and Normal Anatomy

Real-time ultrasonography not only facilitates the examination of the kidney, but also allows interventional procedures such as percutaneous nephrostomy or renal biopsy. A complete renal study should include transverse and longitudinal scans with the patient in both the decubitus and the supine position. The examination of the kidneys usually begins with a modified coronal approach. The right kidney is best imaged through the anterior axillary line in the supine or partial decubitus position, with the liver used as an acoustic window. The renal parenchyma usually is less echogenic than the liver. The right kidney can also be visualized in the prone position via the translumbar route. The left kidney is examined in the right lateral decubitus position, with the spleen used as an acoustic window. A prone position may also be used. Full inspiration may help in visualizing occult upper renal poles. The renal measurements obtained with ultrasound are more accurate than x-ray measurements because of the lack of magnification with ultrasound. The right kidney is between 8 and 14 cm in length and the left between 7 and 12.5 cm. Estimates of renal volume may be obtained by measuring the renal dimensions and using the formula for a prolate ellipse.[6] The outline of an adult normal kidney is smooth, showing a capsule with strong echoes because of the surrounding fat tissue and homogeneous low-intensity echoes corresponding to the renal cortex. The medulla is less echogenic than the cortex. An echogenic distinctive line representing the arcuate vessels may be detected between the cortex and the medulla. The thickness of the cortex and medulla ranges from 1.5 to 2 cm. The central sinus presents high-intensity echoes. The major component of the echoes within the sinus is the fat that surrounds the pelvis, infundibulum, and calyces. The hyperechogenic sinus is normally in continuity with the capsular echoes via a medial insertion. Normal calyces and ureters are not visible by ultrasound. When dilated, however, they can be seen as tubular structures. Vascular structures can also be seen within the sinus echoes (Figure 5–19).

Renal Transplantation

Developments in surgical techniques, immunosuppressive drugs, and modulation of immune reactions have made kidney transplantation the treatment of choice for end-stage renal failure.[7] The success of renal transplantation depends on preparation of the donor and recipient, surgical technique, and manipulation of the immune response. The comprehensive problems of the renal trans-

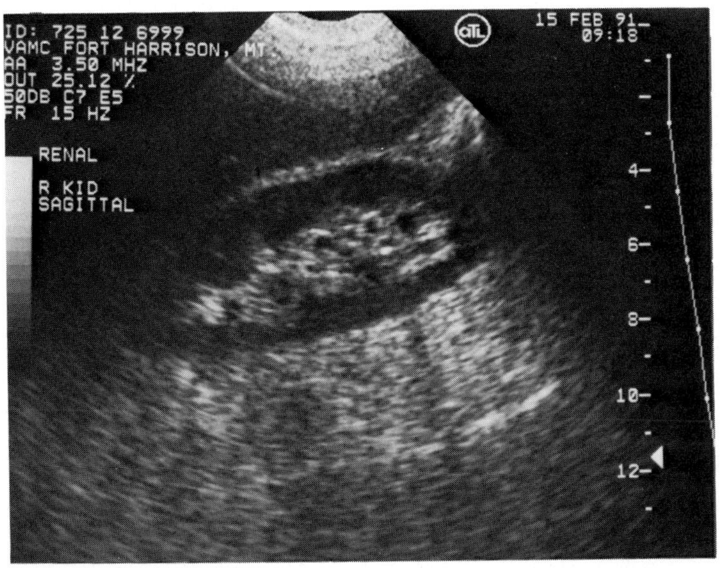

FIGURE 5–19. Sagittal ultrasound image of a normal kidney scanned with a 3.5 mHz transducer. The sinus fat surrounding the renal pelvis appears hyperechoic. The parenchyma of the kidney has a homogeneous low-intensity echo pattern.

plant patient are not addressed here. However, a variety of complications occur in renal transplant patients and ultrasound sometimes facilitates the diagnosis. Prompt diagnosis of complications, which may be difficult because of the immunosuppressed status of the transplant patient, may help preserve the renal function.

The donor kidney is usually placed extraperitoneally in the iliac fossa. This relatively superficial position of the kidney makes sonographic visualization easy. High-frequency transducers produce good-quality images. The normal renal parenchyma shows a poorly echogenic cortex and a distinctive corticomedullary junction. The medullary pyramids are hypoechoic, and a centrally distinct hyperechoic renal sinus is seen. Real-time ultrasound is useful to determine the long axis of the transplanted kidney and to recognize possible bowel loops obscuring the upper pole of the allograft. The wider view field of static B scanners offers a superior evaluation of the entire allograft bed and its length. The allograft undergoes compensatory hypertrophy.[8] Real-time ultrasound is effective in tracing the ureter and detecting the possible site of obstruction. Because of a smaller transducer surface area, a sector scanner allows greater angulation than static scanners.

Nuclear renography and ultrasound are the most commonly used tools for monitoring dysfunction in the posttransplant period. However, other modalities, including computerized tomography (CT) scans and magnetic resonance imaging (MRI), are being used with increasing frequency. Renal allograft rejection is a complex immunologic response of the host following exposure to incompatible donor histocompatibility antigens. With acute rejection, the allograft often becomes enlarged. The allograft becomes globular with distinct, enlarged hypoechoic medullary pyramids. Confluent sonolucencies may be seen in the parenchyma when areas of hemorrhagic infarction occur. The corticomedullary junction may be indistinct, and hilar echogenicity is decreased. These changes are seldom seen in acute tubular necrosis. Although these sonographic findings are not pathognomonic signs of acute rejection, they may be helpful in differentiating rejection from other causes of graft malfunction.[9] Duplex Doppler sonography[10] and renal angiography are useful diagnostic modalities for vascular complications. Duplex Doppler sonography has also been proposed for detection of acute renal transplant rejection. The accuracy varies widely in the literature, with a sensitivity range of 9% to 76%.[11,12]

Urologic complications can be a major cause of morbidity after renal transplantation. Early reports showed a higher incidence of these complications, but currently the incidence is less than 5%.[13] Ureteral obstruction has been reported to occur in 1% to 9.7% of transplant recipients.[14] Its incidence increases with time, reaching nearly 10% 5 years after transplantation. Ultrasonography typically demonstrates hydronephrosis with ureteral ectasia. Straiton and co-workers, in studying 439 renal transplants, verified the sensitivity of sonography in detecting hydronephrosis and found renal calyceal dilation to be a more reliable sign than renal pelvic dilation. In this study calyceal dilation was associated with obstruction in the majority of cases, whereas pelvic dilation was a relatively insignificant finding (Figure 5–20).[15] Urine leak at the ureteroneocystostomy site is a potential early complication of renal transplantation. Bladder fistulas have been reported in 0.6% to 4.4% of transplant recipients,[13] but ischemic injuries of the ureter are more common. Urine extravasation may form a urinoma. Symptoms include a decrease in urine output, swelling over the graft area with or without fever, ileus, and sepsis. The sonographic appearance of urinomas is largely nonspecific and does not differentiate urinoma from other peritransplant fluid collections such as lymphocele, hematoma, or abscess. Ultrasound-guided fluid aspiration may be useful (Figure 5–21).

One of the most common complications following renal transplantation is the development of a pelvic lymphocele. Inadequate ligation of the lymphatic channels around the allograft bed may produce lymph accumulation. Lymphoceles tend to occur 2 to 6 weeks after surgery, although they may develop at any time. Lymphoceles vary in size. When large, they may cause ipsilateral lower extremity edema because of compression on the iliac vein. A mass effect may also induce renal impairment with hydronephrosis and bladder compression. On ultrasonograms lymphoceles are cystic masses, often lobular in shape. They frequently contain thin internal interfaces. Percutaneous aspiration under sonographic guidance can be both diagnostic and therapeutic in some patients (Figure 5–22).

Hematomas may be present during the immediate posttransplant period as a consequence of vascular leak or secondary to tearing of the renal capsule during an episode of severe acute rejection with swelling of the allograft. Recent hematomas can be moderately echogenic because of organized clot. Old hematomas often contain irregular septations with relatively hypoechoic areas corresponding to areas of fibrinolysis (Figure 5–23).

Renal Masses

Renal imaging has been enhanced by the introduction of ultrasound, CT, and MRI. Smith and associates detected an increase of almost five times in the detection rate of renal tumors 3 cm or smaller when they compared the periods 1974-1977 and 1982-1985.[16] MRI offers several advantages, such as the determination of tumor location, assessment of vascular patency, detection of lymph node metastasis, and evaluation of direct tumor extension

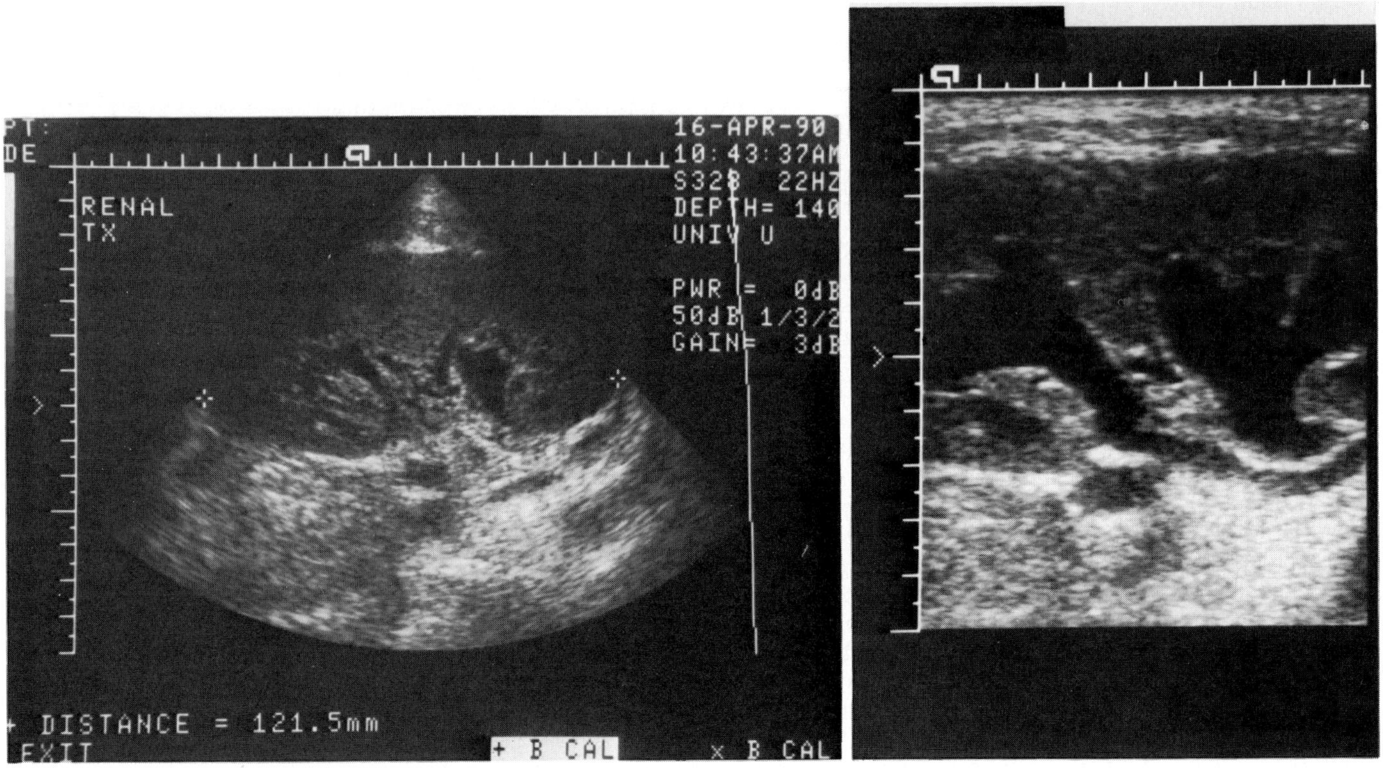

A B

FIGURE 5–20. Progressive hydronephrosis in a transplanted kidney with a duplicated collecting system. **A,** The kidney 1 month after transplant shows no hydronephrosis. **B,** The ultrasound image taken 2 months later shows hydronephrosis with a dilated collecting system and ureter.

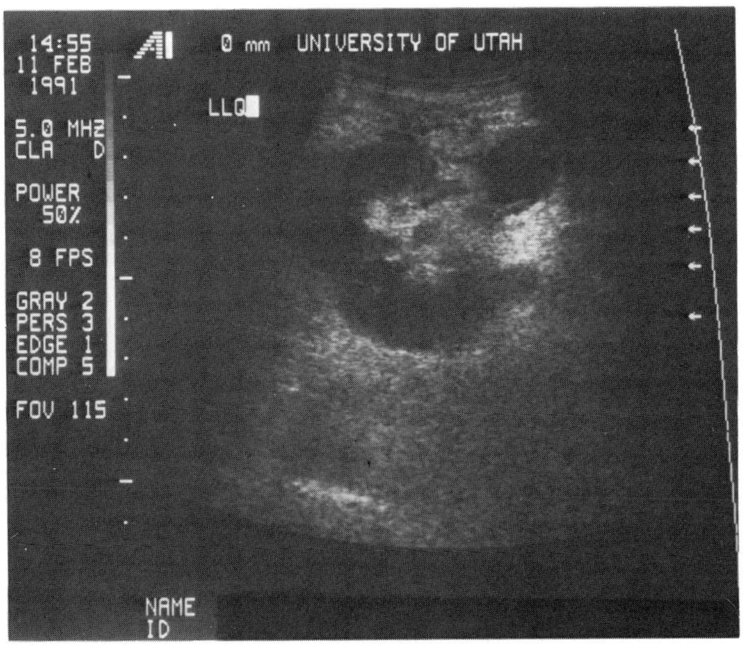

FIGURE 5–21. Transverse image of a transplanted kidney 3 months after surgery. The upper right portion shows an anechoic area from a urinoma produced by a leak at the ureterovesical anastomosis.

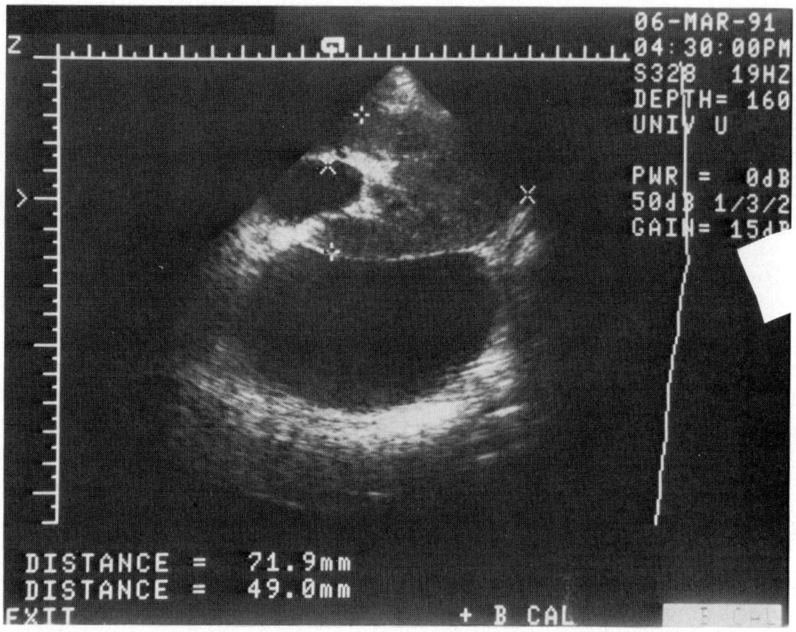

FIGURE 5–22. Large lymphocele surrounding a transplanted kidney. Dilation of the renal pelvis resulting from compression of the ureter is evident.

into adjacent organs. Nevertheless, contrast-enhanced CT is more sensitive than MRI in demonstrating solid lesions less than 3 cm in diameter.[17,18] Recent developments in Doppler ultrasonography have made it useful in the differential diagnosis of hypervascular renal masses. A peak systolic Doppler shift frequency of 2.5 kHz or greater represents neovascularity.[19,20]

Most renal masses prove to be simple renal cysts, but renal tumors must be excluded from the diagnosis. Masses as small as 1 cm are visualized by ultrasound. Simple renal cysts have a characteristic sonographic appearance, including an anechoic internal structure, a round or oval shape, a smooth, sharply defined wall, and acoustic enhancement beyond the posterior wall (Figure 5–24).

Cysts commonly arise from the cortical portion of the kidney, but parapelvic cysts may be confused with hydronephrosis. The identification of normal calyces not communicating with the cyst helps to establish the diagnosis.

Complex cysts are those with cystic and solid components. They may be seen with necrotic hypernephroma, but multilocular cysts, hemorrhagic cysts, and abscess can present the same sonographic appearance. On the ultrasonogram they show mixed internal echoes and a poorly defined

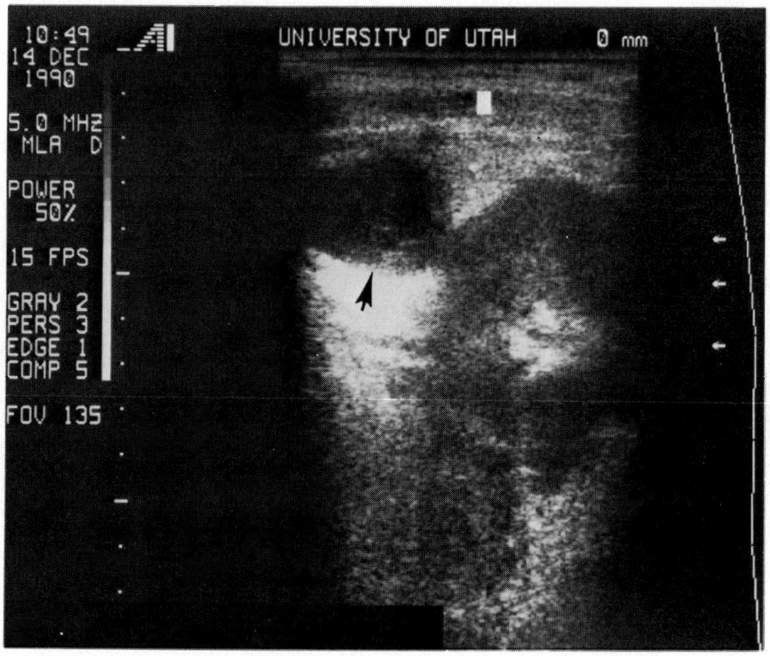

FIGURE 5–23. Transverse view of a transplanted kidney with a hematoma at the lower pole *(arrow)*.

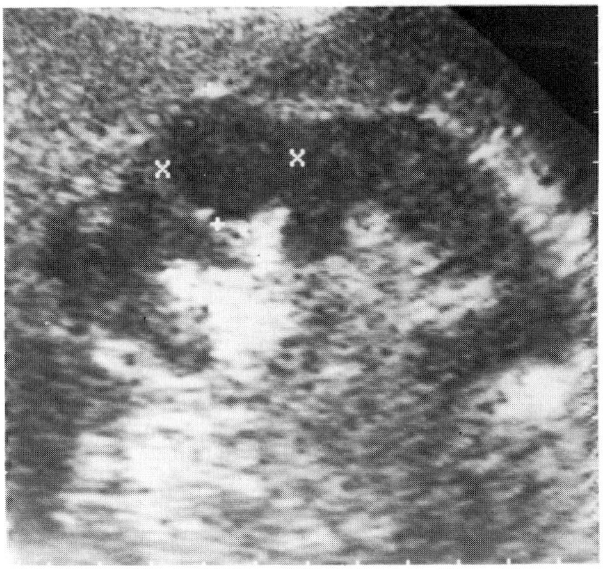

FIGURE 5–24. Simple renal cyst seen in longitudinal projection. There are no internal echo structures, and the wall is smooth and round.

thickened wall that may be calcified or have multilocular septations.

Solid masses can be hyperechoic, isoechoic, or hypoechoic when compared with normal renal tissue. Areas of hemorrhage and necrosis show low echogenicity. Usually, the more vascular a tumor, the greater the number of interfaces and the more echogenicity. Overall, however, the echogenicity of a solid mass does not directly correlate with vascularity. When large masses are present, neoplastic replacement of tissue does not allow echo comparison with normal structures. The outline and size of the kidney, as well as comparison with adjacent structures, facilitates the diagnosis. In a prospective study Warshauer and co-workers found that ultrasonography excretory urography, and linear tomography had similar sensitivity for detection of renal masses 3 cm or more in diameter. For lesions less than 3 cm but greater than 2 cm, ultrasound, unlike excretory urography, maintained a high sensitivity when compared with CT. When lesions between 1 cm and 2 cm were evaluated, ultrasound diagnosed 60% of CT-confirmed lesions (Figure 5–25).[21]

Renal adenocarcinomas are the most common malignancy of the kidney in adults, and their echo structure may vary from hyperechogenic to hypoechogenic. Lymphomas tend to be more hypoechoic than the normal renal parenchyma because of their uniform cellularity. Perirenal masses and retroperitoneal lymphadenopathy are commonly seen.

Angiomyolipomas have some unique sonographic characteristics. The fatty components within the angiomyolipoma often demonstrate a well-defined hyperechoic mass, although this is not always detected and could be confused with an echogenic renal cell carcinoma. CT is useful in diagnosing angiomyolipoma. An intrarenal well-defined mass with a density similar to that of adjacent retroperitoneal fat is pathognomonic.[22]

Oncocytomas are usually considered benign tumors and are often found incidentally. Ultrasound does not differentiate them from renal carcinoma, although oncocytomas are usually well-defined, homogeneous solid masses of moderate echogenicity. CT demonstrates a homogeneous mass that may have a central low-density linear scar.

Stones

Plain film of the abdomen should be the initial study obtained in patients with suspected nephrolithiasis, since more than 90% of urinary calculi are radiopaque. The radiodensity of stones varies with the chemical composition. Magnesium ammonium phosphate (struvite) and cystine stones are

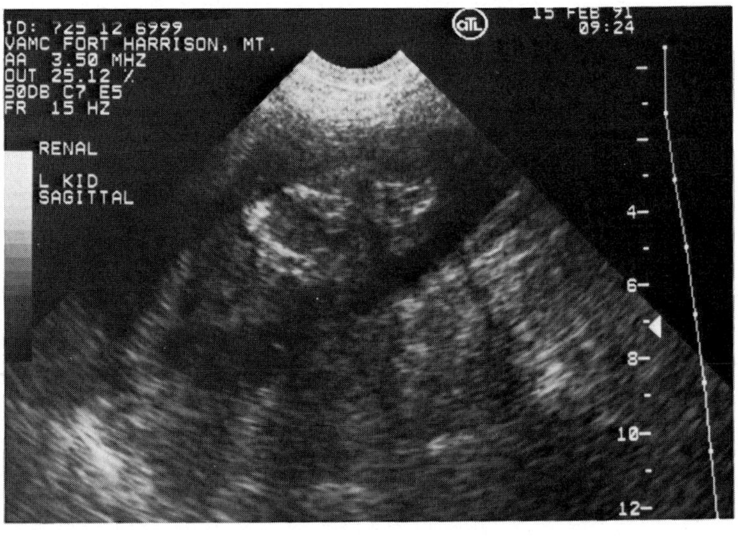

FIGURE 5–25. Solid mass occupying the central portion of the kidney. The mass has a mixed echo pattern, which is characteristic of renal cell carcinoma.

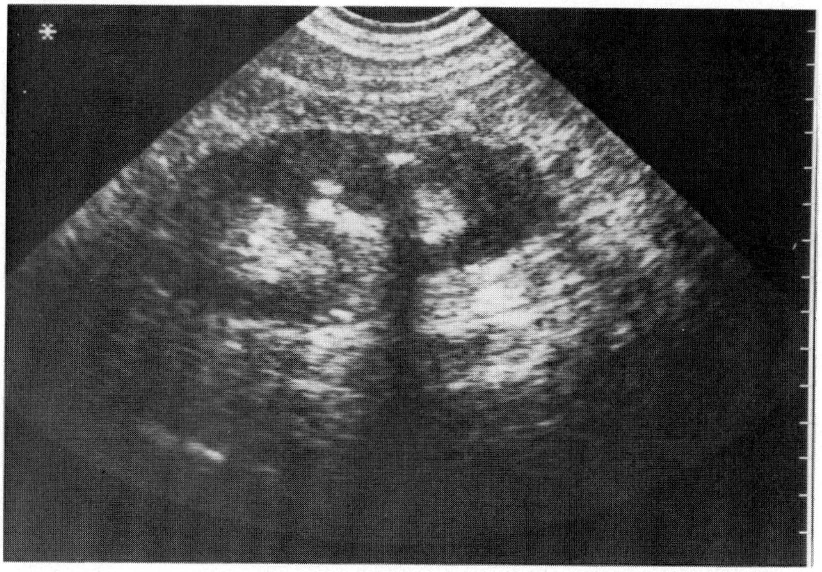

FIGURE 5–26. Small stone in the lower pole of the right kidney. The reflective stone produces obvious shadowing, which makes the diagnosis easier.

often less radiopaque than calcium oxalate or calcium phosphate (apatite) stones. Pure uric acid or matrix calculi are considered truly radiolucent. Kidney-ureter-bladder radiography documents the number, size, and location of all stones. Intravenous pyelography helps determine the exact location of the stone, the presence of hydronephrosis, delay in excretion of the contrast medium, and indirectly, the renal function. Retrograde pyelography can be useful in defining the exact anatomy of the urinary system.

Ultrasonography may provide useful additional information in patients with known or suspected renal stones. The ultrasonographer can assess the amount of parenchyma present in an obstructed kidney, identify radiolucent calculi, and detect perirenal extravasation or perirenal abscesses. Regardless of their chemical composition, calculi are dense and highly reflective of the ultrasound beam, generating an intense echogenic focus associated with a distal acoustic shadow (Figure 5–26). Renal calculi are usually located in the highly reflective central echoes of the renal sinus. If the stone does not reach a sufficient size to produce acoustic shadowing or if no obstruction is present, diagnosis may be difficult. In general, however, most stones within the kidney, even those as small as a few millimeters, are identifiable with ultrasonography. This can be helpful in establishing the diagnosis in patients who have radiolucent filling defects within the renal pelvis.

Some lithotripters use ultrasonography for stone localization. The accuracy, lack of radioactive exposure, and ability to maintain real-time imaging are advantages. Although spreading of the acoustic shadow and motion of the stone with shock waves are helpful indicators, however, adequacy of stone fragmentation is difficult to assess with ultrasound. Moreover, stones in the ureter are difficult to visualize (Figure 5–27).

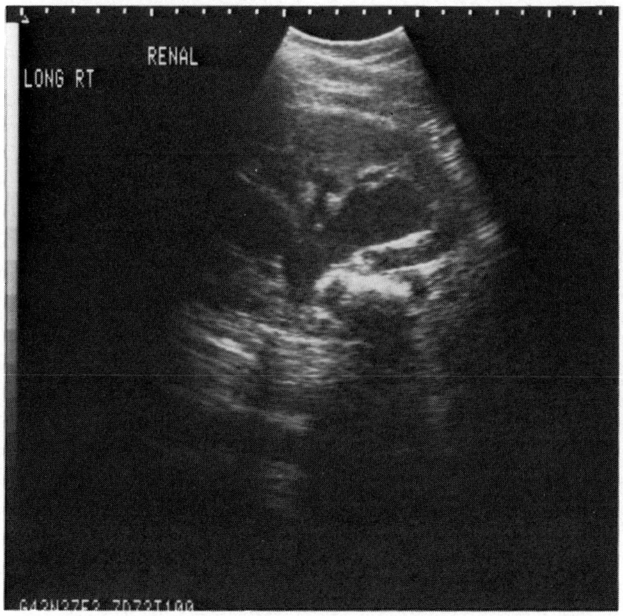

FIGURE 5–27. Large stone in the upper ureter causing hydronephrosis. The dilated collecting system and the intense shadowing behind the stone are evident.

Urinary Bladder

The fluid-filled urinary bladder can be easily visualized with ultrasonography and can be scanned via a transabdominal, transurethral, or transrectal approach. The marked mismatch in acoustic impedance that occurs at the level of the fluid-filled bladder may cause some artifacts such as slice thickness and reverberation. The bladder should always be examined in a distended state unless the postvoiding residual urine is to be measured. The contrast provided by the urine allows visualization of tumors, calculi, blood clots, ureteroceles, and diverticula, as well as volume determinations. Ultrasonography therefore provides useful information about the bladder in a noninvasive manner.

Bladder calculi and blood clots can usually be diagnosed without difficulty. They appear as echogenic structures within the anechoic fluid-filled bladder and change in position as the patient's position is altered. The acoustic shadow from stones differentiates them from blood clots. Detection of a ureterocele should prompt renal scanning to rule out hydronephrosis. Extrinsic masses adjacent to the bladder such as cervical, colon, or prostatic carcinomas, perivesical abscesses, hematomas, or urinomas are well visualized by ultrasonography. With an extravesical neoplasm invading the bladder, the bladder may be fixed in association with the primary tumor. If the trigone is involved, a dilated lower ureter at the site of the ureteral orifice may be seen. With real-time ultrasound a urine jet may be observed when the ureter expels urine into the fluid-filled bladder.

Ultrasonography is valuable in assessment of the bladder neck. Detrusor sphincter dyssynergia appears as a round, narrowed bladder neck that does not open when the detrusor sphincter contracts. This can be assessed by urodynamic studies with ultrasonography. The resected area following transurethral prostatic resection can be accurately determined. The presence of a significant median lobe acting as a valvular mechanism against the bladder neck can be easily diagnosed through a transrectal or transabdominal approach (Figure 5–28).

Noninvasive ultrasound techniques to estimate residual urine can replace catheterization. Urine volume may be accurately estimated by a variety of elaborate planimetric methods. Poston, Joseph, and Riddle[23] assumed the shape of the postmicturition bladder to be a rectangle-based prism and then altered the final coefficient based on catheterization volumes. With the formula $0.7 \times (H \times D \times W)$, where H is the largest superoinferior dimension in the sagittal plane, D is the largest anteroposterior dimension in the sagittal plane, and W is the maximum transverse diameter in the transverse plane, urinary residual volumes can be estimated with an accuracy adequate for most purposes. Birch, Hurst, and Doule noted that geometric formulas are difficult to apply to patients with bladder outflow obstruction because of the variations in bladder shape.[24] Keily and associates found a mean error of 8% of true urinary bladder volume with a standard deviation of 23%, although the mean error was 4.5% with a standard deviation of 23% when the true volume was less than 400 ml.[25] The use of transrectal linear array has been proposed to measure bladder volumes of 5 to 200 ml. In one study the mean error was 16% when two sagittal bladder diameters were used in the formula: Volume in milliliters = $5.3 \times (\text{Height} \times \text{Depth}) - 21$.[26] Several portable ultrasound scanners that automatically determine bladder volume also have proved to be reasonably accurate.[27]

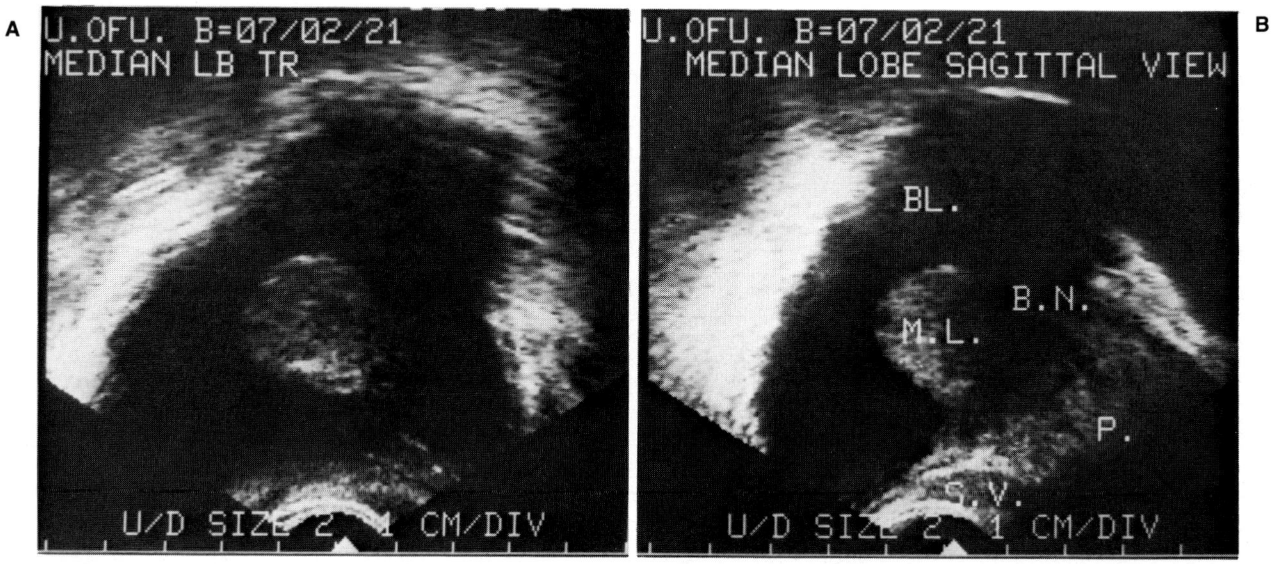

FIGURE 5–28. Large median lobe of the prostate viewed with transrectal ultrasound. **A,** The transverse image shows a floating appearance of the median lobe. **B,** On a sagittal image the median lobe can be seen surrounded by the residual urine in the bladder *(BL)*. The bladder neck *(BN)* and the lateral lobes of the prostate *(P)* are evident.

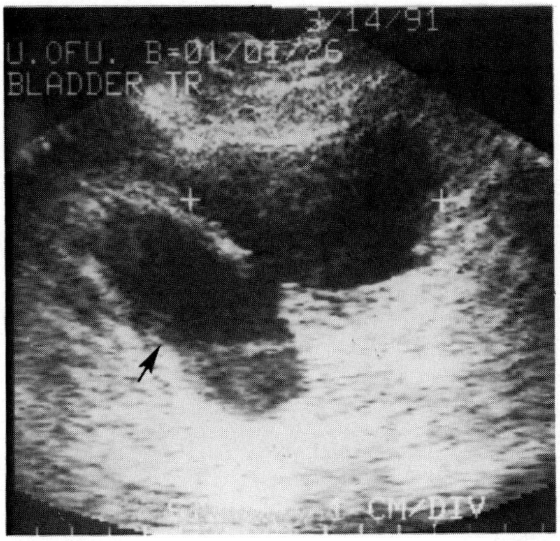

FIGURE 5–29. Large bladder diverticulum *(arrow)*. The ostium is relatively narrow.

Bladder Diverticula

A bladder diverticulum is a sac of variable size that results from herniation of bladder mucosa through the muscular wall. Bladder diverticula can be either congenital or acquired. Congenital diverticula are often large, solitary, and located near the ureteral orifice and usually are not associated with infravesical obstruction or neurologic disease. Acquired diverticula result from lower urinary tract obstruction and can be seen in both adults and children. Diverticula greater than 2 cm in diameter can usually be seen by ultrasound, and occasionally the ostium may be detected (Figure 5–29).

Postvoiding scans demonstrate the emptying capacity of the diverticulum. Since stasis is common, stones may be identified. The incidence of transitional cell carcinoma within diverticula is approximately 3% to 6.7% higher than in the normal bladder.[28] The neoplasms are seen sonographically as intradiverticular echogenic masses without acoustic shadowing and do not move with changes in patient position.

Bladder Tumors

Although ultrasonography is not a primary modality in the evaluation of transitional cell carcinoma of the bladder, it can be useful for detection and staging in some cases. Superficial bladder tumors are usually exophytic and papillary. By ultrasound, they show an increased or mixed echogenic pattern with protrusion from the bladder wall into the distended bladder lumen. The bladder wall is usually well defined, highly echogenic, and 3 to 6 mm thick. With superficial tumors it remains intact and does not change in thickness or echogenicity. The echogenic mass of a bladder tumor remains fixed when the patient's position is altered, which helps to differentiate between tumors and blood clots or debris (Figure 5–30).

The false positive rate for the detection of bladder cancer by transabdominal ultrasound has been reported to be about 10%, with the diagnostic accuracy depending primarily on the size of the tumor, bladder distention, the location of the tumor, and the operator's skill.[29] Tumor size seems to be the most important factor; detection ranges from 33.3% for tumors less than 0.5 cm in diameter to 95% for those larger than 2 cm.[30] In some series, however, size has not been an essential diagnostic factor.[31] Bladder tumors in the anterior wall and in the dome of the bladder may be difficult to recognize with ultrasound.

When the tumor infiltrates the bladder wall, ultrasound may show distortion in the contour of the bladder with fixation, a decrease in wall mobility, and increased thickness of the detrusor muscle at the level of the tumor. If the tumor extends beyond the bladder wall, an echogenic mass may be seen contrasting with the perivesical tissue.

Transrectal ultrasound has been useful in the detection of prostatic involvement with transitional cell carcinoma of the bladder. The prostatic urethra is the area most commonly involved. Endoscopy and biopsy are the most useful methods of examination. However, in many cases the transitional cell carcinoma involves areas not seen by endoscopy such as prostatic stroma, ejaculatory ducts, seminal vesicles, or periprostatic tissues. Terris, Villers, and Freiha found that transrectal ultrasound had a low sensitivity for detection of transitional cell carcinoma of the prostatic urethra.

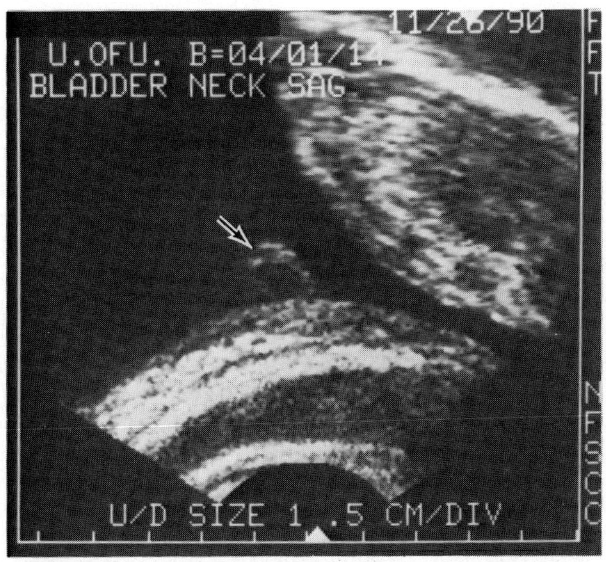

FIGURE 5–30. Superficial bladder tumor arising from the distal trigone near the bladder neck as seen on a transrectal ultrasound image. The bladder wall *(arrow)* shows no distortion or irregularity.

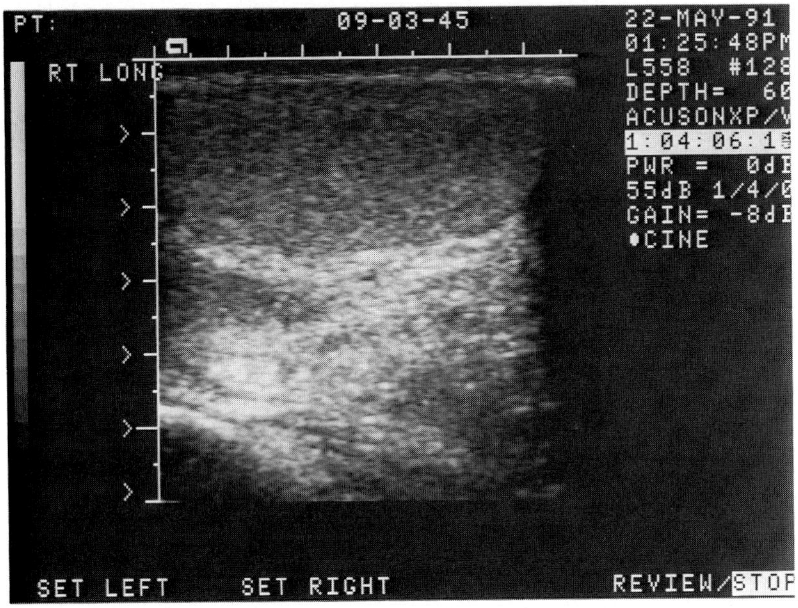

FIGURE 5–31. Normal testis viewed with a longitudinal image. The testicular parenchyma is homogeneous.

However, hypoechoic lesions of the prostate gland in patients undergoing radical cystoprostatectomy must prompt suspicion of either transitional cell carcinoma or prostate adenocarcinoma in patients with known bladder cancer.[32]

Staging of bladder tumors depends on excretory urography, cystoscopy with biopsies, and bimanual examination under anesthesia. Errors with these methods are due mainly to understaging.[33] MRI may be more accurate than CT in staging bladder carcinomas and is therefore probably the best noninvasive imaging technique for staging.[34,35] Transabdominal ultrasound is less useful, and transurethral ultrasound staging of bladder tumors has not fulfilled early promises of accuracy.

Testes

Ultrasound is a sensitive method for detecting testicular abnormalities that could otherwise be clinically dubious. Masses as small as a few millimeters in diameter can be seen with ultrasound. The proximity of the testis to the scrotal skin permits the use of high-frequency real-time transducers with optimal resolution.

The normal testis measures approximately 4 × 3 × 3 cm. In an adult male a small amount of fluid, which is anechoic by ultrasound, is normally found between the visceral and parietal layers of the tunica vaginalis. If excess fluid collects, it forms a hydrocele. Hydroceles may be idiopathic or associated with prior trauma, infection, or neoplasm. Transillumination frequently establishes the diagnosis, but ultrasound helps determine the characteristics of the testis and rule out an intratesticular mass.

The tunica albuginea appears as a thin hyperechoic layer surrounding the testis. In the parenchyma of a normal testis, a homogeneous medium-level echogenicity can be identified (Figure 5–31). However, the echo pattern of the testicular parenchyma is not always homogeneous. The mediastinum of the testis appears as an echogenic line parallel to the epididymis. Axial scans using pulsed Doppler sonography have also described hypoechoic intratesticular bands in the middle third of the testicle. This correlates with a normal variant of intratesticular vessels and has no apparent clinical significance.[36]

The epididymis lies along the posterolateral aspect of the testis and usually has the same or a slightly more echogenic appearance than the testicular parenchyma. The head of the epididymis produces high-amplitude, coarse echoes. Spermatoceles typically arise near the head of the epididymis and are seen as a cystic anechoic mass, clearly separable from the upper pole of the testis. In epididymitis the epididymis is edematous, prominent, and thicker than the normal 7 to 8 mm width. Decreased echogenicity is often observed, and the epididymis is more sonolucent. The inflammatory process may also affect the testicular parenchyma (Figure 5–32). In orchitis, abnormal ultrasound echoes may be present within the testis. The clinical presentation and the ultrasound scan help in the differential diagnosis of testis tumors, although sometimes the findings are not characteristic. In chronic epididymitis, focal or generalized thickening with a coarsened texture and increased echogenicity may make difficult the differential diagnosis with a tumor. If a cleavage plane between the epididymis and the testis is not seen on ultrasound, a neoplasm cannot be excluded.

Varicoceles are dilated veins of the pampiniform plexus that usually lie posterolateral to the testis and are more common on the left side. The normal veins of the spermatic cord are no greater than 2

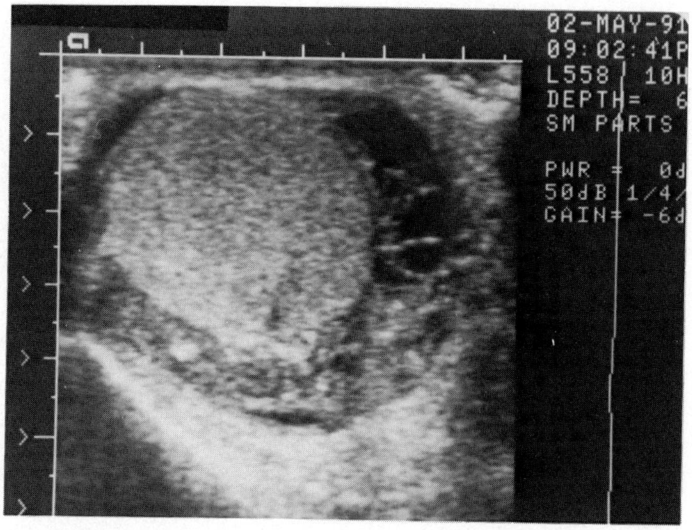

FIGURE 5–32. Ultrasound image showing epididymitis. The epididymis is thickened and has scattered hypoechoic areas.

mm in caliber, whereas varicoceles may distend to 5 or 6 mm in diameter, especially with the Valsalva maneuver or in the upright position. Ultrasound demonstrates tubular and circular sonolucencies that increase in size during the Valsalva maneuver. In addition, duplex Doppler ultrasound can detect venous flow.

Testicular torsion requires prompt diagnosis and treatment. Nuclear scanning has had a paramount role in the evaluation of equivocal cases of acute testicular torsion. However, advances in pulsed Doppler and color-coded duplex sonography provide new technical approaches in the diagnosis of testicular torsion. Doppler sonography was correlated with scintigraphy and surgery in several studies in patients with acute torsion of the scrotum.[37-39] Doppler sonography was shown to be at least as accurate as testicular scintigraphy and provided a rapid and noninvasive method for assessing testicular perfusion.

Testicular ultrasound, when readily available, is indicated in many cases of blunt scrotal trauma. Ultrasound may establish the diagnosis of hematocele, intratesticular hematoma, or testicular rupture in patients with blunt scrotal trauma when scrotal swelling makes the physical examination difficult.[40] Ultrasound may increase the ability to diagnose and treat parenchymal injuries that could otherwise result in loss of the testis.[41]

Testis Tumors

Most testicular malignancies are of germ cell origin. Early diagnosis remains an important factor in survival, and ultrasound may be of value in both the detection of nonpalpable lesions and the evaluation of the contralateral testis. Bilateral tumors have been reported in approximately 2% to 3% of patients with testis tumors.

Ultrasound has a 90% to 100% accuracy in differentiating between intratesticular and extratesticular masses.[42] Intratesticular tumors appear as focal areas of disorganized texture that are usually hypoechoic. All intratesticular lesions should be considered potentially malignant, whereas extratesticular lesions are usually inflammatory or traumatic.

Marth and associates found that ultrasound could distinguish cell type (seminoma versus nonseminomatous) in 70% of tumors. Seminomas typically appear as homogeneous, hypoechogenic, and sharply delineated masses (Figure 5–33). Nonseminomatous tumors are less well circumscribed, inhomogeneous, and hypoechoic. They may have a normal echo pattern or appear as a hyperechoic mass with cysts and calcifications.[43] The sonographic pattern is not always characteristic.[44] Infection and trauma must be excluded when echogenic areas do not show the hypoechogenicity usually associated with tumors. Diffuse testicular tumors may have a homogeneous parenchymal pattern that is incorrectly interpreted as normal unless the normal side is scanned for comparison. Asymmetry in echo amplitude is noted when the two sides are compared (Figure 5–34). Leukemic and lymphomatous involvement of the testis shows decreased echogenicity in a diffuse or focal pattern.

Prostate Gland

Transrectal ultrasonography and MRI have emerged as the best imaging modalities for the prostate gland. Interpretation of transrectal ultrasonography requires a precise understanding of prostate anatomy. The accuracy of ultrasonography depends on demonstration of internal prostatic architecture. In turn, improvements in technology and wider use of ultrasonography have increased knowledge of prostate anatomy.

In 1968 McNeal reported for the first time the existence of histologic heterogeneity in the glandular tissue of the prostate gland.[45] This histologic variation causes differences in the reflection of

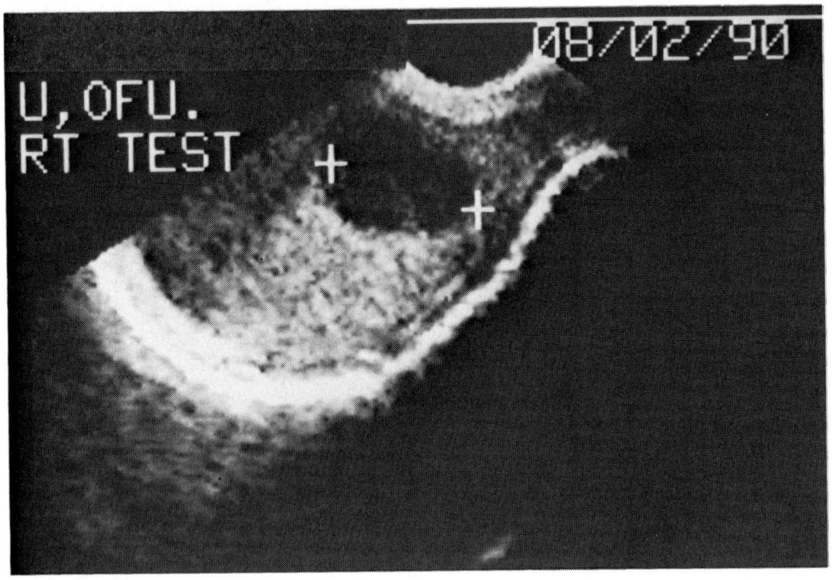

FIGURE 5–33. Hypoechoic intratesticular lesions that proved to be seminoma.

sound waves, allowing identification of these various zones by ultrasonography. The tissue immediately surrounding the ejaculatory duct, referred to as the central zone, consists of large acinar glands with irregular contour, numerous ridges, or septa projecting into the lumen. The epithelial cells appear crowded, with large nuclei at different levels. McNeal proposed that the central zone was embryologically of wolffian duct origin, whereas the remainder of the prostate arose from the urogenital sinus. The central zone corresponds to approximately 25% of the glandular prostate. It appears to be the site of origin of only 5% to 10% of prostate cancers. Lee and associates have stated that the entrance of the seminal vesicles and vasa deferentia into the central zone produces a site of anatomic weakness where a capsular covering is absent.[46] They believe that the absence of capsule in this region allows early extraprostatic dissemination of prostate cancer. This finding has not yet been confirmed.

The peripheral zone of the prostate gland is composed of small, round, regular acini with smooth walls. The epithelium is simple columnar with pale cells and basal small nuclei. The peripheral zone makes up nearly 70% of a normal prostate gland and is the origin of 70% to 80% of prostate adenocarcinomas. McNeal also described a cylindrical sphincter of smooth muscle that surrounds the urethra from the upper end of the verumontanum proximally to the bladder neck. The transition zone is immediately lateral and ventral to this sphincter. The histologic appearance and architecture of the transition zone closely resemble those of the peripheral zone, but the glandular tissue lies anterior and closely follows the course of the sphincter toward the bladder neck. The transition zone constitutes less than 5% of the normal prostate gland and

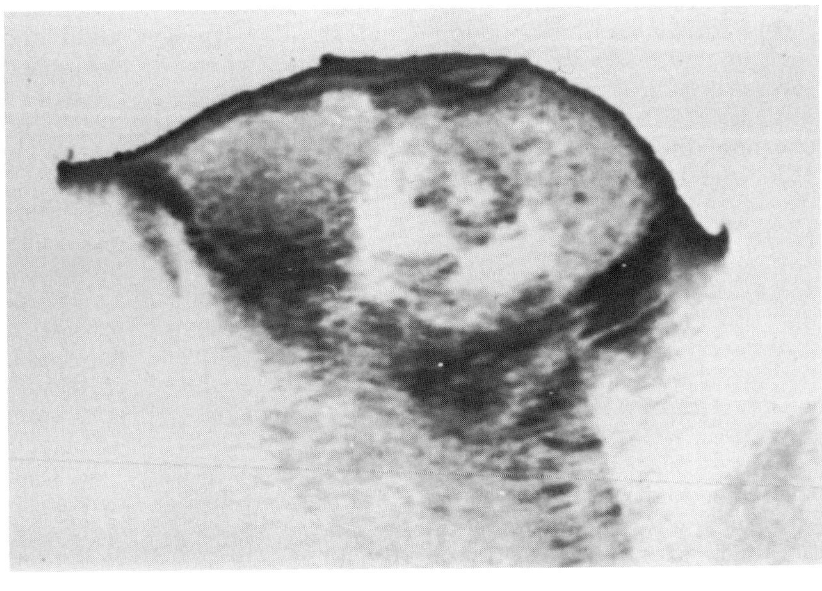

FIGURE 5–34. Intratesticular mass with irregular outline and a mixed echo pattern. Histologic study showed a teratocarcinoma.

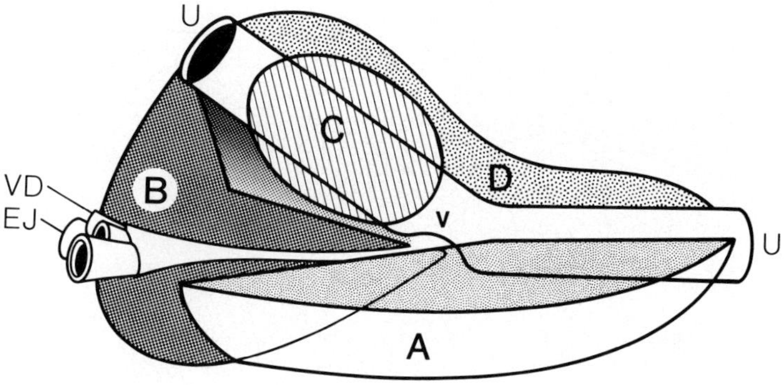

FIGURE 5–35. McNeal's zonal anatomy of the prostate gland in sagittal view. *A*, Peripheral zone; *B*, central zone; *C*, transitional zone; *D*, anterior fibromuscular stroma; *U*, urethra; *v*, verumontanum; *VD*, vas deferens; *EJ*, ejaculatory ducts.

is the site of origin of benign prostatic hyperplasia (BPH). Some 10% to 20% of prostate cancers arise in the transition zone. Because of their central location, transition zone tumors often are nonpalpable and probably account for most stage A tumors.

The final zone described by McNeal corresponds to the anterior fibromuscular stroma. Because this region at the anterior surface of the prostate gland is nonglandular, it is not thought to be a site of origin for prostate cancer (Figure 5–35).

Prostate Volume Calculation

Estimation of prostate size is important in routine urologic practice, since it may influence the selection of therapy for BPH, determine the prostatic response to hormonal, radiation, or drug therapy,[47] or help in the interpretation of prostate specific antigen values. In the follow-up of patients treated for prostatitis, prostatic volume determinations may assist in determining response to treatment.[48] Transrectal ultrasound provides a safe method for repeated assessments of the prostate gland. When used to compare prostatic volume calculations obtained by ultrasound and pathology in 100 cadaveric prostate glands, transrectal ultrasound showed a high degree of correlation unless there was an unconfined prostate cancer with poorly defined boundary echoes.[49]

Transabdominal ultrasound scanning is a simple, noninvasive, relatively accurate method to obtain prostate volumes.[50] In a recent study, different sonographic formulas to estimate prostatic volume were compared and evaluated on 150 pathologic specimens obtained from radical prostatectomies and radical cystoprostatectomies. The prolate spheroid volume calculation, based on the assumption that the prostate gland is a prolate spheroid (oblong), uses the formula pi/6(Major transverse dimension)^2 × Anteroposterior dimension. This formula does not require the cephalocaudal dimension, which generates a large portion of the errors when the ellipsoid formula pi/6(Transverse diameter × Anteroposterior diameter × Cephalocaudal diameter) is used. The same authors correlated the different formulas with different real prostatic volumes and concluded that the prolate spheroid formula was the best one to estimate prostate glands weighing less than 80 g. However, the spherical formula pi/6(Transverse dimension)^3 was most accurate for glands weighing more than 80 g.[51]

Echo Pattern of Normal Prostatic Tissue

The anatomic distinction between the central and the peripheral zone generally is not imaged by ultrasound, despite their histologic differences. Normal central and peripheral zones usually are seen as a homogeneous isoechoic area in the posterior sections of the prostate gland. Their normal echo pattern is used as a reference for defining other structures as hypoechoic or hyperechoic.

When a transrectal probe is used, the anteriorly located transition zone is moderately hypoechoic. Frequently, however, a mixed echo pattern is seen, making interpretation difficult. The transition zone can occupy as much as 90% of the prostate volume in a man with significant BPH. A clear distinction is seen between the peripheral and transition zones, and a sharp, hypoechoic boundary divides the zones. This corresponds to the surgical capsule of the prostate gland and can easily be seen in both transverse and parasagittal planes (Figure 5–36).

Although the capsule of the prostate is not a true anatomic capsule, it is usually defined as a relatively hyperechoic area surrounding the peripheral zone. The capsule has some thickness, usually attributed to a combination of capsular fibers and periprostatic fat. Corpora amylacea are present most often in the acini of the central zone surrounding the ejaculatory duct. They are seen as hyperechoic areas and are important landmarks for locating the verumontanum. Prostatic calculi produce a hyperechoic area with a shadow. The prostatic urethra distal to the verumontanum can be traced with high-resolution transducers as a slightly hypoechoic area compared with the surrounding peripheral zone.

Prostatitis

Acute prostatitis typically produces symptoms of local heat, tenderness, inflammation of the gland, urinary frequency, urgency, fever, and chills. The prostatic fluid contains leukocytes, and the infect-

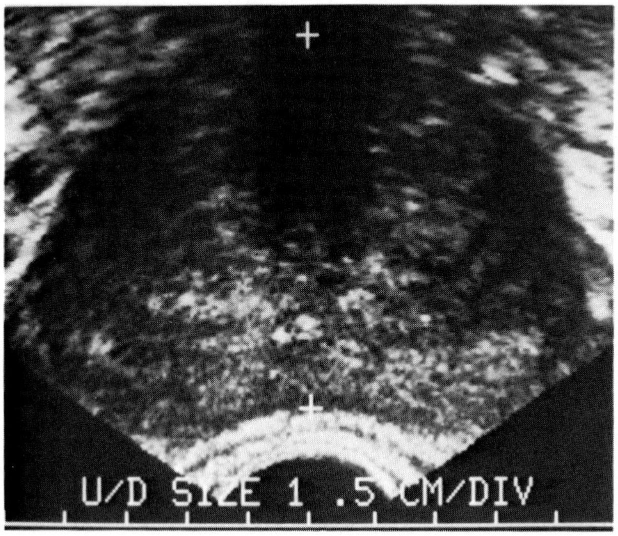

FIGURE 5–36. Transrectal ultrasound image of a normal prostate gland. The gland is symmetric and shows a homogeneous peripheral zone. The transitional zone has a characteristic mixed echo pattern. The urethra appears as a hypoechoic area in the midportion of the prostate.

ing organism can often be grown on culture.[52,53] Transrectal ultrasound of the prostate may show enlargement of the gland but with preservation of symmetry and capsular regularity. The parenchyma may have a markedly low-intensity echogenicity, although this finding is not specific. Ultrasonography may be useful in the follow-up of the treated patient and to rule out abscesses.

Chronic bacterial prostatitis often has a less characteristic clinical presentation and a more indolent course. As with acute prostatitis, no specific sonographic signs establish the diagnosis. However, seven ultrasound features that appear to correlate with a diagnosis of chronic prostatitis have been described: high-density echoes representing corpora amylacea, midrange echoes associated with inflammation, fibrosis, echolucent zones, capsular irregularity and thickening, ejaculatory duct calcification, and periurethral irregularity.[54] Local antibiotic instillation by sonographic needle guidance has been described as a treatment alternative in patients with chronic prostatitis.[55]

Benign Prostatic Hyperplasia

BPH develops primarily from bilateral nodular expansion of the transition zone. In the transition zone most nodules are glandular in origin, whereas those arising in the periurethral tissue are usually derived from stromal tissue. Although periurethral nodules increase in number and volume with age, they grow much more slowly than those originating in the transitional zone.[45] The size of the transition zone has been measured by transrectal ultrasound in patients with or without BPH. In patients without BPH the mean size of the transition zone was 6.14 ± 3.2 g, compared with 24.81 ± 14.4 g in the BPH group.[56]

In patients with BPH, ultrasound shows the prostate gland to be diffusely enlarged with a rounded appearance. The greatest increase in size occurs in the anteroposterior diameter. These anatomic modifications allow use of the spherical formula (transverse dimension^3) to estimate prostatic volumes when the gland weighs more than 80 g.[51] The peripheral zone becomes compressed against the pseudocapsule of the prostatic gland. The transition zone is moderately hypoechoic when compared with the peripheral zone. The proximal periurethral tissues containing longitudinal smooth muscle fibers are highly hypoechoic.

When BPH occurs, the transition zone tends to become progressively distinct and hypoechoic, sometimes presenting a mixed echogenic pattern that makes the differential diagnosis with carcinoma difficult.

The evaluation of a patient with symptomatic BPH should include the diagnostic testing necessary to supplement the clinical examination and select a suitable medical treatment. In the absence of symptoms such as hematuria, elevated creatinine level, history of renal stone disease, or other upper urinary tract disease, contrast imaging of the upper urinary tract probably is not necessary.[57] However, ultrasound can be a simple method to exclude hydronephrosis.[58] Ultrasound not only aids in determining prostate volume but also helps detect the presence or absence of a median lobe, elevated postvoiding residuals in the urinary bladder, or any sonographic evidence of an occult carcinoma.

Echo Pattern of Prostate Cancer

The ultrasonic characteristics of carcinoma of the prostate have changed with the development of higher frequency transducers. There is still controversy regarding the echogenicity of tumors, as well as the sensitivity of ultrasound in detecting cancers in different zones of the prostate. Early investigators using B-mode and initial gray scale imaging reported that prostatic carcinoma appeared as hyperechoic areas. With the development of 5 and 7 MHz transducers, it became evident that most peripheral zone tumors were hypoechoic.[46] If the presence of collagen in the stroma of prostatic tissue determines echogenicity, prostate cancer may appear hypoechoic because the stroma is replaced by infiltrating glandular tumor elements. Waterhouse and Resnick found that smaller tumors tend to be hypoechoic whereas larger lesions rarely are purely hypoechoic.[59] Large prostate cancers can replace all of the normally isoechoic peripheral zone, thereby obliterating any ultrasound reference for contrast with normal tissues (Figure 5–37).

Shinohara and associates reviewed the findings in 70 patients undergoing transrectal ultrasonography using a chair-mounted 5 MHz transducer.

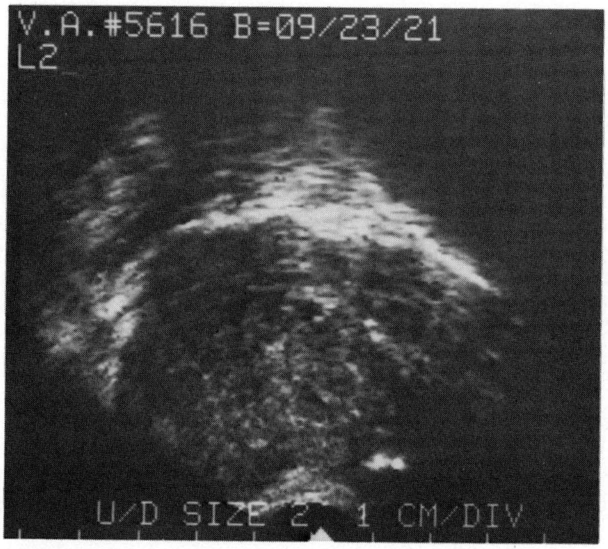

FIGURE 5–37. Large, infiltrative adenocarcinoma of the prostate gland. The tumor obliterates the normal anatomic landmarks and produces a mixed echo pattern to the entire prostate.

Comparison was made with whole-mount histologic sections.[60] Sixty percent of the tumors were hypoechoic; 39% were isoechoic and difficult to distinguish from the surrounding tissue; and only one tumor was hyperechoic. Most hypoechoic tumors were poorly differentiated, whereas isoechoic lesions were better differentiated. The authors suggested that the echo pattern of the prostate gland resulted from reflections of the sound wave at the interface between the prostatic stroma and the fluid-filled acinar lumen. They concluded that the cellular composition of tumors contains few sonographically detectable interfaces, creating a hypoechoic appearance compared with adjacent normal tissues. The higher the grade, the poorer the glandular detail and the more hypoechoic the tumor.

Rifkin, McGlynn, and Choi evaluated 51 histologically confirmed prostate cancers, 40 after needle biopsy and 11 after radical prostatectomy.[61] Somewhat in contrast to the findings of Shinohara's group, low–Gleason grade tumors correlated significantly with hypoechoic lesions, whereas isoechoic or somewhat hypoechoic areas were associated only with anaplastic, high-grade tumors. All of the scans were performed with a transducer whose frequency exceeded 5 MHz. These investigators concluded that the most important factor determining echogenicity was the amount of stromal fibrosis. Tumors with a mixed echo pattern or frankly hyperechoic areas tended to be higher grade and to show extensive fibrotic changes, but considerable overlap was seen among histologic types.

Recent studies with a 7 MHz transducer have shown that the overwhelming majority of peripheral zone prostate cancers are hypoechoic.[62] Cooner and co-workers found prostate cancer in 28 men, and all lesions were hypoechoic compared with the isoechoic peripheral zone.[63] Areas of mixed echogenicity were seen in two tumors that had invaded the transition zone. Biopsies of hyperechoic lesions in the peripheral zone invariably were negative for cancer, showing normal tissue or chronic prostatitis. Stamey and Hodge reported that 94% to 100% of 100 stage B tumors palpable on digital rectal examination were visible as hypoechoic lesions on transrectal ultrasonography.[64] However, 20% of the palpable B_1 and B_2 nodules were associated with a tumor in the contralateral prostate lobe that was not detected by either ultrasonography or digital rectal examination.

We have evaluated 150 patients with carcinoma of the prostate gland by transrectal ultrasonography with a 7 MHz transducer. Whole-mount histologic sections of the prostate gland have been examined after radical prostatectomy, and the specimens have undergone multidimensional computer image analysis. The overwhelming majority of palpable tumors were seen as hypoechoic areas in the peripheral portion of the prostate gland (Figures 5–38 and 5–39).

Although peripheral zone cancers are hypoechoic in the substantial majority of patients scanned with contemporary 7 MHz transducers, tumors in other zones of the prostate gland show more variation. Large tumors that obscure the normal prostate anatomy may appear mixed or even isoechoic. The echo pattern of anteriorly located tumors is more difficult to define, and this difficulty is reflected by the decreased sensitivity and specificity of transrectal ultrasonography in transition zone tumors. The normally hypoechoic tissue texture of the transition zone, enlargement by BPH, calcifications, and previous transurethral instrumentation, and scarring from infections all contribute to the difficulty in interpreting transrectal ultrasonography findings in the transition zone. Therefore increased importance is placed on other sonographic characteristics such as overall prostate shape, symmetry, and the anteroposterior dimension of the gland. Capsular boundary echoes also are important. Distortion and absence of normal internal echoes are significant features in the evaluation of the anterior prostate gland.

Early Detection of Prostate Cancer with Ultrasonography

Undoubtedly, transrectal ultrasonography is capable of imaging some prostate cancers that are not palpable. In addition, most palpable tumors are visible by ultrasonography. This knowledge naturally has led to the evaluation of transrectal ultrasonography for early detection of prostate cancer.

Watanabe and co-workers used ultrasound for screening of prostate cancer in 1396 men.[65] Cancer was identified in only 0.16%. However, these stud-

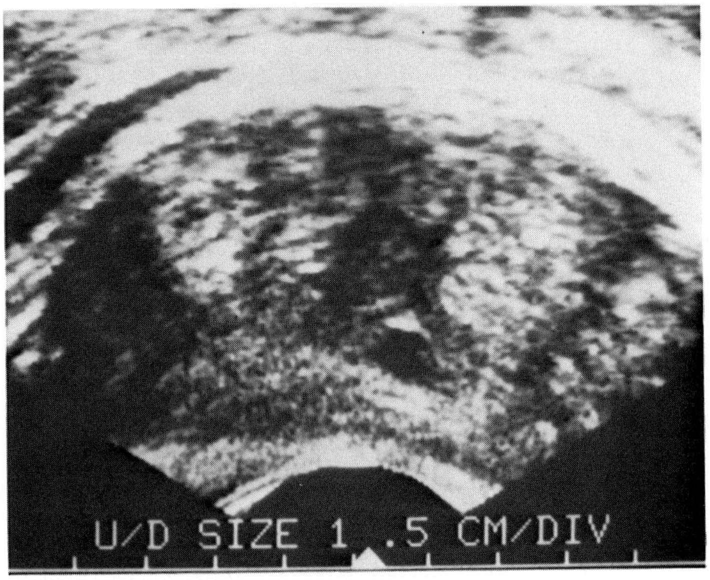

FIGURE 5–38. Transrectal ultrasound examination of the prostate gland showing a hypoechoic area in the right peripheral zone. The pattern is characteristic of adenocarcinoma of the prostate.

ies were performed with a chair-mounted scanner and a 3.5 MHz transducer. Also, given the variations in the clinical expression of prostate cancer in different countries, screening studies in Japan may not be applicable to patient populations in the United States.

There are no good screening studies investigating the value of ultrasonography with 7 MHz transducers on populations of men in the United States. Patients who come for evaluation on their own or through referral probably do not represent a general population. The primary factor influencing the predictive value (both positive and negative) of a test is the disease prevalence. Differences in prevalence between a referral population and an unselected group are incalculable. Nevertheless, information about the sensitivity and specificity of transrectal ultrasonography in clinical practice can be gained from evaluation of several series.

Lee and co-workers used transrectal ultrasonography and digital rectal examination to evaluate 784 self-referred men.[66] Transrectal ultrasonography detected cancer in 2.6% of the patients, compared with 1.3% for digital palpation. Cooner and associates performed transrectal ultrasonography in 1807 men referred in a general urology practice.[67] Biopsy was performed in 835 patients (46%) and 263 cancers were detected, yielding a detection rate of 14.6% of the overall population. Ragde and associates examined 1051 men responding to media solicitation for transrectal ultrasonography.[68] Biopsy was performed in 138 patients (18%) based on sonographic abnormalities. Cancer was found in 50 patients (4.7% of the total).

The preceding data suggest that transrectal ultrasonography detects prostate cancer more often than does digital palpation. In fact, the detection rate almost doubles, from about 2% to almost 4%.

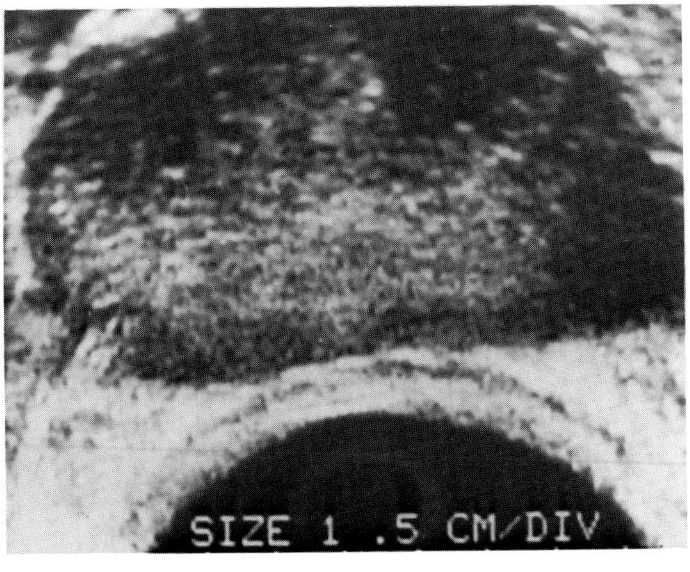

FIGURE 5–39. Hypoechoic area in the left lateral peripheral zone seen on a transrectal ultrasound image in transverse view. The hypoechoic area is contrasted with the homogeneous pattern of the more normal-appearing peripheral zone.

However, two primary issues remain unresolved. The rate of detection of prostate cancer clearly is related to the frequency and number of biopsies, independent of the ultrasound or rectal examination findings. The morbidity and expense of prostate biopsy have decreased with the introduction of automatic guns for transrectal biopsy, and in most contemporary series of ultrasonography the urologists have taken advantage of this by performing biopsies more readily if they suspect prostate cancer. In reported series of digital rectal examination for screening or early detection of prostate cancer, only a small percentage of patients (about 5%) underwent biopsy,[69] whereas in recent ultrasound series as many as 40% to 50% of the patients had biopsies. The impact of this increased frequency of biopsy on the higher detection rates seen with ultrasound studies cannot be ignored or calculated.

Another important consideration is the biologic significance of nonpalpable tumors detected by ultrasonography. Even if ultrasonography detects more cancers than digital rectal examination, the question remains whether the tumors detected by ultrasound are the ones destined to produce morbidity or death if left neglected or untreated.[70]

Transrectal ultrasonography used alone is a relatively imprecise method for early detection of prostate cancer. In the series of Lee and associates only 5% of patients with an abnormal ultrasound examination but a normal prostate specific antigen concentration and digital rectal examination had carcinoma confirmed on biopsy.[62] Furthermore, no patient with a normal marker level, a normal rectal examination, and an ultrasound-detected lesion smaller than 1 cm was found to have cancer. Thus, although ultrasonography clearly is capable of imaging some nonpalpable tumors, the procedure does not seem indicated for early detection of prostate cancer if both prostate specific antigen levels and rectal examination findings are normal. Transrectal ultrasound may be useful in the early detection and biopsy confirmation of pelvic recurrence after radical prostatectomy (Figure 5–40).[71]

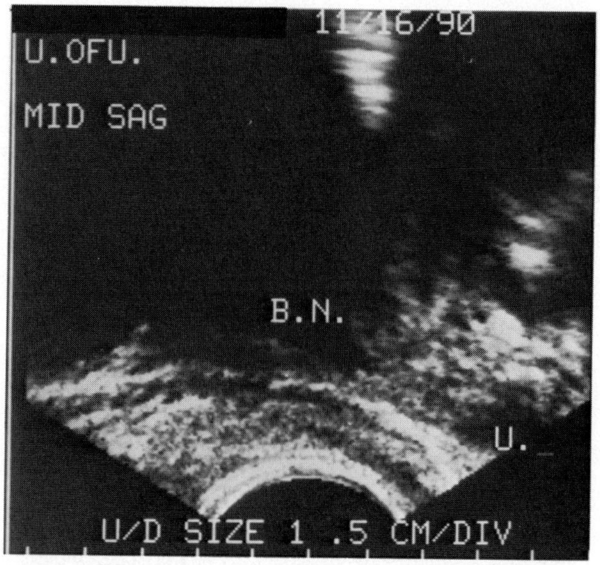

FIGURE 5–40. Sagittal view of the bladder neck *(BN)* and urethra *(U)* in a patient 1 year after radical prostatectomy. Tissue density can be seen surrounding the bladder neck, which biopsy showed to be locally recurrent adenocarcinoma.

Ultrasound Staging of Prostate Cancer

The inaccuracies of digital rectal examination in the staging of carcinoma of the prostate are well known. Nevertheless, other methods for staging, such as CT, have not found widespread acceptance because of inaccuracies and expense. A multiinstitutional cooperative trial involving 230 patients reviewed the usefulness of MRI and transrectal ultrasound in staging early prostate cancer. In this study MRI correctly staged 77% of cases of advanced disease and 57% of cases of localized disease, compared with 66% and 46%, respectively, for transrectal ultrasound. Future studies with intrarectal surface coils for MRI may show an improvement over ultrasound in the evaluation of patients with prostatic cancer, but with currently available equipment, staging has not been highly accurate.[72]

A review of the ultrasonographic findings that have been useful in staging prostate cancer is pertinent. Initially the overall shape and symmetry of the prostate gland should be considered. Tumor volume is an important feature. McNeal and associates have shown that lesions with volume greater than 3 ml usually exhibit capsular penetration or seminal vesicle invasion, whereas tumors less than 1 ml in volume often are confined within the capsule.[73] The recognition that nearly 50% of patients with stage B_2 carcinoma are found to have capsular invasion if whole-mount prostate sectioning is performed limits the comparability between transrectal ultrasonography staging studies and historical series in which rectal examination was used alone. Without the benefit of whole-mount prostate sectioning and "representative" samples of tissue, histologic studies of radical prostatectomy specimens previously showed capsular penetration or seminal vesicle involvement in no more than 20% of patients. Armed with this knowledge, the examiner probably would be less inclined to declare a tumor extracapsular on the basis of the digital rectal examination findings. On the other hand, the contemporary knowledge that most high-volume tumors and half of stage B_2 lesions penetrate the capsule would tend to increase the "sensitivity" of any staging procedure.

The capsular or boundary echoes of the prostate gland can be ascertained in either a transaxial or a sagittal view. Bulging, thickening, irregularity, interruption, and asymmetric contour have all been associated with capsular invasion (Figure 5–41). Lee and associates have described a trapezoidal area whose boundaries on the sagittal image are

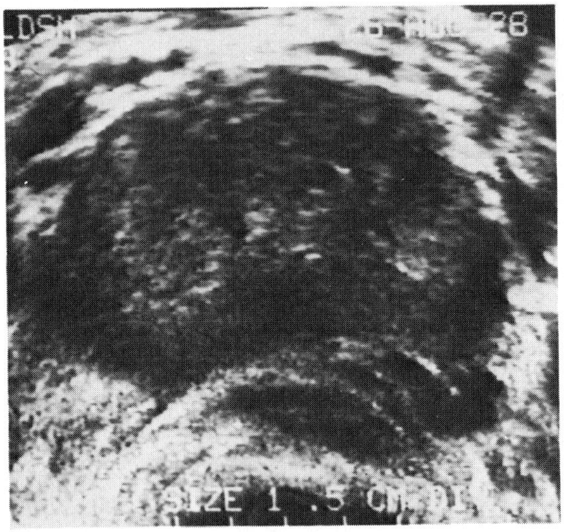

FIGURE 5–41. Transverse image of the prostate gland in a patient with a biopsy-proven adenocarcinoma. The obvious irregularity and interruption of the capsular boundary is consistent with local tumor extension.

the apex of the prostate, the urethra, the rectal wall, and the rectourethralis muscle.[46] They state that obliteration of this area is one of the earliest signs of extracapsular apical tumor extension.

Changes in the seminal vesicles associated with early tumor involvement are not well understood. Certainly, abnormal internal echoes, anterior displacement, or disparity in size and shape may increase the level of suspicion (Figure 5–42). Symmetry is best evaluated on a transaxial scan. Most often, normal seminal vesicles are symmetric and vary little in size, even after ejaculation.[74] The normal fat plane between the seminal vesicle and the base of the prostate is best evaluated on a sagittal image. The entrance of the seminal vesicles into

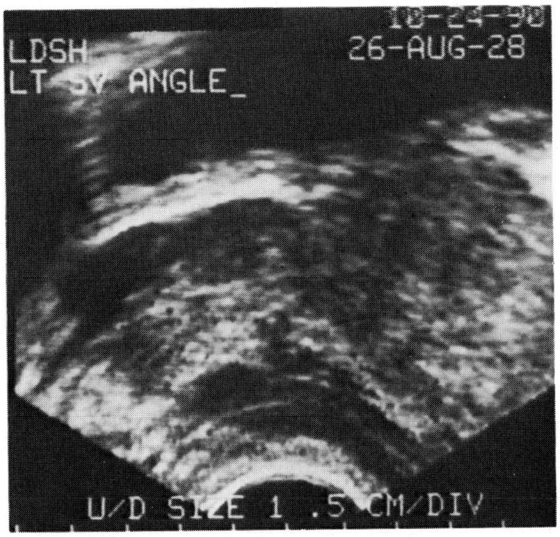

FIGURE 5–42. Sagittal image of the prostate gland showing a hypoechoic area in the peripheral zone that extends into the base of the seminal vesicle. The normal angle between the seminal vesicle and prostate is obliterated.

the ejaculatory ducts forms a beak. The absence of this normal finding has been described as an early sign of seminal vesicle invasion.[46]

Hodge, McNeal, and Stamey performed ultrasound-directed biopsies in 20 ultrasonographically abnormal and 40 normal-appearing seminal vesicles in patients with clinical stages B_2, B_3, and C prostate cancer.[75] Biopsies were positive for cancer in 14 (70%) of the 20 patients with abnormal seminal vesicles. In addition, 18% of the 40 patients with normal-appearing seminal vesicles had tumor invasion noted histologically after radical prostatectomy. Hodge and co-workers concluded that abnormalities of the seminal vesicles on ultrasonography usually indicate gross tumor invasion that may be undetected by digital palpation (Figure 5–43). Andriole and Catalona used transrectal ultrasonography with a 7 MHz transducer to stage cancer in 54 patients undergoing radical prostatectomy for localized disease.[76] Thirteen patients had capsular penetration or seminal vesicle invasion, but transrectal ultrasonography correctly identified this in only five (38%). The intraprostatic extent of the tumor was underestimated in 35% of the patients. Hashimoto and co-workers found an agreement between ultrasonography and pathologic findings of the seminal vesicles in 24 of 28 patients (86%).[77] However, only six of these patients had seminal vesicle invasion, and transrectal ultrasonography accurately predicted this in only two.

Salo and associates used transrectal ultrasonography for preoperative staging in 38 patients undergoing radical retropubic prostatectomy.[78] The study had a sensitivity of 86% for extracapsular extension and a specificity of 94%. For seminal vesicle involvement the sensitivity was only 29% but specificity was 100%.

Several investigators have examined the ability of ultrasound to detect associated unsuspected tumors in specimens from men undergoing radical protatectomy for known adenocarcinoma. Hodge and associates found tumor in the contralateral lobe in 20% of patients despite a normal-appearing ultrasound examination.[75] Carter and colleagues found unsuspected contralateral tumor in 42% of 59 patients undergoing radical prostatectomy.[79] Transrectal ultrasonography was performed preoperatively with either a 5 or a 7 MHz transducer. A positive predictive value was calculated at 54% with a negative predictive value of 66%. Not surprisingly, ultrasonography is not capable of imaging all prostate cancers; the study can depict only gross architectural changes, not microscopic tumor. In addition, some gross cancers undoubtedly are not detected by ultrasonography (Figure 5–44).

Seminal Vesicles

Evaluation of the seminal vesicles is an important aspect of the management of carcinoma of the

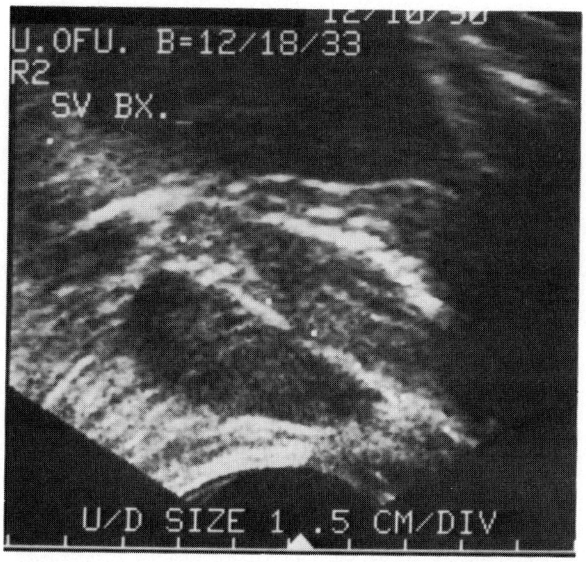

FIGURE 5–43. Sagittal view of a dilated seminal vesicle. The base of the prostate gland can be seen on the right, and the bladder neck is superior. A needle biopsy tract is identifiable. Ultrasonography can facilitate specific anatomic biopsies of the prostate gland and seminal vesicles.

prostate,[80,81] infertility,[82,83] recurrent prostatitis, hematospermia, and perineal and ejaculatory pain.[84] In addition, tumors,[85] abscesses,[86] and cysts[87] occasionally occur primarily in the seminal vesicles. A normal seminal vesicle is virtually nonpalpable on rectal examination, and digital rectal palpation usually provides only suggestive evidence in patients with abnormalities of the seminal vesicles.

Because of difficulties in making an accurate diagnosis of seminal vesicle abnormalities by digital rectal palpation, various imaging methods have been explored. Vasoseminal vesiculography,[88,89] CT,[90] and MRI have been used. However, because of its noninvasive nature, relative inexpensiveness, and excellent visualization of the seminal vesicles, transrectal ultrasonography[91-93] is the preferred method to image the seminal vesicles in most patients.

The normal sonographic appearance of the seminal vesicles has been described as diffuse and homogeneous with a level of echogenicity slightly less than that of the normal adjacent prostate gland. They may be rounded in appearance, elongated, lobulated, or bowtie or dumbbell shaped (Figure 5–45). Importance has been given to their anatomic relationship with the prostate gland in the sagittal view, as well as to symmetry. Alteration in echo pattern or obliteration of normal anatomic planes may indicate seminal vesicle tumor extension in patients with carcinoma of the prostate gland.

ULTRASONOGRAPHY IN PEDIATRIC UROLOGY

In the past decade ultrasonography has become one of the principal diagnostic modalities in pediatric urology, primarily because it is noninvasive and easy to use and does not cause radiation exposure or require contrast agents. Approximately 3% of live newborns examined with ultrasonography are found to have a congenital anomaly associated with a chromosomal abnormality, a single gene defect, or an abnormality of polygenic inheritance.[94] Screening ultrasonography may be indicated in the siblings of patients with congenitally obstructed kidneys, reflux, or other cystic kidney disease. In addition to evaluation of neonates and children with increased family risk, screening of healthy infants has been suggested. Steinhart and co-workers studied 437 asymptomatic infants between 2 and 10 months of age and found that 1.37% had urologic abnormalities requiring surgical correction.[95] In an attempt to establish the prevalence of occult renal abnormalities in school-age children, Chung-Pin Sheih and associates studied 132,686 elementary children.[96] Renal abnormalities were detected in 0.5%, but only 0.037% required surgery. The four most common abnormalities detected were hydronephrosis (39.6%), unilateral small kidney (19.8%), unilateral agenesis (15.9%), and renal cystic disease (13.9%). Although the authors concluded that this incidence justified routine screening, few would recommend ultrasonography for an otherwise healthy infant or child.

Rosendahl performed 4586 fetal ultrasound studies in pregnant women to detect urinary tract malformations.[97] The incidence of abnormalities was 0.48%; hydronephrosis was the most common dis-

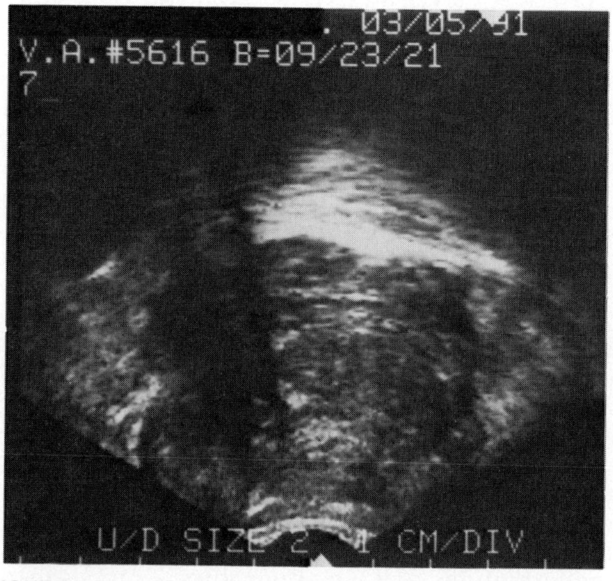

FIGURE 5–44. Transverse image of a high-grade prostate cancer that extends anteriorly away from the peripheral zone. Despite the size of the tumor, digital palpation of the prostate did not detect abnormalities.

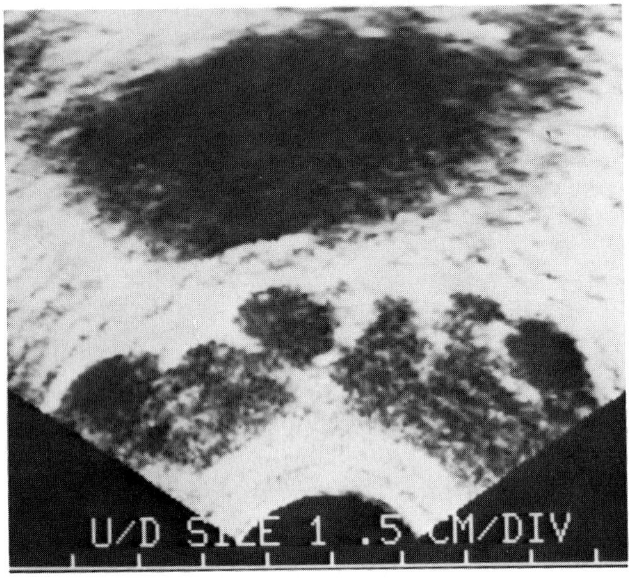

FIGURE 5–45. Normal seminal vesicles seen in transverse image. Usually the seminal vesicles are symmetric in size and shape.

order. The positive predictive value of ultrasound was 81.5%, and the negative predictive value 99.9%. Scott and Renwick found urologic abnormalities in 0.13% of neonates.[98] Of the urinary tract abnormalities suspected antenatally on the basis of ultrasound, more than two thirds were confirmed postnatally.

Prenatal Fetal Ultrasonography

Among the numerous indications for prenatal ultrasound are determination of fetal and placental location, assessment of gestational age, a family history of previous anomalies, and suspicion of gestational abnormalities. Although ultrasound screening programs to detect fetal malformations have been advocated,[99] a consensus conference in 1984 concluded that ultrasound examination during pregnancy should be performed only for a specific medical indication.[100]

Ultrasonography has produced dramatic changes in the prenatal evaluation of the fetus. For antenatal scanning a mild distention of the maternal urinary bladder is needed to serve as an acoustic window. The entire uterus is examined in the longitudinal and transverse planes. Fetal viability, position of the fetus and the placenta, and relative amount of amniotic fluid are documented. With real-time ultrasound a biparietal diameter measurement is recorded for gestational age, as well as the visualization of intracranial structures. A transabdominal section at the level of the umbilical vein is performed to compare head and body size. Fetal organs are scanned to determine their presence and normality. In a normal fetus the bladder may be visualized at 14 weeks' gestation. The kidneys may be visible at 14 weeks and should always be identifiable by 18 weeks. The kidneys are best seen initially on a transverse scan of the fetus just below the level of umbilical vein and located posteriorly and adjacent to the fetal spine (Figure 5–46). Fetal kidneys appear sonographically identical to adult kidneys. They contain a central echodense area representing the pelvocalyceal system surrounded by the less dense renal parenchyma.[101] The renal pelvis may be as great as 1 cm in diameter without indicating any pathologic condition.[102] Hydronephrosis of moderate degree can be noted by 16 to 18 weeks of gestation. Normally the fetal ureter is not seen. The fetal adrenal glands may be recognized after the 30th week as relatively hypoechoic triangular structures located superior to the upper poles of the kidneys. The fetal bladder is usually filled and appears as a sonolucent structure. A bladder that is not detectable after 16 weeks of gestation suggests an abnormality. Compromise of fetal urine production may result in oligohydramnios after 16 to 20 weeks of gestation, which is one of the strongest indicators of poor postnatal outcome in cases of identified fetal genitourinary abnormalities. Fetal sex may also be determined by ultrasonography and is important when there is a risk for X-linked genetic disorders.

Overall, genitourinary anomalies comprise about 50% of prenatal sonographically detectable malformations, with hydronephrosis representing two thirds of these (Figure 5–47). Supravesical obstruction is more frequent than infravesical obstruction, and unilateral hydronephrosis is more common than bilateral (Figure 5–48).[103]

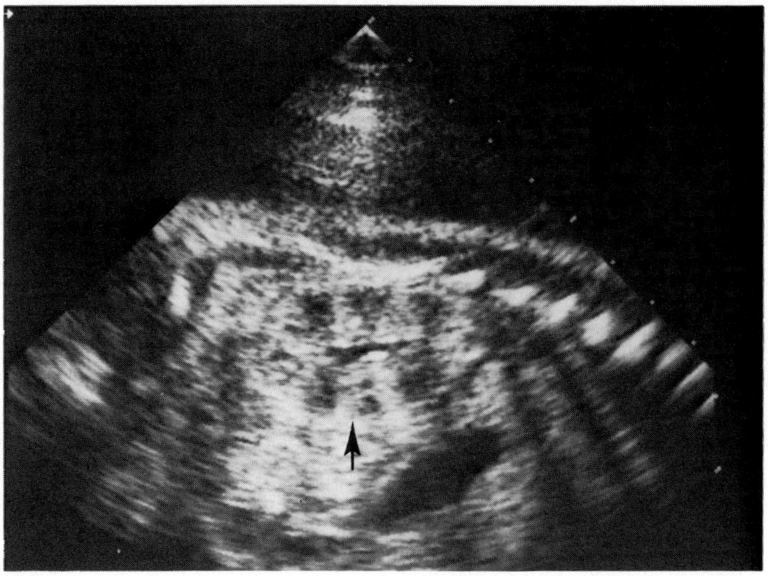

FIGURE 5–46. Fetal kidney at 18 weeks' gestation viewed sonographically. The kidney characteristically shows greater corticomedullary differentiation than does an adult kidney.

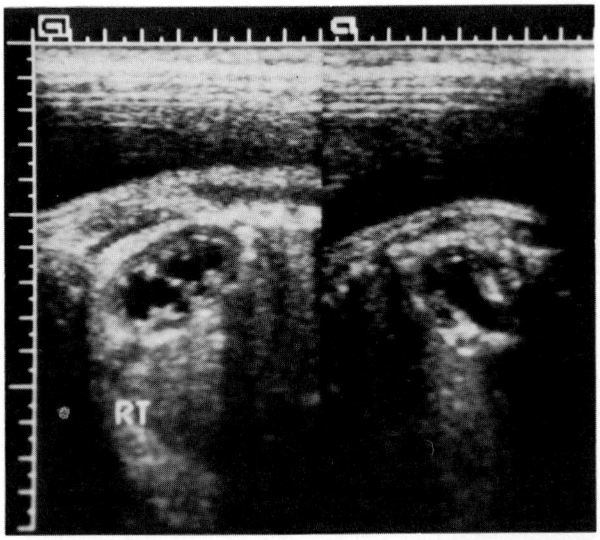

FIGURE 5–47. Hydronephrosis in a fetus at 35 weeks' gestation is caused by ureteropelvic junction obstruction.

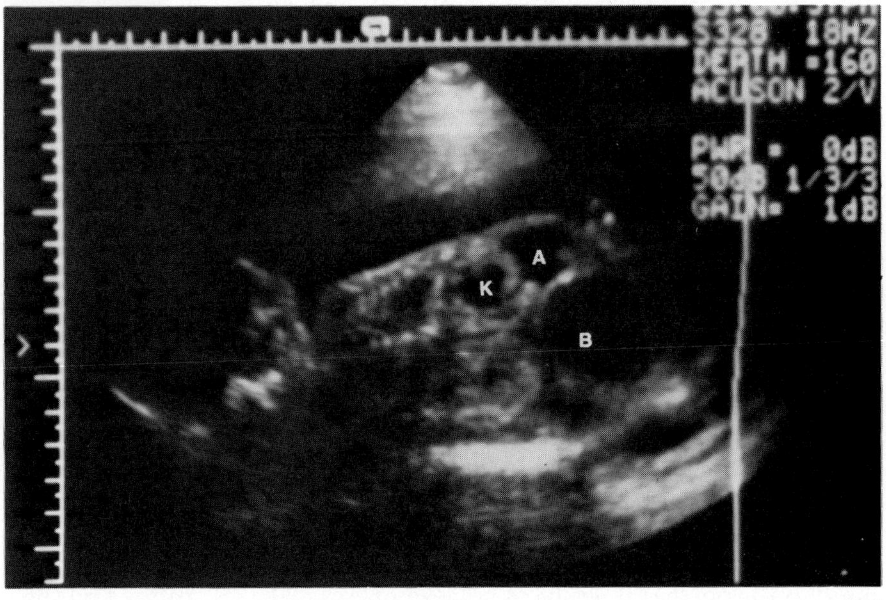

FIGURE 5–48. Ultrasound in a fetus at 26 weeks' gestation with obstructive posterior urethral valves. *A,* Ascites; *B,* bladder; *K,* kidney with hydronephrosis.

Abdominal Masses in Neonates

Ultrasonography is often the first diagnostic step for the evaluation of abdominal masses in children. Ultrasonography reveals both the location and the density of the mass and determines whether it is predominantly cystic, solid, or of a mixed pattern. Cystic lesions of the urinary tract detected by ultrasonography result mainly from hydronephrosis, multicystic kidney, polycystic kidney, duplications, or reflux. The most common solid tumors are mesoblastic nephromas or neuroblastomas. Wilms' tumors rarely occur in the newborn.

The operator performing a pediatric ultrasound study must understand the normal renal ultrasonographic characteristics and the expected size of the kidney. The child is examined in the supine position. The right kidney is viewed longitudinally through an acoustic window provided by the liver. The left kidney is more likely to be visualized longitudinally through the spleen. Up to the sixth month of age the neonate has enhanced corticomedullary differentiation. The cortical echoes increase because of the greater volume occupied by the glomeruli, and the echoes from the renal pyramids decrease. The prominent hypoechoic pyramids may be mistaken for dilated calyces or cysts and have a triangular configuration with their apices pointing toward the central collecting system. The corticomedullary ratio is increased because of the larger volume of the medulla compared with the adult kidney. Indentations of the renal contour called fetal lobulations are prominent up to the second year of age, when the kidney adopts the adult sonographic characteristics.[104]

In a reported series of 560 healthy newborn infants, renal measurements were made by ultrasonography between 48 and 72 hours after delivery. With a median gestational age of 40 weeks and a mean birth weight of 3291 g, the mean renal length was 4.26 cm with a standard deviation of 0.45 cm. This study also showed consistently that the left kidney was longer and thinner than the right. Boys had larger kidneys than girls.[105]

Ultrasound allows renal measurements that are not subject to differences in centering of the x-ray tube and the distance from the patient. To obtain a regression equation for renal length, Rosenbaum and associates used a real-time mechanical sector scan on 203 pediatric patients ranging in age from several hours to 19 years. For children younger than 1 year in age, the renal length was $4.98 + 0.155$ cm $\times$ Age in months. In children older than 1 year in age, renal length was $6.79 + 0.22$ cm $\times$ Age in years. The mean renal length by age in this group of patients is plotted in Table 5–1.

TABLE 5–1. Summary of Grouped Observations—Mean Renal Length

*Average Age**	*Interval**	*Mean Renal Length (cm)*	*SD*	*n*
0 mo	0–1 wk	4.48	0.31	10
2 mo	1 wk–4 mo	5.28	0.66	54
6 mo	4–8 mo	6.15	0.67	20
10 mo	8 mo–1 yr	6.23	0.63	8
1½	1-2	6.65	0.54	28
2½	2-3	7.36	0.54	12
3½	3-4	7.36	0.64	30
4½	4-5	7.87	0.50	26
5½	5-6	8.09	0.54	30
6½	6-7	7.83	0.72	14
7½	7-8	8.33	0.51	18
8½	8-9	8.90	0.88	18
9½	9-10	9.20	0.90	14
10½	10-11	9.17	0.82	28
11½	11-12	9.60	0.64	22
12½	12-13	10.42	0.87	18
13½	13-14	9.79	0.75	14
14½	14-15	10.05	0.62	14
15½	15-16	10.93	0.76	6
16½	16-17	10.04	0.86	10
17½	17-18	10.53	0.29	4
18½	18-19	10.81	1.13	8

*Years unless specified otherwise.
From Rosenbaum DM, Korngold E, Teele RL: Sonographic assessment of renal length in normal children. AJR 142:467, © Am Roent Ray Soc, 1984. Reprinted by authorization.

Hydronephrosis

Hydronephrosis is the most common abdominal mass in the perinatal period. A dilated urinary excretory system could be caused by a broad variety of urologic diseases, including uretropelvic junction obstruction, ureterocele, obstructed duplicated system, posterior urethral valves, or reflux. A prenatal diagnosis of hydronephrosis may represent normal structures, insignificant variants, or physiologically significant anomalies that require treatment.[107]

Ureteropelvic junction obstruction is a common disorder of childhood. Approximately two thirds of newborns with such obstruction are boys, and in 60% the obstruction is on the left side. Approximately 20% are found to have a significant obstruction bilaterally, whereas in older children bilateral involvement is seen in 5%. With unilateral obstruction, contralateral renal anomalies such as duplication or malrotation have been described.[108]

Ureteral obstruction caused by ureterocele can be identified with ultrasound. Normal ureters are rarely visualized sonographically because of overlying bowel gas and their small size. Sonographic visualization of a ureter usually implies pathologic dilation and can be traced distally toward the bladder. In addition, segmental hydronephrosis involving the upper portion of the kidney may be seen with ultrasound. The identification of hydroureteronephrosis requires a careful search of the bladder for an intravesical cystic structure (ureterocele) (Figure 5–49).

When an ultrasound diagnosis of hydronephrosis is established prenatally, it must be confirmed after delivery. VCUG should be performed to rule out reflux and the possibility of ureterocele or posterior

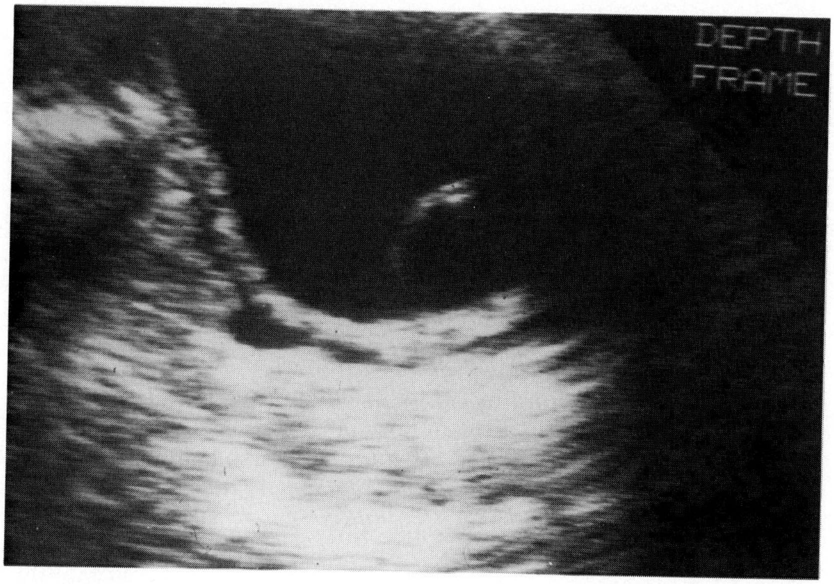

FIGURE 5–49. Bladder ultrasound in a 3-year-old child showing a filling defect consistent with an obstructive ureterocele.

urethral valves. If the VCUG is normal, the identification of the site and cause of obstruction can be assessed by intravenous pyelography or ^{99}Tc DTPA renal scintigraphy.[109,110]

Multicystic Kidney

A multicystic kidney is a congenital entity and the second most common cause of an abdominal mass in the neonate. It represents an extreme form of dysplasia associated with atresia of the ureter. This abnormality should not be confused with polycystic disease of either the infantile or the adult type, in which there is no renal parenchymal dysplasia.[111] The malformation in a multicystic kidney is recognized as a cystic mass with cysts of different sizes that can achieve considerable dimension. Most specimens have a central area with rudimentary renal tissue and dysplastic elements. The initial sign is most often a unilateral abdominal mass with predominance in males and on the left side. Patients have an increased incidence of contralateral renal abnormalities. Ultrasound typically shows noncommunicating cysts of varying shape and size, with a peripheral distribution (nonmedial location) of the largest cysts, interfaces between cysts, absence of identifiable renal sinus, and no surrounding renal parenchyma (Figure 5–50).[112]

Infantile Polycystic Kidney Disease

Infantile polycystic kidney disease is a rare autosomal recessive inherited disease with diffuse involvement of both kidneys. The neonate has bilateral flank masses that are symmetric, tense, hard, and nontransilluminating. The urine output and degree of renal insufficiency are variable, but oliguria is common. In severe cases the child dies in the first few days of life. Pulmonary hypoplasia is a common cause of persistent respiratory distress.

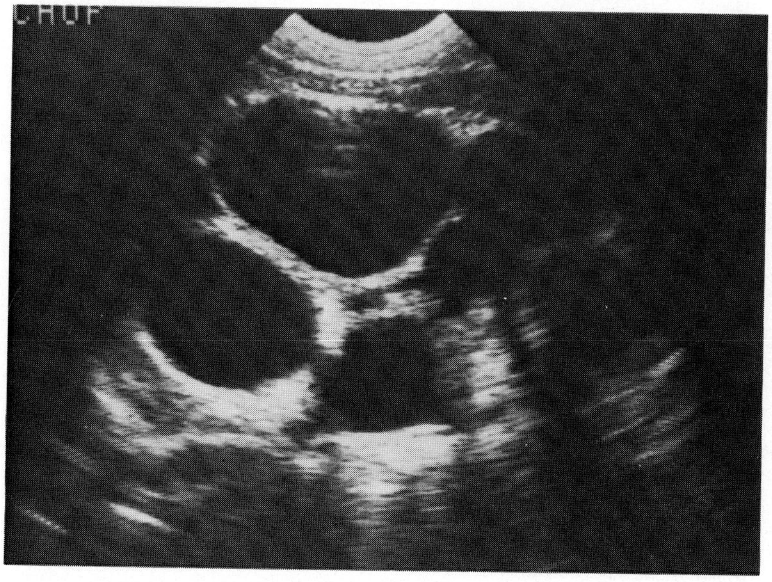

FIGURE 5–50. Multicystic dysplastic kidney. Cysts of various sizes can be seen throughout the kidney without any apparent functional renal parenchyma.

In less severe cases renal insufficiency develops in early childhood and shows variable progression. Systemic hypertension, hepatomegaly, and splenomegaly develop in almost all patients. Growth retardation is common.

Sonographic studies show enlarged kidneys. The ectatic tubules (cysts) are usually so small that they can not be appreciated by ultrasound, but the interfaces produced by the walls of the tubules cause increased echogenicity throughout the parenchyma. The diffuse echogenic renal pattern caused by the increased number of interfaces results in poor definition of the renal sinus, medulla, and cortex. The corticomedullary junction is not visualized because of the increased echogenicity of the parenchyma. The hypoechogenicity of the medulla that occurs with a normal newborn kidney is not observed (Figure 5–51).

Renal Tumors

The renal neoplasm most commonly seen in the first weeks of life is congenital mesoblastic nephroma, also referred to as fetal renal hamartoma, leiomyomatous hamartoma, or fetal mesenchymal hamartoma.[113] These lesions are distinguished from the typical Wilms' tumor by their earlier presentation and their histologic characteristics. The cut surface is firm, homogeneous, and rubbery with a pale yellowish gray appearance. The tumors are unencapsulated and infiltrating, often replacing most of the kidney. Cystic changes, hemorrhage, and necrosis are uncommon.[114] Histologic study shows dysplastic or immature tubules and glomeruli irregularly scattered within a fibrous or mesenchymal stroma. Ultrasonography characteristically shows a solid, poorly defined lesion that has low-level echoes and cannot be readily differentiated from Wilms' tumor. Excretory urography demonstrates an intrarenal mass effect with calyceal distortion. Computerized tomography shows a heterogeneous solid mass arising from the kidney.

Wilms' tumor (nephroblastoma) is the most common malignant neoplasm in the urinary tract of children. This tumor occurs most often during the first 7 years of life, with a peak incidence at 3 years. Genitourinary anomalies (fusion, renal ectopy, renal hypoplasia, duplication, hypospadias, and cryptorchidism) are present in about 4.5% of patients with Wilms' tumor.[115] Overall, 15% of the patients also have other congenital abnormalities (aniridia, hemihypertrophy, musculoskeletal anomalies, and the Beckwith-Wiedemann syndrome).[116]

In patients with Wilms' tumor, intravenous pyelography typically shows an intrarenal mass with distortion of the calyceal system. Real-time ultrasonography is useful for assessing the nonfunctional kidney, the renal vein, the inferior vena cava, and the retroperitoneal space and for detecting the possibility of liver metastases. Most commonly, the sonographic appearance is of an intrarenal mass sharply marginated with compressed renal tissue forming a pseudocapsule. There are variable regions of low to moderate echogenicity with hypoechoic and anechoic areas corresponding to necrotic hemorrhage.

Neuroblastomas have a different origin and clinical characteristics from those of Wilms' tumor. Ultrasound or intravenous pyelography usually shows suprarenal neuroblastomas displacing the kidney inferiorly and laterally with maintenance of a normal calyceal pattern. Infrequently the tumor invades the renal parenchyma, causing calyceal distortion. Calcifications in a characteristically speckled pattern can be seen in 50% of the patients, giving a higher echogenic pattern with occasional shadowing by sonography. Other neuroblastomas may exhibit homogeneous low-level

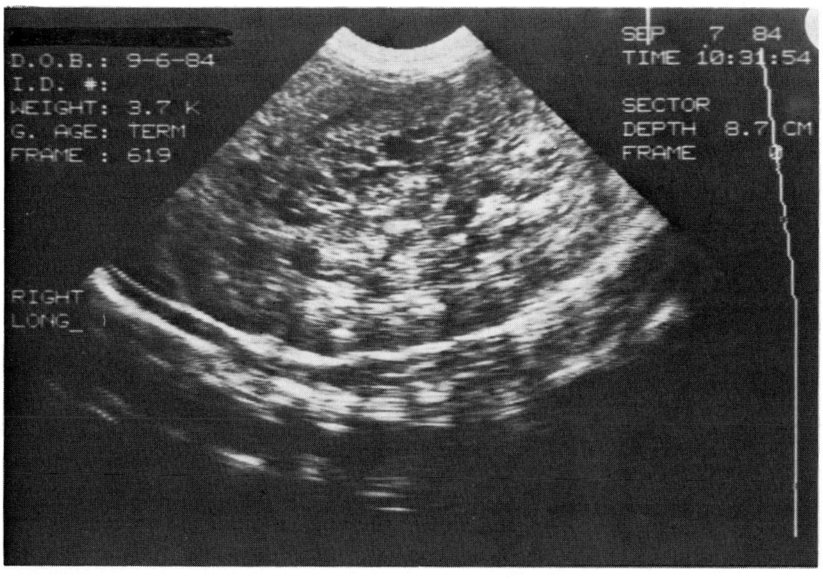

FIGURE 5–51. Infantile polycystic kidney. The renal size is markedly enlarged with increased echogenicity throughout the renal parenchyma.

internal echoes, generating sonographic characteristics similar to those of Wilms' tumors.[117]

ACKNOWLEDGMENTS: We thank William J. Zwiebel, M.D., for providing prenatal ultrasound images and George A. Devault for renal transplant images.

REFERENCES

1. Wicks JD, Howe KS: Fundamentals of ultrasonographic technique. Chicago: Year Book, 1983, pp 1-5.
2. Watanabe H, Igari D, Takahashi Y, et al: Transrectal ultrasonography of the prostate. J Urol 114:734-739, 1975.
3. Harada K, Tanahashi Y, Igari D, et al: Clinical evaluation of inside echo patterns in gray scale prostatic echography. J Urol 124:216-220, 1980.
4. Lee F, Gray JM, McLeary RD, et al: Transrectal ultrasound in the diagnosis of prostate cancer location, echogenicity, histopathology and staging. Prostate 7:117-129, 1985.
5. American Institute of Ultrasound in Medicine: Safety considerations for diagnostic ultrasound. Bethesda, Md: The Institute, 1984.
6. Moskowitz PS, Carroll BA, McCoy JM: Ultrasonic renal volumetry in children. Radiology 134:61-64, 1980.
7. Yoshimura N, Oka Y: Medical and surgical complications of renal transplantation. Med Clin North Am 74(4):1025-1036, 1990.
8. Chinn DH, Hricak H: Ultrasonography of the renal transplant. In Resnick MI, Sanders RC (eds): Ultrasound in urology, ed 2. Baltimore: Williams & Wilkins, 1984, p 335.
9. Venkateswara Rao K: Mechanism, pathophysiology, diagnosis and management of renal transplant rejection. Med Clin North Am 74(4):1039-1057, 1990.
10. Hoskins PR: Measurement of arterial blood flow by Doppler ultrasound. Clin Physiol Measure 11(1):1-26, 1990.
11. Perrella RR, Duerinck AJ, Tessler FN, et al: Evaluation of renal transplant dysfunction by duplex Doppler sonography: a prospective study and review of the literature. Am J Kidney Dis 15(6):544-550, 1990.
12. Townsend R, Tomlanovich SJ, Goldstein RB, Filly RA: Combined Doppler and morphologic sonographic evaluation of renal transplant rejection. J Ultrasound Med 9(4):199-206, 1990.
13. Loughlin KR, Tilney NL, Richie JP: Urologic complications in 718 renal transplant patients. Surgery 95:297-302, 1984.
14. Kinnaert P, Hall M, Janssen F, et al: Ureteral stenosis after kidney transplantation: true incidence and long-term follow-up after surgical correction. J Urol 133:17-20, 1985.
15. Straiton JA, McMillan MA, Morley P: Ultrasound in suspected obstruction complicating renal transplantation. Br J Radiol 62(741):803-806, 1989.
16. Smith SJ, Bosniak MA, Megibow AJ, et al: Renal cell carcinoma: earlier discovery and increased detection. Radiology 170(3 pt 1):699-703, 1989.
17. Baumgartner BR, Chezmar JL: Magnetic resonance imaging of the kidneys and adrenal glands. Semin Ultrasound CT MR 10(1):43-62, 1989.
18. Benson AM, Haaga JR, Resnick MJ: Staging renal carcinoma: what is sufficient? Arch Surg 124(1):71-73, 1989.
19. Kuijpers D, Jaspers R: Renal masses: differential diagnosis with pulsed Doppler U.S. Radiology 170(1 pt 1):59-60, 1989.
20. Kier R, Taylor KJ, Feyock AL, Ramos IM: Renal masses: characterization with Doppler U.S. Radiology 176(3):703-707, 1990.
21. Warshauer DM, McCarthy SM, Street L, et al: Detection of renal masses: sensitivities and specificities of excretory urography/linear tomography, U.S., and C.T. Radiology 169:363-365, 1989.
22. Mostofi FK, Hartman DS, Davis CJ: Radiopathological aspects of benign tumors of the kidney. AUA Update Series, vol VIII:130-135, 1989.
23. Poston JG, Joseph AE, Riddle PR: The accuracy of ultrasound in the measurement of changes in bladder volume. Br J Urol 55:361-363, 1983.
24. Birch NC, Hurst G, Doyle PT: Serial residual volumes in men with prostatic hypertrophy. Br J Urol 62:571-575, 1988.
25. Keily EA, Hartnell GG, Gibson RN, Williams G: Measurement of bladder volume by real-time ultrasound. Br J Urol 60:33-35, 1987.
26. Haylen BT, Parys BT, West CR: Transrectal ultrasound to measure bladder volumes in men. J Urol 143(4):687-689, 1990.
27. Ireton RC, Krieger JN, Cardenas DD, et al: Bladder volume determination using a dedicated portable ultrasound scanner. J Urol 143:909-911, 1990.
28. Droller MJ: Transitional cell cancer: upper tracts and bladder. In Walsh, Gittes, Perlmutter, Stamey (eds): Campbell's urology, ed 5. Philadelphia: Saunders, 1986, p 1402.
29. Malone PR: Transabdominal ultrasound surveillance for bladder cancer. Urol Clin North Am 16(4):823-827, 1989.
30. Jtzchak Y, Singer D, Fischelovitch Y: Ultrasonographic assessment of bladder tumors. J Urol 126:31-35, 1981.
31. Abu-Yousef MM, Narayana AS, Franken EA, Brown RC: Urinary bladder tumors studied by cystosonography, I. Radiology 153:223-226, 1984.
32. Terris MK, Villers A, Freiha FS: Transrectal ultrasound appearance of transitional cell carcinoma involving the prostate. J Urol 143:953-956, 1990.
33. Abu-Yousef MM, Narayana AS, Brown RC, Franken EA: Urinary bladder tumors studied by cystosonography. II. Staging. Radiology 153:227-231, 1984.
34. Hodson NJ, Husband JE, MacDonald JB: The role of computed tomography in the staging of bladder cancer. Clin Radiol 30:389-395, 1979.
35. Rholl KS, Lee JK, Heiken JP, et al: Primary bladder carcinoma: evaluation with MR imaging. Radiology 163:117-121, 1987.
36. Fakhry J, Khoury A, Barakat K: The hypoechoic band: a normal finding on testicular sonography. AJR 153(2):321-323, 1989.
37. Burks DD, Markey BJ, Burkhard TK, et al: Suspected testicular torsion and ischemia: evaluation with color Doppler sonography. Radiology 175(3):815-821, 1990.
38. Lerner RM, Mevorach RA, Hulbert WC, Rabinowitz R: Color Doppler U.S. in the evaluation of acute scrotal disease. Radiology 176(2):355-358, 1990.
39. Middleton WD, Siegel BA, Melson GL, et al: Acute scrotal disorders: prospective comparison of color Doppler U.S. and testicular scintigraphy. Radiology 177(1):177-181, 1990.
40. Kratzik C, Hainz A, Kuber W, et al: Has ultrasound influenced the therapy concept of blunt scrotal trauma? J Urol 142(5):1243-1246, 1989.
41. Fournier GR, Laing FC, Mcaninch JW: Scrotal ultrasonography and the management of testicular trauma. Urol Clin North Am 16(2):377-385, 1989.
42. Carroll BA, Gross DM: High frequency scrotal sonography. Am J Roentgenol 140:511-515, 1983.
43. Marth D, Scheidegger J, Studer UE: Ultrasonography of testicular tumors. Urol Int 45(4):237-240, 1990.
44. Sanders RC: The practical value of diagnostic ultrasound in urology. J Urol 126:283-287, 1981.
45. McNeal JE: Regional morphology and pathology of the prostate. Am J Clin Pathol 49:347-357, 1968.
46. Lee F, Torp-Pedersen ST, Siders DB, et al: Transrectal ultrasound in the diagnosis and staging of prostatic carcinoma. Radiology 170:609-615, 1989.

47. Fehr JL, Knonagel H: Importance of prostatic sonography in the evaluation of conservative therapy of prostatic hyperplasia. Urol Int 45(4):231-233, 1990.
48. Clements R, Griffiths GJ, Peeling et al: Transrectal ultrasound in monitoring response to treatment. Urol Clin North Am 16(4):735-740, 1989.
49. Jones DR, Roberts EE, Griffiths GJ, et al: Assessment of volume measurement of the prostate using per-rectal ultrasonography. Br J Urol 64(5):493-495, 1989.
50. Vilmann P, Hancke S, Strange-Vognsen HH, et al: The reliability of transabdominal ultrasound scanning in the determination of prostatic volume. Scand J Urol Nephrol 21:5-7, 1987.
51. Terris MK, Stamey TA: Determination of prostate volume by transrectal ultrasound. J Urol 145:984-987, 1991.
52. Mears EM, Stamey TA: Bacteriologic localization patterns in bacterial prostatitis and urethritis. Invest Urol 5:491-518, 1968.
53. Drach GW: Problems in diagnosis of bacterial prostatitis: gram negative, gram positive and mixed infections. J Urol 111:630-636, 1974.
54. Doble A, Carter SC: Ultrasonographic findings in prostatitis. Urol Clin North Am 16(4):763-772, 1989.
55. Jimenez-Cruz JF, Boromat Tormo F, Gallego Gomez J: Treatment of chronic prostatitis: intraprostatic antibiotic injections under echography control. J Urol 139:967-970, 1988.
56. Greene DR, Egawa S, Hellerstein DK, Scardino PT: Sonographic measurements of transition zone of the prostate in men with and without benign prostatic hyperplasia. Urology 36(4):293-299, 1990.
57. McClennan BL: Diagnostic imaging evaluation of benign prostatic hyperplasia. Urol Clin North Am 17(3):517-536, 1990.
58. Torp-Pedersen NJS, Nielsen H: Abdominal ultrasound versus intravenous urography in the evaluation of infravesically obstructed males. Scand J Urol Nephrol 23:89-92, 1989.
59. Waterhouse RL, Resnick MI: The use of transrectal prostatic ultrasonography in the evaluation of patients with prostatic carcinoma. J Urol 141:233-239, 1989.
60. Shinohara K, Wheeler TM, Scardino PT: The appearance of prostate cancer in transrectal ultrasonography: correlation of imaging and pathological examinations. J Urol 142:76-82, 1989.
61. Rifkin MD, McGlynn ET, Choi H: Echogenicity of prostate cancer correlated with histologic grade and stromal fibrosis. Radiology 170:549-552, 1989.
62. Lee F, Torp-Pedersen ST, Littrup PJ, et al: Hypoechoic lesions of the prostate: clinical relevance of tumor size, DRE and PSA. Radiology 170:29-32, 1989.
63. Cooner WH, Mosley BR, Rutherford CL, et al: Clinical applications of transrectal ultrasonography and PSA in the search for prostatic cancer. J Urol 139:758-761, 1988.
64. Stamey TA, Hodge KK: Ultrasound visualization of prostate anatomy and pathology. Monogr Urol 9(3):56, 1988.
65. Watanabe H, Ohe H, Inaba T, et al: A mobile mass screening unit for prostatic disease. Prostate 5:559-565, 1984.
66. Lee F, Littrup PJ, Torp-Pedersen ST, et al: Hypoechoic lesions of the prostate: clinical relevance of tumor size, DRE and PSA. Radiology 168:389-394, 1988.
67. Cooner WH, Mosley BR, Rutherford CL, et al: Prostate cancer detection in a clinical urologic practice by ultrasonography, digital rectal examination and prostate specific antigen. J Urol 143:1146-1154, 1990.
68. Ragde H, Bagley CM, Aldape HC, et al: Screening for prostatic cancer with high-resolution ultrasound. J Endourol 3:115-123, 1989.
69. Chodak GW, Schoenberg HW: Early detection of prostate cancer by routine screening. JAMA 252:3261-3264, 1984.
70. Johansson JE, Andersson SO, Krusemo UB, et al: Natural history of localized prostatic cancer. Lancet: April 15, 1989, pp 799-803.
71. Parra RO, Wolf RM, Huben RP: The use of transrectal ultrasound in the detection and evaluation of local pelvic recurrences after a radical urological pelvic operation. J Urol 144(3):707-709, 1990.
72. Rifkin MD, Zerhouni EA, Constantine A, et al: Comparison of magnetic resonance imaging and ultrasonography in staging early prostate cancer. N Engl J Med 323:621-626, 1990.
73. McNeal JE, Kindrachuk RA, Frieha FS, et al: Patterns of progression in prostate cancer. Lancet 1:60-63, 1986.
74. Hernandez AD, Urry RI, Smith JA Jr: Ultrasonographic characteristics of the seminal vesicles after ejaculation. J Urol 144:1380-1382, 1990.
75. Hodge KK, McNeal JE, Stamey TA: Ultrasound guided transrectal core biopsies of the palpably abnormal prostate. J Urol 142:66-70, 1989.
76. Andriole GI, Catalona WJ: Transrectal ultrasonography in the staging of prostate cancer. In Resnick MR, Watanabe H, Karr JP (eds): Diagnostic ultrasound of the prostate. New York, 1989, Elsevier Science, pp 25-30.
77. Hashimoto T, Saito T, Kobayashi H, et al: Detection of cancer invasion into the seminal vesicles by ultrasound and puncture. In Resnick MR, Watanabe H, Karr JP (eds): Diagnostic ultrasound of the prostate, New York, 1989, Elsevier Science, pp 41-47.
78. Salo J, Kivisaari L, Rannikko S, et al: Computerized tomography and transrectal ultrasound in the assessment of local extension of prostatic cancer before radical retropubic prostatectomy. J Urol 137:435-438, 1987.
79. Carter HB, Hamper UM, Sheths S, et al: Evaluation of transrectal ultrasound in the early detection of prostate cancer. J Urol 142:1008-1010, 1989.
80. Smith JA and Middleton RG: Staging of prostate cancer. In Smith JA Jr and Middleton RG (eds): Clinical management of prostatic cancer. Chicago, 1987, Year Book, pp 103-120.
81. Wajsman A and Klimberg IW: Staging evaluation and follow-up of patients with advanced prostatic cancer. Semin Urol 6:249, 1988.
82. Urry RL and Cockett ATK: Male infertility, workup, treatment and research. New York, 1976, Grune & Stratton.
83. Colpi GM, Ballerini G, Zanollo A: Ultrasonography of the seminal vesicles in infertility. Prog Reprod Biol Med 12:124, 1985.
84. Littrup PJ, Lee F, McLeary RD, et al: Transrectal US of the seminal vesicles and ejaculatory ducts: clinical correlation. Radiology 168:625, 1988.
85. Kawahara M, Matsuhashi M, Tajima M, et al: Primary carcinoma of seminal vesicle: diagnosis assisted by sonography. Urology 32:269, 1988.
86. Lee SB, Lee F, Solomon MH, et al: Seminal vesicle abscess: diagnosis by transrectal ultrasound. J Clin Ultrasound 14:546, 1986.
87. Walls W, Linn F: Ultrasonic diagnosis of seminal vesicle cyst. Radiology 114:693, 1975.
88. Banner MP and Hassler R: The normal seminal vesiculogram. Radiology 128:339, 1978.
89. Beck PH, Whitlock MW, McAninch JW, et al: Vasoseminal vesiculography in staging adenocarcinoma of the prostate. Urology 11:239, 1978.
90. Stanley RJ, Sagel SS, Fair WR: Computed tomography of the genitourinary tract. J Urol 119:780, 1978.
91. Tanahashi Y, Watanabe H, Igari D, et al: Volume estimation of the seminal vesicles by means of transrectal ultrasonotomography: a preliminary report. Br J Urol 47:695, 1975.
92. Ronnberg L , Ylostalo JP: Estimation of the size of the seminal vesicles by means of ultrasonic B-scanning: preliminary report. Fertil Steril 30:474, 1978.
93. Jimenez-Cruz JF, Mayayo T, Lovaco F, et al: Transabdominal sonography of seminal vesicles. J Urol 127:260, 1982.
94. Gillenwater JY, Grayhack JT, Howards SS, Duckett JW: Adult and pediatric urology, vol 2. 1987, pp 1501-1508.

95. Steinhart JM, Kuhn JP, Eisenberg B, et al: Ultrasound screening of healthy infants for urinary tract abnormalities. Pediatrics 82(4):609-614, 1988.
96. Sheih CP, Liu MB, Hung CS, et al: Renal abnormalities in school children. Pediatrics 84(6):1086-1089, 1989.
97. Rosendahl H: Ultrasound screening for fetal urinary tract malformations: A prospective study in general population. Eur J Obstet Gynecol Reprod Biol 36(1-2):27-33, 1990.
98. Scott JES, Renwick M: Antenatal diagnosis of congenital abnormalities in the urinary tract. Br J Urol 62:295-300, 1988.
99. Helin I, Persson P: Prenatal diagnosis of urinary tract abnormalities by ultrasound. Pediatrics 78(5):879-883, 1986.
100. Frigoletto F, Auerbach R, Brickler A, et al: Consensus conference: the use of diagnostic ultrasound imaging during pregnancy. JAMA 252(5):669-672, 1984.
101. Canty TG, Leopold GR, Wolf DA (eds): Ultrasonography of pediatric surgical disorders. New York, 1982, Grune & Stratton, p 14.
102. Arger PH, Coleman BG, Mintz MC, et al: Routine fetal genitourinary tract screening. Radiology 156:485, 1985.
103. Mandel J, Peters CA, Retik AB: Current concepts in perinatal diagnosis and management of hydronephrosis. Urol Clin North Am 17(2):247-262, 1990.
104. The urinary tract. In Mittelstaedt CA (ed): Abdominal ultrasound. New York, 1987, Churchill-Livingstone, pp 229-230.
105. Scott JE, Hunter EW, Lee RE, Matthews JN: Ultrasound measurement of renal size in newborn infants. Arch Dis Child 65:361-364, 1990.
106. Rosenbaum DM, Korngold E, Teele RL: Sonographic assessment of renal length in normal children. AJR 142:467-469, 1984.
107. Hartman GE, Shochat SJ: Abdominal mass lesions in the newborn: diagnosis and treatment. Clin Perinatol 16(1):123-135, 1989.
108. Elder JS, Duckett JW: Perinatal urology. In Gillenwater JY, Grayhack JT, Howards SS, Duckett JW (eds): Adult and pediatric urology. Chicago, 1987, Year Book, pp 1554-1563.
109. Kass EJ, Fink-Bennett D: Contemporary techniques for the radioisotopic evaluation of the dilated urinary tract. Urol Clin North Am 17(2):273-289, 1990.
110. Zerin JM, Lebowitz RL: Pediatric uroradiology. AUA Update Series, lesson 28, vol 8, 1989.
111. Bernstein J, Gardner KD: Renal cystic disease and renal dysplasia. In Campbells urology. ed 5, 1986, p 1760.
112. Peters CA, Mandel J: The multicystic dysplastic kidney. AUA Update Series, lesson 7, vol 8, 1989, p 52.
113. Gilchrist GS, Kelalis PP: Tumors and related disorders, kidney and ureter. In Kelalis PP and King LR (eds): Clinical pediatric urology, vol 2. Philadelphia, 1976, Saunders, p 915.
114. Yambao TJ, Schwartz D, Henderson R, et al: Prenatal diagnosis of a congenital mesoblastic nephroma. J Reprod Med 31:257-259, 1986.
115. Kramer SA, Kelalis PP: Pediatric urologic oncology. In Gillenwater JY, Grayhack JT, Howards SS, Duckett JW (eds): Adult and pediatric urology, vol 2. Chicago, 1987, Year Book, p 2001.
116. Snyder HC, D'Angio GJ, Evans AE, Raney RB: Pediatric oncology. In Walsh, Gittes, Perlmutter, and Stamey (eds): Campbell's urology, vol 2, ed 5. Philadelphia, 1986, Saunders, p 2245.
117. The retroperitoneum. In Canty TG, Leopold GR, Wolf DA (eds): Ultrasonography of pediatric surgical disorders. New York, 1982, Grune & Stratton, p 169.

CHAPTER 6

PHOTOGRAPHY AND VIDEO UROLOGY

RICHARD K. BABAYAN

No textbook of urologic innovations would be complete without referring to the rapid technologic advances in endoscopic imaging that have occurred in the last decade. Video monitoring, recording and taping, and digitized storage and retrieval of freeze-frame video images have significantly broadened and enhanced traditional urologic endoscopy. Endoscopic photography and videotaping have progressed from an expensive and cumbersome, occasionally used novelty to a practical and affordable daily utility. The key to this video technologic explosion has been the development of high-resolution, lightweight, compact, and affordable charge-coupled device (CCD) cameras, which can be universally adapted to virtually all urologic endoscopes.

ENDOSCOPIC PHOTOGRAPHY

Still photography using 35 mm slide film with specially adapted endoscopic camera mounts has been used as a teaching and documentation tool throughout the history of modern urologic endoscopy. It is mentioned in this chapter for its historical significance and its current utility, but as is made evident later in this chapter, digitized imaging and freeze-frame video reproduction will probably replace endoscopic photography as we know it today. In its earliest applications, photographic technique was limited by the inadequate illumination provided by primitive light sources and by the poor quality of the early endoscopic lens systems. The introduction of high-intensity light sources and the improved optical quality of both rod lens and fiberoptic imaging bundles have enabled excellent quality color reproduction of still endoscopic images. The use of high-speed 35 mm color slide film with automatic light source synchronization has also eliminated many of the previous difficulties in obtaining truly representative endoscopic photographs (Figure 6–1).

Unfortunately, problems remain with endoscopic photography. Most endoscopy involves constant movement and manipulation of the instrument to position the viewing port on an area of interest. Even with the best state-of-the-art photographic equipment, it is the rare urologist who can obtain images of consistent quality while performing an endoscopic procedure. Virtually all 35 mm cameras are cumbersome and unwieldy when mounted on the eyepiece of either a rigid or a flexible endoscope. Cameras hinder the urologist's ability to perform an endoscopic procedure because of the weight and imbalance they add to the endoscope. In addition, urologists frequently need to take a dozen or more shots to obtain a single image that adequately represents the endoscopic finding they wish to capture on film. Some endoscopic findings, such as a bladder tumor, lend themselves well to still photography, whereas others are better represented by dynamic serial images such as those seen with videotaping.

Modern endoscopic video does not have the same limitations as still endoscopic photography. A running documentation of the endoscopic procedure may be obtained without sacrificing the surgeon's time or taxing his or her endoscopic abilities. Modern video cameras tend to be lighter and less obtrusive than 35 mm cameras when attached to endoscopes. Video monitor–based endoscopy may actually enhance the endoscopist's view and obviate the need to assume awkward positions in order to peer into the endoscope; thus it may spare the endoscopist much of the fatigue inherent in the performance of urologic endoscopy. The limitation of video endoscopy is in obtaining still images comparable to the best 35 mm photographic images. This apparent deficit may be overcome in the near future. Whereas endoscopic slide photography has reached an apparent technologic plateau, the development of video technology has been paralleling that of computer microchip memory technology. At the current growth trajectory in video technology,

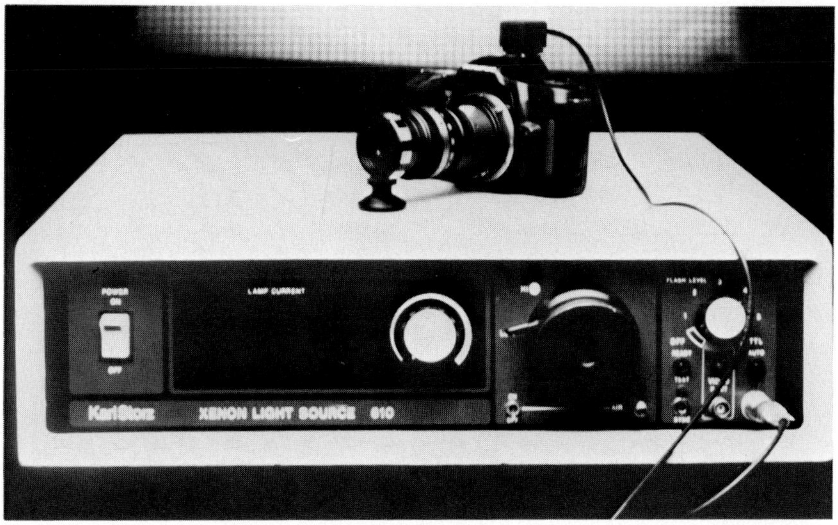

FIGURE 6–1. A 35 mm camera with endoscopic lens mount and light synchronization cord.

a quadrupling of the number of picture elements per CCD can be anticipated every 3 years. The results of the video technology explosion have been rapid miniaturization of camera size and continued improvement in image quality and reproduction.

TECHNICAL ASPECTS OF VIDEO ENDOSCOPY

The application of video techniques to urologic endoscopy has been an attractive concept for decades, but the enormous size, weight, and expense of earlier tube cameras made their use both difficult and impractical. A gradual reduction in the size of tube cameras during the 1970s and early 1980s resulted in hand-held cameras of some practicality (Figure 6–2). The true medical video revolution, however, began with the development of CCD video cameras with microchip technology, which replaced the previously cumbersome Vidicon and Saticon tube cameras.

All current urologic video cameras are of the CCD type. These cameras are typically compact and lightweight, some as small as 3 ounces. They can be adapted to the eyepieces of urologic endoscopes regardless of whether the endoscope is rod-lens or fiberoptic, rigid or flexible. These video cameras may be either gas sterilized or submerged and soaked in disinfectants. Many have built-in beamsplitters (Figure 6–3). These are optical devices that permit video monitor projection and simultaneous direct endoscopic visualization. The beamsplitter literally divides the light into two optical paths of varying proportion. Typically 70% to 85% of the light goes for the camera and monitor projection and 15% to 30% is available for direct viewing. Beamsplitter cameras have been popular as initial video purchases because of their versatility and because they allow standard endoscopic viewing while simultaneously videotaping and allowing others to observe the procedure on the monitor. As urologists become more accustomed to monitor-based endoscopy, beamsplitters are giving way to direct-coupled cameras of smaller size and equal or superior image quality (Figure 6–4).

The CCD camera operates by converting light from optical images into electronic energy, which

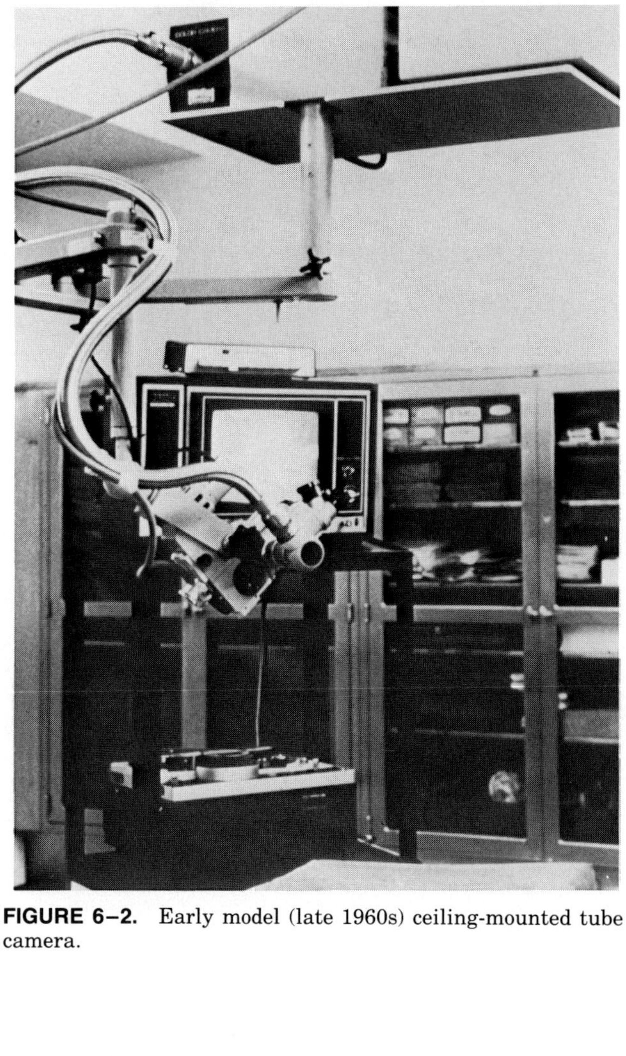

FIGURE 6–2. Early model (late 1960s) ceiling-mounted tube camera.

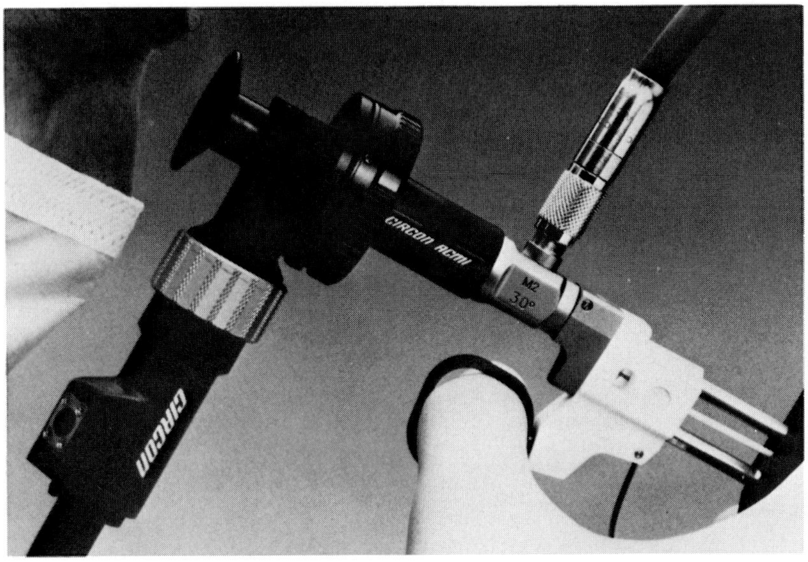

FIGURE 6–3. Compact CCD beamsplitter video camera mounted on the eyepiece of a resectoscope.

is processed, transferred, and reconverted into light energy for image reconstruction on a TV monitor. To understand this process, even in simplistic, nonoptical engineering terms, the reader needs a few electronic definitions. These are listed in Appendix A.

The heart of the chip camera is the charge-coupled device, which is a solid-state sensor composed of individual picture elements or pixels, which are light sensitive and self-scanning. As the visual image changes before the sensor, variability in the light energy perceived by the pixels is converted into an electronic signal frequency.

Color translation and reproduction are accomplished in a similar manner. Single-chip cameras divide the pixels into three catagories to scan either for one of the primary colors (red, green, or blue) or for one of the so-called complementary colors (cyan, yellow, or magenta). Color is translated to the monitor through a complex series of transfers and reconstructions of electronic signals. Noise distortion in translation can often lead to color variability. Recently a compact three-chip camera was introduced (Figure 6–5). This type of camera uses three separate CCDs linked together by a prism. As light images are focused through the prism, each individual CCD receives and has responsibility for scanning only one primary color. This results in three times the input of electronic color signals to the monitor for translation. Signal distortion is less likely, and thus color resolution is much improved. The current cost of this camera, however, is roughly double that of the single CCD camera, and the three-chip camera is somewhat larger and heavier. Whether the difference in color resolution at this time is worth the additional expense is debatable. Probably this multichip camera will become more practical and cost effective as smaller and more compact CCDs are developed.

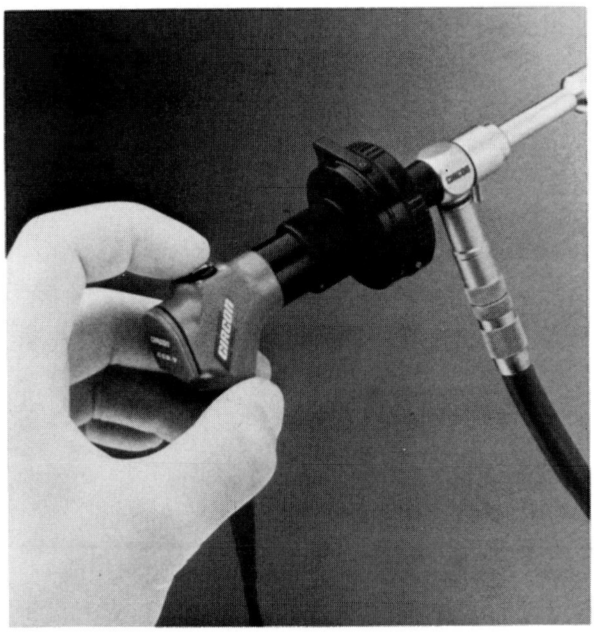

FIGURE 6–4. Direct-coupled CCD camera without beamsplitter.

Video chip cameras will not gain further significant improvement in resolution of image quality until the current TV scanning systems, NTSC (National Television System Committee), used in North America and Japan, and PAL (Phase Alternating Line), used throughout Europe, are replaced by a new high-definition TV system. Under the NTSC system, color video signal translation is limited to 525 lines per frame at 30 frames/sec (60 Hz). The European PAL system constructs monitor images based on a scanning rate of 625 lines per frame at 25 frames/sec (50 Hz). Thus the two systems are incompatible. The hope for the future is a high-definition system that achieves worldwide acceptance for color image reconstruction. High-

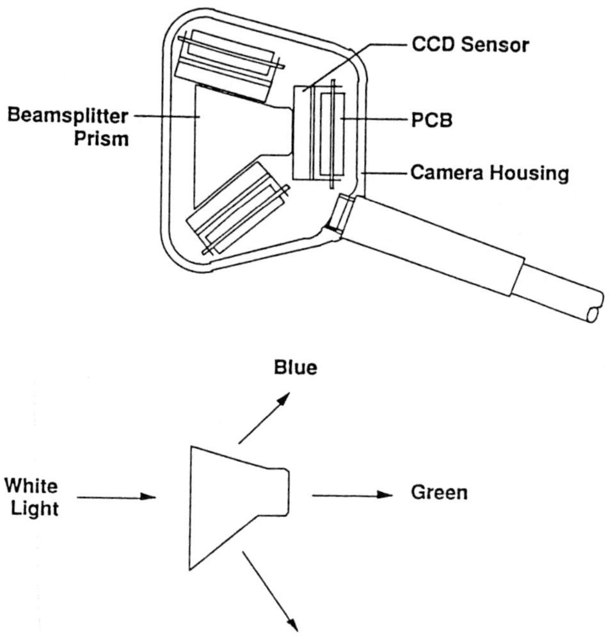

FIGURE 6–5. Schematic representation of three-chip camera. The prism and filters separate light into primary colors.

definition TV is expected to more than double the scan lines per frame and increase the luminescence bandwidth to 20 MHz. This will result in a fivefold increase in the number of effective pixels and a dramatic improvement in picture quality.

Once the light image has been scanned by the camera, captured, and translated into electronic impulses for video monitor imaging, it can also be transferred to tape for storage and review. Videotape recorders use magnetic tape traveling across a recording head to imprint the electronic impulses captured by the CCD camera. The type of magnetic tape used ranges from 3/4 inch to 1/2 inch to 8 mm, depending on individual preferences or desires. The larger 3/4 inch tape is advantageous for editing and still frame reproduction but is bulky and cumbersome for everyday use and storage. The 8 mm videotapes are quite compact and economical but lack the quality of image reproduction of 3/4 inch or super VHS tapes.

Recent advances in digital image storage and retrieval systems have given rise to video floppy disk systems capable of storing up to 50 still images on a single video floppy disk (Figure 6–6). These can be retrieved and viewed on a video monitor or linked to a color hard copy printer for image reproduction (Figure 6–7). The quality of the resulting color hard copy is similar to that of a Polaroid instant photo. Color images are reproduced with more than 500 lines of horizontal resolution. These images are printed on sheets of 5½ × 4 inch paper. One, four, or 24 video still images can be printed per page. Computer-linked systems now available even allow digitized endoscopic images to be incorporated into an operative report, yielding a laser printer–quality color endoscopic image inserted within the text of the endoscopic report. Both visual and written documentation of the findings of an endoscopic procedure can thus be cataloged for future reference and review.

CURRENT APPLICATIONS

Although video cameras have been a mainstay in arthroscopy and gastrointestinal endoscopy for years, urologists have been reluctant to convert from traditional direct-vision endoscopic viewing to video monitor–based urologic endoscopy. They argue that they have managed quite nicely looking directly through the eyepiece of cystoscopes, ureteroscopes, nephroscopes, and the like, so why change? There are a number of logical reasons

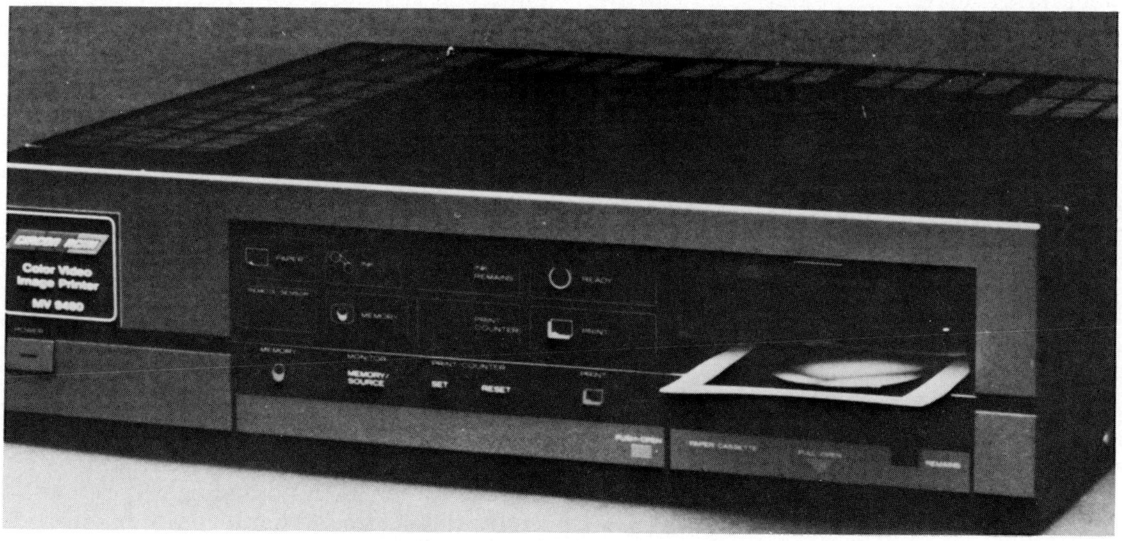

FIGURE 6–6. Video floppy disk recorder.

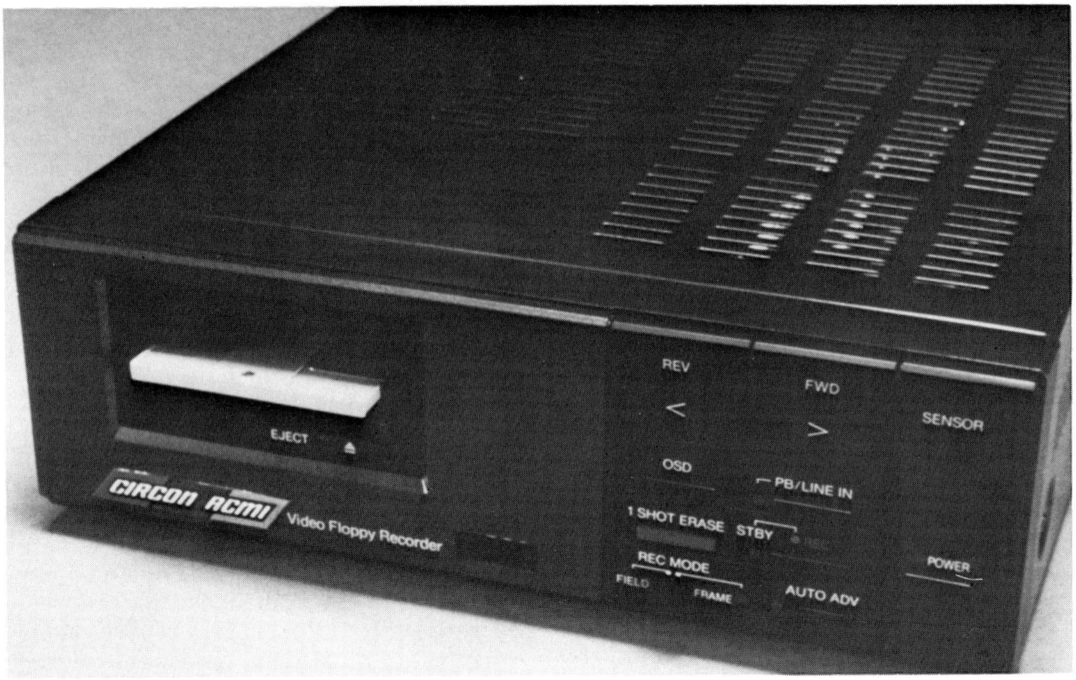

FIGURE 6–7. Color video image printer capable of producing hard copies within 80 seconds.

to make the switch to video endoscopy, as well as driving forces that will inevitably bring this about.

Medical Education and Acquisition of New Skills

Endoscopic skills involve hand-eye coordination and fine manual dexterity. Whether one is involved in resident education or attempting to master a new endoscopic skill, having the best possible view of the operative field is of utmost importance. It would be foolish to limit oneself to peering with one eye through a small eyepiece when technology can provide a clear large magnified image that can be viewed not only by the primary endoscopist but also by assistants and students. In the case of resident education, video is far superior to previous teaching attachments, which were notorious for decreasing available light and allowed only one individual the opportunity of viewing the endoscopic field. The use of video has significantly decreased the learning curve in acquiring new skills and refining endoscopic technique. Guidance can be given throughout an endoscopic procedure. This results in more rapid performance of a procedure and decreases the potential for morbidity. This is especially true in the case of endourologic procedures such as ureteroscopic stone manipulation, which often requires two pairs of hands, one to maneuver the scope and the other to manipulate the accessories. The monitor is an invaluable aid in the performance of such procedures. Group viewing and discussion of the endoscopic procedure can occur, and videotaping with later review can reinforce technical nuances acquired during the performance of a previous procedure.

Safety and Efficiency

Given the variety of endoscopes at the urologist's disposal and the difficulties of passing these instruments through the urinary tract, the urologist must often work for a long time in an awkward position to complete an endoscopic procedure (Figure 6–8). In addition, urologists commonly come in contact with blood, urine, or irrigation solutions during a routine procedure because of the proximity of the urologist's head to the endoscope. To make matters worse, patients are also subjected to extremes in positioning so that the urologist has room to squeeze his or her head in place to peer through the scope. When a compact microchip camera is applied to the eyepiece of the endoscope, neither the urologist nor the patient need be subjected to the routine contortions of years past. The attachment of the camera to the scope allows the urologist to assume a natural and comfortable position, well away from the operating table, thus sparing the neck and shoulders from fatigue (Figure 6–9). The elimination of neck strain and fatigue often shortens the endoscopic procedure and thus benefits the patient by decreasing anesthesia time. In the case of ureteroscopy, where C-arm fluoroscopy is commonly employed, an additional safety benefit is the distance the surgeon can remain from the radiation source without compromising endoscopic technique.

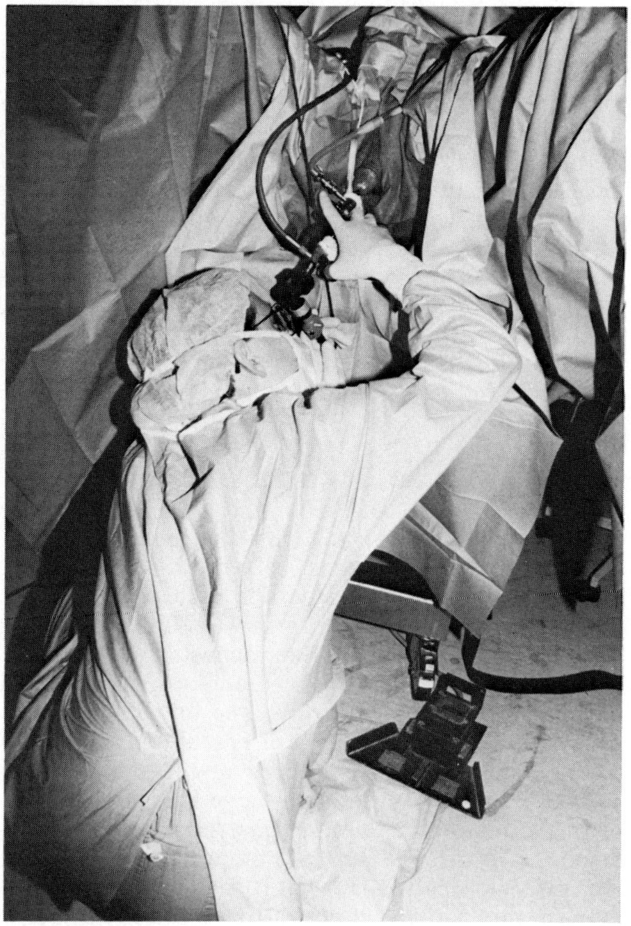

FIGURE 6–8. Urologist kneeling at the base of the cystoscopy table to look directly into the eyepiece of the cystoscope.

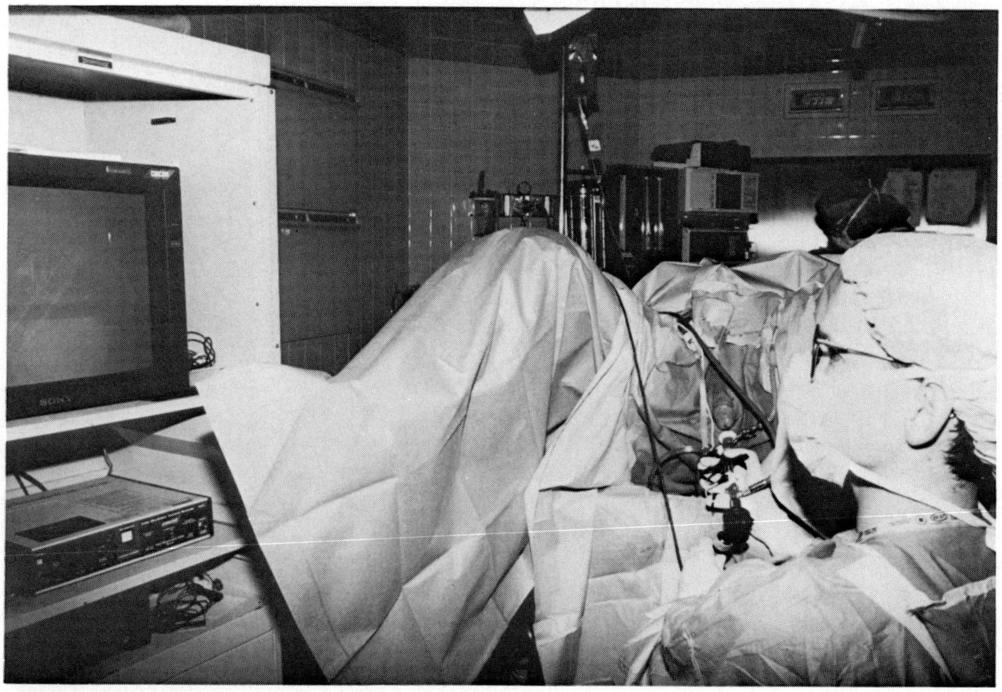

FIGURE 6–9. Monitor-based cystoscopy, which allows the urologist to assume a comfortable posture while viewing high-quality magnified endoscopic image.

Operating Room Staff Coordination

One of the most universal and frustrating experiences of urologists is the inability to communicate their needs rapidly during an endoscopic procedure. The operating room (OR) staff has no way of anticipating the surgeon's needs because they have no concept of what the surgeon is doing through the endoscope. Monitor-based endoscopy allows all OR personnel to view the procedure. This leads not only to a better informed staff, but also to a more interested one. Video monitor endoscopy allows the OR staff to participate in the case, which results in improved attention and better assistance.

Case Documentation

The video camera not only improves visualization and technical performance but also is a superb documentation tool. Videotape records of individual cases may be kept for review or used to generate hard copy photos of pertinent aspects of a case. Still video images can be captured and stored for future reference on video floppy disks or on the newer optical disks. Video mapping of urothelial tumors for sequential comparison and review has been advocated. Computer-enhanced video images have become commonplace among gastrointestinal endoscopists. As video technology expands and the costs continue to decline, the digitized video endoscopy record may replace paper in the medical records of the future.

PRACTICAL CONSIDERATIONS

A number of driving forces are responsible for the recent interest in video endoscopy within the urologic community. First and foremost are the size reduction and improved image quality that have been achieved by video manufacturers within the last decade. A number of recent publications have extolled the benefits of state-of-the-art CCD video cameras during transurethral resection and endourologic procedures.[1-3] These reports reiterate the points brought out in the previous section with regard to medical education, safety, staff coordination, and documentation. Surgeons increasingly recognize that video-assisted endoscopy improves operative efficiency and shortens procedure time. A recent review of transurethral resections performed at University Hospital in Boston has indicated that the routine use of video during the performance of transurethral prostatic resection (TURP) has increased the volume of prostatic chips resected in a shorter operative time than was possible before the use of monitor-based endoscopy.

Another driving force toward the adoption of video endoscopy has been the emergence of laparoscopic techniques in urology. The video camera and monitor-based endoscopy are inherent in the use of laparoscopy. As urologists strive to replace traditional open urologic operations with laparoscopic procedures, they must become adept at working while watching the video monitor. This skill naturally translates to applications in other urologic endoscopic procedures. Conversely, urologists interested in acquiring laparoscopic skills find that if they perform traditional urologic endoscopic procedures, such as the TURP, while viewing the video monitor, the transition to monitor-based laparoscopy is easier.

LIMITATIONS OF VIDEO ENDOSCOPY

Although video endoscopy is likely to become commonplace for routine urologic endoscopy in the near future, there are significant obstacles in the path of general acceptance of this technology. Foremost is the initial cost of purchase and maintenance of equipment. A good-quality compact video system including a CCD camera, video recorder, and TV monitor costs approximately $10,000. Purchase of accessories, such as floppy disk recorders, hard copy printers, and sophisticated video mobile carts (Figure 6–10), can more than double the initial in-

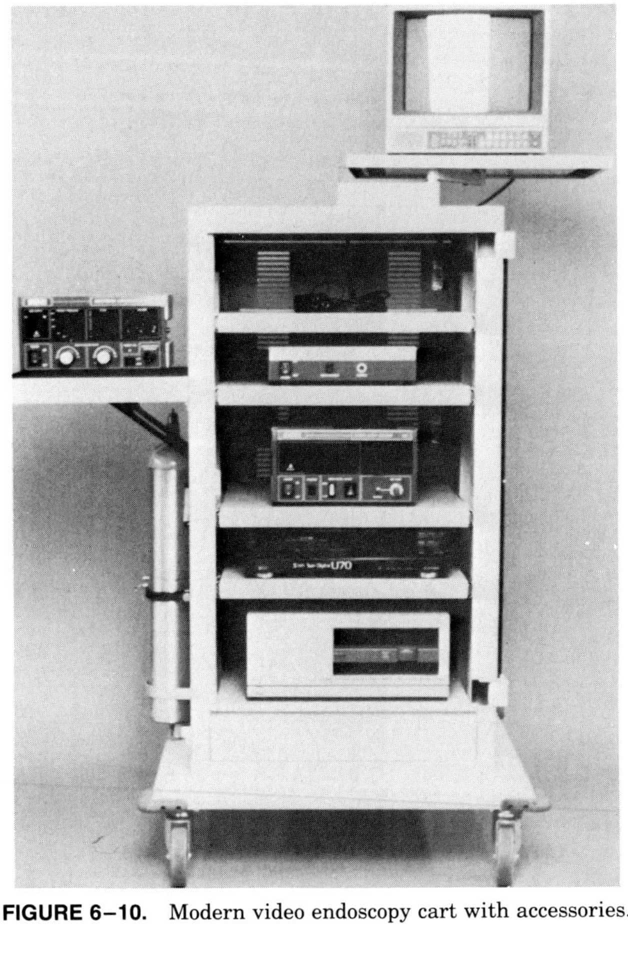

FIGURE 6–10. Modern video endoscopy cart with accessories.

vestment. No video camera is as sensitive to light accommodation as the human eye. Therefore, even with the best automatic light-shuttering systems, combined with high-intensity light sources, some degree of "bleaching" of an image occurs because of light reflection, or dampening of an image because of inadequate illumination. Color distortion has been a problem with video cameras in the past, although this has become less an issue with each new camera generation. The ultimate limitation to video endoscopy in urology has been the reluctance of urologists themselves to embrace this technology. This, however, appears to be a transient phenomenon. Traditionally, urologic surgeons have been innovative and quick to adopt technologic advances that enhance their ability to deal with urologic diseases. As video technology advances and its current limitations are overcome, a widespread application in urology will undoubtedly emerge.

FUTURE CONSIDERATIONS

The trend in video technology is toward smaller cameras of lower cost that use more compact yet powerful electronic sensors. At the current rate of technologic advancement in the video microchip industry, within a decade electronic miniaturization will make standard optical lens technology obsolete. In other medical specialties such as gastroenterology, which uses large-bore flexible instruments, fiberoptic bundles have already been replaced by CCD chips placed at the distal end of the scope. The image picked up by the CCD is electronically transmitted to the monitor without the need of relay through a fiberoptic bundle or series of lenses. These instruments have no eyepiece and are potentially more durable, since there are no fiberoptic bundles to break or lenses to come out of alignment. Of potential advantage in the future is the possibility of creating an endoscope with a small CCD at the end that would allow incorporation of a much larger working channel than is possible today in direct optic endoscopes. The video endoscope would, of course, require that the operator use a monitor-based viewing technique.

Clearly, any advances in camera or video endoscope design would require parallel improvement in video image processing and reproduction. As technology shifts from optical to digital image acquisition and reproduction, better techniques will be developed to display the by-product. High-definition TV has the potential for enhancing current TV reproduction by a factor of five. When a universal decoding and translation system is finally adopted in the next few years, a variety of competing reproduction and recording technologies will emerge and probably replace videotaping as we know it today. Whether the system will be digital tape cassettes or laser disk technology is still unclear. What is certain, however, is that video is a rapidly advancing technology. These advances have received widespread and rapid acceptance within both the medical community and the general population. With continuing improvement in image quality, associated with decreasing size and cost, video will continue to have a tremendous impact on urologic endoscopy and will probably become the driving force in endoscopic technology of the future.

REFERENCES

1. Preminger GM: Video-assisted transurethral resection of the prostate. J Endourol 5:161, 1991.
2. Widran J: Video transurethral resection using controlled continuous flow resectoscope. Urology 31:382, 1988.
3. Allhoff E, Bading R, et al: The chip camera: perfect imaging in endourology. World J Urol 6:8, 1988.

CHAPTER 7

URODYNAMICS

RICHARD C. LABASKY

Urodynamics refers to a broad range of tests used to evaluate the morphologic, neurophysiologic, pharmacologic, and hydrodynamic characteristics of the lower urinary tract. Urodynamics tests are intended to provide objective data about lower urinary tract characteristics that clinicians consider significant. The technical characteristics of the tests are based on specific physical laws and a range of facts and assumptions about the function of the lower urinary tract. The tests are used to supplement the other data obtained in the urologic evaluation, especially the history and the physical and neurologic examinations. Most have been used in one form or another for over a century.[1,2]

This chapter is a broad review of the basic principles and techniques of urodynamics. It shows why and how urodynamics equipment is selected and used, how the tests can be selected and performed properly, and what the abnormalities shown on the tests imply for a urodynamics diagnosis. More specifically, the chapter should provide the urologist with a basic core of information for three purposes:

1. To understand the basic principles and technologic state of the equipment used for urodynamics tests so that equipment can be purchased and used with a better understanding of its strengths, weaknesses, and inherent sources of error, as well as its requirements for support staff and maintenance
2. To select the most appropriate tests for obtaining specific urodynamics data that will delineate the pathophysiology of the lower urinary tract, thereby limiting unnecessary or inappropriate testing
3. To interpret the results of the various urodynamics tests, understand the limitations and caveats inherent in the results, and make the urodynamics diagnosis of the lower urinary tract dysfunction

Abnormalities on urodynamics tests are not diagnostic of specific diseases, nor do they necessarily indicate the specific site of a lesion causing the lower urinary tract dysfunction. As with any diagnostic test, the urologist must fit the urodynamics diagnosis with the knowledge of the clinical situation and the attendant differential diagnosis to make the final diagnosis.

This chapter does not review the details of the anatomy, neurophysiology, and pharmacology of the lower urinary tract.[3-9] Furthermore, it does not delineate all the testing abnormalities specific to particular diseases or syndromes, nor the complete differential diagnosis applicable to the urodynamics diagnosis. For this information the reader should consult other sources as needed. He or she can then apply the basic information on technique and interpretation of urodynamics testing that is given in this chapter.

BASIC PRINCIPLES OF URODYNAMICS

Urodynamics tests are designed to evaluate the three main elements of the lower urinary tract—the bladder, the urethra, and their sensation—while urine is filling the bladder, being stored, and being voided from the bladder through the urethra. This chapter reviews the primary urodynamics tests used today: urinary flow rate measurement (uroflowmetry), cystometry, electromyography, urethral pressure measurement, simultaneous cystometry and uroflowmetry (pressure/flow study), and video urodynamics (Table 7–1, Figure 7–1). The tests provide either direct or indirect (implied) data about the bladder, urethra, or sensory function. For many years the terminology used to describe the testing procedures and results represented a return of the Tower of Babel. Finally, over several years the International Continence Society (ICS) standardized the terminology for lower urinary tract function.[10] The ICS terminology is used in this chapter, and urologists are encouraged to learn it so they can communicate the findings of urodynamics testing in the most consistent, convenient, accurate, and understandable fashion. According to the ICS terminology the function of each

TABLE 7–1. Urodynamics Tests and the Data Provided

Test	*Filling/Voiding*	*Detrusor*	*Urethra*	*Sensation*
Uroflowmetry	−/+	I	I	I
Cystometry	+/−	D	I	D
Pressure/flow	−/+	D	I	I
Urethral pressure	+/+	—	D	—
Electromyography	+/+	—	I	—
Video urodynamics	+/+	*	*	*

D, Direct measurement; *I*, indirect measurement; *, depends on specific tests performed with fluoroscopy.

component of the lower urinary tract can be normal, overactive, or underactive during filling and storage or voiding; specific ICS terms therefore fall into one of those three categories (Tables 7–2 and 7–3).

Just as the clinician must understand the basic principles, techniques, and capabilities of urodynamics tests, the urodynamicist must ensure that the tests are conducted properly so that the results are meaningful and interpretable. Each test, and the pattern of the findings of the tests, should reproduce as thoroughly as possible the patient's symptoms, and be repeated within reason until such reproduction is achieved. If the urodynamics tests produce findings unrelated to the patient's complaints, the results are probably artifacts, clinically unrelated and irrelevant, or fortuitous and possibly related yet clinically unexplainable at that point. In rare circumstances, as when surgery or treatment might alter the lower urinary tract, urodynamics testing may be performed on a patient without known dysfunction to obtain baseline in-

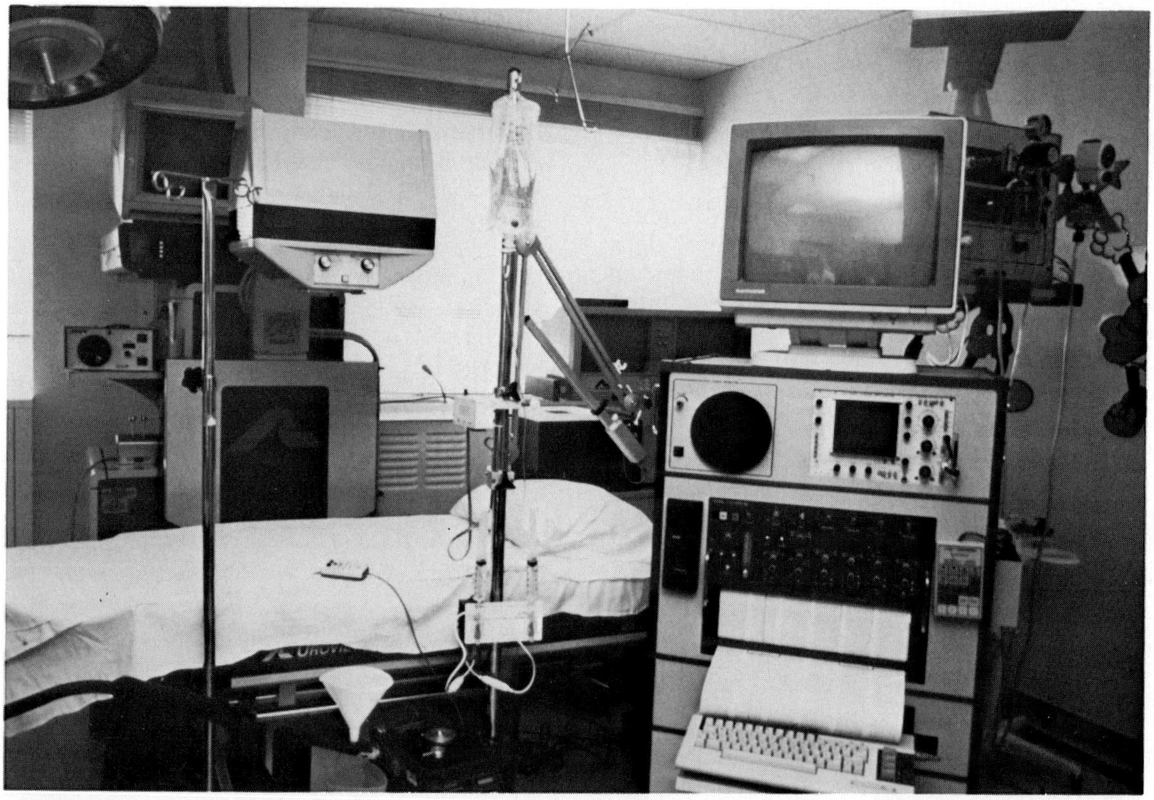

FIGURE 7–1. A complete urodynamics laboratory with the data monitoring and recording unit on the right with a six-channel paper strip chart recorder in the middle. Just above the strip chart are an audio speaker and an oscilloscope to observe the output of the electromyography. Below the strip chart is a keyboard used to input data pertinent to the test to be performed and recorded on a videotape machine. The monitor displays the urodynamics data in real time and serves as a playback screen for tests recorded on the videotape. To the left of the main unit is an intravenous (IV) pole holding, from the bottom of the picture up, the infusion pump, the pressure transducers, the articulating arms of the urethral pressure profilometry pulling device, and the infusion fluid. To the left of the IV pole is the fluoroscopy unit and table, with the electromyography amplifier resting on the table. In the foreground of the table is the funnel to direct urine flow into the urinary flowmeter. Except for the fluoroscopy machine, the unit is completely mobile so that it can be set up in any arrangement, depending on the patient and testing situation.

TABLE 7–2. Urodynamic Classification of Lower Urinary Tract Dysfunction

Component	Activity	Dysfunction
Detrusor	Overactivity	Detrusor instability Detrusor hyperreflexia Low compliance
	Underactivity (Absolute or Relative)	Acontractility Areflexia
Urethra	Overactivity	Obstruction
	Underactivity	Total incompetence Anatomic incompetence
Sensation	Overactivity Underactivity	

formation before the intervention is performed. To obtain the most valid, useful data and interpretation, the urologist must bring three assets to urodynamics tests: (1) a thorough understanding of the patient's history and physical examination; (2) a genuine interest in and familiarity with the pathophysiology of the lower urinary tract and urodynamics techniques, terminology, and test interpretation; and (3) personal, direct supervision, observation, and interpretation of the tests.

URINARY FLOW RATE MEASUREMENT (UROFLOWMETRY)

Measuring the flow rate of urine from the bladder provides some of the most basic but useful data about lower urinary tract function.[2] The concept of the flow rate is a simple one. The detrusor must elevate intravesical pressure enough to allow expulsion of the urine past any resistance by the urethra. Optimally, the active and passive resistance components of the urethra are reduced maximally to provide the least obstruction to the urine being

TABLE 7–3. International Continence Society Symbols Used in This Chapter

BASIC SYMBOLS	
Pressure	P
Volume	V
Flow rate	Q
Time	T
Length	L
SPECIFIERS	
Bladder	ves
Detrusor	det
Abdominal	abd
Urethra	ura
VALUES	
Maximum	max
Minimum	min
Average	ave

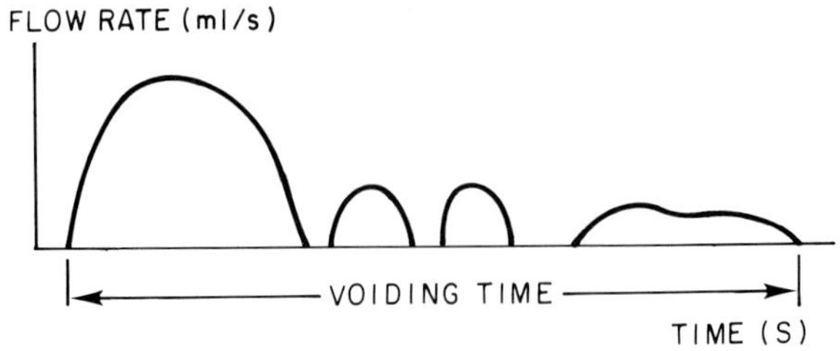

FIGURE 7–2. Normal urinary flow curve with the major parameters designated according to International Continence Society definitions. In this case of an uninterrupted flow curve, the voiding time equals the flow time.

compressed within the bladder. Ideally and normally, the bladder and urethra are coordinated, the urethra relaxing as the detrusor contracts. The sensation the individual feels throughout the process of detrusor contraction, urethral relaxation, and urine flow should be acceptable and comfortable or "normal." To whatever extent these "normal" conditions are met, urine flows out of the urethra and the rate and pattern of the flow can be observed.

Determining the flow rate does not directly assess the bladder, urethral, and sensory characteristics; rather, an abnormal flow rate or pattern indicates that some component in the lower urinary tract is abnormal, at least during the voiding process. Unfortunately, the converse, that a normal flow rate means that lower urinary tract function is completely normal, is not always true. Some situations illustrating these concepts are presented later.

Flow rate is the volume of urine expelled from the bladder through the urethra per unit time, measured in milliliters per second (ml/sec). The flow rate is plotted against time to produce a curve similar to that shown in Figures 7–2 and 7–3. Such flow rate–time curves permit description of the rate and pattern of the urinary flow according to ICS terminology.

Urinary flow may occur in one of two patterns, as a single bolus (continuous flow; Figure 7–2) or in several boluses (intermittent flow; Figure 7–3).

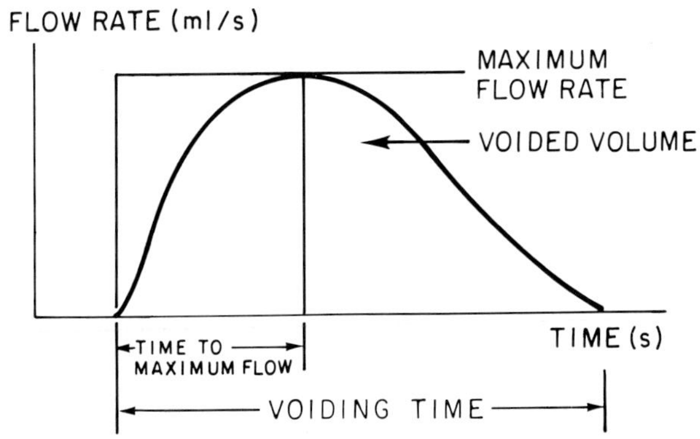

FIGURE 7–3. Intermittent flow pattern. In this case the flow time would be less than the voiding time.

Voiding time is the total duration of the voiding effort; flow time is the time during which measurable urine flow occurs. When voiding is continuous, flow time equals voiding time; for intermittent flow, voiding time is greater than flow time.

Voided volume is the total volume expelled through the urethra and is the integration of the area beneath the volume-time curve(s). Maximum flow rate is the maximum measured flow rate. Average flow rate is voided volume divided by the flow time. Time to maximum flow is the elapsed time from onset of flow to maximum flow. One major caveat is that average flow rate is meaningful only if flow is continuous and without terminal dribbling.

Equipment

The simplest technique for approximating urinary flow rates requires only a stopwatch and a measuring cup.[2] The clinician directly observes, or listens nearby, as the patient voids, and records the volume voided and the voiding time. The clinician may also attempt to grade the force or caliber of the stream and note any terminal dribbling. This technique provides only average flow rate data and invades the patient's privacy, a condition that is especially important in women. Also, the ability to repeat the test and record and compare data uniformly is less than ideal.

A variety of other techniques have been developed, some more useful than others; these are reviewed well by a number of authors,[2,11-17] especially Ryall and Marshall.[2] Attempts to measure flow by observing the distance the urine stream can be projected horizontally (the casting distance) or vertically mistake the velocity energy available in the stream for the volume of flow. The former is related to both urinary voiding pressure and the diameter of the urethral meatus; the smaller the meatus, the greater the velocity and casting distance, although the volume voided (flow rate) may not be as much as that associated with an equal pressure but larger meatus. Besides this basic limitation created by the laws of fluid flow, the technique is useless with female patients.[15]

Somewhat more advanced are simple hand-held devices that measure maximum flow rate and voided volume, such as the flowmeter developed by Drake and Binard, the peakometer.[18] Such devices are inexpensive and reusable by an individual patient, but they do not record the flow pattern, do not allow detection of a brief, unrepresentative flow rate rise caused by abdominal straining, and are inaccurate in the lower flow ranges (about 10 ml/sec) where flow rate measurements are of greatest value.

A more sophisticated but more cumbersome system collects the urine in a separate tube each second as the tubes rotate past the patient on a carousel.[19] Other techniques measure the rate of air displacement from a container as urine is directed into it[13,20,21] or the rate of radioisotope elimination from the bladder.[22] Among the more complex techniques are drop spectrometry[23-25] and electromagnetic[26,27] and ultrasonic measurements of flow.[28] These methods, as well as modifications of the techniques discussed below,[29] have been attempts at better instantaneous measurements of flow without the error of the time lag as the urine passes from the meatus to the measuring device. They are used primarily in research and require more refinement before they can be used widely in clinical settings.

Very reliable, accurate, reproducible, and useful flow measurements are obtained in privacy with the rugged, commercially available flowmeters. Such flowmeters are scientifically sound, since they use one of several principles of physics to provide flow rate data essentially instantaneously.[30] One technique, the gravimetric method, uses a weight transducer to measure the mass of urine voided. The mass is proportional to the volume of urine, and electronically differentiating volume with respect to time yields flow rate. Potential errors with such systems are insignificant (the velocity energy of urine falling directly upon the transducer) or can be prevented or corrected (measurements with fluids of densities widely different from urine, such as radiographic contrast material; mechanical disturbances such as vibrations or knocking). A simple pressure transducer could be used in a similar fashion by converting the hydrostatic pressure of the accumulating column of voided urine to volume and then to a flow rate.[14,16,31-35]

In the rotating disk method the power needed to keep a horizontal disk rotating at a constant speed is measured. As urine falls upon the disk and remains there until it is spun off by centrifugal force, the disk's inertia and therefore the power requirement increase. The power requirement is proportional to the flow rate, and electronic integration yields voided volumes. These systems respond rapidly and are not affected by mechanical disturbance. However, fluid densities widely different from urine and where the urine stream strikes the disk can cause errors, so a special funnel is needed to guide the urine to the disk.[36-38]

A third measurement technique, the capacitance method, uses a metal strip dipped into the urine collection vessel. The strip's electrical capacitance decreases as the vessel fills with urine, since the urine contains electrolytes that conduct electrical current. Thus the volume voided is proportional to the capacitance change; differentiation of the volume with respect to time yields flow rate. These devices have no moving parts, making them reliable and relatively inexpensive. However, calibration variations can be significant.[12]

The flowmeter should have technical characteristics that ensure reasonable accuracy and precision in the range of data acquisition, as well as convenience and safety in use, cleaning, calibration, and maintenance.[30] The commercially available flowmeters generally meet these criteria. Accuracy for flow rates and volume should be within ±5% throughout the range of the flowmeter, with good linearity of response from 0 to 50 ml/sec up to volumes of 1000 ml. The greatest accuracy is needed at low flow rates, about 10 to 20 ml/sec. For example, an accuracy of 5% based on the full scale of 50 ml/sec is 2.5 ml/sec. This same absolute accuracy level applied to a flow rate of 10 ml/sec is 25% of the measured value, not the 5% that would presumably apply.[12,36,38] The rate of response for data acquisition display (the time constant) must be such that the device detects significant flow fluctuations, yet damps out irrelevant, abrupt, brief changes that are considered "noise"; rates of 0.5 to 0.75 second are appropriate.[12,30,32,38]

The flowmeter should be convenient to use and set up; automatic start and stop functions are particularly useful. Both male and female patients should be able to use the device. It should be compact enough to be used in a place offering reasonable privacy to the patient. It should be durable and safe enough for patients to use without direct supervision. At the minimum the data output format should be easily interpreted, be permanent, and show the flow curve on a graph; basic strip chart pen recorders are adequate in terms of frequency response and quality of the display. Further data printout capability, providing such information as flow rates and volume voided, is useful but not essential; in fact, such data printouts can be misleading or contain artifacts as "data," so the clinician must examine the flow curve itself to confirm that the printed numerical data are valid. The flowmeter should be easily cleaned, have minimal and easily accomplished calibration and maintenance requirements, and allow paper or printer changing with ease. Finally, the flowmeter selected should be compatible with other urodynamic equipment already in use.

Technique

The clinician does not actually perform the flow test—the patient and the flowmeter do. However, the clinician insures that the test is conducted properly. Patient nervousness, unintended inhibition of the flow, artificial straining, movement of the urinary stream around the flowmeter's funnel (wag artifact), and urethral instrumentation before the test can affect results and are preventable with proper attention to technique.

As with all urodynamics testing, uroflowmetry should duplicate the symptoms and situation the patient routinely experiences. The patient should have as much privacy as possible during the test; this is particularly true for women, who sometimes cannot complete the test in the clinic even in the best of circumstances. The bladder should be adequately full, meaning that the patient should have at least the usual sense of bladder fullness and need to void that is present in a routine situation away from the clinic. To produce this situation, the patient may need to drink fluids in the clinic, or beforehand, to fill the bladder. If the patient voids only a small volume for the test, an output chart recorded at home for several days may show that such small volumes truly represent the patient's normal efforts. The patient should void in the manner typical for him or her, without preliminary advice or coaching, whether this involves straining, sitting, standing, or any other variation of "normal." The patient should be asked if the flow rate and pattern during the test are similar to those produced away from the clinic; if not, the test may have to be repeated one or more times until the patient feels that routine voiding characteristics are being recorded. The flowmeter's curve should be generated with a paper speed that allows easy examination of the flow pattern and determination of maximum flow.

Normal and Abnormal Flow Rates and Patterns

Apart from the testing environment and the patient's lower urinary tract dysfunction, several factors affect the normal urinary flow rate (Figures 7–4 to 7–10), including patient age and sex, the bladder volume at the time of voiding, and voided volume.[12,13,17,18,20,36,39-56] A number of authors have attempted to adjust for these variables, but the resulting normal values are not in total agreement. However, several broad conclusions are consistent in these studies. Flow decreases through the adult years in men and slightly so in women. Men's flow rates are lower than women's after volume and age are taken into account. Bladder and voided volumes are significant because the detrusor functions most efficiently and flow rates are maximum when the bladder volume is about 300 to 400 ml. Flow rates are significantly lower with lesser or greater bladder volumes.

Several other practical generalizations can be made.[12,13,17,18,20,27,36,39,41-53,56] For voided volumes of at least 200 ml in adults and 150 ml in children over 4 years old, (1) maximum flow rates less than 10 ml/sec are abnormal, probably because of urethral overactivity (obstruction) unless bladder underactivity (acontractility or areflexia [see later discussion]) is a possible cause; (2) maximum flow rates from 10 to 15 ml/sec are equivocal and require repeat or possibly simultaneous cystometry and uroflowmetry (pressure/flow) studies; and (3) maximum flow rates above 15 ml/sec are usually normal and rarely associated with obstruction except in situations of abnormally high voiding pressures

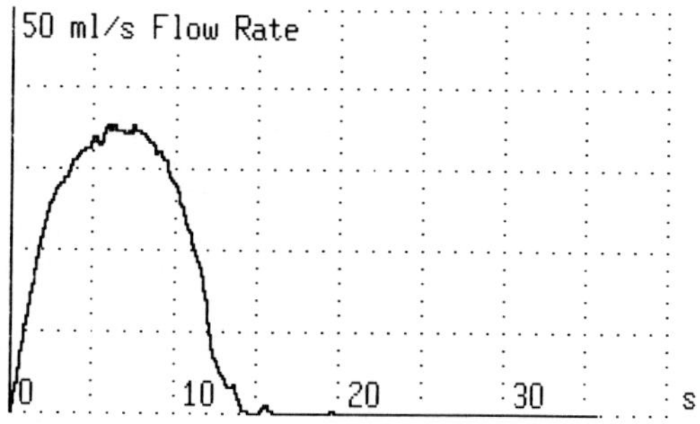

Results of UROFLOWMETRY

Voiding Time	T100	16	s
Flow Time	TQ	15	s
Time to max Flow	TQmax	6	s
Max Flow Rate	Qmax	35.3	ml/s
Average Flow Rate	Qave	22.5	ml/s
Voided Volume	Vcomp	330	ml

FIGURE 7–4. Actual flow curve from a urologically normal patient. Included on the machine's automatic printout are the major parameters used to describe the flow curve. The volume, flow rates, and curve shape are normal.

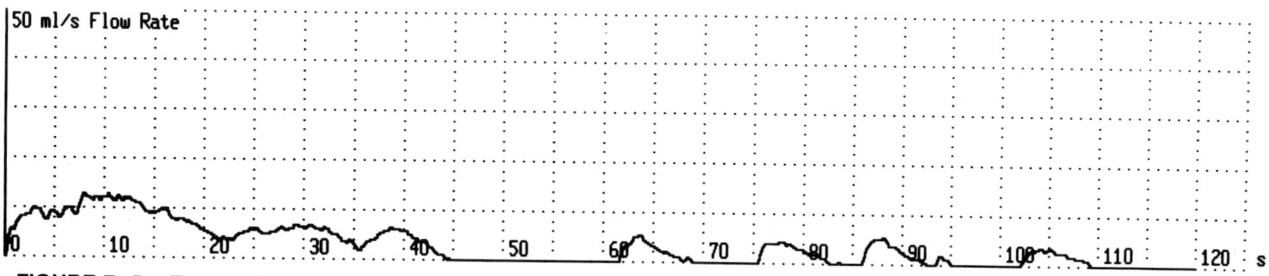

FIGURE 7–5. Extended, intermittent flow pattern seen with both severe urethral overactivity and detrusor underactivity.

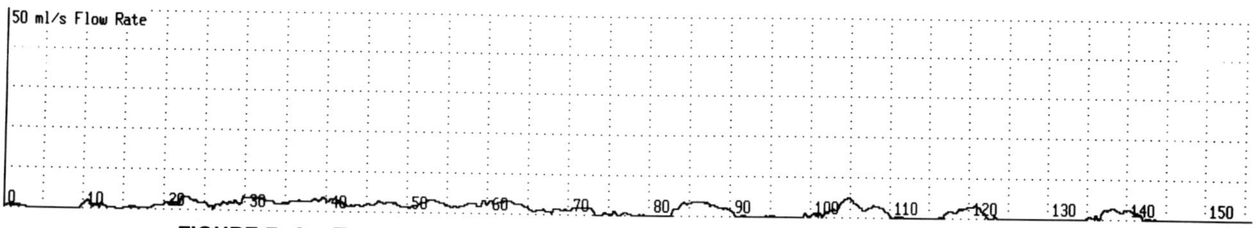

FIGURE 7–6. Extreme example of severe urethral overactivity or detrusor underactivity.

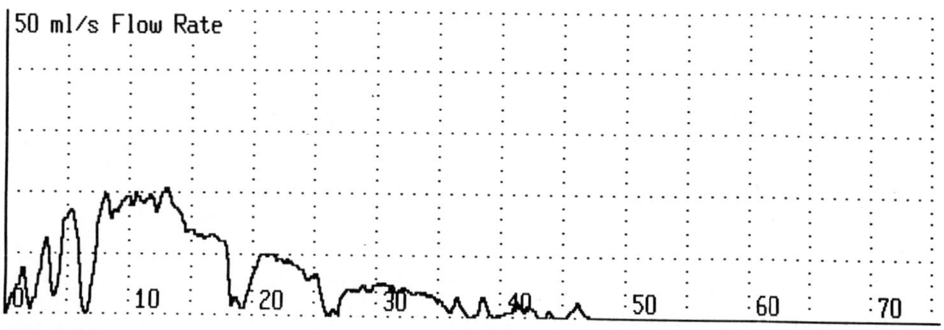

FIGURE 7–7. Intermittent flow pattern with flow augmented by straining to assist voiding in a patient with urethral overactivity caused by benign prostatic hyperplasia. This pattern can also be seen in a patient who strains to void but has detrusor underactivity (acontractility), although the flow periods would probably be more widely spaced. Simultaneous cystometry and uroflowmetry with abdominal pressure measurement elucidates the extent of detrusor contraction versus straining, although the patient can also be asked to repeat the flow rate measurement but without straining.

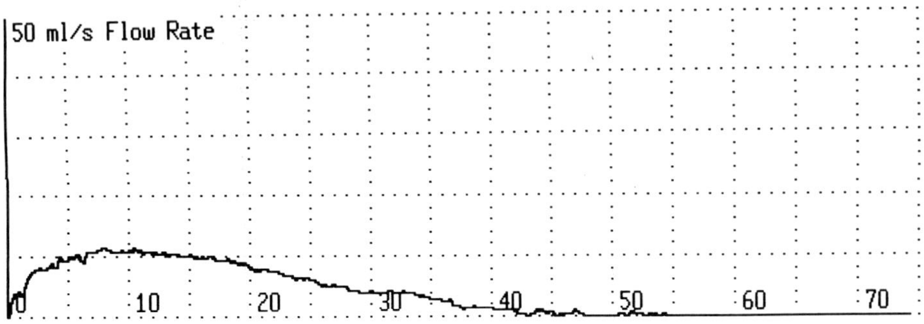

FIGURE 7–8. Flow curve in a patient with urethral overactivity (obstruction). The maximum flow rate is reached soon after flow begins, and the rate declines steadily until completion. This patient has benign prostatic hyperplasia.

with normal flow.[57] These flow rate guidelines can be about 2 to 4 ml/sec greater for men between 15 and 45 years old and for women of any age. Because these practical guidelines are imprecise, detailed flow analyses should be consulted, especially when flow rates are equivocally normal, voided volumes are consistently low (less than 200 ml, a common problem with older men),[17,58] or the patient is a child.[12,13,17,18,20,27,36,39,41-53,56]

In addition to the flow rate value, the flow curve shape is significant. A normal shape is smooth, with a maximum flow reached at about one third of the total voiding time so that the curve is not quite symmetric about the maximum flow point. No interruption to the flow pattern and no initial or terminal dribbling should be apparent (Figures 7–4 to 7–10).

Abnormal flow rates and patterns usually result from abnormalities of bladder, urethral, or sensory function, but factors such as psychic inhibition or flow patterns not average or routine for the patient must be considered. Since none of these elements is evaluated directly with uroflowmetry, however, this test does not indicate the cause of the abnormality in most situations. With absolute or relative detrusor underactivity, the maximum flow rate is low; the patient often aids voiding by intermittent abdominal straining, making the flow pattern intermittent or irregular with brief, sudden increases in the maximum flow rates (Figures 7–5 to 7–7). Sometimes straining may produce a normal flow rate and curve, obscuring the true abnormal function. With urethral overactivity (obstruction [see later discussion]) the flow rate is also low and the flow curve can be either continuous or intermittent (Figures 7–8 to 7–10). A continuous flow curve in a patient with obstruction usually results from such processes as benign prostatic hyperplasia, stricture, or even cystocele. An intermittent flow curve with obstruction is usually caused by detrusor-sphincter dyssynergia, dysfunctional voiding (e.g., nonneurogenic neurogenic bladder), and even the inhibition of voiding caused by the patient's anxiety and nervousness in the testing situation; these flow curves can resemble those associated with bladder underactivity. The supervoider produces extremely high flow rates (often greater than 50 ml/sec); this in itself is not abnormal, although it is sometimes associated with bladder overactivity (detrusor instability) in bladder filling and storage (see later discussion), or with the patient straining hard to help an already adequate detrusor contraction in an effort to "please" the physician. Artifacts in the flow curve most commonly appear as irregular, sharp peaks; these are often caused by direct, sudden impact of the urinary stream on the flowmeter's disk or scale or by the patient's attempt to achieve a high flow rate by brief sudden straining (Figure 7–11).

Although abnormal uroflowmetry rates and patterns can indicate that lower urinary tract dysfunction is present, the test is not specific enough to allow a certain or specific diagnosis of the cause of the abnormality. Other types of urodynamic tests are often necessary for a final correct diagnosis.

Indications

Several primary indications for urinary flow testing exist:

1. Investigation of suspected urethral overactivity or detrusor underactivity of any cause

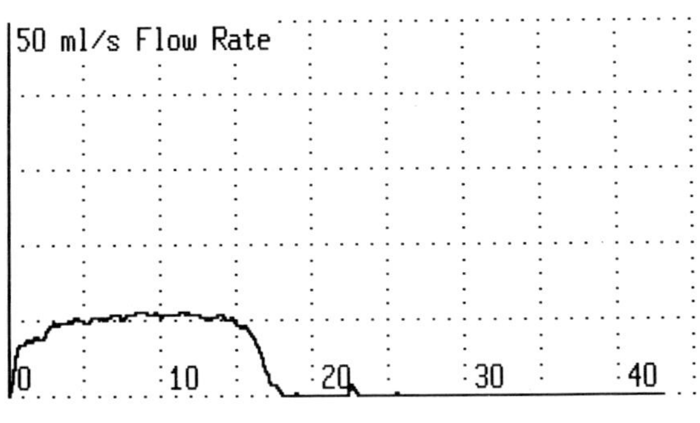

FIGURE 7–9. Flow curve in a patient with urethral overactivity caused by a urethral stricture. The maximum flow rate is reached soon after flow begins and remains stable until completion of voiding.

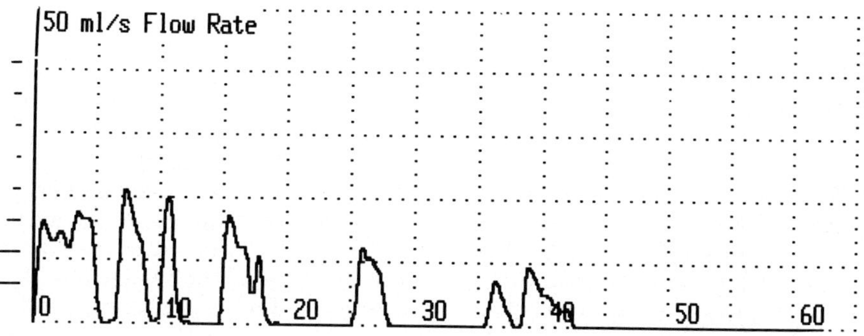

FIGURE 7–10. Intermittent flow pattern with relatively rapid changes in flow rate commonly seen in urethral overactivity from detrusor-sphincter dyssynergia. The pattern is difficult to distinguish from that produced by straining to void (see Figure 7–8). This patient has severe multiple sclerosis, which explains the dyssynergia pattern, but a cystometrogram with electromyography of the periurethral muscles and simultaneous cystometry and uroflowmetry with electromyography are necessary to confirm the diagnosis.

2. Before and after any surgical procedure intended to modify voiding function (e.g., prostatectomy)
3. Before and after any surgical procedure that might alter the voiding function (e.g., bladder neck suspension or radical pelvic surgery)
4. Before and after pharmacologic treatment of the lower urinary tract

CYSTOMETROGRAM

The urologist commonly wants to obtain objective data about lower urinary tract characteristics during the period of bladder filling and urine storage.[1] Normally the bladder fills to an appropriate volume with urine and stores it at low pressures; the urethra is competent and prevents any urinary leakage; and the person feels no discomfort, pain, or urgency to void, only a sensation of filling that increases gradually and comfortably until the bladder is full and, if the circumstances permit, leads to voiding to empty the bladder. The cystometrogram (CMG) is the urodynamics test that provides information about this period of bladder filling and urine storage. The CMG evaluates how the active (detrusor muscle) and passive (collagen and elastic tissue) elements of the bladder wall respond to filling.

The CMG provides direct data about the bladder's capacity and storage pressures. By knowing whether and how any fluid leaks from the bladder during the CMG, the urologist can draw conclusions about the competence of the urethra, although nothing about the urethra is directly measured. Direct data about sensation are provided by the patient, whose subjective impressions are recorded in relation to the bladder volumes and pressures and the urethral competence.

The inability to achieve normal bladder capacity, maintain normal bladder pressures and continence, and have normal bladder sensation is indicative of a disorder of the lower urinary tract during storage and filling, but only if, like other urodynamics tests, the CMG supports the clinical findings. A normal CMG in the face of lower urinary tract symptoms or signs should be considered normal only if the clinician is convinced that everything possible was done to replicate the patient's problems, and even then doubt about this conclusion may remain. Significantly, normal CMG findings are rare if the study was carefully performed and a thorough history and physical examination suggest a lower urinary tract disorder. (After all, for what reason

FIGURE 7–11. Artifact at the start of the flow curve produces a brief rapid flow as a result of straining by the patient at the start of voiding. Although his true maximum flow rate is about 10 ml/sec, the artifact causes the flow machine's printout to indicate a maximum flow of 20 ml/sec, pointing out the need for the urologist to review the flow pattern before reaching conclusions based only on the automatically generated numerical data.

would the test have been ordered or performed in the first place?) Since the CMG is a test of lower urinary tract function during filling and storage, extrapolation of CMG results to voiding function is inappropriate.

Bladder volume or capacity has several specific definitions related directly to the patient's sensation.[10] Bladder sensation is based on the patient's subjective report of what he or she feels during the bladder filling process. Record is made of bladder volume at the time of the first desire to void, a feeling that normally is comfortably suppressed. The volume at the normal desire to void is recorded when the patient would normally void at the next available opportunity but can delay without distress. Bladder volume is also recorded at a strong desire to void (the desire to void is persistent but without a fear of leakage); this volume corresponds to the maximum cystometric capacity (MCC). Urgency is a strong desire to void accompanied by fears of leakage or pain. Pain may occur with bladder filling and is abnormal; when present, its site and character should be described.

Clearly, sensation dictates the cystometric volumes. When sensory function is underactive (decreased or absent), MCC is the volume at which the clinician decides to stop filling and so is arbitrary. In a case of urethral underactivity (incompetence), the MCC can be varied again by the clinician's decision about when to stop the filling process as related to the degree of leakage of fluid; it can even be artificially increased by occluding the bladder outlet with a Foley catheter balloon to stop the leakage. The functional bladder capacity (FBC) is obtained by direct measurement of the voided volume by the patient at home and so is more clinically relevant. The maximum (anesthetic) bladder capacity (MABC) is measured by filling the bladder with the patient under deep general or spinal-epidural anesthesia.

Three important pressure measurements are made during cystometry.[10] The intravesical pressure (P_{ves}) is the measured pressure within the bladder; it is the sum of the pressures created by the bladder itself plus the pressures of the abdominal cavity. The intraabdominal pressure (P_{abd}) is the pressure within the abdomen assumed to be acting on the external surface of the bladder; practically, it is estimated by measuring intrarectal, vaginal, or rarely intraperitoneal or extraperitoneal pressures. Detrusor pressure (P_{det}) is the portion of intravesical pressure created only by the active and passive forces of the bladder wall exclusive of intraabdominal pressure; it is approximated by subtracting intraabdominal from intravesical pressure, which makes measurement of intraabdominal pressure an important element for accurate interpretation of the intravesical pressure measurements. Any of the measured pressures can remain stable or fluctuate during the CMG.

Equipment

Three technical requirements for performing cystometry are (1) a method for measuring the pressure within the bladder; (2) a method for infusing a fluid into the bladder; and (3) a method for recording the pressure and volume data (Figures 7–12 to 7–14).[30,59] The early development of these methods has been summarized well by Ek and Bradley.[1] The simplest method of obtaining a CMG would be to place one catheter with a single lumen into the bladder, allow normal bladder filling with urine to occur, and measure intravesical pressure with the catheter. This approach has the advantage of using a physiologic filling process but the disadvantage of being lengthy and tedious. A more rapid approach would employ a single-lumen catheter through which the bladder is filled by pouring water into it; intravesical pressure is approximated by observing the height of the fluid in the catheter. Alternatively, a manometer could be attached to the filling line with a Y connector and the pressure measured intermittently or constantly[60,61]; this pressure, however, is influenced by the column of filling fluid, which must be taken into account if the filling line is not temporarily disconnected from the catheter.

The disadvantages of these single catheter approaches are obvious. The pressure measurements without a manometer are only approximations of detrusor pressure and are performed intermittently so that much of the activity of the bladder during the filling process is missed while the tubing is connected to the filling fluid source. Even with a Y connector and manometer, delay and damping effects may alter the pressure measurements. The

FIGURE 7–12. A 7F catheter tip transducer system with one transducer mounted at the tip of the catheter just distal to a fluid infusion port. A second transducer is mounted about 6 cm more proximally. This configuration can be used for simultaneous intravesical and intraurethral pressure measurements and bladder filling.

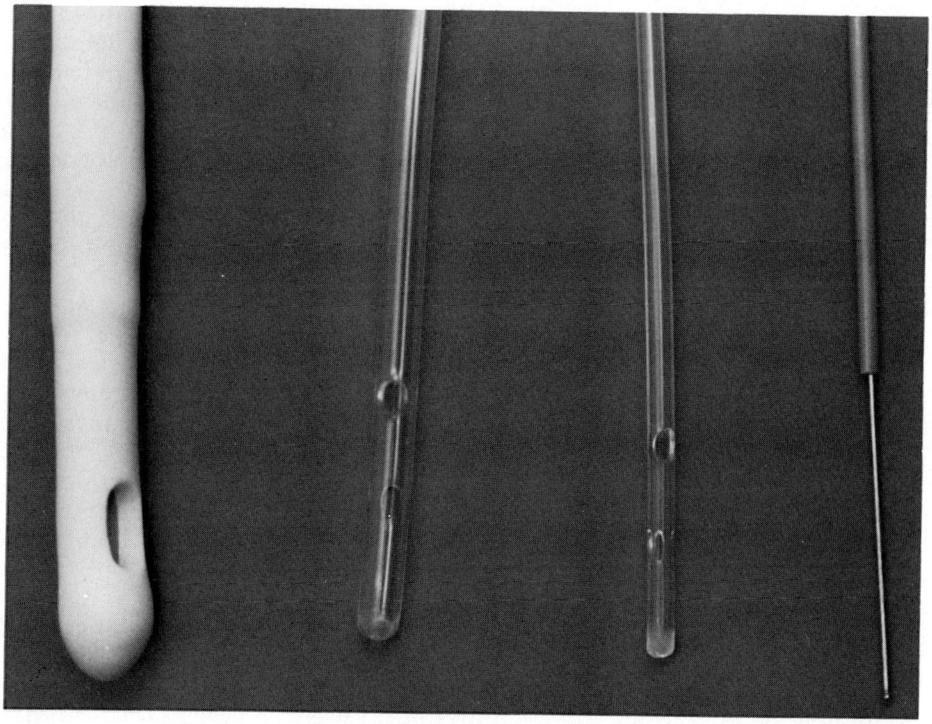

FIGURE 7–13. Single-lumen catheters that can be used for pressure measurement or fluid infusion. *Left to right:* 14F Foley balloon catheter; 8F and 5F infant feeding tubes with two distal side holes; and 4F tube (with removable guidewire for easier insertion) for intravesical pressure measurements, which is particularly useful with simultaneous cystometryuroflowmetry evaluations because of its small size.

filling process is not physiologic because it is rapid, uneven, and at an uncertain rate; even with an automatic infusion pump to fill the bladder, the process remains cumbersome, requiring simultaneous data measurements, recording, and bladder filling. Despite these drawbacks, however, such simple "bedside" or "eyeball" CMGs can detect gross abnormalities and can be useful as screening tools.[62-64]

State-of-the-art cystometry is now based on more functional and accurate techniques that use separate access routes to the bladder for simultaneous

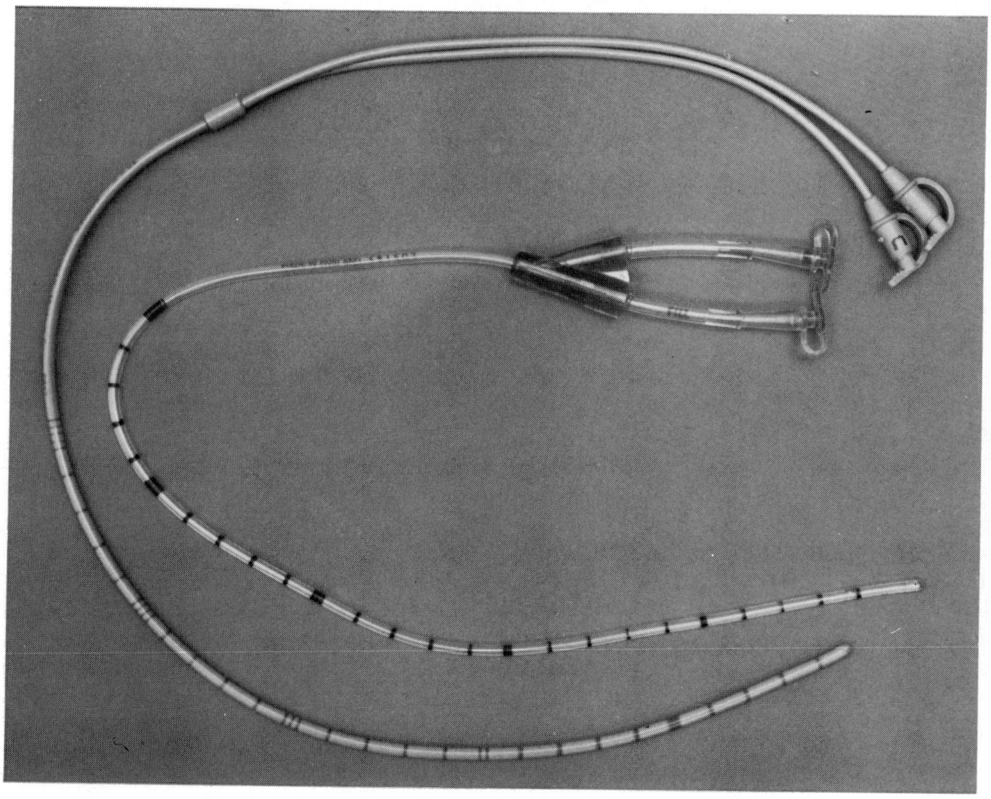

FIGURE 7–14. Double-lumen catheters. The inner tube shown has side holes within 1 cm of the end of the tube so that it can be used for simultaneous pressure measurement and infusion. The outer tube has a side hole at the tip of the catheter and another about 6 cm from the end; it can be used for pressure measurements from two locations if desired.

pressure measurement and filling, measure intraabdominal pressure, provide a method to control and measure filling rates and volume, and have an automatic data recording system. Most of the drawbacks of the simpler techniques are eliminated, and the measurements are more accurate and efficient. Physiologic filling can also be used with these approaches, if desired (see "Ambulatory Urodynamics").

Pressure Measurement Techniques

Although a manometer can provide accurate pressure measurement, acquisition of the pressure data has been simplified by pressure transducers that electronically transform the pressure measurement into digital or analog form for data display and recording systems.[30,59] Pressure transducers and the attached pressure detection system, including tubing and fluids, should provide data over pressure ranges from 0 to 300 cm H_2O with a frequency response for most intravesical and intraabdominal measurements of up to about 15 Hz. The standard, commercially available transducers reliably provide accurate, meaningful data if used properly. They prevent or limit the most common sources of error inherent in transducers: zeroing errors, calibration errors, and artifact.[30,65,66]

Zeroing errors occur when during measurement the transducer changes position relative to the zero pressure reference point (the pubic symphysis for the ICS system) because of transducer or patient movement.

Calibration refers to the process of establishing the correct electronic relationship between the transducer and the signal processing equipment; it confirms that the transducer transmits accurate data about the pressures it is measuring. The two main sources of calibration error are drift of the zero point (also called zero offset) and change in the amplification factor. The operator can periodically check zero point drift by opening the dome of the transducer to the atmosphere; the transducer and processing equipment should be adjusted so that the pressure reads zero. The zero point can drift slightly with temperature, ideally less than 0.1 cm $H_2O/°C$, and with time over several hours; the latter change is usually small enough (1% to 2%) not to affect the readings over an extended period, but this too should be tested (see "Ambulatory Urodynamics"). A properly zeroed transducer should then have its output, or amplication factor, checked by comparison of the output to the pressure produced by columns of water of known height from 0 (atmospheric pressure) to 100 cm.[65] The transducer's output along these pressures should be quite linear, that is, directly related to the applied pressure, although the output with pressure increasing and decreasing will be slightly different, a phenomenon called hysteresis. Together the linearity and hysteresis error should be less than $\pm 1\%$ over the 100 cm pressure range. Ideally calibration is performed each day that the urodynamics equipment is used, and if calibration or linearity errors are greater than 1%, the transducer should be replaced. Air bubbles in a liquid system, or liquid in a gas system, may cause signal damping and give a slow or reduced pressure response, affecting all aspects of a transducer's accuracy; therefore foreign elements should be kept totally from the system.

Artifacts can occur from movement of, or vibration to, the transducer, the bladder measurement points, or the connection between the two. Cracks in connecting tubing and fluid leaks can also cause artifacts. Intravesical pressure data by itself must be interpreted cautiously, taking into account changes in intraabdominal pressure; conversely, changes in measured intraabdominal pressure may not represent true changes but may be caused by artifacts from rectal contraction and relaxation, stool in the vault that may change the pressure readings or damp the signal in an open tube system, or tube position at the anal sphincter, which itself may show pressure fluctuations or possibly be incompetent, making it difficult to keep the tube within the rectum.

Pressure transducers can be located in one of several locations: external to the patient on a stand placed at the zero reference point, attached to the patient at the zero reference point, or at the site of desired pressure measurement mounted on a catheter, the catheter tip transducer.[59,67] Catheter tip transducers, the most compact type, are usually strain gauges mounted flush to the catheter surface.[68] One or more gauges are mounted on a catheter to allow positioning at the site(s) of pressure measurement. Because of the transducer location, for instance, within the bladder, the device has a built-in zeroing error, since the transducer always reads the absolute hydrostatic pressure of the bladder without relation of the gauge to the zero reference point; as the patient changes position, the pressure reading varies because of the weight of the abdominal contents on the viscus where the catheter is placed. Differences between catheter tip transducer measurements in the bladder and rectum are not the same as when external transducers are used. For these reasons catheter tip transducers should be used very cautiously when detrusor pressure measurements are desired.[30,59]

The catheter tip transducer is connected to the data processing unit by insulated cable, which presents no electrical hazard to the patient and does not cause artifact. The frequency response of catheter tip transducers is excellent, so they are particularly valuable if rapid changes in pressure are to be expected, a quality of little significance for cystometry but of critical importance when measuring certain urethral pressures (see "Urethral Pressure Measurements"). Disadvantages of catheter tip transducers are that they are expensive, fragile, and somewhat more difficult to handle and calibrate than other transducer types.

Transducers mounted outside the bladder are the most durable, least expensive, and easiest to handle of the options available. The most common location for these external transducers is on a stand away from the patient. Such transducers have a fluid-filled (liquid or gas) tube connecting the bladder and the transducer, increasing the risk for movement artifacts and damping effects. The tube may have an open end or side holes near the tip, or it may have a closed balloon end.[59] Since the transducer and patient are not physically connected, the potential for zeroing errors increases; it is necessary (but unlike the situation with catheter tip transducers, possible) to readjust the zero location whenever the patient moves.

Zeroing errors are less likely with external, body-mounted transducers fixed at the zero reference point. Such transducers are compact, and the relatively short tubing length from the bladder to the transducer reduces movement artifacts. These qualities are valuable for extended, ambulatory patient monitoring. Unfortunately, fixing the transducer securely and stably to the patient can be difficult.

Generally, any transducer should be durable enough to withstand relatively rough handling, frequent use, and for catheter tip transducers, sterilization after each use. Operators must avoid causing overload damage to the transducer by applying excess pressure, as when flushing the system. Overall, the level of care and attention required to mount, clean, and maintain the transducer and the staff available to perform such functions must be considered.

Adequate location and response of the measurement system can be checked by having the patient cough. The pressure change should be prompt, pronounced, and brief. The changes of the intravesical and intraabdominal pressures should be about the same; if they are not, the systems should be checked for the possible sources of error noted previously.

Fluids and Infusion Systems

Bladder filling can occur by normal urinary diuresis or be induced by diuretics.[69] More rapid and measurable filling is achieved with externally supplied fluids, either liquid or gas. Gas (in the form of carbon dioxide [CO_2]), and liquid (whether sterile water, physiologic saline solution, or radiologic contrast medium) are the two types of fluids used for cystometry. Liquid medium in any form is the more physiologic choice, since it is a liquid like urine and behaves in a similar fashion. Liquid is better if the CMG is needed for the diagnosis of urinary incontinence. Liquid is essential in the evaluation of the pressure/flow relationship between the bladder and urethra in the voiding process and when the CMG is obtained under direct fluoroscopic observation (video urodynamics; see later discussion), when liquid radiologic contrast medium is used.

Despite certain advantages and situations in which they must be used, liquids present some drawbacks not present with gas systems. The measurement system must be completely sterile, and separate catheters or lumens are necessary, one for filling and one for pressure measurement. Zeroing problems are of greater concern with external transducers, and artifacts can occur when the tubing is moved or shaken. Liquids are messier to handle, must be sterile, and can create a problem for cleanup and safety when spilled around the examination area. The time required to obtain a CMG with liquid is greater than that required for a gas CMG, and the equipment is usually more complex.

The use of gas presents certain drawbacks. The fluid is unphysiologic. CO_2 can cause pain, probably by going into solution in the urine and being converted to carbonic acid, resulting in mucosal inflammation. Unlike the liquid media, gas cannot be used to document incontinence, pressure/flow relationships, or the fluoroscopic appearance of the bladder and urethra in the filling process. Gas may leak undetected through the urethra inadvertently, creating inaccuracies in volume measurement. Unlike liquid, gas cannot duplicate the real increase in bladder mass that occurs during bladder filling, a point that has at least theoretical importance.

Measurable differences between liquid and gas exist. The volumes at which first sensation and MCC occur are 20% to 50% lower than capacities measured with liquid cystometry.[70] Repeated CO_2 cystometry shows varying results in these same volumes, which generally makes the findings of the presence of sensations of filling with CO_2 more valuable than the volumes at which they occur.[70-72] The compliance can vary by as much as 30% on repeated testing with gas.[71,72] Repeated water cystometry also shows changes in volumes for sensation levels but no other changes in pressure data.[70]

Some technical points must be considered in arranging the tubing and pressure systems for CO_2 cystometry. The systems should have narrow, short tubing lengths for optimal speed and amplitude of the pressure response, as well as a valve to prevent backflow of urine into the CO_2 tubing when the gas flow is off. The transducer should be placed above the level of the patient so that urine will not flow into the tubing by gravity. The zero level for the gas transducer is not critical, since the gas itself has no weight to affect the pressure reading.

Despite the uncertainty about the specific numerical data on pressures and volumes from CO_2 cystometry, there seem to be few major qualitative differences between the findings with water and CO_2 cystometry; both techniques detect the same types of detrusor filling and storage abnormalities, although the specific numerical data that describe the abnormalities may differ.[70] Overall, the characteristics of CO_2 cystometry make it more useful in providing gross, general qualitative screening cystometric data on detrusor function and the presence or absence of sensation during filling and storage than the more detailed quantitative information that is often desired from urodynamics. Regardless of which fluid is used, the major caveat of urodynamics testing applies: the test's findings and the patient's clinical situation must be compatible.

The infusion system depends on the fluid selected. If liquid is used, infusion by a simple gravity method of hanging the bottle above the bladder is adequate. However, measuring and controlling infused volumes accurately with this technique can be frustrating and difficult. Also, depending on the height of the liquid bottle and intravesical pressures, the infusion pressures and rates vary. Thus pump-driven infusion systems are much more functional in all respects, and most include automatic shut-offs when the measured bladder pressure exceeds a preset limit, usually 100 to 150 cm H_2O. Furthermore, the infused volume can usually be displayed automatically as part of the output data recording both in real time and for later review.

Most high-volume pump infusion systems count revolutions or cycles of the pump and assume that for each revolution a fixed fluid volume has been infused. Thus for accuracy, the tubing system must be open, without obstruction, free of air, which can be pumped but not with the same volume relationship to revolutions as liquid.

Another way of measuring infused volume is to measure the change in weight of the liquid source bottle with a scale. This technique is without the difficulties present in the pump revolution technique, but it can present problems when liquid of density different from water, such as radiographic contrast material, is used. Such a scale system is relatively delicate, so appropriate precautions must be taken not to damage the scale.

Gas infusion systems rely on the storage of the gas under pressure with pressure-regulating and flow control valves to set and control infusion rates, as well as flowmeters along the infusion line. These systems require automatic displays of infused volumes. The pressure relief valves are set at about 150 cm H_2O. The intravesical pressure can be recorded through a transducer attached to the infusion line or through a separate measurement line.

For a given fluid infusion rate with a display system advancing at a constant speed, volume is plotted on the horizontal or x-axis and pressure on the vertical or y-axis.

Data Recording and Display

Whatever type of transducer is used, the pressure data must be displayed and recorded clearly for both immediate and later review. Two basic types of data display and recording equipment configurations are used. The most basic type of equipment employs a paper strip chart recorder display in which the pressure data from a transducer are printed on the graph paper. The lines can be drawn by a heated or ink stylus, ink jets, or even ultraviolet light. Each recording system requires paper unique to that system. This practical concern affects not only initial equipment cost but also the costs of paper and maintenance through the years for the writing device.

The paper chart recorder simultaneously provides the instantaneous data from the transducer in a graphic display and the permanent record of the evaluation. Over the past several years there has been a growing trend among manufacturers of urodynamics equipment to provide graphic and digital data display on a cathode ray tube (CRT). Such CRT displays must be backed up by some type of paper output generation system, whether a paper strip printer or an x-y plotter, to provide a hard copy of the evaluation. Also, the data must be recorded by computer hardware memory or magnetic tape that can be played back immediately or stored.

Basic paper chart recorders offer the advantage that real-time data are accessible to the clinician, who can make written comments on the data sheet as the test is proceeding. In this fashion clinical observations can be more clearly correlated with the test results at the moment they are occurring. Unfortunately, such immediate recording of observations is not as easy with the CRT display units. Instead the CRT may allow the clinician to make "marks" or "tags" at certain points during the evaluation, after which he or she must still record the significance of those points on the permanent record.

Ease and accuracy in reading numerical data from the hard copy immediately after the test or in the future must be taken into account. For the CRT displays, having the computer temporarily store the evaluation so that it can be replayed is useful. The stored information can then be reexamined so that the "tagged" points can be evaluated more closely or the position of the "tags" moved. In this way data of true interest can be retrieved, rather than just the data where the "tag" happened to fall or where the computer happened to mark it. Although the possibility of blindly accepting printed digital data is a greater likelihood with the CRT/computer-based units, blindly accepting the printed data or curve from any urodynamics machine without closely examining the entire test record and clinical situation can lead to erroneous or absurd conclusions. With computer-based storage systems, the amount of time the data are stored should be adjustable depending on what the test is intended to show; if the test extends beyond a certain time, the computer's memory may overflow and the data may be lost.

Regardless of the system used to provide the permanent copy of the evaluation, the clinician must be aware of the durability and clarity of the copies when in long-term storage.

A major issue is selecting the type of recording unit is how many channels of data it should display. Manufacturers offer up to 11 channels in some configurations, although units with up to six channels are the most practical and useful. The simplest systems display one channel, with pressure on the horizontal axis and volume infused (or time, which can be related to volume) on the vertical axis. The pressure in such basic systems is usually intravesical pressure rather than detrusor pressure. More channels are needed for more thorough, accurate cystometry so that all three pressures (intravesical, intraabdominal, and detrusor) are displayed on separate channels versus time. Additional channels can display simultaneous uroflow, electromyography, urethral pressure data (see later discussion), or volume infused, in various combinations as the number of channels is increased.

Regardless of the type of recording unit selected, the frequency response and paper speed or CRT display speed must be appropriate for the study being performed. Displays producing data at 0.25 to 5 mm of display (paper or CRT) per second are adequate for routine cystometry purposes, although ranges of 0.5 to 1 mm/sec are the most useful. The transducer, amplifiers, processors, and recording equipment must be compatible technically and electronically; manufacturers have generally ensured this in their configurations. If more than one channel of data is being displayed or recorded and the writing devices or data can overlap from one channel to another, it is vital that this not damage the instrument and that the overlapping curves of the data can be detected and accurately identified.

The controls on the recording equipment must be easy to operate and understandable with the instruction booklets supplied. The manufacturer must supply adequate technical support and answer questions promptly when problems arise. Test variables such as paper or display speed, flow rate, and data obtained must be easily changed to meet the circumstances; in computer-based systems this means that reprogramming must be simple, "user friendly," and amenable to inspection to confirm that the correct program is being used before the test is started. Finally, the purchaser of the equipment must know whether repair or adjustment can be performed by an in-house or locally available biomedical equipment technician, whether the device must or can be returned to the company, or whether a company representative can offer service on site. The promptness of service capability and the availability of temporary replacement components must be established.

Technique

Besides selecting the equipment for cystometry, the clinician plays the primary role in conducting the test. Before the evaluation the urologist must establish several parameters that affect the results and the interpretation: the method of bladder access for intravesical pressure measurement and bladder filling, the use of anesthesia for urethral catheterization or of other medications for patient sedation, fluid temperature, rate of bladder filling, sterilization, patient position, pharmacologic bladder testing, abdominal pressure and its measurement, detection of fluid leakage, and performing the test itself.

Bladder Access

Catheters may be placed into the bladder either suprapubically or transurethrally (Figures 7–12 to 7–14). The ideal method of intravesical pressure measurement is the suprapubic approach, which avoids the potential artifact of a transurethral catheter. However, placement of the suprapubic tube can be uncomfortable even with local anesthetic and may be unsuccessful or unsafe depending on bladder anatomy, obesity, and prior surgery, injury, or radiation treatment. Despite the probable advantages of the suprapubic catheter approach, it is usually impractical, especially in a busy urodynamics clinic. Also, many children may need a general anesthetic for tube placement, which is expensive and has risks. Anesthesia is generally unnecessary for urethral catheterization as long as the child is kept comfortable, informed, and distracted as needed. Having the parents in the room can be helpful with younger children. Mild sedatives can be used in the few circumstances when the other basic techniques fail. For all of these reasons the transurethral catheter placement has been accepted as a reasonable, safe, and accurate technique assuming that catheter size and urethral anesthesia are kept in mind.

Obviously, the smallest catheter that can be used is the most physiologic; such size concerns are particularly important to maintain flow when measuring pressures while voiding (see "Simultaneous Cystometry and Uroflowmetry"). Catheters 5F or smaller have little effect on the flow rate or bladder pressure in virtually all circumstances. The material for the catheter matters little as long as the catheter can consistently be passed into the bladder easily and safely; a possible exception to this is patients with myelomeningoceles who may have allergic and even anaphylactic reactions to latex in catheters and gloves.[73]

The catheters used may have one to three lumens, depending on what the catheter must do in terms of bladder filling, and as part of a fluid-coupled/external transducer or catheter tip transducer system.[59] Some catheters have radiodense markers at key points along their lengths so that these points can be located easily under fluoroscopy. In general, double- and triple-lumen catheters are most useful when repeated filling cystometry is necessary but pressure/flow studies are not, since the multiple-lumen catheters usually have larger calibers and a greater potential of creating obstruction artifacts. Alternatively, separate single-lumen catheters can be placed for each specific function of measurement or filling.

Foley balloon catheters are useful in filling CMGs because they remain in the bladder reliably. The balloon can also be useful in patients with urethral incompetence, since intentionally pulling on the catheter with filling occludes the bladder neck. This allows the bladder to hold more urine so that bladder capacity and pressures can be better assessed.

Urethral catheters can usually be easily, safely, and comfortably placed in both men and women with adequate lubrication alone. An anesthetic gel may improve comfort, especially in a patient with a relatively sensitive or painful urethra or in an anxious patient, especially a male, in whom catheterization may create enough discomfort or anxiety that the remainder of the test may be performed only under duress. In children local anesthesia can be valuable for obvious reasons. In general, moderate amounts of anesthetic do not seem to affect the remainder of the cystometric evaluation. The anesthesia may increase bladder capacity and residual urine in the presence of outflow obstruction, and initiation of micturition may be difficult. However, pressure/flow relationships are apparently not altered by urethral anesthesia.

The clinician should check correct catheter placement and patency of tubes by having the patient strain and cough to demonstrate appropriate pressure responses and by freely irrigating the tubes.

Rate of Bladder Filling

The ICS has defined three categories of fill rates.[10] A fast fill rate is greater than 100 ml/min, a medium fill rate is 10 to 100 ml/min, and a slow fill rate is below 10 ml/min. Most studies are performed at a medium fill rate.

The bladder pressure response in a CMG might be modified by the rate at which the bladder is filled.[74] Although physiologic fill rates are ideal, this technique is impractical in most situations or clinics. Furthermore, although physiologic fill rates may be best at illustrating what happens in "normal" circumstances, the cystometry is being performed on a patient who is presumably "abnormal" and the test is conducted in such a way that the patient's symptoms are replicated; to achieve such replication quickly, accurately, and reproducibly, faster than physiologic fill rates may be necessary.[69,75,76] As emphasized previously, urodynamics test findings that have nothing to do with the patient's clinical situation and that might be artifacts of the fill rate should generally be ignored or at least interpreted with caution.

When abnormal pressure changes are suspected but fill rate artifact must be limited, the fill rate should be as low as 10 to 20 ml/min in adults or less than about 5% of functional bladder capacity in children. Conversely, with a bladder that has a very high capacity or little to no likelihood of abnormal pressure changes, a high fill rate might be used.

Filling should not be started until the bladder has been drained and proper functioning of all monitoring equipment has been confirmed.

Fluid Temperature

Although warming the filling fluid to body temperature is the best means of evaluating the patient's sensory function in a nonprovocative way, such an approach is generally difficult or impractical, and room temperature fluid is adequate. Ice-cold saline solution can be instilled as a test of bladder contractility, but this test is rarely used and is primarily of historical interest in the evaluation of patients with spinal cord injury.

Sterilization

Tubing inserted into the bladder should always be sterile and placed with sterile technique. Catheter tip transducers can be reused if they are sterilized according to manufacturer's recommendation between patients. Disposable catheters are used only once. The external transducers need not be replaced or resterilized for each patient unless fluid could have been transferred from within the bladder to the device, contaminating the system.

Patient Position

The patient is usually in the supine position when catheters and other measurement instruments are being placed. At least one filling study should be performed with the patient in the supine position; this allows an easy check of all the equipment and modification in case some component is not functioning perfectly, and the disorder may become evident without further testing. When the patient is undergoing simultaneous cystometry and fluoroscopy, the supine position may be adequate to observe the bladder and urethra and determine whether vesicoureteral reflux is present. This is also an easy position for observation of stress incontinence, especially in female patients. However, in many instances the patient should be standing or sitting during cystometry to truly replicate the symptoms of the voiding problem. Provocative maneuvers such as coughing, straining, squatting, or jumping may be necessary to provoke the symptoms. Such maneuvers are essential in the evaluation of stress incontinence and sometimes in the evaluation of urge-type incontinence. To quantify urine loss, the clinician can place the patient over the urine flowmeter. The patient must be in the normal voiding position, whether sitting or standing, for the most accurate demonstration of the pressure/flow relationship of the bladder and urethra. If the patient has significant neurologic disease or is otherwise severely disabled, supine may be the safest and most practical position during the evaluation.

Pharmacologic Bladder Testing

The most commonly performed test in cystometry with pharmacologic agents is a test to determine the reason that the detrusor does not contract (acontractility or areflexia; see later discussion). This test, the bethanechol supersensitivity test described by Lapides,[61] relies on Cannon's principle of denervation supersensitivity to circulating receptor agonists. A baseline storage pressure is established at a fixed volume of about 100 ml. Bethanechol 2.5 mg is injected subcutaneously, and the pressure is observed for 30 minutes. Pressure rises of greater than 15 cm H_2O indicate that denervation is a likely cause of the acontractility. Care must be taken that the systemic cholinergic response which may include sweating, abdominal cramping, or diarrhea, is not too uncomfortable for the patient. Cholinergic agents should not be used in patients with asthma or hypertension. Although the test can help distinguish between detrusor acontractility caused by muscle failure and that caused by denervation, the false negative and false positive rates are high and the practical problems in performing the test limit its usefulness.[77,78]

Anticholinergic drugs, such as propantheline 15 mg intramuscularly, can also be given to test their effects on the detrusor. Such tests are used primarily for research.[79]

Alpha-adrenergic agents have been used in urodynamics to evaluate their effects on the urethra, especially in spinal cord–injured patients.[80,81]

In patients with autonomic dysreflexia the use of medications is essential not for diagnosis of the abnormality, but to prevent potentially fatal consequences of the autonomic dysreflexia that occasionally arise during bladder filling. Although intravenous agents may be necessary, sublingual, fast-acting calcium channel blockers such as nifedipine are usually adequate to reduce the serious and acute changes caused by the autonomic dysreflexia.

Intraabdominal Pressure Measurement

Intraabdominal pressure is an important datum in accurate cystometry and in pressure/flow measurements (see "Simultaneous Cystometry and Uroflowmetry"), since pressure changes caused by abdominal straining are reflected in the intravesical pressure (Figure 7–15). True detrusor pressure is obtained by subtracting the intraabdominal from the intravesical pressure. This subtraction is most easily performed automatically by the electronically based data processing and display systems used in most urodynamics

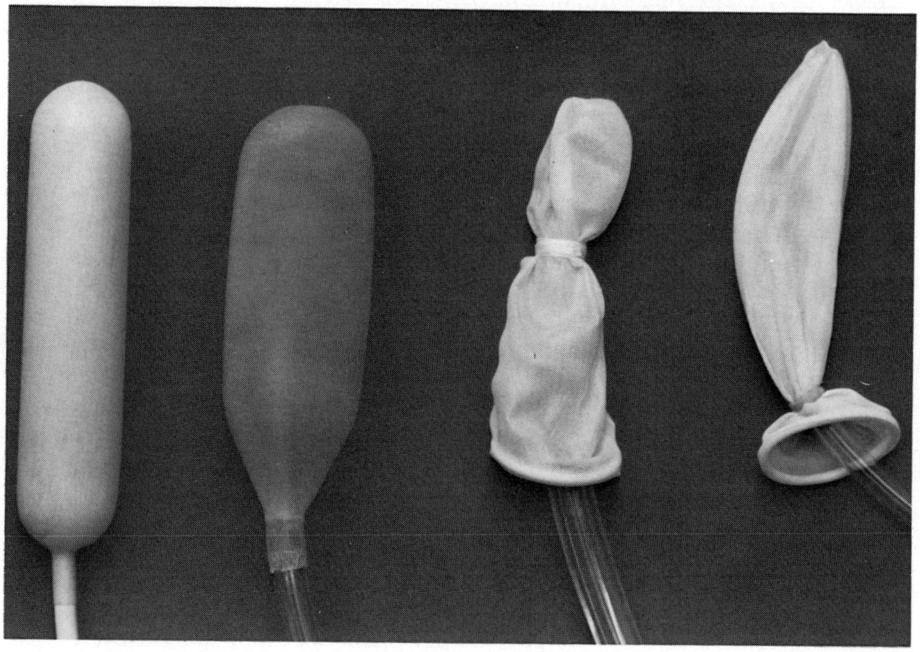

FIGURE 7–15. Tubes for measuring intraabdominal pressures within the rectum. *Left to right:* Two commercially available balloon-type catheters and two "homemade" rectal tubes using finger cots, tubing, and either string or rubber bands to secure the cots. Cost is the primary factor leading to the development of the homemade varieties.

systems. Visual observation or palpation can give only qualitative, not quantitative, indications of straining activity.[82] Without direct intraabdominal measurements, accurate conclusions about detrusor function cannot be reached. Intraabdominal pressure measurements are particularly valuable when the intravesical pressure has small increases, which may or may not be accompanied by intraabdominal pressure increases. Most commonly, measurements of intrarectal pressure substitute for true intraabdominal pressure measurements; some authors have proposed intravaginal measurements.[83]

Caveats apply to the use of rectal tubes for intraabdominal pressure measurements. The measuring portion of the tube, commonly a fluid-filled balloon of some type (often homemade by the urodynamics unit staff), must be placed into the rectal vault and not into the sphincter area. The catheter may have to be taped into place so that it will not be dislodged if the patient moves or strains. The precautions already mentioned regarding pressure measurement catheters also apply to intraabdominal catheters.

Anyone who has performed cystometry with intraabdominal pressure measurements for some time has been faced with the situation of negative or falling intraabdominal pressures after proper zeroing and calibration. This phenomenon can be frustrating and has never been explained. When it occurs, as with any other aberrant or unusual data during urodynamics testing, the details of evaluation at that moment and the patient's clinical condition must be used to guide interpretation of the test results. For example, it may be necessary simply to ignore the intraabdominal pressure measurements for that period and to believe only the intravesical pressures and not the detrusor pressures. Again, the most important aspect of urodynamics evaluations is the clinician's direct observation and understanding of the patient and the technical aspects of the test.

Detection of Fluid Leakage

During CMG the occurrence and magnitude of liquid leakage can be visually observed and perhaps correlated with the patient's history of incontinence. Leakage may also be detected by the urine flowmeter if the leakage is directed into the device during the CMG. Electronic napkins that allow automatic detection and measurement of leakage have been developed[84,85]; such devices have been used in outpatient settings for ambulatory urodynamics testing (see later discussion). The fluid-bridge test detects equilibration of pressures between the bladder and points along the urethra during coughing to confirm urethral patency.[86] Finally, the presence and extent of incontinence for outpatients have been assessed by a number of pad-weighing tests in which the patient performs specific maneuvers in an attempt to produce leakage.[10,87] Unfortunately, these pad-weighing tests show some weaknesses in reproducibility and reliability.[87]

Performing Cystometry

Once the variables and issues just described have been settled, cystometry can be performed to obtain data directly on bladder capacity and pressures and sensation and to infer urethral competence. Since the test must replicate the patient's symptoms and the variables of the test may have to be changed to do so, a universal CMG protocol may not be useful. Direct physician involvement is crucial in avoiding wasteful, misdirected testing and in obtaining accurate, useful conclusions rapidly the first time the test is performed by adjusting the variables of the evaluation as needed.

Most of the discussion in the preceding section applies to the formal, complex electronic CMG. The technique of the "bedside" urodynamics test mentioned earlier is simple.[62-64] The patient is placed in the supine or lithotomy position. A catheter is placed into the bladder, and a catheter-tip syringe is attached to the end of the catheter. The bladder is slowly filled with room temperature saline solution or water in fixed increments of about 50 ml. The volumes at which first sensation, urgency, and capacity occur are noted. The rate at which the syringe empties is observed. Any reversal of the process may indicate an involuntary bladder contraction. If the bladder filling is relatively slow, the clinician can conclude that the bladder capacity is quite small or that the bladder has a low compliance. When capacity is reached, the catheter is removed and the patient is asked to perform a number of stress maneuvers to produce incontinence. The patient can then void, and because the volume infused is known, the amount of residual urine can be checked quite accurately if the bladder was emptied before the test.

Normal Cystometry

The data from the CMG related to bladder function are capacity and storage pressure (Figure 7–16). The normal maximum cystometric capacity (MCC) varies with the patient's age and somewhat with the patient's sex. Generally an MCC of about 400 to 600 ml is normal for an adult man and about 100 ml less for a woman. For a child, formulas such as Volume in ounces = Patient age in years + 2 give good approximations.[88] To be considered truly normal, capacities must be reached with normal sensation and with little or no leakage.

With the bladder empty the detrusor pressure may have a range of values depending on the relative values of the intravesical and intraabdominal

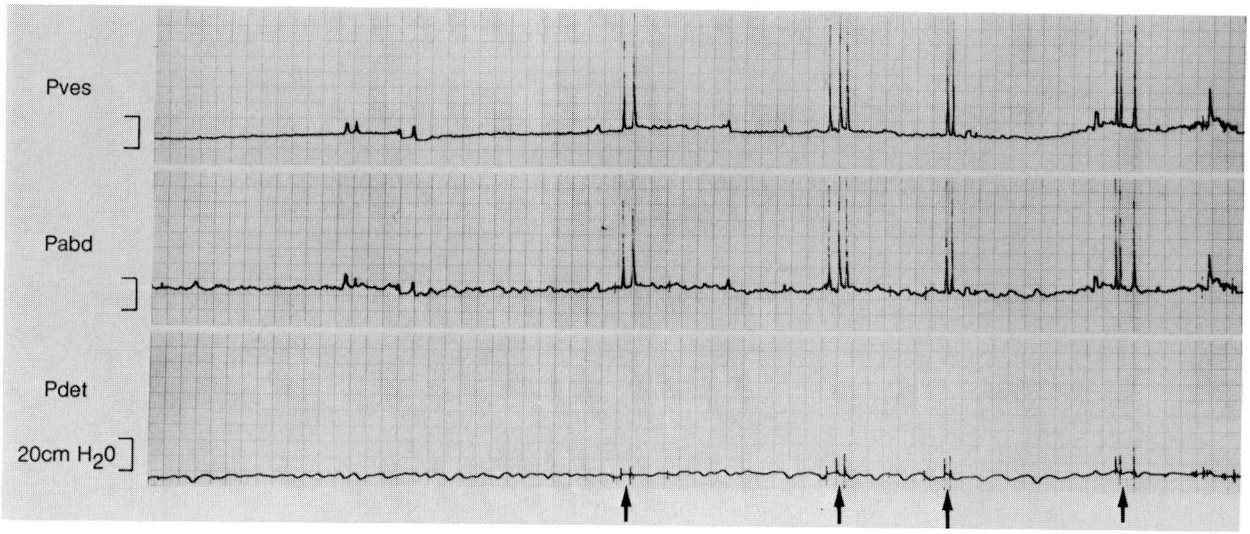

FIGURE 7–16. Normal filling cystometrogram. The detrusor pressure increases only about 6 cm H_2O throughout the filling process to normal capacity. The brief pressure rises *(arrows)* are points at which the patient coughs, significantly raising the intravesical and intraabdominal pressures but not appreciably affecting the detrusor pressures.

pressures. This initial pressure is called the resting or initial filling pressure, and all other pressures in the CMG are referred to this value. In the first 100 to 150 ml of volume, the detrusor pressure may rise to 5 cm, but this is inconstant and occurs most often with CO_2 infusion systems, probably as a result of flushing of liquid from the gas line. With further filling the detrusor pressure rises steadily but only a small amount (Figure 7–16); that is, it accommodates the added volume. Accommodation is also expressed as normal compliance (change in volume divided by change in detrusor pressure) (ml/cm H_2O). Although the ICS has yet to define normal compliance, the detrusor pressure change to 400 to 600 ml should be less than 15 cm H_2O, so the ratio of volume to pressure should be greater than about 30 ml/cm H_2O. For smaller MCCs the allowable pressure rise is also proportionally reduced, although this too is without clear ICS definition.

Besides accommodating properly, the normal bladder during filling shows no phasic pressure increases that are greater than 15 cm H_2O or that cause urgency or fluid leakage.[10] A change from the supine to the sitting or standing position may result in a pressure change of 50 cm or more, a consequence of the pressure of the intraabdominal organs resting on the bladder and rectum. Often this change is eliminated by replacing external transducers at the zero reference point; with catheter tip transducers the change may persist.[59]

Normal urethral function during cystometry means that the urethra should be competent; that is, no leakage of fluid should occur through the urethra.

With normal sensory function during cystometry the first desire to void should occur at about 100 to 200 ml, a normal desire should be sensed at about 300 ml, and the strong desire to void should occur at a normal MCC.

Abnormal Cystometry

Abnormal cystometry is a result of overactivity or underactivity of the bladder, urethra, or sensation. If the detrusor contracts during the filling process, phasic pressure increases may occur that cannot be suppressed despite a sense of urgency or a need to empty the bladder (Figure 7–17). Such abnormal contractions indicate bladder overactivity and are called detrusor hyperreflexia (DH) with a known neurologic abnormality as their cause or detrusor instability (DI) otherwise.[10] In most conventions, such involuntary contractions must be greater than 15 cm H_2O to be considered true contractions; practically speaking, however, if such contractions replicate the patient's symptoms (usually urgency), they are clinically and urodynamically significant.[10,89-91]

The second cause of bladder overactivity is low compliance, abnormal gradual increases in bladder pressure during the filling process without phasic pressure changes (Figures 7–18 to 7–19).[10,92-94] Sometimes low compliance is difficult to distinguish from a slowly rising phasic pressure increase. To differentiate the two, the clinician can stop the fluid infusion: with low compliance the detrusor pressure remains unchanged or decreases only slightly, whereas with the contractions of DH or DI the pressure continues to fluctuate, rising or falling several centimeters from the pressure attained at the infusion stop point (Figure 7–19). Combinations of DI or DH and low compliance can occur, as can abnormalities during filling and storage with abnormalities during voiding.[95]

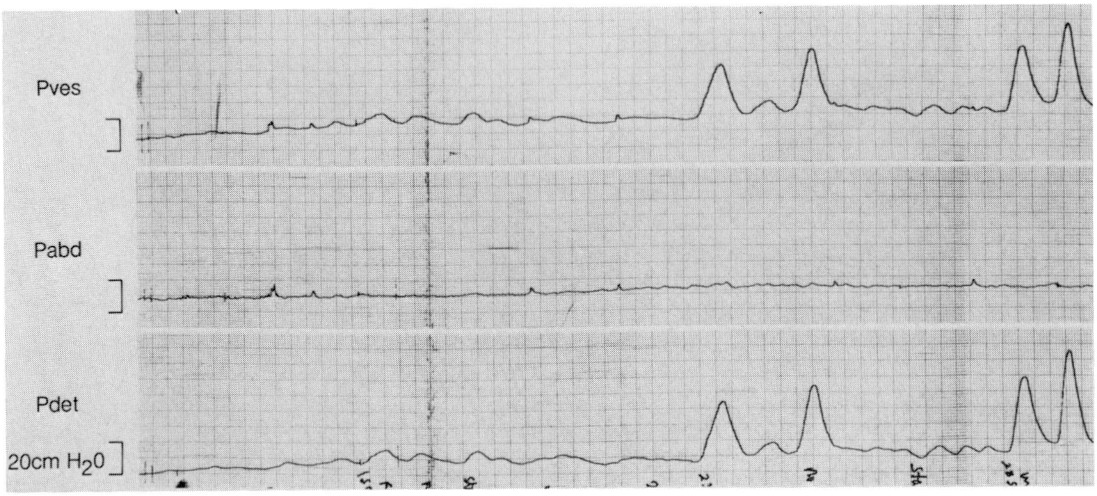

FIGURE 7–17. An abnormal cystometrogram showing phasic detrusor pressure increases consistent with detrusor overactivity (detrusor instability or hyperreflexia). Intraabdominal pressure does not change during the intravesical pressure increases.

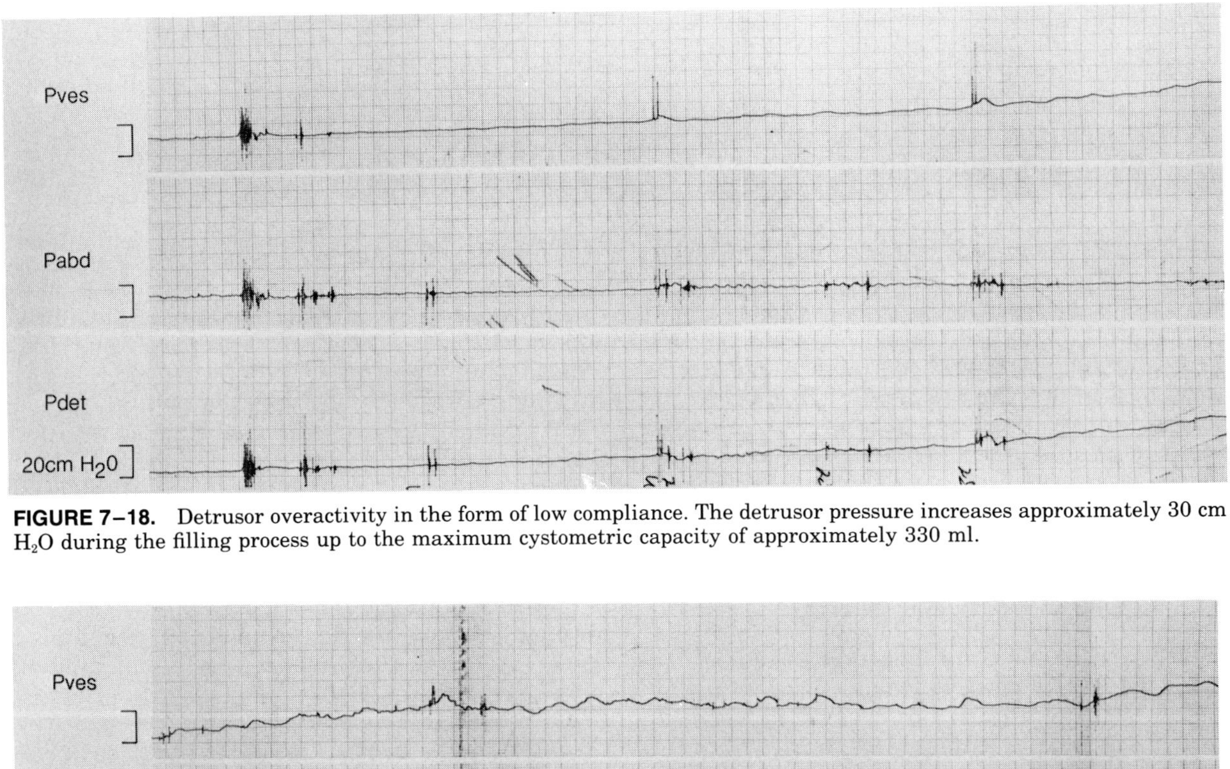

FIGURE 7–18. Detrusor overactivity in the form of low compliance. The detrusor pressure increases approximately 30 cm H_2O during the filling process up to the maximum cystometric capacity of approximately 330 ml.

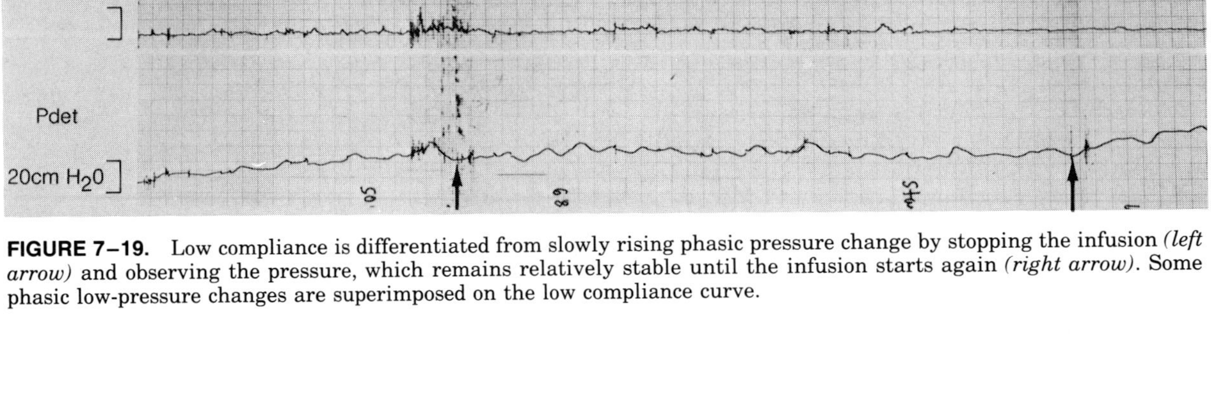

FIGURE 7–19. Low compliance is differentiated from slowly rising phasic pressure change by stopping the infusion *(left arrow)* and observing the pressure, which remains relatively stable until the infusion starts again *(right arrow)*. Some phasic low-pressure changes are superimposed on the low compliance curve.

Detrusor underactivity cannot be diagnosed during cystometry, since such diagnoses can be made only during attempts at voiding.

Normal urethral function (competence) during filling, the urethra's ability to maintain continence, is assessed indirectly during cystometry by an observation of whether leakage occurs. If leakage does occur, the other significant data to note are the detrusor pressure and what the patient's activity and sensory status are at that moment. For leakage (incontinence) to occur from any mechanism, the detrusor pressure must exceed the maximum urethral pressure. The detrusor pressure at which involuntary leakage occurs is called the leak point pressure (LPP). The LPP is especially important in the presence of neurologic disease because it well defines the often fixed urethral resistance characteristics. A pressure of 40 cm H_2O has been recognized as the critical LPP above which upper urinary tract changes and damage are almost certain to occur with high-pressure bladder dysfunction from low compliance or detrusor hyperreflexia.[92-94,96,97] Clearly, the higher the LPP, the greater the competence of the urethra.

Leakage can occur with low LPP when the urethra is underactive (incompetent). Genuine stress urinary incontinence (GSUI) is involuntary leakage occurring when the intravesical pressure exceeds the maximum urethral pressure in the absence of a detrusor contraction.[10,98] Such intravesical pressure rises are commonly associated with provocative stress maneuvers (Figure 7–20). Total urethral incompetence in a woman whose urethra provides no closure capability is called type III urethra/incontinence. This diagnosis is confirmed with simultaneous cystogram demonstrating an open, or nearly open, bladder neck and urethra without detrusor contraction (see later discussion).[98]

Simultaneous intraabdominal pressure measurements are essential to confirm that no detrusor contraction and pressure increase are induced by the stress maneuvers to cause leakage; such a phenomenon is called stress-induced detrusor instability.

In an uncommon form of urethral incompetence, incontinence during cystometry can occur without detrusor pressure change, stress maneuvers, a type III urethra, or even patient awareness. Such incontinence is due to intermittent, spontaneous drops in urethral closure pressure, a condition called urethral instability (see "Urethral Pressure Measurements").[99-110] Detrusor instability may follow the urethral relaxation, creating a mixed problem. Generally, urethral sphincter electromyography and urethral pressure measurements are necessary to confirm this diagnosis, which still lacks precise definition.

Except for the LPP, no objective data about the urethra are obtained during cystometry, and even the LPP is actually a bladder characteristic from which urethral properties are extrapolated. Other conclusions about urethral competence are general, qualitative descriptions.

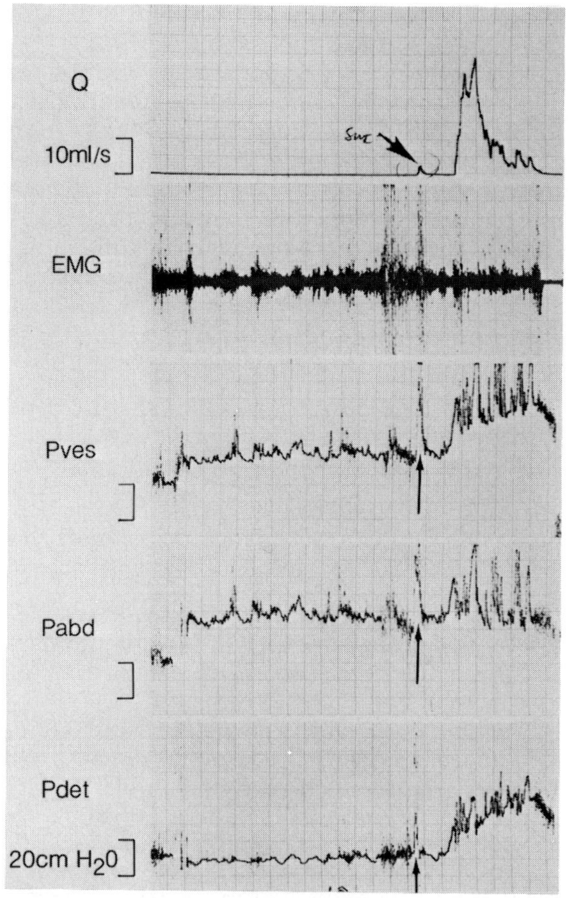

FIGURE 7–20. This figure demonstrates a number of urodynamic findings applicable to several sections in this chapter. The patient is seated on the commode over the urinary flowmeter with perianal electromyographic (EMG) electrodes. The flow pattern is normal, with two brief low spikes resulting from straining maneuvers that are obvious on the intraabdominal pressure. Before the normal urinary flow curve is a brief flow spike *(arrow)* caused by the patient's coughing. Since no increase in detrusor pressure occurs, this is genuine stress urinary incontinence. The EMG display shows an increase in activity associated with the coughing, as well as some increase in activity just prior to the cough as the patient adjusted herself on the commode chair, resulting in motion artifact. During the voiding portion of the tracing a normal detrusor pressure increase occurs characteristic of a normal pressure/flow relationship in terms of pattern and pressure and flow parameters. At the end of the flow is a persistent elevation in the detrusor pressure, a normal variant called an aftercontraction.

Urethral overactivity cannot be diagnosed during cystometry because this property can be observed only during voiding.

Increased, or overactive, sensation reduces the normal volumes at which the patient reports the various types of voiding desires, and decreased, or underactive, sensation increases them. Urgency is a desire to void with a fear of impending leakage or pain; it is abnormal. Pain is also abnormal. Overactive sensation can be caused by almost any inflammatory, infectious, neoplastic, or noxious stimulus. Overactive sensory function without evident cause is termed sensory instability.

The CMG commonly demonstrates combinations of detrusor, urethral, and sensory abnormalities, especially GSUI and detrusor instability.[89,111] Thus the CMG must investigate these possibilities adequately before the test is considered complete. Whatever the urodynamics findings, they are not diagnostic of a specific lesion; rather, they must be used with other available information to make the final diagnosis. Again, correlation of the urodynamics test with the patient's clinical situation is vital, especially before invasive therapy is attempted.

Indications

The CMG is indicated in several situations to evaluate storage characteristics when more basic clinical studies do not yield the diagnosis:

1. To confirm the cause of incontinence
2. To evaluate pain or irritative symptoms (urgency, frequency, and nocturia) of the lower urinary tract
3. In a patient with known or suspected neurologic disease or injury, in whom diagnoses based on clinical grounds alone are unreliable
4. In a patient who has not been helped by therapy based on clinical information alone, especially before further invasive therapy is carried out
5. To investigate the cause of otherwise unexplainable abnormalities such as hydronephrosis, reflux, or postoperative changes
6. To obtain functional data on the lower urinary tract before and after any type of therapy, but especially invasive, nonreversible therapy
7. When the basic evaluation does not suggest the diagnosis or contains conflicting information.

ELECTROMYOGRAPHY

Most urodynamics tests are assessments of the effects the detrusor sphincter or muscles produce; also valuable is an assessment of what a muscle is actually doing, that is, measurement of the electrical activity associated with muscle depolarization, a process called electromyography (EMG). In urodynamics, EMG of the urethral, periurethral, or perineal striated muscles is practical, routine, and occasionally essential, providing direct data about electrical activity of the striated muscles but only indirect information about the urethra's effective functional activity.[112-118] The standard urodynamic EMG provides no data about the detrusor muscle or sensation (except perhaps about whether the patient noticed placement of the electrodes) but refers only to the activity of the urethral sphincter striated muscle.

The basic unit of muscle activity is the motor unit, which has two components, a single motor neuron, extending from the cell body in the anterior horn of the spinal cord to the synapse at the muscle cell wall, and the associated muscle fibers. Depolarization of the motor unit produces the basic EMG signal, the motor unit action potential. Normal motor unit action potentials have a characteristic configuration, amplitude, and duration. As motor units are "recruited" to act together, the EMG increases in intensity until all associated motor units are depolarizing together to create the maximum EMG signal, the full recruitment or full interference pattern.

Normally a person can contract the striated muscle of the external sphincter voluntarily and on command at any point during the filling, storage, or voiding process. Such complete, sudden contraction of the sphincter rapidly produces a full interference pattern, which remains without decay for as long as the person contracts the muscle. Pressure on the glans penis or clitoris, or pressure of a Foley balloon on the bladder neck caused by briskly pulling on a catheter, causes a brief contraction of the same external sphincter muscle, a response called the bulbocavernosus reflex. The efferent limb of this reflex uses the pudendal nerve, and the afferent pathways differ: glans or clitoral pressure uses the pudendal nerve, and the Foley catheter pull uses the pelvic nerve. However, each technique provides an indication of the status of the sacral reflex arc. The bulbocavernosus reflex is usually a weaker EMG signal than the full interference pattern. As the bladder fills, the sphincter gradually contracts more to ensure continence; as a reflection of this contraction the EMG signal gradually increases in activity, sometimes reaching the level of the full interference pattern when the bladder is very full and the patient is feeling a strong urge to void. This EMG increase with filling is called the guarding response and is normal. Straining or coughing causes a burst of EMG activity approaching or equaling the full interference pattern. Finally, when voiding occurs, the EMG is silent just before the detrusor contraction, indicating complete relaxation of the striated muscle of the external sphincter, which allows synergistic voiding.[113-119]

Equipment

Several different EMG techniques are used in urodynamics,[30,112-116,120-123] each providing a different level of precision in directly measuring the electrical activity of the urethral sphincter muscles. Measurement of electrical activity from muscles requires two separate electrodes and a neutral ground electrode. The ground electrode is usually placed on the thigh, and the two other electrodes can be placed in a variety of locations, each of which affects the nature of the information gathered from the EMG study.

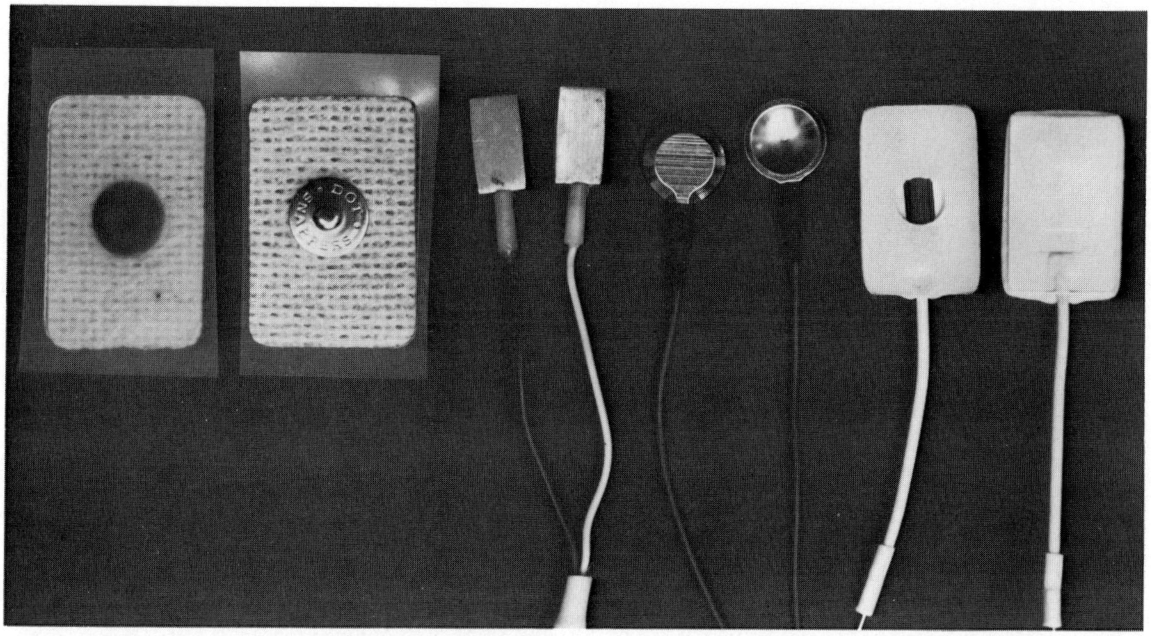

FIGURE 7–21. Pairs of skin surface electromyographic electrodes. On the left and right ends of the photograph are electrodes with their own adhesive for attaching to the skin. The two electrode pairs in the middle require taping to the skin.

The most basic EMG technique, in which two surface electrodes are attached to the skin or tissue near the muscles to be tested, provides an overall impression of average muscle activity of large groups of muscles. The simplest approach employs patch electrodes that are attached on opposite sides of the anterolateral perianal skin.[121,122] The method used to stick the electrodes to the skin depends on the electrode type; some are more adherent and convenient to apply (Figure 7–21).

Perianal skin electrodes provide an approximation of the electrical activities of the urethral sphincter muscles, since these electrodes actually detect overall perineal and perianal sphincter muscle activity rather than specific periurethral activity. Such a gross approximation is accurate enough for most routine urodynamics evaluations except in cases of neurologic disease (especially demyelinating disease and pelvic injury) or after urethral surgery or injury.[113,117,121,122,124-126] Furthermore, the perianal electrodes are practical, since they are inexpensive, easy and painless to apply, and well tolerated by patients.

Surface electrodes have also been placed on urethral catheters in such a way that the electrodes contact the urethral sphincter area more directly (Figure 7–22).[123,127] The catheter provides bladder filling and pressure measurement capability. Vaginal and rectal EMG electrodes are also available (Figure 7–23). These internal electrodes can provide EMG quality at least as good as the skin electrodes, but the disposable types are more expensive and sometimes difficult to position properly. The rigid anal plug types are also less comfortable for the patient than other options; they may be accidentally expelled with straining, make rectal pressure measurements more difficult, and induce artifactual increases in the EMG signal because the patient squeezes the rectal sphincter to keep the plug in. As a result, these electrode types are less commonly used for most urodynamics tests.[121]

When more precise information about smaller or more specific bundles of muscles is needed, needle or wire electrodes must be used (Figure 7–24). Two thin wire electrodes are passed within guiding needles (about 27 gauge) into the periurethral muscle area to lie about 1 cm apart with a grounding pad on the skin; after placement the two wires are left in the muscle and the guiding needles removed. Needle tip electrodes of about the same size can be used in a similar fashion.

In the concentric needle, about 23 to 29 gauge, the sheath of the needle acts as one electrode and a thin wire mounted within the sheath serves as the second electrode; a ground lead is also needed. Of similar size is a bipolar needle that has two wires within an outer sheath needle; the sheath can serve as the ground. Because concentric and bipolar needles are so compact, they are capable of detecting electrical activity of muscle within a diameter of about 1 mm, so that the activity of a single or a few motor units can be evaluated. However, because the range of focus is so narrow, the needle position often must be modified so it can be placed in the most appropriate location for an accurate EMG.

The primary advantages of needle electrodes are less artifact and greater ability to detect activity in specific muscles and to obtain raw EMG data. Such advantages are useful in patients with known or suspected neurologic or urethral disease or injury that necessitates gathering the more precise information available with the more invasive tech-

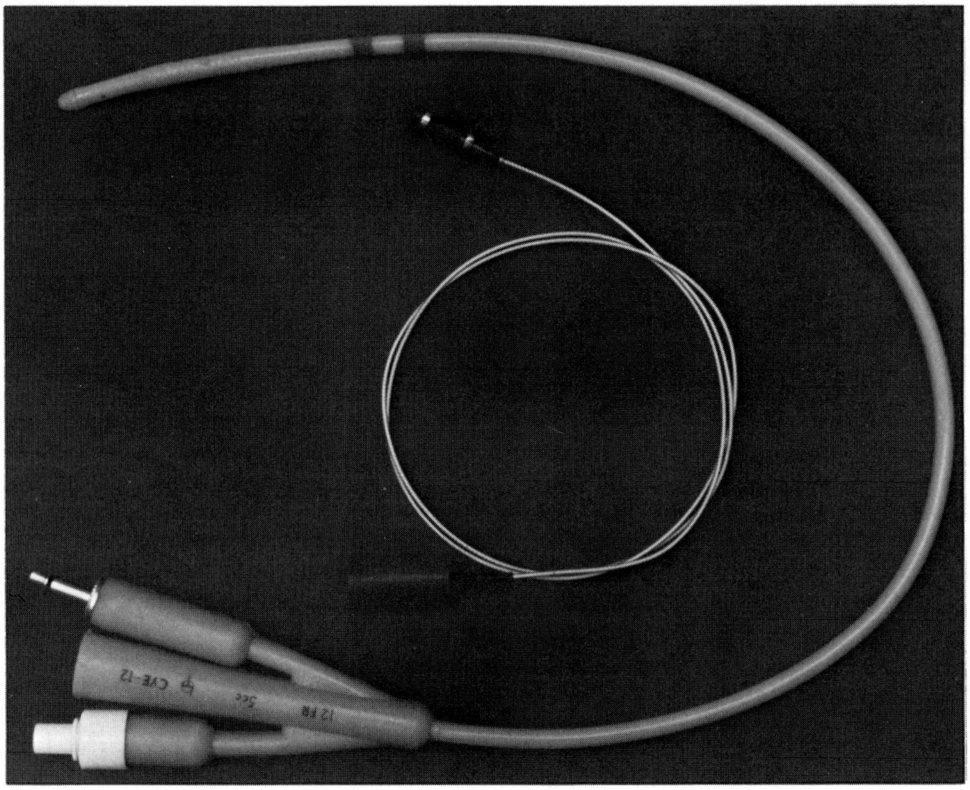

FIGURE 7–22. Catheter-mounted intraurethral electromyographic electrodes. In the center is a coiled electrode that can be placed on a Foley catheter. On the outer portion of the figure is a catheter with the electrodes already built into it.

nique. Because placement of the needles and wires is painful, neurologically intact patients, especially children, have difficulty accepting needle electrodes. Skill and patience are needed for accurate placement, and the electrodes, especially the rigid type, may be dislodged if the patient changes position. The concentric and bipolar electrodes are delicate and expensive. The surface electrodes are inexpensive, can be placed painlessly with much less expertise, and are not easily dislodged; however, they can become wet, they are more likely to generate artifacts, and the EMG signal is only an imprecise approximation of specific sphincter muscle signal. However, as noted previously, for most

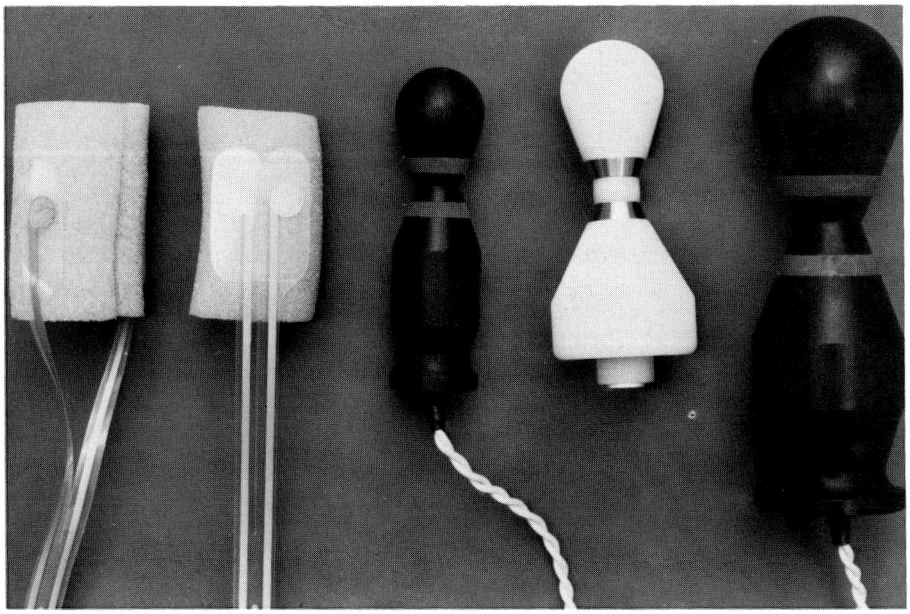

FIGURE 7–23. Internal surface electromyographic electrodes. *Left to right:* Intrarectal sponge electrode with electrodes mounted on opposite sides of the sponge; intravaginal sponge electrode with electrodes placed close together to locate sphincter activity on the anterior vaginal wall; three intrarectal plug electrodes in various sizes.

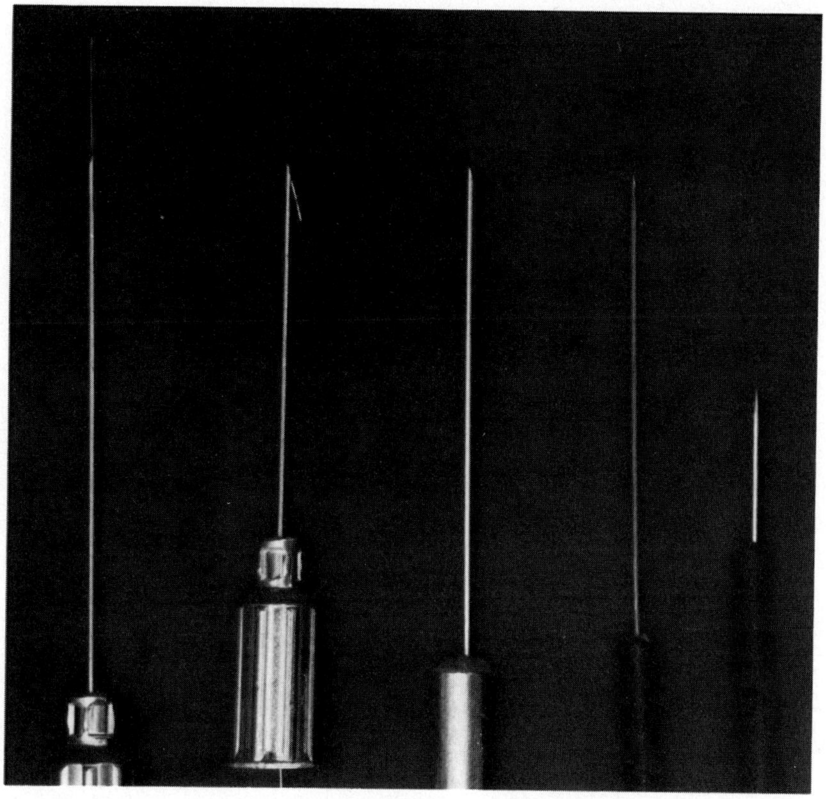

FIGURE 7–24. Needle electromyographic electrodes. *Left to right:* Thin wire electrodes with a barbed end and insulated main shaft within the 27-gauge needle guides with a longer male needle introducer on the left and a shorter female introducer needle on the right; a coaxial needle electrode (in the middle of the figure); and two needles that are monopolar needle electrodes without barbed ends.

urodynamics testing the surface electrodes provide the gross data needed to make the urodynamics diagnosis.

The ground lead and the electrodes, regardless of type, send their electrical signal of muscle activity to an amplifier unit. The amplified signal is then transmitted as raw EMG data or is modified through rectification and integration to produce average or integrated EMG signals for final output or display.

Several options for EMG signal display or output are available. The most basic output modes are the strip chart recorders and CRTs used for standard CMG recording. However, these devices have frequency responses in the range of 100 Hz, too slow to provide a permanent record of individual motor unit action potentials with frequencies between 1000 and 10,000 Hz. Thus the standard urodynamics output modes give the urologist only a gross impression of the character of the total, unprocessed, raw EMG signal during urodynamics testing. By processing the EMG signal, the standard urodynamics equipment more easily displays the EMG activity with less electrical noise despite the inherent frequency response problems. One way of processing the raw EMG signal is to rectify and average the signal, producing a slowly varying line on the display. If a 5 or 10 Hz sine wave is added to the signal, the pattern more closely resembles a true EMG pattern. A second way of processing the raw EMG signal is to sum, or integrate, the total potential changes, positive and negative, over a specific time interval. With this integrated method the magnitude and duration of the potentials affect the display. Still another method involves converting the EMG signal frequency to voltage and producing a signal with a magnitude proportional to the counted number of potentials. The counted and integrated signals are similar on a standard urodynamics display unit. Any of these processed EMG signal displays is only an approximation of the gross muscle activity and lags behind the true activity by as much as a few seconds. For most urodynamics testing this lag is not of great significance but must be recognized. An audio output complements the visual output and is valuable when the clinician is directly observing the evaluation (Figure 7–25).

To qualify the nature of EMG activity and detect abnormal motor unit potentials (e.g., polyphasic waves, fibrillations, giant waves, and positive sharp waves), needle electrodes and an oscilloscope are necessary. On the oscilloscope a freeze-frame mode, perhaps with photographic or videotaping capability, is valuable for longer examination of specific motor unit waveforms.

The basic principles of highly specific needle EMG techniques can be applied to study nerve conduction times (e.g., dorsal penile nerve conduction), reflex latencies (e.g., bulbocavernosus reflex times), evoked potentials, and sensory thresholds.[115,128,129] Such detailed evaluations are performed only in cases of known or suspected neurologic disease in which the details of the motor unit EMG or con-

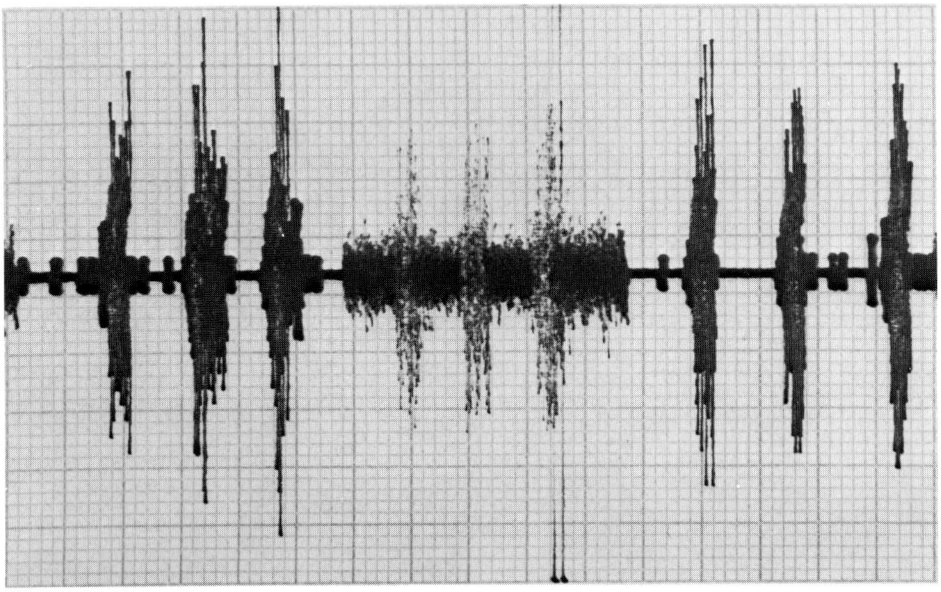

FIGURE 7–25. Electromyographic (EMG) display using both a direct and an integrated output on a strip chart recorder with a paper speed of 0.5 mm/sec. Each small box is equivalent to 1 mm, or 2 seconds of time. The patient has skin surface electrodes placed on the perianal skin and is intermittently voluntarily contracting and relaxing the perianal muscles. In the middle of the figure is the EMG pattern with the machine on the direct setting. At rest, some baseline activity occurs, but with voluntary contraction the magnitude of the response (vertical height at the display) increases and the tracing becomes more feathery, followed by relaxation and return to the baseline output. Flanking the direct EMG output on both sides is the output on the integrated setting. The density of the lines of the display is greater because the pen motion is slower. At rest, essentially no baseline activity occurs. With voluntary contraction the height of the display increases dramatically until relaxation again occurs.

duction-type studies may affect the diagnosis or prognosis. Such situations are unusual in the context of urodynamics evaluations, and few urologists have the knowledge, experience, interest, or time to become proficient in these techniques; instead, the assistance of an interested neurologist is valuable in these situations. For these reasons such special and unusual studies are not discussed further in this chapter.

In most urodynamics testing, raw EMG data and specific muscle or nerve studies provided by wire and needle electrodes are unnecessary, since the basic surface electrodes and strip chart or CRT display units usually provide the gross EMG (kinesiologic) data needed to make a urodynamics diagnosis. Regardless of the equipment used, the quality of EMG data available for later review will be no better than its quality during the original study. In the case of many strip charts and most CRT displays, the data for delayed review are often impossible to interpret accurately, especially if even a mild amount of artifact was present on the original study. There is no substitute for real-time observation of EMG data by the clinician.

Technique

The most important aspect of the EMG technique is accurate placement of the EMG electrodes. For the skin surface electrodes the skin must be carefully prepared with alcohol, gentle abrasion may create good contact between the electrode surface and the skin, and shaving of hair may be necessary. Appropriate electroconductive gels should be applied to ensure good electrical contact between the electrode and the skin. The anal, vaginal, and urethral catheter electrodes are placed so that the electrodes are oriented properly relative to the sphincter areas.

Needle electrodes can be inserted into several muscles to produce the desired EMG data about urethral sphincter activity. In increasing order of precision, the perianal sphincter, the perineal or bulbocavernosus muscles, and the periurethral muscles provide approximations of the true urethral sphincter activity.

If the needle electrodes are placed in the perianal muscles, the needles are passed about 1 cm into the muscle through the skin near the anterior midline at the anal verge. For bulbocavernosus muscle placement, the muscle can be palpated and the needle passed into the body of the muscle. For periurethral muscle placement in a male patient, the clinician places the wire and electrodes about 1 to 2 cm distal to the apex of the prostate gland, penetrating the skin of the perineum for about 3 to 4 cm near the midline between the anal verge and scrotum with a finger placed in the rectum to palpate the apical prostate area. In a female patient the clinician guides the needles into the anterior periurethral tissues 1.5 to 2.5 cm deep into the proximal to middle urethra by passing the needles about 0.5 cm anterolateral to the urethral meatus on each side of the midline, palpating through the vagina as necessary to feel the approximate position of the bladder neck and midurethra. Needle electrodes are placed in a fashion similar to that for the thin wires with finger guidance through the vagina or rectum, although they can be more accurately placed wherever the discrete muscle activity is to be monitored, including the perianal, bulbocavernosus, or periurethral muscles. For most urodynamics purposes, placing the needles in the periurethral area provides the most accurate, specific, and useful information about the striated muscle of the urethral sphincter. When a unilateral lesion may be present (as with a herniated disk or pelvic nerve injury), the needles or wires can be placed to evaluate each side of the midline separately.

A relaxed, cooperative patient is important in yielding useful, interpretable EMG data. The patient should be warm and comfortably positioned, with as little of the physical exposure inherent in the techniques as possible. Since EMG needle insertion is usually painful, the patient should be warned about this but reassured that the discomfort will be brief and is generally well tolerated.

The examiner can confirm accurate electrode placement by checking the quality of the full interference pattern and the bulbocavernosus reflex before initiating other urodynamic tests (Figure 7–25).[113-115,117,118] The entire EMG system should be turned on and the sensitivity adjusted so that minimal activity is detected when the patient is at rest but a good signal is seen when the patient contracts the periurethral and perianal muscles as strongly as possible to generate a full interference pattern. The full interference pattern reflects the maximum recruitment of individual motor units. This signal is a reference point as the maximum signal that would be expected during the remainder of the urodynamics testing. Sometimes patients have difficulty understanding how to contract to create a good full interference pattern, but most neurologically normal patients eventually provide some increase in the EMG signal lasting as long as the contraction is held. Failure to elicit a normal full interference pattern in a neurologically normal patient usually means that the command to contract the muscles was not understood or properly executed or that the electrodes are poorly placed or improperly connected or grounded. Rarely the poor or absent full interference pattern indicates a genuine, occult neurologic deficit. Besides the full interference pattern, other voluntary contraction responses can be tested with Valsalva, Credé, and coughing maneuvers, each of which should produce an increase in the EMG signal. The bulbocavernosus reflex is then tested as discussed previously. Absence of a good bulbocavernosus reflex can have the same causes as an abnormal full interference pattern, especially after any technical problems of electrode placement, grounding, and connections are corrected.[130]

During the various urodynamics tests the EMG signal is carefully monitored for changes from the baseline, especially as they relate to the simultaneous pressure measurements and sensation reports from the patient. Again, because the significance of the EMG signals may be impossible to put into proper perspective after the testing is completed, depending on the mode of storage and output or display, there is no substitute for direct observation of the tests by the clinician.

Normal and Abnormal Electromyographic Patterns

The normal and abnormal nature of the full interference pattern and bulbocavernosus reflex are discussed previously. During the bladder filling process the EMG signal may remain stable or increase in intensity. A gradual, steady increase in signal intensity is the normal guarding response. EMG overactivity in the form of a rapid, significant increase in EMG activity preceding or accompanying an increase in detrusor pressure from an involuntary bladder contraction is also a guarding response. If the patient feels the pressure increase and is merely attempting to suppress the bladder contraction to prevent leakage, the guarding response is normal even if the detrusor pressure increase is not.[113,118,119] If the patient does not feel the pressure increase, which is almost always due to significant neurologic deficit such as spinal cord injury, the simultaneous detrusor pressure and EMG signal (and urethral pressure) increase is termed detrusor-sphincter dyssynergia (DSD).[3,115,125,131-134] DSD is pathologic EMG overactivity, an abnormality that, like a high leak point pressure, can adversely affect the upper urinary tract (Figures 7–26 to 7–29).[92,97,133] DSD has been classified into three main types based on the relationship between the EMG and detrusor pressure signals[132] or on the nature of the neurologic lesion.[133]

Artifactual increases in the EMG also can occur because of tube or wire motion; wetting or dislodgement of the electrodes; electrical bridging between electrodes (shorting out); patient actions such as movement, coughing, lifting the head, or tightening the muscles near the electrodes; or external influences such as in-line 60-cycle artifact from other electrical equipment operating nearby. Other sources of artifact include poor patient contact with the electrodes; dirty electrodes; broken or loose wires, connections, or insulation; and incorrect sensitivity of the processing equipment. Careful attention to technique is vital in obtaining a meaningful EMG study.

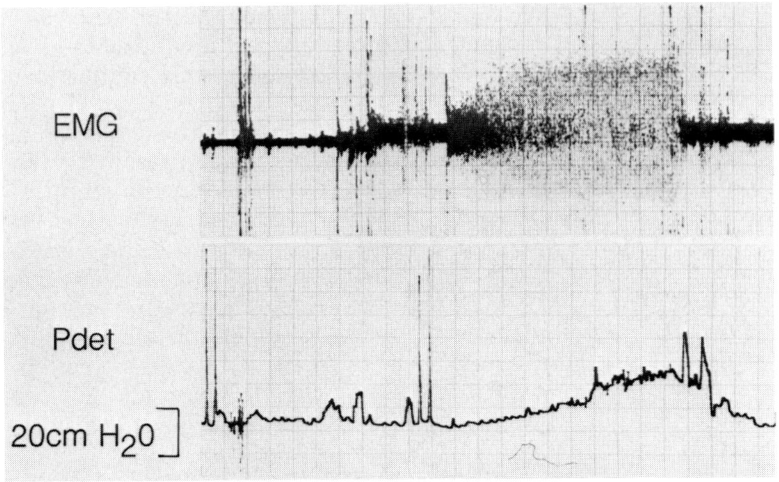

FIGURE 7–26. A direct electromyogram (EMG) during filling cystometry. With the gradual phasic pressure increase a corresponding gradual increase in the intensity of the EMG signal occurs. The signal increase is not only an increase in height of the display but also a more feathery display because of the more rapid pen motion associated with the increased EMG signal intensity. This EMG pattern may correspond to either voluntary guarding by a patient in response to the detrusor pressure increase or detrusor-sphincter dyssynergia. The differentiation between these two depends on the patient's sensation and neurologic status.

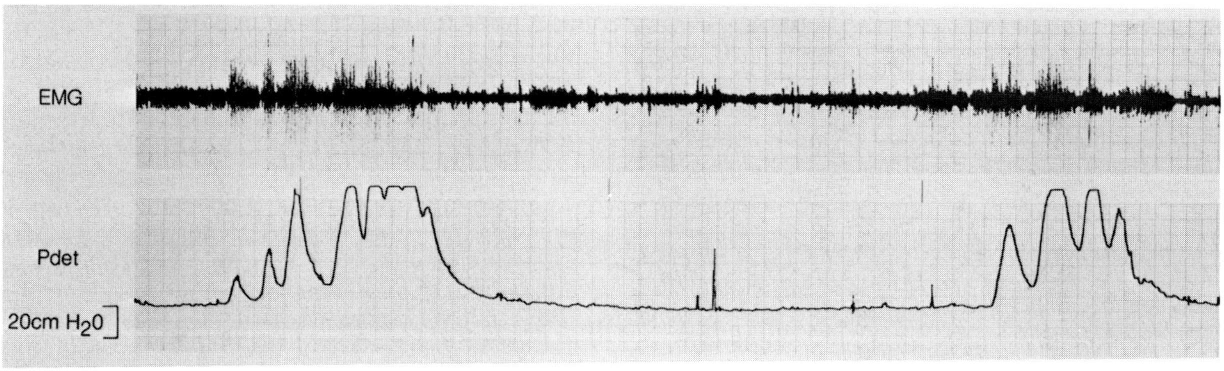

FIGURE 7–27. Direct electromyogram (EMG) obtained during filling cystometry. The EMG pattern is consistent with either normal guarding or detrusor-sphincter dyssynergia.

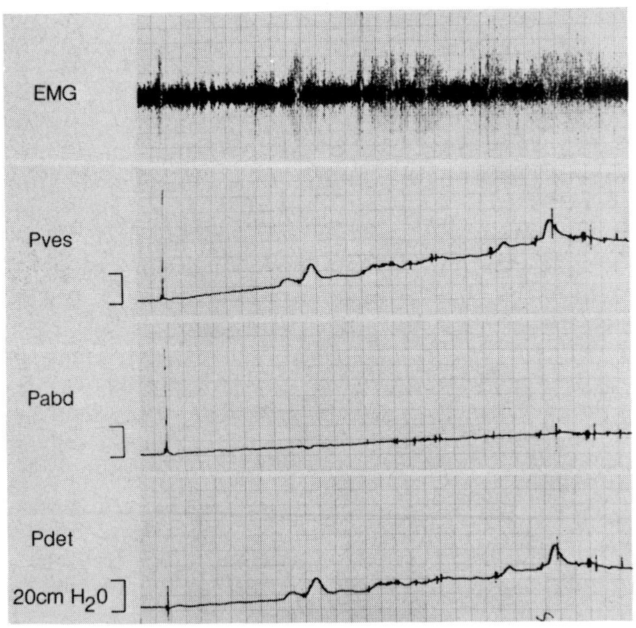

FIGURE 7–28. Direct electromyogram (EMG) obtained during filling cystometry. With the steady pressure increases associated with low compliance, the baseline EMG signal steadily increases. With the intermittent phasic pressure increases, a more pronounced increase occurs in the EMG activity, both associated with a normal guarding response or detrusor-sphincter dyssynergia.

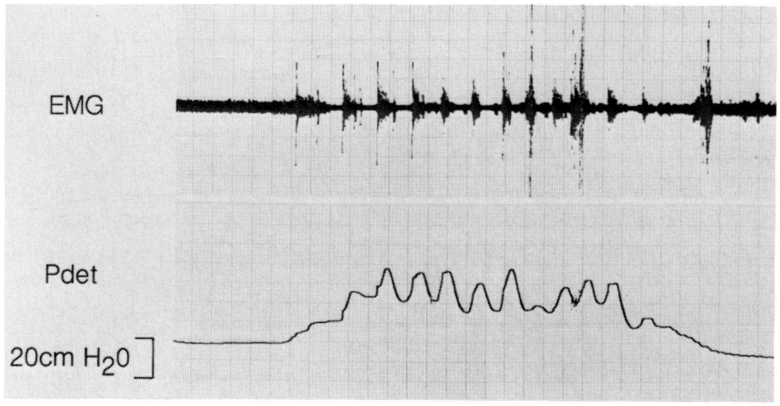

FIGURE 7–29. Direct electromyogram (EMG) obtained during filling cystometry shows intermittent increases and decreases in EMG signal intensity in association with phasic detrusor increases in a case of detrusor-spincter dyssynergia in a paraplegic patient.

Brief underactivity of the EMG can also occur during filling. These decreases may correspond to relaxation of the urethra, called urethral instability, a process that may lead to incontinence (see "Urethral Pressure Measurements").

During voiding the normal EMG activity should show complete silence just before detrusor contraction and urine flow.[82,113,115,118,135,136] EMG overactivity with corresponding decrease in flow rate indicates an inappropriate increase in the urethral muscular activity and is indicative of an obstructive process such as DSD, a voluntary patient contraction, or dysfunctional voiding.[3,10,82,113,115,119,125,128,131,132,135-139] If no decrease in flow rate occurs with the EMG signal increase, the EMG signal change is probably artifact and of no clinical significance[3,119,131,132,135]; this emphasizes the rare need for EMG monitoring of neurologically normal patients with no evidence of voiding dysfunction by history, uroflowmetry, or residual urine measurement. Disparity of EMG activity among the perineal muscle groups is reported in patients with known neurologic injury[113,117,122,124-126]; this may cause some problems with accurate interpretation of the EMG signals, depending on what types of electrodes are placed and where. If the data fit the clinical situation, they are probably accurate; if not, the clinician must use judgment about how much more precise the EMG monitoring or other testing must be to make the diagnosis.

Artifactual causes of the abnormal increases in the EMG signal with voiding are the same as those that can occur during bladder filling. Also, the embarrassment or discomfort of the EMG or the voiding process can cause artificial increases in the EMG signal. Many of these misleading artifacts can be detected only by careful observation of the equipment and the patient at the time of the test, making retrospective reviews of the EMG of limited validity.

Indications

EMG is most useful in delineating sphincter activity in the following situations:

1. Known or suspected neurologic disease or injury that may cause an abnormality of sphincter muscle activity during storage or voiding
2. Incontinence that seems to be spontaneous and in which the patient has no sensation of an impending detrusor contraction or of the leakage itself
3. Abnormal voiding patterns or emptying, which may be due to abnormal sphincter activity whether from neurologic or nonneurologic causes (e.g., dysfunctional voiding)

URETHRAL PRESSURE MEASUREMENT

Normal urethral function requires that the urethra remain closed during the storage and filling process to maintain continence, and then relax and open as completely as possible when voiding is attempted. Such closing and opening functions would seem to relate directly to pressures the urethra might produce through the actions of its mucosal, vascular, collagen, elastin, and muscular components and has led to the development of urethral pressure measurement techniques.[140-144] Measurement of urethral pressure provides direct data on urethral function but no information about detrusor or sensory function. Unfortunately, as discussed later, the intuitive value of the urethral pressure measurements has not been borne out in practice because of the great overlap between "normal" and "abnormal" and the challenges involved in properly using the equipment and techniques.

Intraurethral pressure varies along the urethral length, being equal to the bladder pressure at the internal urethral meatus, reaching a point of zero (atmospheric pressure) at the external urethral meatus, and depending on the patient and circumstance, having a range of values above zero between these two locations (Figure 7–30). In female patients the pressures are measured from internal to external meatus; in male patients they are taken from the internal meatus to just beyond the external striated sphincter. If the pressures are plotted along the vertical axis with the corresponding po-

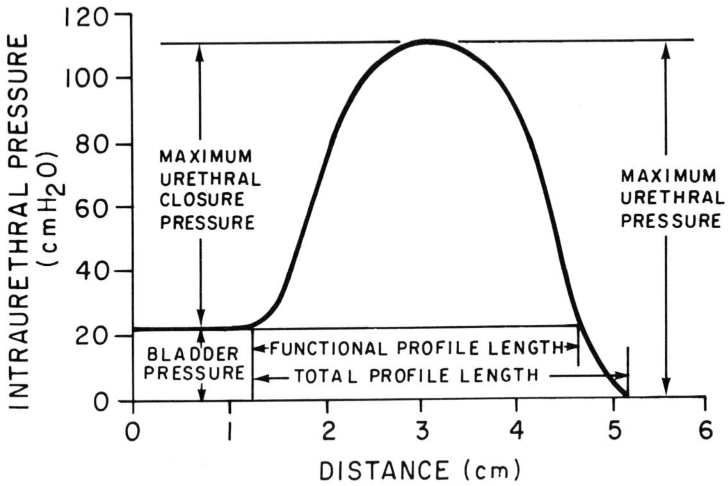

FIGURE 7–30. Normal female urethral pressure profile showing the key parameters and normal shape according to International Continence Society criteria.

sitions along the length of the urethra, or at a specific point over time, as the horizontal axis, a profile of the urethral pressure is produced, the urethral pressure profile (UPP). The profile measurements obtained during bladder filling and storage with the patient, urethra, and bladder at rest are resting UPPs; measurements obtained while the patient performs stress maneuvers such as coughing and straining are called stress profiles. A voiding UPP is obtained while the patient voids. The measurements can be obtained not only at various points along the urethral length, but also at points around the urethral circumference.

Simultaneous measurement of intravesical pressure is essential during stress and voiding UPPs to take detrusor pressure changes from contractions or stress maneuvers into account. Subtracting simultaneously measured intravesical pressure from urethral pressure yields the urethral closure pressure; when measurements are performed along the urethral length, the urethral closure pressure profile is obtained. The closure pressure is a reflection of the excess urethral pressure available to exceed the intravesical pressure at that moment and location.

Maximum urethral pressure is the highest pressure of the UPP. The maximum urethral closure pressure is the maximum difference between simultaneously measured intravesical and urethral pressures. Functional profile length, at rest or during stress, is the urethral length along which the urethral pressure exceeds intravesical pressure; like the maximum urethral closure pressure, this gives some impression of the urethral length available to maintain continence against the bladder pressure. The total pressure profile length is the urethral length along which any positive urethral pressure occurs; it has no clear clinical usefulness.

Middle-aged and older men have a zone of elevated pressure called the prostatic plateau before the region of the maximum urethral pressure (Figure 7–31). Within the plateau region may be a

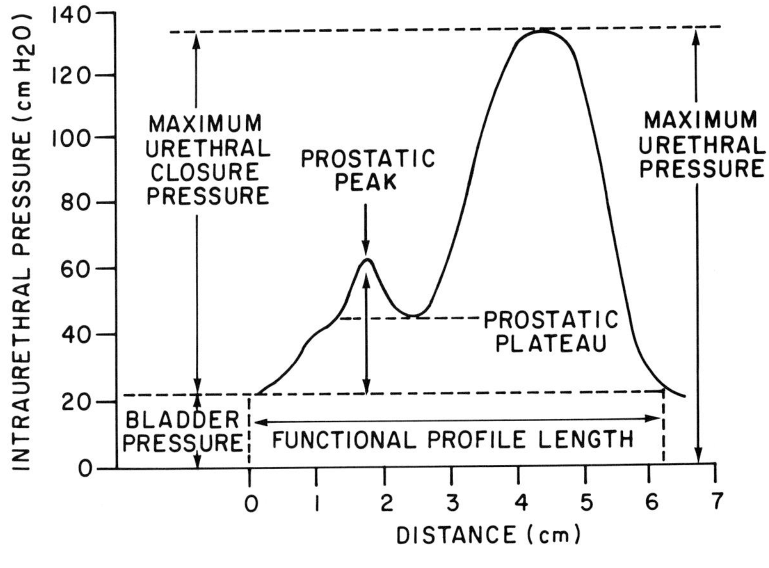

FIGURE 7–31. Urethral pressure profile showing the key parameters and normal shape for an elderly man with a typical prostatic peak according to International Continence Society criteria. In a younger man the prostatic peak might be absent and only a prostatic plateau present as a relatively horizontal pressure line before the more distal pressure increase.

smaller zone of further elevated pressure called the prostatic peak.[145-147]

The pressure transmission ratio is the quotient of urethral pressure change divided by intravesical pressure change during a stress maneuver; the quotient is multiplied by 100 to create a percentage. Pressure transmission ratios can be obtained along the urethral length, producing a transmission profile. When a single transmission value is stated, the point along the urethra must be specified. Although the term "transmission" is now in standard use, it may be misleading because it implies a totally passive process. A passive process has not yet been proved and active muscular activity may be a contributing factor.[148]

Equipment

Regardless of other variations in technique the urethral pressures are measured with transducer systems having the same characteristics as those discussed in the section on the CMG[59]; the reader should refer to that section as necessary to complement the following discussion. The type of pressure measurement catheter is the most significant variable affecting the UPP technique and results. The three primary catheter and technique types[59,149] are fluid perfusion,[99,141,143-147,150-158] intraurethral balloon,[140,159-161] and catheter tip transducer.[59,67,73,101,123,142,162-172]

In the fluid perfusion technique the urethral pressure is considered equal to the pressure needed to perfuse a catheter at a constant rate with either liquid (water) or gas (CO_2).[59,99,141,143-147,150-152,154-158,173] The technique measures the cumulative effects of the occlusive pressure or tension of the urethral wall in the region of the perfusing fluid plus the resistance to flow in the urethra and the perfusion catheter. The perfusion catheter has one or more holes at the end or along the side of the tube through which the fluid flows at a constant rate into the urethral lumen. The catheter is pulled through the urethra by hand (clumsy and imprecise) or by a catheter withdrawal machine (controlled and precise),[152,174] so that the measured pressures can be correlated with urethral position. If the pulling speed is the same as a simultaneous display or paper printout speed, urethral positions correspond directly with the printout positions. Once the fluid perfusion pressure exceeds the pressure of the urethra distal to the point of perfusion, the perfusion fluid leaks out of the urethra and the pressure measurement becomes somewhat less precise.

The accuracy of any perfusion profilometry method can be affected by simple physical problems such as the presence of gas in a liquid line, liquid in a gas line, or a leak at any connection point along the system. Several technical variables can also significantly affect the accuracy of the fluid perfusion profilometry: catheter size, number of catheter eye holes, rates of perfusion and catheter withdrawal, and the dynamic response time of the entire system.[59,141,143,144,146,150,151,175] A catheter size from 4F to 10F yields the most consistent results. Larger sizes are more likely to inappropriately measure elastic elements as part of the urethral pressure. A single side exit hole is inaccurate, so a catheter with an end exit or at least two radially directed opposing holes set back from the catheter tip is most appropriate. There is some directionality to the UPP measurements with fewer holes, a concern also present with catheter tip transducers. Fluid perfusion rate must be constant and is best controlled with a syringe pump machine.[152] Liquid perfusion rates between 2 and 10 ml/min are appropriate. With faster rates the pressures are artificially high; with slower rates extremely slow withdrawal rates are necessary to give accurate results. The catheter withdrawal rates compatible with the perfusion rates of 2 to 10 ml/min are 5 to 40 cm/min and are best maintained with mechanical catheter withdrawal devices.

The dynamic response time of the fluid perfusion profilometry system is important.[59,142,143,150,151] This value is related to the system's ability to respond to rapid changes in urethral pressure, in other words, whether the system is physically able to detect the pressure changes within the urethra as the catheter is moved through it. The dynamic response time is determined by the length and diameter of the tubing between the transducer and the patient, the perfusion rate, and the catheter withdrawal speed. A simple way of determining that the response time is inadequate is to note the appearance of the pressure profile. If the curve is relatively straight on the upstroke and even more abrupt and straight on the downstroke, the response is inadequate and the infusion rate should be increased or the withdrawal rate decreased to allow accurate measurement.

These general physical characteristics limit perfusion techniques to resting UPP measurements unless special care is taken in designing and operating the entire UPP system, in which case stress profiles can be obtained.[59,148,176] Another variation of the technique, in which water-filled tubing without active perfusion is used, has been employed in voiding profile studies.[133,177-179] This approach has technical limitations that have not yet been fully analyzed, which must be considered before the approach is used widely.

If gas is used as the fluid,[123,154,155,173] perfusion rates of 150 to 300 ml/min are necessary to correspond to flow rates of 2 to 10 ml of water per minute; corresponding catheter pull rates are 3 to 5 cm/min. The infusion rate of the gas is not constant, since it decreases when intraurethral pressures are high. The gas is also compressible, which alters the dynamic response characteristics. Furthermore, when such high fill rates are required, the UPP must be completed rapidly to prevent changes in bladder behavior resulting from rapid bladder filling. In general, gas pressure profilometry is not recommended unless the investigator is experienced with the technique.[59,123,155]

Balloon or membrane catheters have one or more small balloons or membranes mounted on the catheter.[59,140,159-161] The balloon is filled with fluid (usually water) attached to a transducer. These catheters produce quite accurate UPPs, and the response time is rapid so that they can be used for resting, stress, and voiding UPPs. The balloons are delicate and somewhat more difficult to use than the perfusion profilometry catheters, and the operator must frequently calibrate the system and remove any air bubbles from it.[59] Unfortunately, the very size of the balloon affects the urethra's physical characteristics and the spatial resolution of the measurements, reducing the pinpoint accuracy that might be desired in the measurements. Balloon catheters cannot be used for voiding profilometry.

The most modern, accurate, dependable, and practical pressure profilometry technique for reproducible resting, stress, and voiding measurements employs catheter tip transducers.[59,67,73,101,123,142,162-165,167,169,170-172] Dynamic response time variables or concerns with large volumes of fluid filling the bladder, tubing, leakage, air bubbles, or zeroing errors are eliminated with this type of transducer. Catheter tip transducers have several potential drawbacks besides their cost. Theoretically, movement and contact or "sticking" artifact can occur between the urethral mucosa and the transducers. Also, the older, stiffer catheters can induce an artifact by distorting the urethra; newer, more flexible catheters do not present this difficulty. Of benefit, but a drawback in some situations, is the spatial resolution of the transducers, which is small because of their lengths. Finally, since the transducer is oriented in a specific direction on the catheter, circumferential differences in the measured pressures must be considered.[59,164,166,167,171,180,181] Attempts have been made to rectify the concerns about spatial resolution, mucosal contact, and circumferential differentials and also to "smooth out" the dynamic response curves by covering the catheter tip transducer with a balloon.[168,172] Despite these concerns the catheter tip transducer is the best overall system for obtaining any type of UPP.

Technique

While the technique of urethral pressure measurements depends largely on the equipment, several general aspects of technique deserve special mention. Whatever technique is used, the specifications of the equipment and technique used in the test must be described in detail, including such items as catheter type, size, and configuration; orientation, pull speed; infusion rates; bladder volume; patient position and maneuvers performed; and recording apparatus.[10] Urethral pressure measurements must be repeated until a consistent, similar pattern is produced. This concept is a correlate of the one applicable to other urodynamics tests, which are repeated until the patient's clinical situation is reproduced. Intravesical pressure measurement is always valuable and is essential for stress and voiding profiles. At the beginning of the measurements the urethral and intravesical probes should be placed in the bladder and the pressure values should be identical. Although not obtained routinely, intraabdominal pressures can be measured if enough transducers and recording channels are available, allowing analysis of abdominal pressure transmission apart from any detrusor effects; these are especially valuable when the patient is upright or for stress UPP.

Catheter withdrawal rates vary with technique in the perfusion method to provide an adequate dynamic response as discussed previously. With the balloon and catheter tip transducer techniques, withdrawal rates are usually about 1 to 2 mm/sec but can be as slow as 1 cm/min. These rates meet the dynamic response criteria discussed previously and allow the clinician to set a rate that provides a direct correlation between the urethral position and the display. Alternatively, the catheter can be withdrawn in increments of about 5 mm, the pulling stopped, and measurements taken while the patient performs the stress maneuvers, the nature and force of which should be recorded.

The circumferential orientation of the catheter's pressure sensing point can be significant with perfusion catheters that have only one exit hole and with catheter tip transducers, so the orientation must be specified because no standard orientation has yet been accepted. When voiding UPPs are obtained, precise localization of the pressure measurement point is essential. When stress or voiding UPPs are obtained without pulling the catheter, the urethral pressure is usually measured at the point of maximum resting urethral pressure or at a fixed position from the bladder neck. Synchronous fluoroscopy is useful for localization in these situations.

The UPP is easier to obtain with the patient supine rather than sitting or standing. However, the supine position may not allow testing for the patient's complaint. There is no standard amount of fluid with which the bladder should be prefilled during the pressure measurements, but the amount should be related to the patient's clinical complaints and be clearly recorded and reproduced with each test on that patient.

The effects of drugs, especially adrenergic agents, on the urethra can be tested with the UPP techniques.[81,160,182]

Although most of the causes of artifact have been discussed, the effect of the patient must not be ignored. The patient may modify urethral pressures by contracting or relaxing the urethral and pelvic floor muscles, sometimes without being aware of doing so, and sometimes because the urethra is sensitive or tender. Repeating the test several times is vital because much of the confidence in the test's accuracy comes with reproducibility.

Normal and Abnormal Urethral Pressure Measurements and Patterns

Specific values and general characteristics for normals in UPP testing have a wide range and come from a variety of sources.[117,143,156-158,160,162,164,165,167,170-172,180,181,183-187] Summaries of these ranges of normal follow.

The normal resting UPP in women is relatively symmetric about a maximum pressure at the mid-urethra of 40 to 80 cm H_2O (Figure 7–30); asymmetry usually results from artifacts of the technique, especially poor dynamic response times. The functional profile length in the female is about 2.5 to 4 cm. Maximum urethral pressure values for the female decrease slightly with age. Small-magnitude rhythmic pressure variations with the catheter static and the patient at rest usually correspond to vascular pulsations and are normal.[187,188] During stress maneuvers the urethral pressure increases just before the increase in intravesical pressure and the normal pressure transmission is greater than 100% so the urethral closure pressure remains positive[148,164,165,172,180]; surgery should effect the same results[183,189] even if resting pressures do not change.[184,190,191] Excellent graphic descriptions of the various normal and abnormal patterns of the UPP are given by Hilton and Stanton,[164] Hilton,[165] Asmussen and Ulmsten,[142] Bunne and Obrink,[181] Constantinou,[192] and Constaninou and Govan.[193]

To maintain continence at any time, a person should have a urethral pressure greater than the corresponding intravesical pressure increases. Urine fills the urethra to the point at which the intraurethral pressure exceeds the intravesical pressure; if such a higher pressure point is not reached, incontinence or voiding occurs. Thus a negative urethral closure pressure or a low pressure transmission ratio or delayed urethral contraction may correspond to the patient's history of incontinence and support the diagnosis.[148,164,172,180]

In men[145-147] the UPP normally is not symmetric but has a maximum pressure of about 80 to 90 cm H_2O in the region of the external sphincter at the membranous urethra (Figure 7–31). In a young male the UPP is the same shape as that of a female. At puberty the prostatic plateau appears, followed later by the prostatic peak. The peak's pressure is usually less than the maximum pressure at the external sphincter area. With age the maximum pressure does not change much (10 to 20 cm H_2O), but the profile's length and the pressure of the plateau and peak area usually rise because of prostatic growth. The normal functional profile length is about 4 to 6 cm. Pressures in the bulbous and penile urethra are not usually measured. Even strictures in the urethra distal to the sphincter are not usually measured for pressures, since this measurement requires that the catheter be the same diameter as the stricture. In both males and females no notable pressure rise occurs at the bladder neck.

As the bladder fills, the urethral pressures usually increase. When the patient changes from the supine to sitting to standing positions, the urethral closure pressure rises slightly. During sleep the urethral pressure falls.[194]

In voiding UPPs the pressure at the point of measurement should drop and equal the intravesical pressure in female patients; the same pressure equilibration occurs in male patients unless the urethral pressure measurement is made distal to the membranous urethra. When an obstruction is proximal to the measurement point, the urethral pressure is lower than the intravesical pressure. This technique may be useful in confirming a diagnosis and in locating the region of obstruction.[177-179]

Overactivity (increases) in membranous urethral pressure coincident with involuntary rises in detrusor pressure may indicate appropriate guarding in a neurologically normal person or detrusor-sphincter dyssynergia in a neurologically impaired one. Overactivity can occur from obstruction in such conditions as benign prostatic hyperplasia or detrusor–bladder neck dyssynergia or after surgery such as bladder neck suspensions, pubovaginal slings, or artificial urinary sphincters. The patient may artifactually increase the urethral pressure through urethral contraction or spasm, but these findings are not easily or consistently duplicated.

Spontaneous drops in urethral pressure (underactivity) can occur without an associated change in detrusor pressure and sometimes lead to incontinence.[10] Although no formal definition is available, a pressure drop greater that 15 cm H_2O is termed urethral instability.[99-108,195] Some authors contend that the variations are merely physiologic.[109,110] Steady, uniform urethral pressure underactivity in segments or throughout the urethra may result from atrophy, surgical or accidental trauma, or neurologic changes causing denervation and sometimes the totally incompetent urethra of type III stress incontinence. No pressure level defines the incompetent urethra, but maximum urethral pressures of less than about 10 cm H_2O are clearly well below normal.[196]

Indications

Unfortunately, resting urethral pressure measurements have never fulfilled the dreams of clinicians in providing the unique and unequivocal data about urethral function that would allow definitive diagnoses, particularly in the assessment of stress urinary incontinence.[117,143,156,157,161,162,164,167,171,181,183-187,191,197,198] Several factors have caused this disappointment. First, UPPs are difficult to perform and reproduce for a clinician not familiar with the technique. Different techniques have yielded slightly different results, which makes comparison and standardization difficult. Many "normal" values in the literature were obtained with patients supine and bladders empty, hardly clinically significant situations. Measured with catheter tip transducers and single hole perfusion catheters, the urethral pressure has been found to vary circumferentially at a specific point along the urethra, which underlines the need for careful catheter orientation during the test. Finally and most important, although many patients with incontinence have resting maximum urethral pressures below those of "normals," overlap of the values is significant, making the specificity of the test low. Because of these real limitations the stress UPP is much more useful than the resting UPP for the evaluation of stress incontinence but even then is not essential. The relatively uncommon clinical conditions in which urethral pressure measurements may be useful include the following:

1. Determining the occlusive effect of malfunctioning artificial urinary sphincters
2. Supplementing other studies that are *equivocal* in the diagnosis of such conditions as complex incontinence, including possible type III stress incontinence (resting and stress UPPs), urethral instability (resting UPP), or outflow obstruction (voiding UPP)
3. Evaluating obstruction in a patient who can void only very small volumes
4. Ambulatory urodynamics
5. Research, especially in such areas as drug and surgical therapies and basic research on the function of the urethra

SIMULTANEOUS CYSTOMETRY AND UROFLOWMETRY: THE PRESSURE/FLOW STUDY

Despite their usefulness, uroflowmetry and filling cystometry alone cannot provide information about two key aspects of the voiding process: the level of detrusor contractile capability and the level of detrusor activity needed to produce the flow curve. Simultaneous measurement of the detrusor pressure (cystometry) and urinary flow rate (uroflowmetry) while voiding is the pressure/flow (PF) study. It is the basic technique for obtaining information about the independent and the interactive functional characteristics of the bladder and urethra during voiding, with attempts made to express their functions in terms of bladder work and urethral resistance. The PF study provides direct data about detrusor function during voiding not provided by any other urodynamic technique. It also provides indirect data about the urethra and sensation.

The normal voiding process was described in the uroflowmetry section. The normal flow curve of routine uroflowmetry would describe the normal curve of the PF study. The normal detrusor pressure curve has a smooth but relatively brisk increase and decrease, shows a slight plateau in the midportion, and reaches the baseline at the end of voiding. The most important terms used to describe the results of the PF study are shown in Figure 7–32. Opening time is the time from the initial increase in detrusor pressure to the initiation of flow. Opening pressure is the pressure at the initiation of flow. Maximum pressure is the highest pressure occurring during flow. The pressure at maximum flow is the pressure at the maximum flow rate. The latter two pressures have clear clinical significance; opening pressures and times are of less clinical value. The voiding process should be comfortable for the patient to be considered normal.

Equipment

PF measurements require the same equipment used for cystometry and uroflowmetry. A few caveats are needed. The first major issue is the route of bladder access. A suprapubic catheter approach

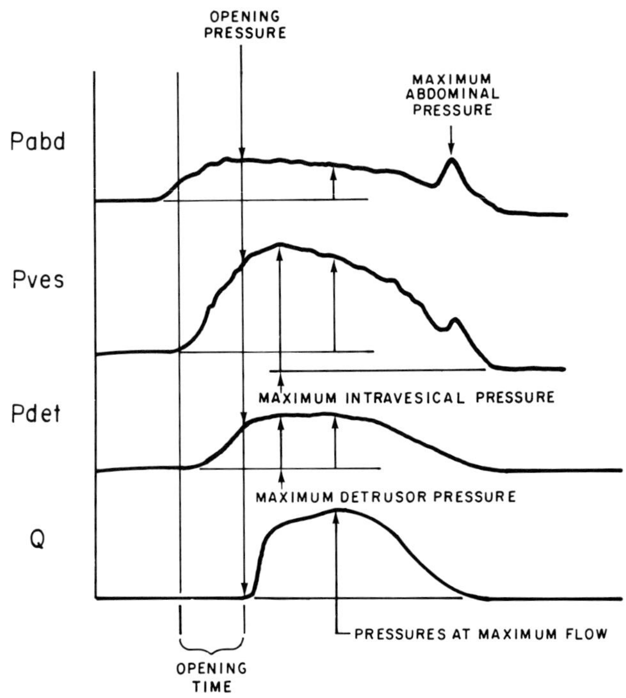

FIGURE 7–32. Simultaneous cystometry and uroflowmetry (pressure/flow study) showing the key parameters and normal curve shapes according to International Continence Society criteria.

eliminates the potentials of added urethral obstruction[179,199] and subjective patient irritation or distraction that occur with a transurethral catheter. A 5F urethral catheter also causes little to no change in the detrusor voiding pressure,[179,200,201] although flow rate is decreased slightly.[179,199-201] In general, urethral catheters 5F or less present no added obstructive component except in a patient who is already severely obstructed, in which case the severity of the obstruction is enhanced during the study.[179,202] The obstructive nature of the catheter can be put into perspective in two ways: (1) by comparing the PF testing flow rate with the flow rate before instrumentation; if they are similar, the PF value probably represents the normal situation; and (2) by repeating the study as necessary to make the diagnosis. In still equivocal cases clinical judgment or other tests (video urodynamics, voiding urethral pressure measurements) may be needed.

Use of a catheter long enough to allow some curling of excess length in the bladder helps prevent the patient from voiding the tube out during the test, as does taping the tube securely to the penis or labia. PF studies should include intraabdominal pressure measurements to allow determination of detrusor pressure.[82]

Some delay occurs between the detrusor pressure event and the resulting flow pattern (time lag), a result of the physical distance from the bladder to the flowmeter. Minimizing this distance and the lag time is useful,[23-29] but this should not be done at the expense of creating an environment even less comfortable for the patient than that already present for the standard urodynamics tests. The difficulty in having the patient relaxed enough to void in a standard fashion may prevent many patients from voiding normally or even at all.

Technique

Since most PF studies are performed after filling CMGs, the PF study is usually produced by having the patient assume the normal voiding position at some point during or after the CMG. External transducers must be at the appropriate zero level. The only urethral tube in place should be the small-diameter pressure catheter. Obviously a PF study can be performed only with liquid. Care must be taken when interpreting flow rates with the gravity and momentum type flowmeters when radiologic contrast material is used, since its density is greater than that of water.

After voiding, the residual urine should be measured and the patient asked whether the voiding effort accurately reflected what occurs routinely, and if not, what was different. The study should be repeated until the patient's routine pattern is replicated. Similarly, if residual urine levels before the PF study were low but the residual after a study was high, the test should be repeated until that discrepancy is explained. The sum of residual urine and voided volume may exceed infused volume because of urine production.

The test can be repeated by refilling the bladder through the pressure measurement catheter until the patient has a normal to strong desire to void, at which point the catheter is reattached to the transducer line. The patient should cough before voiding to ensure that pressure transmission is not damped and that the tube has not been displaced from the bladder.

A stop-flow test can be performed to assess the isovolumetric detrusor pressure, an indication of the maximum detrusor power.[203,204] The test is performed by having the patient interrupt voiding as rapidly as possible and observing the resulting detrusor pressure rise. If the patient cannot contract the urethra rapidly enough, or relies on a suppression of the detrusor contraction to stop voiding, the balloon of a Foley catheter can be pulled down abruptly and held against the bladder neck to occlude the flow. The stop-flow test has two uses: (1) as a research tool to assess the detrusor's power and its response to obstruction and (2) to assess the detrusor voiding power available after surgery to correct incontinence, since patients with low isovolumetric detrusor pressures may have problems voiding postoperatively. Whether the latter application is of practical value (what would be done differently except to warn the patient of the possibility?) is still in question. Other concerns about the usefulness of the test are that the pressure is a function of bladder volume; that anatomy, especially with neuropathic bladders, alters the results; and that a low isometric pressure may be due to inhibition or a slow occlusion.

Normal Pressure/Flow Studies

When interpreting PF studies the clinician must actually review the flow and pressure curves to obtain an accurate and complete impression of the voiding process, rather than simply accepting any data or calculations that might be produced by a computer data system. Normal flow rates during PF tests are the same as those that apply to free-flow states, taking into account all the variables discussed in the preceding section on urine flow rate measurements (Figure 7–33).

For women normal pressures are 50 to 70 cm H_2O at maximum flow rates of 25 ml/sec, with only some variation with age.[204,206-208,257] Sometimes, however, a woman voids with a normal flow curve and rate and leaves no residual urine, yet has no elevation of detrusor or abdominal pressures; such situations are normal and not indicative of detrusor underactivity (Figures 7–34 to 7–36).

Normal voiding pressures at maximum flow rates for males are more difficult to establish, especially in older men because of the range of obstructive

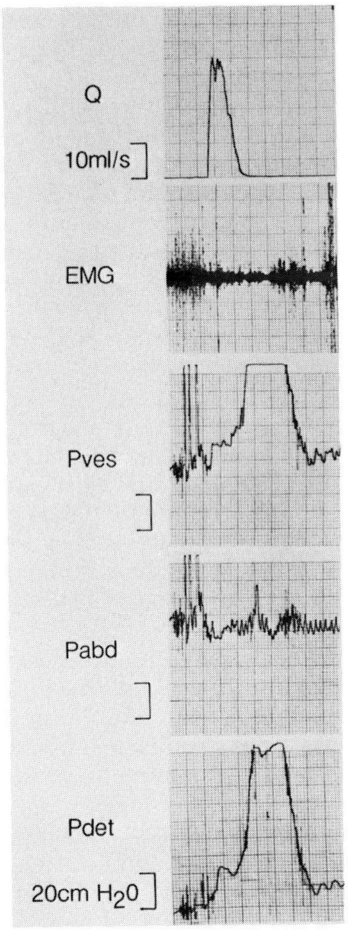

FIGURE 7–33. Normal pressure/flow study demonstrating an excellent flow rate and pattern. With voiding the detrusor pressure increases only approximately 20 cm H_2O. At the end of voiding is a significant increase in detrusor pressure, a normal variant called an aftercontraction. (See also Figure 7–20).

effects the prostate gland may have in different individuals. Obstruction can sometimes cause a compensatory increase in detrusor pressure to maintain a relatively normal flow rate. However, pressures of 60 to 80 cm H_2O with maximum flow rates of 20 ml/sec can be considered normal as a first approximation.[201,203,206,208-211,257]

Sometimes, after normal voiding is complete, the detrusor contracts again, producing an aftercontraction (Figures 7–20 and 7–33). This phenomenon is of uncertain clinical significance but is found in patients with no urologic abnormalities.

Normal pressure and flow values define the PF relationship as normal. However, normal values for detrusor voiding pressures should be applied to a specific patient only if the patient has signs or symptoms of abnormal voiding function. The most common example of this is the one discussed previously of women who void normally but without detrusor pressure increase; such patients are normal. The other extreme is the patient who cannot relax enough in the testing situation to generate a detrusor contraction or void at all. This is not uncommon, especially among women or children, and such patients should not necessarily be considered abnormal.

Abnormal Pressure/Flow Studies

The line between normal and abnormal in PF studies is imprecise, and the clinician's understanding of the clinical situation can make a significant difference in performance and interpretation of the study. The primary abnormalities during voiding are detrusor underactivity and urethral overactivity. Detrusor overactivity is addressed later in the context of urethral overactivity. Urethral underactivity during voiding is the ideal circumstance and so is actually normal.

The detrusor can be absolutely underactive in that it never contracts either voluntarily or involuntarily. In most cases this abnormality is called acontractility; it is called areflexia when a neurologic abnormality causes the absence of contractility. The PF data for absolute acontractility show no detrusor pressure increase, although some low flow may be generated by straining maneuvers (Figure 7–37). As noted previously, normal flow and emptying can be generated without a detrusor contraction, especially in women; this is *not* detrusor underactivity.

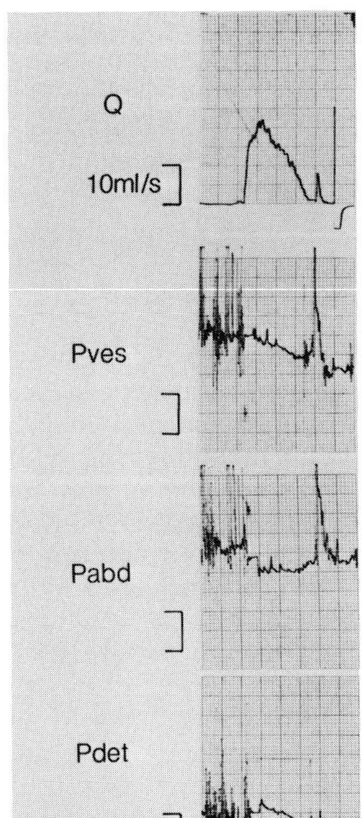

FIGURE 7–34. Pressure/flow study. The flow rate and pattern are normal with essentially no detrusor pressure increase. This is not detrusor acontractility but instead is a normal variant of a pressure/flow study in a woman.

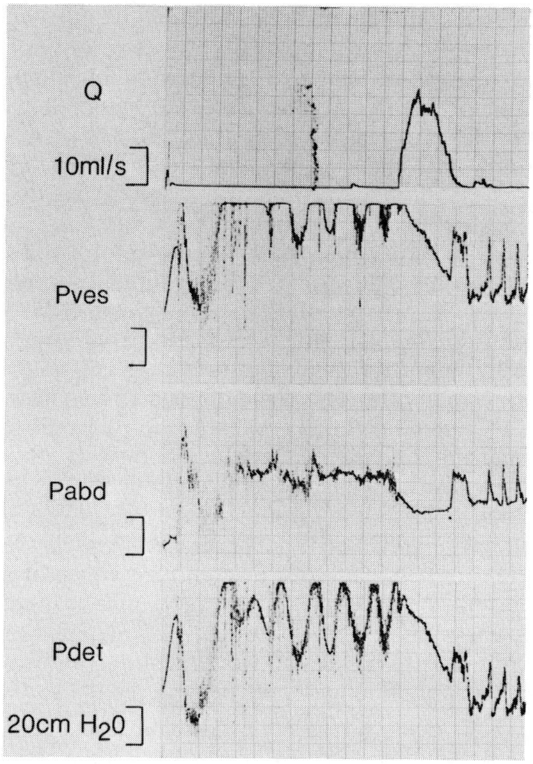

FIGURE 7–35. Pressure/flow study. This patient has significant detrusor instability during the filling portion of the cystometrogram. Finally the urge is strong enough that voiding cannot be delayed and a normal flow rate and curve are produced as the detrusor pressure falls with sphincter relaxation. With the voiding process a slight decrease in the intraabdominal pressure occurs, the result of overall relaxation as the patient contracts strongly to prevent urinary leakage associated with the detrusor instability.

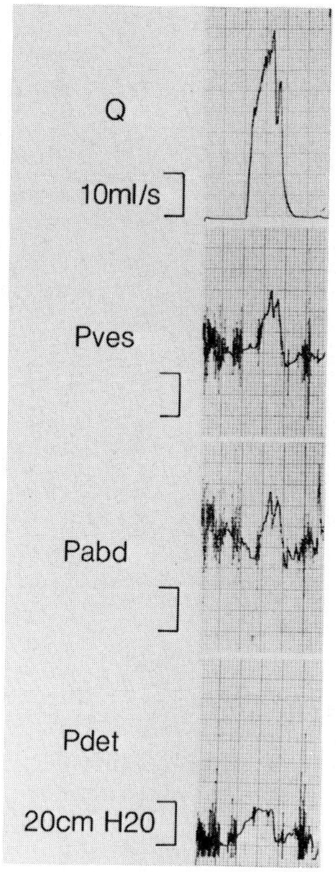

FIGURE 7–36. Pressure/flow study. A normal flow rate and pattern are generated by this patient with a combination of a slight increase in detrusor pressure of about 20 cm H_2O supplemented by some abdominal strain as noted on the intraabdominal pressure measurement.

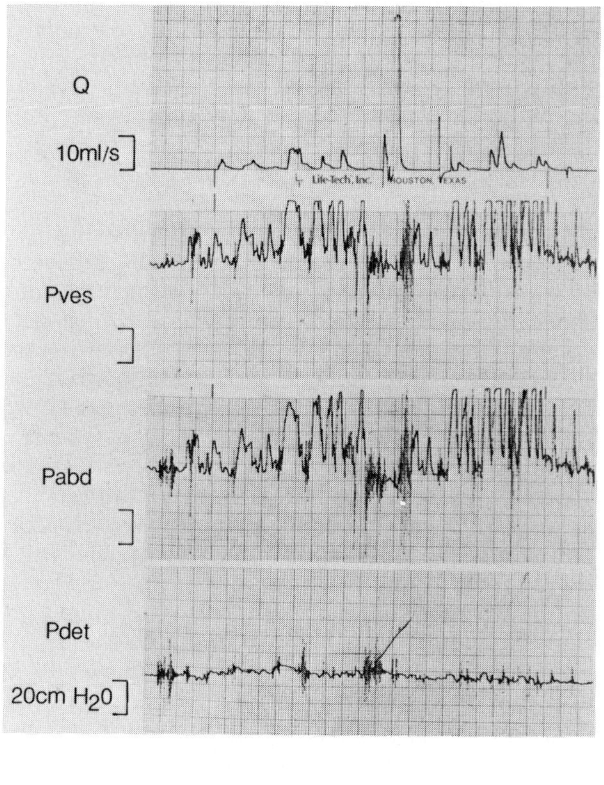

FIGURE 7–37. Pressure/flow study. Total detrusor acontractility in which the patient voids only by straining, resulting in the intermittent low flow rate.

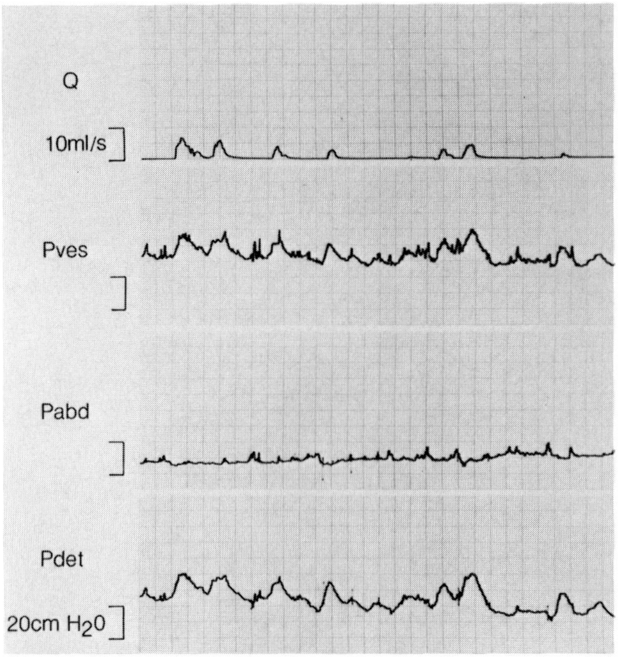

FIGURE 7–38. Pressure/flow study. Fluctuating low-pressure detrusor contractions are consistent with relative detrusor acontractility. The result is a low flow rate with an intermittent pattern.

Somewhat closer to normal from the extreme of absolute underactivity is the relatively underactive detrusor that generates a low-pressure contraction inadequate to empty the bladder; the contraction may also be short in duration or fluctuating. The corresponding flow is low or absent (Figure 7–38).[10,42,212-214] The minimum acceptable detrusor pressure has never been strictly defined, but patients with maximum detrusor voiding pressures below 30 cm H_2O are generally considered to have relative detrusor underactivity (low contractility or relative acontractility) if the flow rate is less than 12 ml/sec.

Conversely, the bladder may generate high voiding pressures to overcome the obstruction created by some type of urethral overactivity or to maintain a normal detrusor voiding pressure despite a subnormal flow rate.[42,57,138,139,212-218] Causes of obstruction can be static, such as strictures, benign prostatic hyperplasia, or detrusor–bladder neck–proximal urethral dyssynergia, or dynamic, such as detrusor-sphincter dyssynergia or dysfunctional voiding (nonneurogenic neurogenic bladder) (Figures 7–39 and 7–40). In this case the detrusor is not overactive per se, but merely compensating for the decreased flow by increasing its pressure, a simple shift in position along its long-established pressure/flow curve relationship in which the amount of work the detrusor can do is fixed but the pressure and flow vary inversely.[8,206,215,219,220] Thus obstruction can be loosely defined as high detrusor pressure with inappropriately low flow (Figure 7–39), but more specific definitions of obstruction vary. In some reports obstruction is defined as sustained voiding pressures greater than 30 cm H_2O (young men), 60 cm H_2O (older men), or 20 cm H_2O (women), all with peak flow rates below 12 ml/sec,[139,213,214,216,218] although the same flow rate with the higher normal detrusor pressures is always an acceptable guideline. Others have attempted to relate pressure and flow through some type of urethral resistance parameter. Despite extensive efforts to do this, no single parameter is considered clinically useful and accurate enough to be consistently applicable. The ratio of pressure to flow P_{det}/Q_{max}[219,221] is useful only in laminar (nonturbulent) flow through a rigid tube; since the urethra is distensible and urine flow is turbulent, this ratio is not accurate.[203,219,222] The ratio P_{det}/Q_{max}^2 is a somewhat more refined approximation, with values greater than 0.5 in older men, and greater than 0.2 in women, children, and younger men, considered obstructive.[51,145,203,205,209,214,219,222-226,258] Even this approximation is not always adequate clinically and must be applied cautiously, especially in borderline

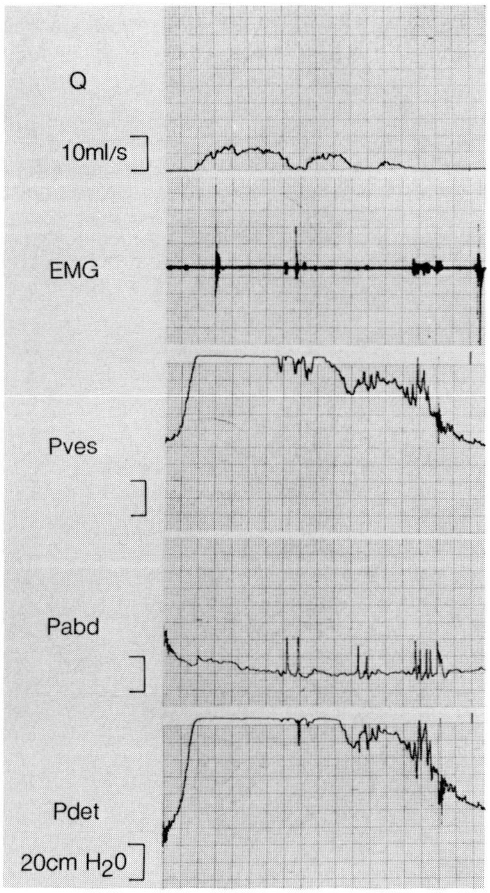

FIGURE 7–39. Pressure/flow study. A man with benign prostatic hyperplasia shows an extremely high voiding pressure, greater than 80 cm H_2O above his storage baseline with no abdominal straining and with an extremely low unextended flow curve, all consistent with obstruction.

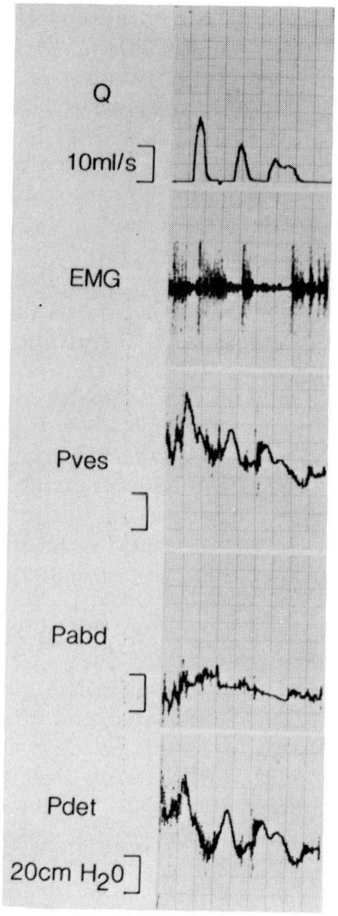

FIGURE 7–40. Intermittent voiding pattern with normal increases in detrusor pressure. The intermittency is a consequence of abnormal increases in the electromyographic (EMG) signal and increases in urethral closure pressure. This circumstance could be considered detrusor-sphincter dyssynergia; however, the patient is a neurologically normal child. The EMG pattern is characteristically found in patients with the voiding dysfunction nonneurogenic neurogenic bladder.

cases, for patients with low voided volumes, or for those with low flow rates with a urethral catheter in place. Research is being done to describe the pressure/flow relationship mathematically and graphically (Figure 7–41) with more than one or two parameters in terms of urethral resistance and detrusor work and power in fashions that will be more clinically useful, especially in equivocal cases.[10,55,56,212,215,219,220,222,227-233]

Indications

The PF study is the most useful test for assessing the detrusor and urethra during voiding. It can provide information to confirm the roles of the bladder and urethra in the following cases:

1. Obstructive voiding symptoms, elevated residual urine levels, and equivocal uroflowmetry findings in the absence of a clinically reasonable cause or in cases in which either urethral overactivity (obstruction) or detrusor underactivity (acontractility or areflexia), or both, may be causing the voiding dysfunction
2. Overflow incontinence
3. Detrusor instability associated with obstructive symptoms, as in a male patient with benign prostatic hyperplasia
4. A child with incontinence, upper urinary tract damage, or lower urinary tract dysfunction that may be a result of a dysfunctional voiding pattern
5. Neurologic diseases clearly or potentially affecting lower urinary tract function
6. Failed prior treatment for presumed obstruction

VIDEO URODYNAMICS

Although each of the urodynamics tests discussed provides some information about how the lower urinary tract functions, none provides information about what the tract looks like. Of particular interest in lower urinary tract dysfunction is the anatomic appearance of the bladder neck and urethra concurrent with other urodynamics data. An ideal way to obtain this information in real time is by performing the urodynamics tests under simultaneous fluoroscopic observation, a process commonly called video urodynamics (VUD). VUD provides the same data as whatever other urodynamics tests are performed, plus the anatomic information otherwise missed.[76,140,234-238] An evolving alternative to

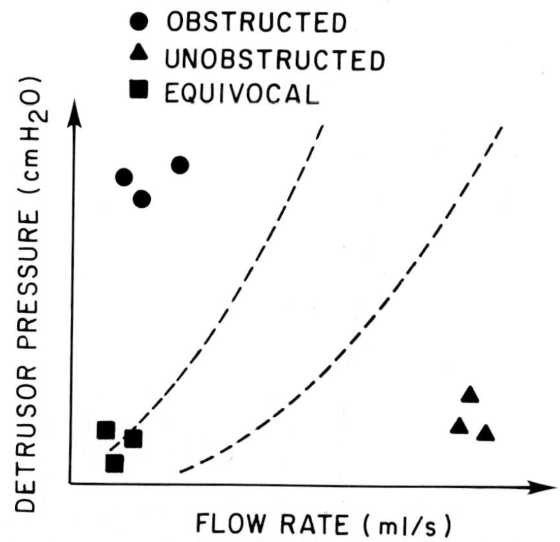

FIGURE 7–41. Pressure/flow diagram according to the recommendations of the International Continence Society. A pressure/flow diagram helps to classify patient in terms of detrusor and urethral function in the voiding process. Although classifying patients as unobstructed or obstructed is relatively easy, many patients fall in an equivocal zone as illustrated by the space between the dotted lines. Also, there are no definitive numbers that unequivocally describe the location of the dotted lines, so a number of approximations are used to describe urethral resistance as discussed in the text.

fluoroscopic observation of the bladder and urethra is ultrasonography.[176,239-243]

Equipment

The VUD unit has three primary elements: the basic urodynamics unit, a fluoroscopy unit, and hardware, which allows visually clear synchronization of the urodynamic tracings with the fluoroscopic image of the bladder on a single television display unit. An associated video recorder allows recording of the test for storage and later viewing. A number of solutions to the hardware problems have allowed VUD to become reality. Early systems used synchronized, mixed signals from a television camera and an image intensifier.[76,140,235,236,244] Later, analog to video converters produced clearer images with easy operation but at significantly greater cost. Analog to digital converters based on microcomputers are now available and allow some later analysis of the test results. Perhaps the most important features of the VUD unit are clear, easily interpretable urodynamic and fluoroscopic images in real time and in playback, applicability to any fluoroscopic imaging system and any combination of urodynamics studies, and reliability.

If ultrasonography is used to visualize the anatomy, the ultrasound probe is intrarectal for male patients and can be intrarectal, intravaginal, or perineal for female patients. The perineal approach is obviously the least invasive and, theoretically at least, the least likely to alter the anatomy inappropriately as measurements are performed. The probes can be sector or linear array scanners with frequencies from 3.5 to 7.5 MHz.[176,239-243] The advantages of ultrasound over fluoroscopic imaging are less radiation exposure; simpler, more mobile equipment; less space requirement and expense; and the ability to use plain fluids rather than radiographic contrast medium. With the ultrasonographic techniques, voiding and Credé maneuvers can be observed before and after treatment without the need for catheter placement, radiographic contrast material, or radiation.[240,241] The probe in position, even in the rectum or vagina, apparently does not alter the urodynamics data, although the perineal location seems optimum.[241,245]

The arrangement of the equipment used during PF studies may have to be modified to allow proper imaging. For example, the normal voiding chair or commode may interfere with the fluoroscopic image, necessitating some modification of the chair or having the patient void in the standing position into a funnel.

Technique

The technique of VUD alters the steps of the other urodynamics tests being performed in only a few simple ways. With fluoroscopy the patient is examined in positions best able to display the bladder and urethra; thus the imaging may have to be done with the patient in the anteroposterior, oblique, or lateral position and supine, standing, or sitting as needed. Depending on the clinical problem, the images must be obtained intermittently with the bladder empty, slightly filled, and at other levels of interest up to capacity. During voiding, the entire process is usually visualized. The patient may be asked to stop voiding momentarily to perform the stop-flow test (see "Simultaneous Cystometry and Uroflowmetry").

Stress and Credé maneuvers should be observed as needed. When incontinence is evaluated, leaking can easily be observed directly at the meatus but mild or moderate volumes of leakage may not be easily seen on the fluoroscope. Reflux can also be detected with fluoroscopy, and recording the pressures at which the reflux begins may have some effect on therapy.

With ultrasound imaging the position of the probe relative to the patient does not change, but the patient can be examined in the supine, standing, and sitting positions. Also, the anatomy of the soft tissues near the bladder and urethra can be observed, although incontinence, reflux, and the bulbous or penile urethra cannot be visualized.[176,240,241,243]

Normal and Abnormal Video Urodynamics

The imaging tools provide views of the anatomy to be correlated with the other urodynamics tests.[73,76,234,237,244] VUD can be useful in the evaluation of incontinence. In women a bladder neck and urethra that are incompetent and open at rest, or nearly so, with leakage and no detrusor pressure change confirms type III GSUI (Figures 7–42 and 7–43). In male patients, contrast material may be retained up to the external sphincter by voluntary contraction of the sphincter, but leakage may occur if the patient relaxes. In a patient with neurologic disease or injury the internal or external sphincter, or both, may be affected. For each of the conditions the points of continence can be easily visualized during VUD with the benefit that simultaneous detrusor contraction can be eliminated as the cause of the urethral opening. VUD can also help visualize incontinence not demonstrable with other tests.

Visualizing the zone or point of urethral narrowing or closure in conjunction with other urodynamics data during voiding confirms the site and cause of obstruction in such conditions as benign prostatic hyperplasia, dysfunctional voiding, and detrusor-sphincter dyssynergia (Figures 7–44 to 7–46). Performing the stop-flow test with VUD in the normal patient should show a "milk-back" of the contrast

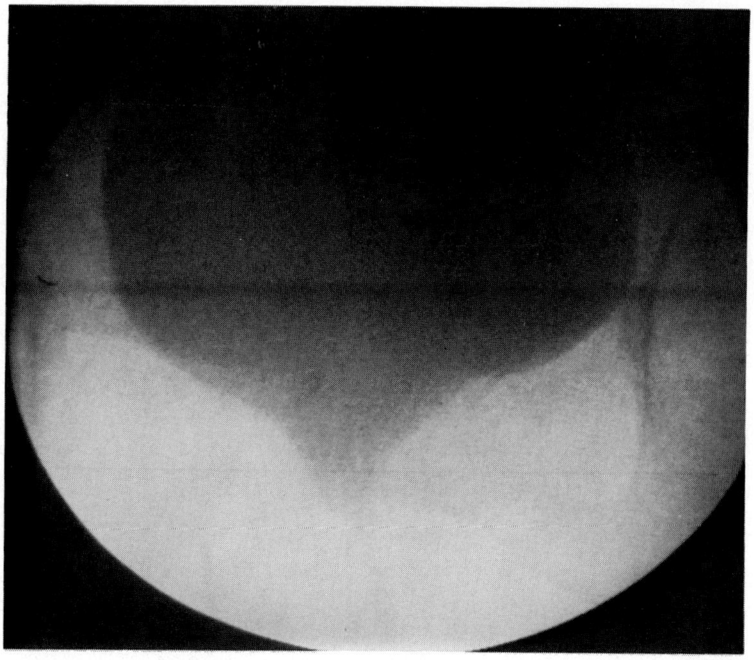

FIGURE 7–42. Standing cystometrogram in anteroposterior position. The bladder neck and urethra are open, and fluid is slowly leaking through the urethra.

material from the sphincter to the bladder neck. This milk-back does not occur in many patients with type III GSUI, after prostate or bladder neck resection, or in men with a detrusor–bladder neck dyssynergia.[76] VUD allows the clinician to draw accurate conclusions about detrusor and urethral function that could not have been made if the urodynamics tests and imaging were performed separately. Confirmation of these complex diagnoses has a tremendous impact on the selection and ultimate success of therapy.

Indications

VUD is particularly valuable in the evaluation of the following conditions[73,76,98,234,237,244,246]:

1. Incontinence, especially the totally incompetent urethra (such as type III GSUI in a woman or postprostatectomy incontinence in a man), which should always be considered in a patient with prior surgery of the urethra and bladder neck, trauma, or neurologic injury
2. Urethral obstruction with the site not dis-

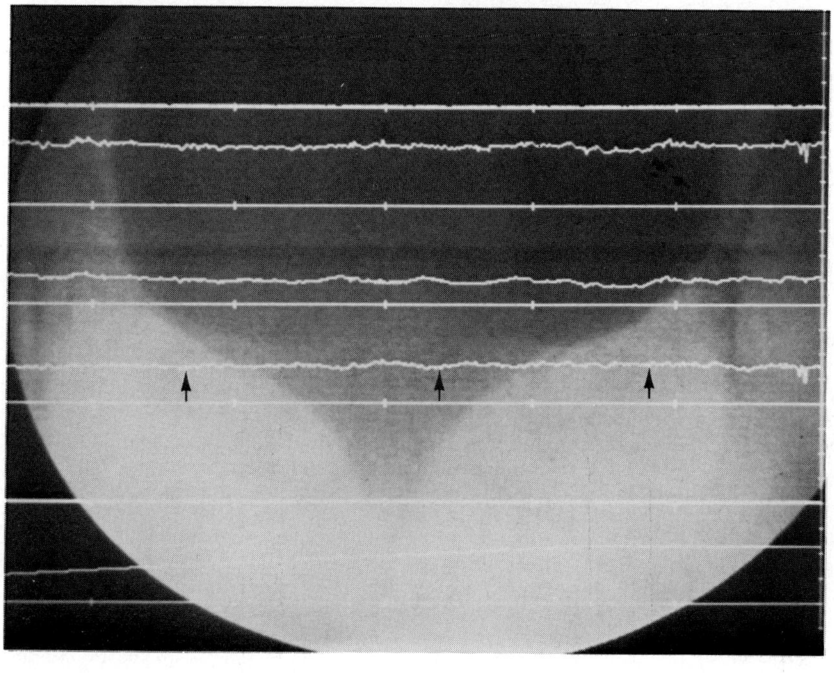

FIGURE 7–43. Video urodynamics. The cystometrogram of Figure 7–42 has the pressure curves superimposed on it. The detrusor pressure *(arrow)* shows no change, and thus the bladder neck and urethra are open not because of an act of bladder contraction but because of urethral underactivity (total urethral incompetence, or type III stress urinary incontinence). Without the combination of the fluoroscopic image and the pressure measurements it would be impossible to confirm that this abnormality was related to detrusor or urethral dysfunction.

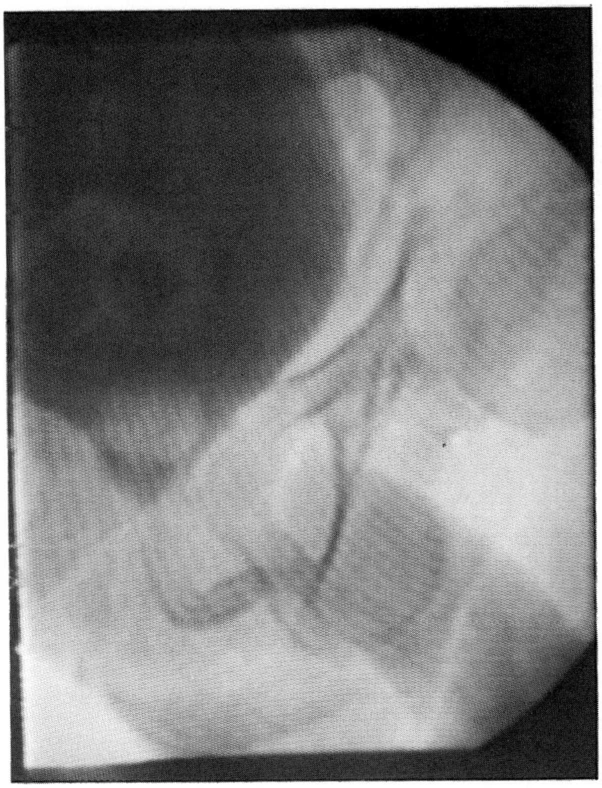

FIGURE 7–44. Video urodynamics. The fluoroscopic image shows an open bladder neck and open urethra with good flow of contrast material and a detrusor pressure of about 55 cm H_2O. The electromyographic signal is relatively quiet. The patient is a quadriplegic who had undergone a sphincterotomy.

cernible clinically, especially in patients with detrusor–bladder neck dyssynergia, dysfunctional voiding, and previous sphincterotomy

3. The patient who has not been helped by presumably correct therapies for the same persisting problem
4. Complicated urinary incontinence not adequately diagnosed by simpler tests, or incontinence associated with voiding dysfunction such as high residual urine levels
5. When detecting the pressure at which vesicoureteral reflux occurs is necessary
6. When the clinical evaluation and simpler tests are inadequate to confirm the diagnosis, or when they lead to disparate diagnoses

AMBULATORY URODYNAMICS

All the urodynamics tests discussed in the preceding sections are attempts to describe round-the-clock lower urinary tract function in an extremely brief period by proper equipment selection and use and careful attention to the details of sometimes provocative testing techniques. Despite the quality of these attempts, however, such tests are not conducted under the most physiologic conditions and so may not always allow an accurate diagnosis because they are mere snapshots of the lower urinary tract function rather than full-length motion pictures. Furthermore, the standard urodynamics techniques restrict the patient physically and psychologically, something that may be important in the diagnosis of incontinence and voiding dysfunction. Thus there may be a role for round-the-clock evaluations of lower urinary tract function, an approach called ambulatory urodynamics.[100,233,247-252]

The same limitations of and definitions for the measurement techniques present in routine urodynamics tests also apply to ambulatory urodynamics. For example, the filling and storage portion of bladder function evaluated with CMG in which intravesical measurements are obtained is still a direct measurement of bladder and sensory function, but an indirect measure of urethral function. Since the clinician will not be present to record the patient's comments about sensation or to note episodes of voiding or incontinence, the patient keeps a diary of such information.

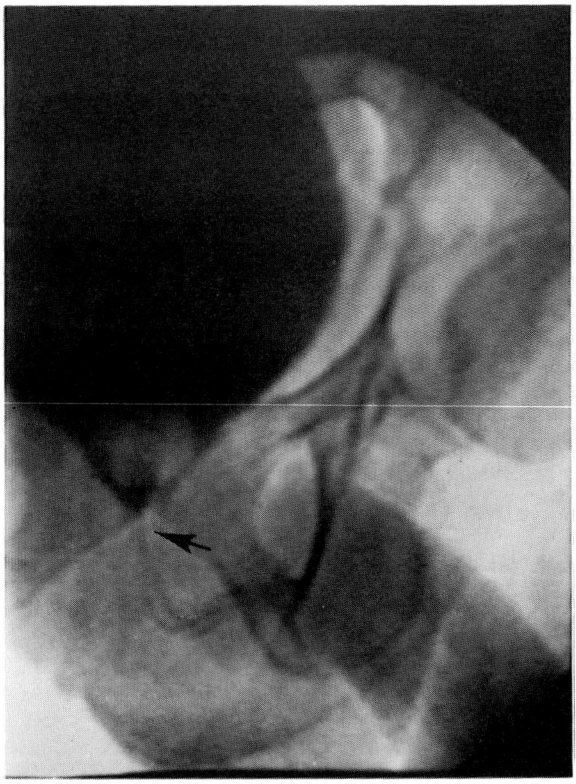

FIGURE 7–45. Moments after the image shown in Figure 7–44, the same patient has a burst of electromyographic activity coincident with closure of the external urethral sphincter *(arrow)* and cessation of the contrast flow. Detrusor pressure arises to approximately 90 cm H_2O at the same moment. The findings are consistent with persistence of detrusor-sphincter dyssynergia with obstruction, which accounts for the patient's problems with recurrent autonomic dysreflexia and incomplete emptying. Without video urodynamics the cause of the patient's persistent urinary tract dysfunction would be impossible to determine.

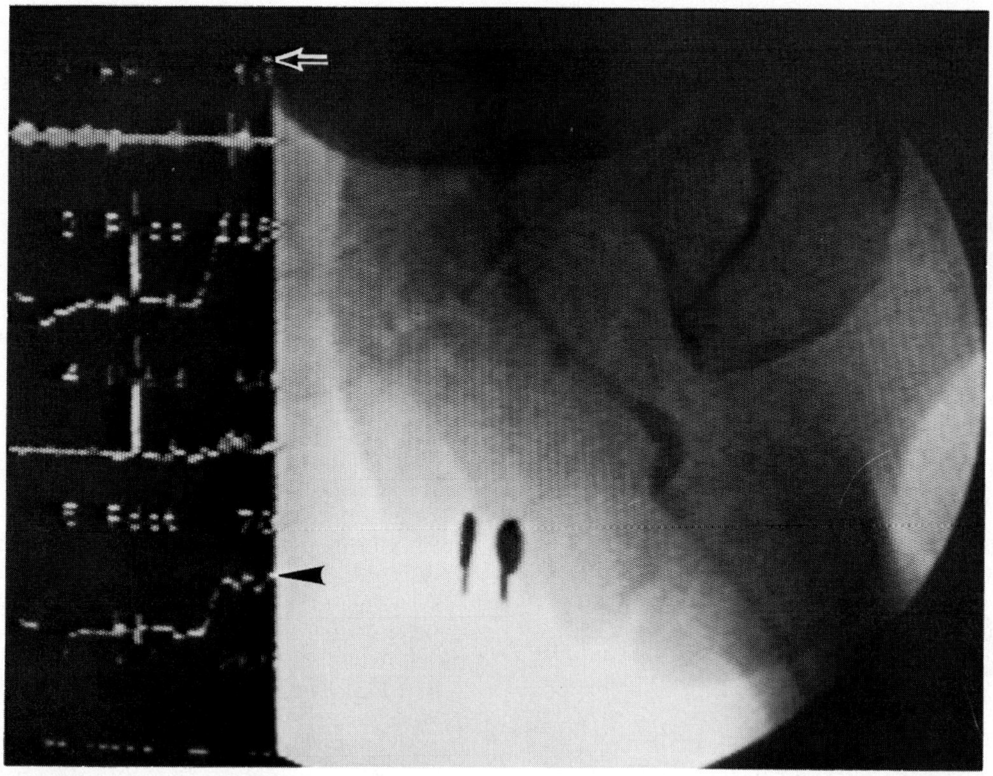

FIGURE 7–46. Video urodynamics of a 50-year-old man with severe obstructive voiding symptoms and low flow rate. The voiding detrusor pressure is about 70 cm H_2O *(arrowhead)* with a barely perceptible flow rate *(arrow)* and a poorly opening bladder neck and prostatic urethra, all consistent with obstruction from benign prostatic hyperplasia.

Equipment

The most basic attempt at physiologic monitoring is urodynamics testing performed with physiologic filling, perhaps modified with an induced diuresis. So that the patient has the mobility to perform routine daily activities, two technical challenges had to be overcome: unobtrusively and reliably obtaining data and either storing or transmitting the data. Probably the earliest attempt at this was the use of the bladder pressure telemetry capsules.[248] Although an excellent concept, these proved too cumbersome, irritating to the bladder, and unreliable. Similarly, the inherent weaknesses of air- or liquid-filled transducers become evident when ambulatory data are desired. Thus the first major step toward successful ambulatory urodynamics came with the development of catheter tip microtransducers to allow unobtrusive data acquisition with relatively easy-to-handle, rugged, reliable transducers. The second development was a way to record the data for later review while still allowing the patient complete freedom of activity. Portable cassette tape recording units[100] and data telemetry techniques[250,251,253] provided the answer initially. More recently, microcomputer technology has permitted the data to be converted from analog to digital and then stored in the computer's memory for later display and review.[247,252] Thus ambulatory urodynamics employs the most sophisticated aspects of the technology of urodynamics data acquisition and recording.

The most commonly measured parameters in ambulatory urodynamics are intravesical and urethral pressures with one catheter and intraabdominal (rectal) pressures with another. The catheters are attached to the microcomputer through appropriate amplifiers and filters so that the data can be converted and processed for storage in the computer. Data points are recorded at least once per second in each channel, even though many more data points may be processed (perhaps 50 per second) to obtain the final data point. Depending on the storage technique, the device can usually store data for 4 to 24 hours, with accuracy of about ±2 cm H_2O.[100,247,252]

The data are ultimately displayed or printed out when the ambulatory device is connected to a small computer. The data are correlated with a diary of symptoms and activities kept by the patient as requested by the clinician. The most modern devices also permit the patient to indicate an event already determined to be significant, such as urgency or incontinence, by pushing a button on the ambulatory device. These event marks are then displayed with the other computer-processed data.

The primary drawbacks with the catheter tip transducers during lengthy ambulatory urodynamics are noise and thermal and baseline drift. Noise is considered the degree of activity of the measured bladder and rectal pressures with normal activity. This noise is acceptably small when the subtracted true detrusor pressure is examined, which emphasizes the importance of using intraabdominal pressure measurements, especially in ambulatory urodynamics.[247] Drift is a characteristic of the transducers and appears to be acceptably small.[247]

The pressure data are also affected by shifts in the relative positions of the zero point for the different transducers, a problem always inherent in catheter tip transducers and discussed previously in the section on the basic cystometrogram. When the catheters are zeroed with the patient supine, the difference in the zero points for the bladder and rectal transducers is the vertical distance between them. When the patient is upright, this difference is less, but the weight of urine in the filling bladder changes the intravesical pressure without changing the intraabdominal pressure.

A final drawback with ambulatory techniques is that bladder volumes or postvoiding residual urine volumes are not measured.

Technique

The most important part of the technique of ambulatory urodynamics is placing the catheter tip transducers and keeping them in place for the duration of the study. The catheters are most easily placed with the patient supine. The intravesical and urethral transducers should be placed in the bladder and the intraabdominal transducer in the rectum, usually after the tip is covered with a finger cot or condom. The transducers should then be zeroed simultaneously. The urethral transducer can be positioned with fluoroscopic guidance or by being placed in the location of maximum urethral pressure. The intravesical measurements remain quite accurate; the urethral measurements are hampered by the slight catheter movement, catheter rigidity, and the orientation of the transducer in only one sector of the entire urethral circumference, problems that can usually be overcome in the carefully controlled, relatively brief studies done for routine urethral pressure measurements but cannot be eliminated in ambulatory measurements. The rectal transducer's position may be threatened by defecation, so planning is in order to prevent this by a routine or induced bowel movement before catheter placement. Also, both catheters should be fixed in place in the most secure fashion possible. After catheter placement and activation of the recording unit, the patient need only maintain the diary, activate the event button as instructed, and avoid dislodging the catheters.

Data Interpretation

The data are interpreted in the same fashion as with standard urodynamics testing. A horizontal time axis allows adequate pinpointing of events and pressures. Ambulatory monitoring is expected to be more sensitive and specific in diagnosing lower urinary tract dysfunction than standard urodynamics testing.[100,248,247,250-254]

Indications

The indications for ambulatory urodynamics are limited because the technology is expensive and only now becoming refined enough for easier data analysis. Possible uses include the following[100,247,250-254]:

1. Patients in whom standard urodynamics tests do not yield a diagnosis, as with incontinence not demonstrated in the simpler urodynamics tests, or in whom the diagnosis must be confirmed, as in acontractility
2. Patients in whom therapy based on simpler urodynamics evaluations has failed and for whom more invasive therapy is planned
3. Research in which the function of the lower urinary tract over several hours must be monitored to better understand normal and abnormal storage and voiding function, specific disease pathophysiology,[100,211,254] therapy effects (e.g., medications, behavioral modification, stimulation techniques), changes with sleep, and so on.

URODYNAMICS IN THE FUTURE

The technologic capabilities for the evaluation of the lower urinary tract enable clinicians to obtain a significant amount of data. The future of urodynamics is not limited to developing newer, better technologic tools, nor does it lie in expanding the use of those tools without clear value. Rather, the future of urodynamics lies in better understanding how to use the tools we have and how the data they produce truly relate to lower urinary tract function and dysfunction. Examples of the directions being taken are more extensive use of ambulatory urodynamics, development of computer-assisted analysis of urodynamic data such as flow rate and pressure/flow studies,[255] better modeling and analysis of bladder and urethral function in voiding,[53,55,219,220,222,256] and better understanding and measurement[59] of urethral pressures and their relationship to anatomy.[167] Continual efforts must be made to educate clinicians about the proper applications of the technology and to warn them against unnecessary or inappropriate applications tried on the basis of spurious reports, research, or medical marketing. More research is needed to refine urodynamics technology, techniques, and knowledge so that urologists will have even greater success in treating patients with lower urinary tract dysfunction.

REFERENCES

1. Anders EK, Bradley WE: History of cystometry. Urology 22:335-350, 1983.
2. Ryall RL, Marshall VR: Measurement of urinary flow rate. Urology 22:556-564, 1983.
3. Blaivas JG: The neurophysiology of micturition: a clinical study of 550 patients. J Urol 127:958-963, 1982.
4. Bottaccini MR, Gleason DM: Fluid mechanics of micturition. In Krane RJ, Siroky MB (eds): Clinical neuro-urology, ed 2. Boston: Little, Brown, 1991, Ch 5, pp 93-108.
5. Elbadawi A: Anatomy and innervation of the vesicourethral muscular unit of micturition. In Krane RJ, Siroky MB (eds): Clinical neuro-urology, ed 2. Boston: Little, Brown, 1991, Ch 2, pp 5-23.
6. Kinder RB, Mundy AR: Neurotransmitters. In Krane RJ, Siroky MB (eds): Clinical neuro-urology, ed 2. Boston: Little, Brown, 1991, Ch 4, pp 83-92.
7. Van Arsdalen K, Wein AJ: Physiology of micturition and continence. In Krane RJ, Siroky MB (eds): Clinical neuro-urology, ed 2. Boston: Little, Brown, 1991, Ch 3, pp 25-82.
8. Schafer W: Detrusor muscle mechanics in clinical urodynamics. In Krane RJ, Siroky MB (eds): Clinical neuro-urology, ed 2. Boston: Little, Brown, 1991, Ch 6, pp 109-149.
9. Wein AJ, Levin RM, Barrett DM: Voiding function: relevant anatomy, physiology and pharmacology. In Gillenwater JY, Grayhack JT, Howards SS, Duckett JW (eds): Adult and pediatric urology, ed 2. St Louis: Mosby–Year Book, 1991, Ch 28, pp 933-1000.
10. Abrams P, Blaivas JG, Stanton SL, Andersen JT: Standardisation of terminology of lower urinary tract function. Neurourol Urodynam 7:403-427, 1988.
11. Griffiths DJ: Urodynamics, ed 1. Bristol: Adam Hilger, 1980, Ch 9, p 97.
12. Rollema HJ: Uroflowmetry. In Krane RJ, Siroky MB (eds): Clinical neuro-urology, ed 2. Boston: Little, Brown, 1991, Ch 11, pp 201-244.
13. Susset JG, Picker P, Kretz M, Jorest R: Critical evaluation of uroflowmeters and analysis of normal curves. J Urol 109:874-878, 1973.
14. Drake WM Jr: The uroflowmeter: an aid to the study of the lower urinary tract. J Urol 59:650-658, 1948.
15. Smith JC: Urethral resistance to micturition. Br J Urol 40:125-156, 1968.
16. von Garrelts B: Analysis of micturition: a new method of recording the voiding of the bladder. Acta Chir Scand 112:326-340, 1956.
17. Ryall RL, Marshall VR: Normal peak urinary flow rates obtained from small voided volumes can provide a reliable assessment of bladder function. J Urol 127:484-488, 1982.
18. Drach GW, Binard W: Disposable peak urinary flowmeter estimates lower urinary tract obstruction. J Urol 115:175-179, 1976.
19. Koontz WW Jr, Rowan GA: A uroflowmeter recording changes in rate each second. Invest Urol 5:35-41, 1967.
20. Holm HH: A uroflowmeter and a method for combined pressure and flow measurement. J Urol 88:318-321, 1962.
21. Palm L: A new uroflowmeter for combined continuous pressure-flow measurement. Dan Med Bull 15:175-179, 1968.
22. Winter CC: Radioisotope uroflowmetry and bladder residual test. J Urol 91:103-106, 1964.
23. Zinner NR, Ritter RC, Sterling AM, Harding DC: Drop spectrometer: a non-obstructive, non-interfering instrument for analyzing hydrodynamic properties of human urination. J Urol 101:914-918, 1969.
24. Zinner NR, Ritter RC, Sterling AM, Harding DC: High-speed cinematography of human urination. Invest Urol 6:605-610, 1969.
25. Gallandat Huet RCG, Kramer AEJL, Sterling AM, Donker PJ: The variability of normal male voiding patterns measured by drop spectrometry. Br J Urol 52:196-203, 1980.
26. Cardus D, Quesada EM, Scott FB: Use of an electromagnetic flowmeter for urine flow measurements. J Appl Physiol 18:845-847, 1963.
27. Scott BF, Quesada EM, Cardus D: Studies on the dynamics of micturition: observations on healthy men. J Urol 92:455-463, 1964.
28. Rollema HJ: Ultrasonic volumetry, a new principle for uroflowmetry: comparison with the DISA mictiometer. Urol Int 33:88-100, 1978.
29. Ask P, Engberg A, Oberg PA, Spangberg A: A short-time delay urinary flowmeter. Neurourol Urodynam 4:247-256, 1985.
30. Rowan D, James ED, Kramer AEJL, et al, and International Continence Society Working Party on Urodynamic Equipment: Urodynamic equipment: technical aspects. J Med Eng Technol 11:57-64, 1987.
31. Kaufman JJ: A new recording uroflowmeter: a simple automatic device for measuring voiding velocity. J Urol 78:97-102, 1957.
32. von Garrelts B, Strandell P: Continuous recording of urinary flow-rate. Scand J Urol Nephrol 6:224-227, 1972.
33. Roy RR: A direct reading uroflowmeter for male and female use. Br J Urol 43:239-242, 1971.
34. Backman KA, von Garrelts B: Apparatus for recording micturition. Acta Chir Scand 126:167-171, 1963.
35. Bowley AR, Legg WCR: Technical note: a new uroflowmeter—an instrument for the estimation of liquid volume and rate flow. Med Biol Eng 9:139-142, 1971.
36. Kondo A, Mitsuya H, Torii H: Computer analysis of micturition parameters and accuracy of uroflowmeter. Urol Int 33:337-344, 1978.
37. Meyhoff HH, Griffiths DJ, Nordling J, Hald T: Accuracy and interpretation of results from the DISA momentum flux meter. Urol Res 8:37-41, 1980.
38. Rowan D, McKenzie AL, McNee, SG, Glen ES: A technical and clinical evaluation of the Disa uroflowmeter. Br J Urol 49:285-291, 1977.
39. von Garrelts B: Micturition in the normal male. Acta Chir Scand 114:197-210, 1957.
40. Gleason DM, Bottaccini MR: Urodynamic norms in female voiding. II. The flow modulation zone and voiding dysfunction. J Urol 127:495-500, 1982.
41. Haylen BT, Ashby D, Sutherest JR, et al: Maximum and average urine flow rates in normal male and female populations—the Liverpool nomograms. Br J Urol 64:30-38, 1989.
42. Siroky MG: Interpretation of urinary flow rates. Urol Clin North Am 17:537-542, 1990.
43. Siroky MG, Olsson CA, Krane RJ: The flow rate nomogram. I. Development. J Urol 122:665-668, 1979.
44. Siroky MG, Olsson CA, Krane RJ: The flow rate nomogram. II. Clinical correlation. J Urol 123:208-210, 1980.
45. Toguri AG, Uchida T, Bee DE: Pediatric uroflow rate nomograms. J Urol 127:727-731, 1982.
46. Toguri AG, Bee DE, Uchida T: Normal pediatric uroflow rates in nonclinical setting. J Urol 127:732-735, 1982.
47. Drach GW, Ignatoff J, Layton T: Peak urinary flow rate: observations in female subjects and comparison to male subjects. J Urol 122:215-219, 1979.
48. Drach GW, Layton T, Bottaccini MR: A method of adjustment of male peak urinary flow rate for varying age and volume voided. J Urol 128:960-962, 1982.
49. Drach GW, Steinbronn DV: Clinical evaluation of patients with prostatic obstruction: correlation of flow rates with voided, residual or total bladder volume. J Urol 135:737-740, 1986.
50. Gierup J: Micturition studies in infants and children: normal urinary flow. Scand J Urol Nephrol 4:191-208, 1970.
51. Gierup J, Ericsson NO: Micturition studies in infants and children: urodynamics in boys with disorders of the lower urinary tract. Scand J Urol Nephrol 5:1-16, 1971.
52. Hjalmas K: Micturition in infants and children with normal lower urinary tract. Scand J Urol Nephrol 37(suppl):1-106, 1976.
53. Rollema HJ, Griffiths DJ, van Duyl WA, et al: Flow rate

versus bladder volume: an alternative way of presenting some features of the micturition of healthy males. Urol Int 32:401-412, 1977.
54. Fantl JA, Smith PJ, Schneider F, et al: Fluid weight uroflowmetry in women. Am J Obstet Gynecol 145:1017-1024, 1983.
55. Griffiths DJ, Rollema HJ: Urine flow curves of healthy males: a mathematical model of bladder and urethral function during micturition. Med Biol Eng Comput 17:291-300, 1979.
56. Schafer W, Rubben H, Noppeney R, Deutz FJ: Obstructed and unobstructed prostatic obstruction: a plea for urodynamic objectivation of bladder outflow obstruction in benign prostatic hyperplasia. World J Urol 6:198-203, 1989.
57. Gerstenberg TC, Andersen JT, Klarskov P, et al: High flow infravesical obstruction in men: symptomatology, urodynamics and the results of surgery. J Urol 127:943-945, 1982.
58. Marshall VR, Ryall RL, Austin ML, Siknclair GR: The use of urinary flow rates obtained from voided volumes less than 150 ml in the assessment of voiding ability. Br J Urol 55:28-33, 1983.
59. Ask P, Hok B: Pressure measurement techniques in urodynamic investigations. Neurourol Urodynam 9:1-15, 1990.
60. Edwards L, Thomas D: A simplified system for urodynamic observations. Br J Urol 43:226-232, 1971.
61. Lapides J, Friend CR, Ajemian EP, Reus WS: Denervation supersensitivity as a test for neurogenic bladder. Surg Gynecol Obstet 114:241-244, 1962.
62. DuBeau CE, Resnick NM: Evaluation of the causes and severity of geriatric incontinence. Urol Clin North Am 18:243-256, 1991.
63. Bavendam TG: Geriatric female incontinence. Probl Urol 5:42-71, 1991.
64. Ouslander J, Leach G, Abelson S, et al: Simple versus multichannel cystometry in the evaluation of bladder function in an incontinent geriatric population. J Urol 140:1482-1486, 1988.
65. O'Donnell PD: Pitfalls of urodynamic testing. Urol Clin North Am 18:257-269, 1991.
66. Lindstrom K, Ulmsten U: Some methodological aspects on the measurement of intraluminal pressures in the female urogenital tract in vivo. Acta Obstet Gynecol Scand 57:63-68, 1978.
67. Erlandson BE, Fall M: Urethral pressure profile studied by two different microtip transducers and an open catheter system. Urol Int 33:79-82, 1978.
68. A stable ultraminiature catheter-tip pressure transducer: technical note. Med Biol Eng 86-89, 1973.
69. van Venrooij GEPM, Kamphuis ET, Wolfhagen MJHM: Diuresis cystometry versus filling cystometry: the diagnostic value of diuresis cystometry in patients with frequency, urgency and/or urge incontinence complaints. Neurol Urodynam 6:29-36, 1987.
70. Jorgensen L, Lose G, Andersen JT: Cystometry: H_2O or CO_2 filling medium? A literature survey of the influence of the filling medium on the qualitative and the quantitative cystometric parameters. Neurourol Urodynam 7:343-350, 1988.
71. Nordling J, Walter S: Repeated, rapid fill CO_2-cystometry. Urol Res 5:117-127, 1977.
72. Wein AJ, Hanno PM, Dixon DO, et al: The reproducibility and interpretations of carbon dioxide cystometry. J Urol 120:205-206, 1978.
73. Meunier P, Mollard P: Urethral pressure profile in children: a comparison between perfused catheters and microtransducers, and a study of the usefulness of urethral pressure profile measurements in children. J Urol 120:207-210, 1978.
74. Klevmark B: Motility of the urinary bladder in cats furing filling at physiological rates. I. Intravesical pressure patterns studied by a new method of cystometry. Acta Physiol Scand 90:565-577, 1974.
75. Ramsden PD, Smith JC, Pierce JM, Ardran GM: The unstable bladder—fact or artefact? Br J Urol 49:633-639, 1977.
76. Webster GD, Older RA: Video urodynamics. Urology 16:106-114, 1980.
77. Blaivas JG, Labib KB, Michalik SJ, Zayed AAH: Failure of bethanechol denervation supersensitivity as a diagnostic aid. J Urol 123:199-201, 1980.
78. Wein AJ, Raezer DM, Malloy TR: Failure of the bethanechol supersensitivity test to predict improved voiding after subcutaneous bethanechol administration. J Urol 123:202-203, 1980.
79. Blaivas JG, Labib KB, Michalik SJ, Zayed AAH: Cystometric response to propantheline in detrusor hyperreflexia: therapeutic implications. J Urol 124:259-262, 1980.
80. Olsson CA, Siroky MB, Krane RJ: The phentolamine test in neurogenic bladder dysfunction. J Urol 117:481-485, 1977.
81. Yalla SV, Rossier AB, Fam BA, et al: Functional contribution of autonomic innervation to urethral striated sphincter: studies with parasympathomimetic, parasympatholytic and alpha-adrenergic blocking agents in spinal cord injury and control male subjects. J Urol 117:494-499, 1977.
82. Koff SA, Kass EJ: Abdominal wall electromyography: a noninvasive technique to improve pediatric urodynamic accuracy. J Urol 127:736-739, 1982.
83. James ED, Niblett PG, MacNaughton JA, Shaldon C: The vagina as an alternative to the rectum in measuring abdominal pressure during urodynamic investigations. Br J Urol 60:212-216, 1987.
84. James ED, Flack FC, Caldwell KPS, Martin MR: Continuous measurement of urine loss and frequency in incontinent patients. Br J Urol 43:233-237, 1971.
85. Stanton SL, Ritchie D: Communications in brief. Urilos: the practical detection of urine loss. Am J Obstet Gynecol 128:461-463, 1977.
86. Sutherst JR, Brown MC: Detection of urethral incompetence in women using the fluid-bridge test. Br J Urol 52:138-142, 1980.
87. Kromann-Andersen B, Jakobsen H, Andersen T: Pad-weighing tests: a literature survey on test accuracy and reproducibility. Neurourol Urodynam 8:237-242, 1989.
88. Berger RM, Maizels M, Moran GC, et al: Bladder capacity (ounces) equals age (years) plus 2 predicts normal bladder capacity and aids in diagnosis of abnormal voiding patterns. J Urol 129:347-349, 1983.
89. Coolsaet BLRA, Elhilali MM: Detrusor overactivity. Neurourol Urodynam 7:541-561, 1988.
90. McGuire E: Bladder instability and stress incontinence. Neurourol Urodynam 7:563-567, 1988.
91. McGuire EJ, Savastano JA: Stress incontinence and detrusor instability/urge incontinence. Neurourol Urodynam 4:313-316, 1985.
92. Galloway NTM, Mekras JA, Helms M, Webster GD: An objective score to predict upper tract deterioration in myelodysplasia. J Urol 145:535-537, 1991.
93. Hackler RH, Hall MK, Zampieri TA: Bladder hypocompliance in the spinal cord injury population. J Urol 141:1390-1393, 1989.
94. Ghoniem GM, Bloom DA, McGuire EJ, Stewart KL: Bladder compliance in meningomyelocele children. J Urol 141:1404-1406, 1989.
95. Resnick NM, Yalla SV: Detrusor hyperactivity with impaired contractile function. JAMA 257:3076-3081, 1987.
96. McGuire EJ, Woodside JR, Borden TA, Weiss RM: Prognostic value of urodynamic testing in myelodysplastic patients. J Urol 126:205-209, 1981.
97. Bauer SB, Hallett M, Khoshbin S, et al: Predictive value of urodynamic evaluation in newborns with myelodysplasia. JAMA 252:650, 1984.

98. Blaivas JG, Olsson CA: Stress incontinence: classification and surgical approach. J Urol 139:727-731, 1988.
99. Colstrup H, Lose G, Jorgensen L: Pressure variations in the female urethra measured by the infusion technique: is it an artifact? Neurol Urodynam 7:457-460, 1988.
100. Kulseng-Hanssen S, Klevmark B: Ambulatory urethro-cysto-rectometry: a new technique. Neurourol Urodynam 7:119-130, 1988.
101. Venema PL, Kramer AEJL: The clinical implication of continuous urethral pressure measurement in women with incontinence. Acta Urol Belg 52:207-215, 1984.
102. Vereecken RL, Cornelissen M, Das J, Grisar P: Urethral and perineal instability. Urol Int 40:325-330, 1985.
103. Vereecken RL, Das J: Urethral instability: related to stress and/or urge incontinence? J Urol 134:698-701, 1985.
104. Penders L, deLeval J, Petit R: Enuresis and urethral instability. Eur Urol 10:317-322, 1984.
105. Low JA, Armstrong JB, Mauger GM: The unstable urethra in the female. Obstet Gynecol 74:69-74, 1989.
106. Kulseng-Hanssen S: Prevalence and pattern of unstable urethral pressure in one hundred seventy-four gynecologic patients referred for urodynamic investigation. Am J Obstet Gynecol 146:895-900, 1983.
107. Sand PK, Bowen LW, Ostergard DR: Uninhibited urethral relaxation: an unusual cause of incontinence. Obstet Gynecol 68:645-648, 1986.
108. Weil A, Miege B, Rottenberg R, Krauer F: Clinical significance of urethral instability. Obstet Gynecol 68:106-110, 1986.
109. Tapp AJS, Cardozo LD, Versi E, Studd JWW: The prevalence of variation of resting urethral pressure in women and its association with lower urinary tract function. Br J Urol 61:314-317, 1988.
110. Kulseng-Hanssen S, Kristoffersen M: Urethral pressure variations in females with and without neurourological symptoms. Scand J Urol Nephrol 114(suppl):48-52, 1988.
111. McGuire E: Bladder instability and stress incontinence. Neurourol Urodynam 7:563-567, 1988.
112. Petersen I, Franksson C: Electromyographic study of the striated muscles of the male urethra. Br J Urol 27:148-153, 1955.
113. Blaivas JG, Labib KL, Bauer SB, Retik AB: A new approach to electromyography of the external urethral sphincter. J Urol 117:773-777, 1977.
114. Jesel M, Isch-Treussard C, Isch F: Electromyography of striated muscle of anal and urethral sphincters. In Desmedt JE (ed): New development in electromyography and clinical neurophysiology, vol 2. Basel: Karger, 1973, pp 406-420.
115. Dibenedetto M, Yalla SV: Electrodiagnosis of striated urethral sphincter dysfunction. J Urol 122:361-365, 1979.
116. Mayo ME: The value of sphincter electromyography in urodynamics. J Urol 122:357-360, 1979.
117. Vereecken RL, Verduyn H: The electrical activity of the paraurethral and perineal muscles in normal and pathological conditions. Br J Urol 42:457-463, 1970.
118. Diokno AC, Koff SA, Bender LF: Periurethral striated muscle activity in neurogenic bladder dysfunction. J Urol 112:743-749, 1974.
119. Wein A, Barrett DM: Etiologic possibilities for increased pelvic floor electromyography activity during cystometry. J Urol 127:949-952, 1982.
120. Evans AR, Felker JR, Shank RA III, Sugarman SR: Pitfalls of urodynamics. J Urol 122:220-222, 1979.
121. Maizels M, Firlit CF: Pediatric urodynamics: a clinical comparison of surface versus needle pelvic floor/external sphincter electromyography. J Urol 122:518-522, 1979.
122. Barrett DM: Disposable (infant) surface electrocardiogram electrodes in urodynamics: a simultaneous comparative study of electrodes. J Urol 124:663-665, 1980.
123. Andersen JT, Bradley WE: Urethral pressure profilometry. Urol Int 33:40-49, 1978.
124. Nordling J, Meyhoff HH: Dissociation of urethral and anal sphincter activity in neurogenic bladder dysfunction. J Urol 122:352-356, 1979.
125. Koyanagi T, Arikado K, Takamatsu T, Tsuji I: Experience with electromyography of the external urethral sphincter in spinal cord injury patients. J Urol 127:272-276, 1982.
126. Sundin T, Petersen I: Cystometry and simultaneous electromyography from the striated urethral and anal sphincters and from levator ani. Invest Urol 13:40-46, 1975.
127. Nordling J, Meyhoff HH, Walter S, Andersen JT: Urethral electromyography using a new ring electrode. J Urol 120:571-573, 1978.
128. Siroky MB, Sax DS, Krane RJ: Sacral signal tracing: the electrophysiology of the bulbocavernosus reflex. J Urol 122:661-664, 1979.
129. Rockswold GL, Bradley WE: The use of evoked electromyographic responses in diagnosing lesions of the cauda equina. J Urol 118:629-631, 1977.
130. Blaivas JG, Bhimani G, Labib KB: Vesicourethral dysfunction in multiple sclerosis. J Urol 122:342-347, 1979.
131. Blaivas JG, Sinha HP, Zayed AAH, Labib KB: Detrusor–external sphincter dyssynergia. J Urol 125:542-544, 1981.
132. Blaivas JG, Sinha HP, Zayed AAH, Labib KB: Detrusor–external sphincter dyssynergia: a detailed electromyographic study. J Urol 125:545-548, 1981.
133. Yalla SV, Blunt KJ, Bam BA, et al: Detrusor–urethral sphincter dyssynergia. J Urol 118:1026-1029, 1977.
134. Siroky MB, Krane RJ: Neurologic aspects of detrusor-sphincter dyssynergia, with reference to the guarding reflex. J Urol 127:953-957, 1982.
135. Barrett DM, Wein AJ: Flow evaluation and simultaneous external sphincter electromyography in clinical urodynamics. J Urol 125:538-541, 1981.
136. Rudy DC, Woodside JR: Non-neurogenic neurogenic bladder: the relationship between intravesical pressure and the external sphincter electromyogram. Neurourol Urodynam 10:169-176, 1991.
137. Hinman F Jr: Nonneurogenic neurogenic bladder (the Hinman syndrome)—15 years later. J Urol 136:769-777, 1986.
138. Siroky MB, Goldstein I, Krane RJ: Functional voiding disorders in men. J Urol 126:200-204, 1981.
139. Webster GD, Lockhart JL, Older RA: The evaluation of bladder neck dysfunction. J Urol 123:196-198, 1980.
140. Enhorning G, Miller ER, Hinman F Jr: Urethral closure studied with cineroentgenography and simultaneous bladder-urethra pressure recording. Surg Gynecol Obstet 118:507-516, 1964.
141. Brown M, Wickham JEA: The urethral pressure profile. Br J Urol 41:211-217, 1969.
142. Asmussen M, Ulmsten U: Simultaneous urethro-cystometry with a new technique. Scand J Urol Nephrol 10:7-11, 1976.
143. Edwards L, Malvern J: The urethral pressure profile: theoretical considerations and clinical application. Br J Urol 46:325-336, 1974.
144. Abrams PH, Martin S, Griffiths DJ: The measurement and interpretation of urethral pressures obtained by the method of Brown and Wickham. Br J Urol 50:33-38, 1978.
145. Abrams PH: Sphincterometry in the diagnosis of male bladder outflow obstruction. J Urol 116:489-492, 1976.
146. Abrams PH: Perfusion urethral profilometry. Urol Clin North Am 6:103-110, 1979.
147. Djurhuus JC, Hansen RI, Nerstrom B: Urethral pressure profile in prostatic surgery. Scand J Urol Nephrol 9:87-88, 1975.
148. Constantinou CE, Govan DE: Spatial distribution and timing of transmitted and reflexly generated urethral pressures in healthy women. J Urol 127:964-969, 1982.
149. Teague CT, Merrill DC: Laboratory comparison of urethral profilometry techniques. Urology 8:221-228, 1979.
150. Brown M: In-vivo determination of error in the measure-

ment of urethral pressure by the method of Brown and Wickham. Br J Urol 47:445-448, 1975.
151. Gilmour RF, James DF, Toguri AG, Churchill BM: Analysis of the urethral pressure profile using a mechanical model. Invest Urol 18:54-58, 1980.
152. Harrison NW, Constable AR: Urethral pressure measurement: a modified technique. Br J Urol 42:229-233, 1970.
153. Rivard DJ, Woodruff MW: Modern urodynamic evaluations in the urologist's office. J Urol 120:732-737, 1978.
154. Raz S, Kaufman JJ: Carbon dioxide–urethral pressure profile in female incontinence. J Urol 117:765-769, 1977.
155. Shawer M, Brown M, Sutherst JR: Comparative examination of female urethral pressure profiles measured by CO_2 and H_2O infusion techniques. Br J Urol 55:326-331, 1983.
156. Awad SA, Bryniak SR, Lowe PJ, et al: Urethral pressure profile in female stress incontinence. J Urol 120:475-479, 1978.
157. Toews HA: Intraurethral and intravesical pressures in normal and stress-incontinent women. Obstet Gynecol 29:613-624, 1967.
158. Glen ES, Rowan D: Continuous flow cystometry and urethral pressure profile measurement with monitored intravesical pressure: a diagnostic and prognostic investigation. Urol Res 1:97-100, 1973.
159. Tanagho EA, Miller ER, Meyers FH, Corbett RK: Observations on the dynamics of the bladder neck. Br J Urol 38:72-84, 1966.
160. Karol JB, Anderson RU: Neuropharmacologic evaluation in spinal cord injury patients using membrane catheter cystosphincterometry. J Urol 124:395-396, 1980.
161. Low JA, Kao M: Intravesical and intraurethral pressure as a measure of urethral sphincter function. Obstet Gynecol 40:627-633, 1972.
162. Asmussen M, Ulmsten U: A new technique for measurements of the urethra pressure profile. Acta Obstet Gynecol Scand 55:167-173, 1976.
163. Asmussen M: Intraurethral pressure recording. Scand J Urol Nephrol 10:1-6, 1976.
164. Hilton P, Stanton SL: Urethral pressure measurement by microtransducer: the results in symptom-free women and in those with genuine stress incontinence. Br J Urol 90:919-933, 1983.
165. Hilton P: The urethral pressure profile under stress: a comparison of profiles on coughing and straining. Neurourol Urodynam 2:55-62, 1983.
166. Van Geelen JM, Doesburg WH, Martin CB Jr: Female urethral pressure profile; reproducibility, axial variation and effects of low dose oral contraceptives. J Urol 131:394-398, 1984.
167. Constantinou CE: Urethrometry: considerations of static, dynamic, and stability characteristics of the female urethra. Neurourol Urodynam 7:521-539, 1988.
168. van der Kooi JB, Kornelis JA, deJonge MC, et al: Urethral pressure recording—an alternative: balloon-covered microtransducer catheter detection. Neurourol Urodynam 7:447-455, 1988.
169. Shelley T, Warrell DW: Measurement of intravesical and intra-urethral pressure in normal women and in women suffering from incontinence of urine. J Obstet Gynecol 72:926-929, 1965.
170. Rud T: Urethral pressure profile in continent women from childhood to old age. Acta Obstet Gynecol Scand 59:331-335, 1980.
171. Cadogan M, Awad S, Field C, et al: A comparison of the cough and standing urethral pressure profile in the diagnosis of stress incontinence. Neurourol Urodynam 7:327-341, 1988.
172. Thind P, Lose G, Jorgensen L, Colstrup H: Urethral pressure increment preceding and following bladder pressure elevation during stress episode in healthy and stress incontinent women. Neurourol Urodynam 10:177-183, 1991.
173. Raz S, Kaufman JJ: Carbon dioxide urethral pressure profile. J Urol 115:439-442, 1975.
174. Lowe PJ, Saunders GTAB, Downie JW, Awad SA: A catheter withdrawing apparatus for clinical urethral pressure profile studies. J Urol 116:626-628, 1976.
175. Ghoneim MA, Rottembourg JL, Fretin J, Susset JG: Urethral pressure profile: standardization of technique and study of reproducibility. Urology 5:623-637, 1975.
176. Fellows GJ: Dynamic ultrasonography for voiding dysfunction. Urol Clin North Am 16:809-814, 1989.
177. Yalla SV, Sharma GVRK, Barsamian EM: Micturitional static urethral pressure profile: a method of recording urethral pressure profile during voiding and the implications. J Urol 124:649-656, 1980.
178. Yalla SV, Blute R, Waters WB, et al: Urodynamic evaluation of prostatic enlargements with micturitional vesicourethral static pressure profiles. J Urol 125:685-689, 1981.
179. Yalla SV, Waters WB, Snyder H, et al: Urodynamic localization of isolated bladder neck obstruction in men: studies with micturitional vesicourethral static pressure profile. J Urol 125:677-684, 1981.
180. Constantinou CE: Resting and stress urethral pressures as a clinical guide to the mechanism of continence in the female patient. Urol Clin North Am 12:247-258, 1985.
181. Bunne G, Obrink A: Urethral closure pressure with stress—a comparison between stress-incontinent and continent women. Urol Res 6:127-134, 1978.
182. Awad SA, Downie JW, Lywood DW, et al: Sympathetic activity in the proximal urethra in patients with urinary obstruction. J Urol 115:545-547, 1976.
183. Faysal MH, Constantinou CE, Rother LF, Govan DE: The impact of bladder neck suspension on the resting and stress urethral pressure profile: a prospective study comparing controls with incontinent patients preoperatively and postoperatively. J Urol 125:55-60, 1981.
184. Obrink A, Bunne G, Ulmsten U, Ingelman-Sundberg A: Urethral pressure profile before, during and after pubococcygeal repair for stress incontinence. Acta Obstet Gynecol Scand 57:49-61, 1978.
185. Henriksson L, Ulmsten U, Andersson KE: The effect of changes of posture on the urethral closure pressure in healthy women. Scand J Urol Nephrol 11:201-206, 1977.
186. Henriksson L, Andersson KE, Ulmsten U: The urethral pressure profiles in continent and stress-incontinent women. Scand J Urol Nephrol 13:5-10, 1979.
187. Enhorning G: Simultaneous recording of intravesical and intra-urethral pressure. Acta Chir Scand 276(suppl):1-68, 1961.
188. Raz S, Caine M, Zeigler M: The vascular component in the production of intraurethral pressure. J Urol 108:93-96, 1972.
189. Hilton P, Stanton SL: A clinical and urodynamic assessment of the Burch colposuspension for genuine stress incontinence. Br J Urol 90:934-939, 1983.
190. Henriksson L, Asmussen M, Lofgren O, Ulmsten U: A urodynamic comparison between abdominal urethrocystopexy and vaginal sling plasty in female stress incontinence. Urol Int 33:111-116, 1978.
191. McGuire EJ, Lytton B, Pepe V, Kohorn EI: Stress urinary incontinence. Obstet Gynecol 47:255-264, 1976.
192. Constantinou CE: Urethrometry: considerations of static, dynamic, and stability characteristics of the female urethra. Neurourol Urodynam 7:521-539, 1988.
193. Constantinou CE, Govan DE: Spatial distribution and timing of transmitted and reflexly generated urethral pressures in healthy women. J Urol 127:964-969, 1982.
194. Sorensen S, Norgaard JP, Knudsen LM, et al: Urethral pressure variations in healthy females during rest and sleep. J Urol 137:1287-1290, 1987.
195. Ulmsten U, Henriksson L, Iosif S: The unstable female urethra. Am J Obstet Gynecol 144:93-97, 1982.
196. McGuire EJ, Lytton B, Kohorn EI, Pepe V: The value of

urodynamic testing in stress urinary incontinence. J Urol 124:256-258, 1980.
197. Aagaard J, Bruskewitz, R: Are urodynamic studies useful in the evaluation of female incontinence? Probl Urol 5:11-22, 1991.
198. Zinner NR, Susset JG, Coolsaet BLRA, et al: The great debate—resolved: the urethral closure pressure profile should be used for diagnosis and management of female stress incontinence. Neurourol Urodynam 2:81-99, 1983.
199. Ryall RL, Marshall VR: The effect of urethral catheter on the measurement of maximum urinary flow rate. J Urol 128:429-432, 1982.
200. Gierup J, Ericsson NO, Okmian L: Micturition studies in infants and children: influence of an indwelling urethral catheter and of rectal pressure recording. Scand J Urol Nephrol 4:209-215, 1970.
201. Neal DE, Rao CVS, Styles RA, et al: Effects of catheter size on urodynamic measurements in men undergoing elective prostatectomy. Br J Urol 60:64-68, 1987.
202. Griffiths DJ, Scholtmeijer RJ: Precise urodynamic assessment of anatomic urethral obstruction in boys. Neurourol Urodynam 1:97-104, 1982.
203. Smith JC: Urethral resistance to micturition. Br J Urol 40:125-156, 1968.
204. Susset JG, Brissot RB, Regnier CH: The stop-flow technique: a way to measure detrusor strength. J Urol 127:489-494, 1982.
205. Gierup J: Micturition studies in infants and children: intravesical pressure, urinary flow and urethral resistance in boys without infravesical obstruction. Scand J Urol Nephrol 4:217-230, 1970.
206. Griffiths DJ: Urodynamic assessment of bladder function. Br J Urol 49:29-36, 1977.
207. Zinner NR, Paquin AJ Jr: Clinical urodynamics. I. Studies of intravesical pressure in normal human female subjects. J Urol 90:719-730, 1963.
208. Schafer W: Analysis of active detrusor function during voiding with the bladder working function. Neurourol Urodynam 10:19-35, 1991.
209. Bryndorf J, Sandoe E: The hydrodynamics of micturition. Dan Med Bull 7:65-71, 1960.
210. Scott BF, Quesada EM, Cardus D: Studies on the dynamics of micturition: observations on healthy men. J Urol 92:455-463, 1964.
211. Webb RJ, Griffith CJ, Zachariah KK, Neal DE: Filling and voiding pressures measured by ambulatory monitoring and conventional studies during natural and artificial bladder filling. J Urol 146:815-818, 1991.
212. Blaivas JG: Multichannel urodynamic studies in men with benign prostatic hyperplasia. Urol Clin North Am 17:543-552, 1990.
213. Chancellor MB, Blaivas JG, Kaplan SA, and Axelrod S: Bladder outlet obstruction versus impaired detrusor contractility: the role of uroflow. J Urol 145:810-812, 1991.
214. Massey JA, Abrams PH: Obstructed voiding in the female. Br J Urol 61:36-39, 1988.
215. Schafer W: Principles and clinical application of advanced urodynamic analysis of voiding function. Urol Clin North Am 17:553-566, 1990.
216. Axelrod SL, Blaivas JG: Bladder neck obstruction in women. J Urol 137:497-499, 1987.
217. Mayo ME: Primary bladder neck obstruction in men: variation in detrusor response. J Urol 128:957-959, 1982.
218. Norlen LJ, Blaivas JG: Unsuspected proximal urethral obstruction in young and middle-aged men. J Urol 135:972-976, 1986.
219. Susset JG, Rabinovitch HH, Rosario F, Nackinnon KJ: Measurement of urethral resistance. J Urol 96:746-755, 1966.
220. Griffiths DJ: Assessment of detrusor contraction strength or contractility. Neurourol Urodynam 10:1-18, 1991.
221. Gleason DM, Lattimer JK: The pressure-flow study: a method for measuring bladder neck resistance. J Urol 87:844-852, 1962.
222. Spangberg A, Terio H, Engberg A, Ask P: Quantification of urethral function based on Griffiths' model of flow through elastic tubes. Neurourol Urodynam 8:29-52, 1989.
223. Bruskewitz R, Jensen KME, Iversen P, Madsen PO: The relevance of minimum urethral resistance in prostatism. J Urol 129:769-771, 1983.
224. Frimodt-Moller C, Hald T: Clinical urodynamics: methods and results. Scand J Urol Nephrol 6(suppl 15):144-155, 1972.
225. Claridge M, Shuttleworth KED: The dynamics of obstructed micturition. Invest Urol 2:188-199, 1964.
226. Whitaker J, Johnston GS: Estimation of urinary outflow resistance in children: simultaneous measurement of bladder pressure, flow rate, and exit pressure. Invest Urol 4:379-389, 1966.
227. Griffiths DJ: The mechanics of the urethra and of micturition. Br J Urol 45:497-507, 1973.
228. Snyder JA, Westmacott R: Treatment of mild, moderate, and severe cystoceles. Probl Urol 5:85-93, 1991.
229. Griffiths D, van Mastrigt R, Bosch R: Quantification of urethral resistance and bladder function during voiding, with special reference to the effects of prostate size reduction on urethral obstruction due to benign prostatic hyperplasia. Neurourol Urodynam 8:17-27, 1989.
230. Spangberg A, Terio H, Ask P, Engberg A: Pressure/flow studies preoperatively and postoperatively in patients with benign prostatic hypertrophy: estimation of the urethral pressure/flow relation and urethral elasticity. Neurourol Urodynam 10:139-167, 1991.
231. Abrams PH, Griffiths DJ: The assessment of prostatic obstruction from urodynamic measurements and from residual urine. Br J Urol 51:129-134, 1979.
232. Schafer W: Urethral resistance? Urodynamic concepts of physiological and pathological bladder outlet function during voiding. Neurourol Urodynam 4:161-201, 1985.
233. Bhatia NN, Bradley WE, Haldeman S: Urodynamics: continuous monitoring. J Urol 128:963-968, 1982.
234. Barton EJ, Sherwood T: Video urodynamic studies and clinical outcome. Br J Urol 56:805-807, 1983.
235. Bates CP, Whiteside CG, Turner-Warwick R: Synchronous cine/pressure/flow/cysto-urethrography with special reference to stress and urge incontinence. Br J Urol 42:714-723, 1970.
236. Bates CP, Corney CE: Synchronous cine/pressure/flow cystography: a method of routine urodynamic investigation. Br J Radiol 44:44-50, 1971.
237. Blaivas J: Multichannel urodynamic studies. Urology 23:421-438, 1984.
238. McGuire EJ: Combined radiographic and manometric assessment of urethral sphincter function. J Urol 118:632-635, 1977.
239. Nishizawa O, Moriya I, Satoh S, et al: A new video urodynamics: combined ultrasonotomographic and urodynamic monitoring. Neurol Urodynam 1:295-301, 1982.
240. Shapeero LG, Friedland GW, Perkash I: Transrectal sonographic voiding cystourethrography: studies in neuromuscular bladder dysfunction. AJR 141:83-90, 1983.
241. Shabsigh R, Fishman IJ, Krebs M: The use of transrectal longitudinal real-time ultrasonography in urodynamics. J Urol 138:1416-1419, 1987.
242. Kohorn EI, Scioscia AL, Jeanty P, Hobbins JC: Ultrasound cystourethrography by perineal scanning for the assessment of female stress urinary incontinence. Obstet Gynecol 68:269-272, 1986.
243. Koelbl H, Bernashek G: A new method for sonographic urethrocystography and simultaneous pressure-flow measurements. Obstet Gynecol 74:417-422, 1989.
244. Blaivas JG, Fisher DM: Combined radiographic and urodynamic monitoring: advances in technique. J Urol 125:693-694, 1981.
245. Richmond DH, Sutherst J: Transrectal ultrasound scanning in urinary incontinence: the effect of the probe on urodynamic parameters. Br J Urol 64:582-585, 1989.

246. Rose DH, Eaton AC: Observations in micturating cystourethrography. J R Soc Med 76:121-125, 1983.
247. Griffiths CJ, Styles RA, Ramsen PD, Neal DE: Ambulatory monitoring of bladder and detrusor pressure during natural filling. J Urol 142:780-784, 1989.
248. Gleason DM, Lattimer JK, Bauxbaum C: Bladder pressure telemetry. J Urol 94:252-256, 1965.
249. Burgio KL, Engel BT, Locher JL: Normative patterns of diurnal urination across 6 age decades. J Urol 145:728-731, 1991.
250. Vereecken RL, Puers B, Das J: Continuous telemetric monitoring of bladder function. Urol Res 11:15-18, 1983.
251. Miyagawa I, Nakamura I, Ueda M, et al: Telemetric cystometry. Urol Int 41:263-265, 1986.
252. van Waalwijk van Doorn ESC, Remmers A, Janknegt RA: Extramural ambulatory urodynamic monitoring during natural filling and normal daily activities: evaluation of 100 patients. J Urol 146:124-131, 1991.
253. Thuroff JW, Jonas U, Frohneberg D, et al: Telemetric urodynamic investigations in normal males. Urol Int 35:427-434, 1980.
254. Styles RA, Neal DE, Ramsden PD: Comparison of long-term monitoring and standard cystometry in chronic retention of urine. Br J Urol 58:652-656, 1986.
255. van Mastrigt R: A computer program for on-line measurement, storage, analysis and retrieval of urodynamic data. Comput Prog Biomed 18:109-118, 1984.
256. Rollema HJ, van Mastrigt R: Objective analysis of prostatism: a clinical application of the computer program CLIM. Neurourol Urodynam 10:71-76, 1991.
257. Frimodt-Moller C: A urodynamic study of micturition in healthy men and women. Dan Med Bull 21:41-48, 1974.

CHAPTER 8

UROLOGIC ACCESSORY DEVICES

LAURENCE B. KANDEL

A wide variety of instruments are used in urologic surgery, from a urethral sound to an extracorporeal lithotripter. Often, especially with descriptions of major pieces of equipment, insufficient attention is directed toward supplemental items and instruments that not only facilitate performance but also often are essential to it. This chapter discusses diverse accessory devices, some of which are used only in conjunction with other items but many of which may be the sole instrument used for a particular purpose.

VEHICLES

The standard vehicle for access to the urinary tract is the cystoscope. Various companies produce a wide array of such instruments. This chapter mentions many companies in providing examples of devices, but not every manufacturer is listed. The major manufacturers of cystoscopic equipment are the American Cystoscope Manufacturing Company, Olympus Company, Storz Company, and Wolf Company. They each produce endoscopes in a variety of French sizes and lengths and even provide cystoscopes sized for children (Figure 8–1).

Although the cystoscope was designed as a diagnostic instrument, users quickly recognized that it would be even more valuable as a working instrument. Thus several working ports (channels) were quickly adapted to this lighted lens system. Working bridges facilitated biopsies, x-ray studies, tissue removal, and orifice catheterization (Figure 8–2). Similarly, as the incandescent light source was replaced with a fiberoptic system, various rigid lens systems were devised, including the standard foroblique (30-degree) lens, the straight-ahead (zero-degree) lens, the lateral (70-degree) lens, and the retrograde (120-degree) lens (Figure 8–3).

Later, flexible (as distinct from rigid lens) fiberoptic systems were devised. At first these vehicles were also strictly diagnostic devices. The rigid accessory equipment previously developed for the rigid cystoscopes could not be used inside these flexible instruments. By necessity, in time, this also changed. Today each of the companies manufacturing rigid cystoscopes also produce flexible fiberoptic cystoscopes (Figure 8–4).

Next came miniaturization. Downsizing of the cystoscope permitted the development of devices that functioned in a similar fashion yet could be used in children. Diameter miniaturization also made possible the first true ureteroscopes (Figure 8–5). Originally designed on the order of 12F to 13F, these scopes have been downsized to as small as 6F to 7F.

The ureter's unique anatomic and pathologic problems demanded more than a ureteroscope that was just a diagnostic instrument.[1] Ureteral tumors required the production of biopsy devices and small electrocautery probes (Figure 8–6). More significant was the need for instrumentation to manage ureteral calculi. These devices are covered in detail later.

Although urologists worked diligently with the early ureteroscopes, it soon became clear that the ureter was not easy to enter, even under direct vision. Furthermore, it was not straight, as were the metal ureteroscopes, and it was not a forgiving structure. The issue of ureteral anatomy quickly became evident. The gentle (or sometimes not so gentle) curve of the intramural ureter, its narrow and pulsatile section as it crosses the iliac vessels, and its ventral and dorsal course over the psoas muscle dictated a more flexible device. As miniaturization in rigid instrumentation progressed, parallel advances were made in flexible fiberoptic scopes. The flexible ureteroscopes with small diameter and functional working ports have helped urologists deal with the peculiarities of the ureter.

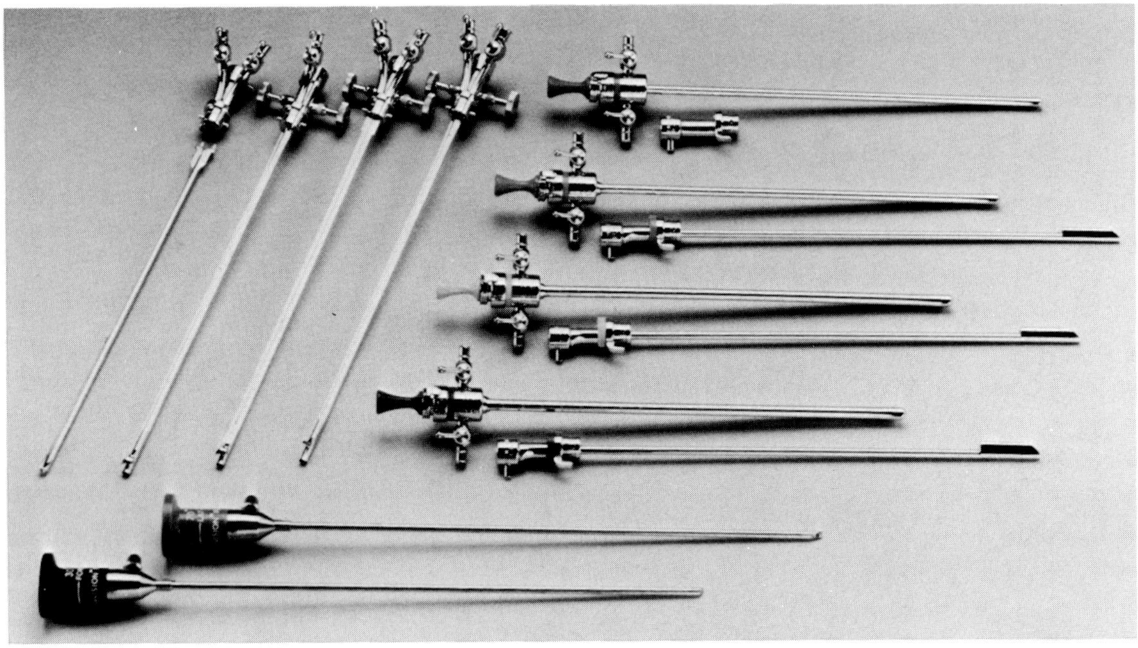

A

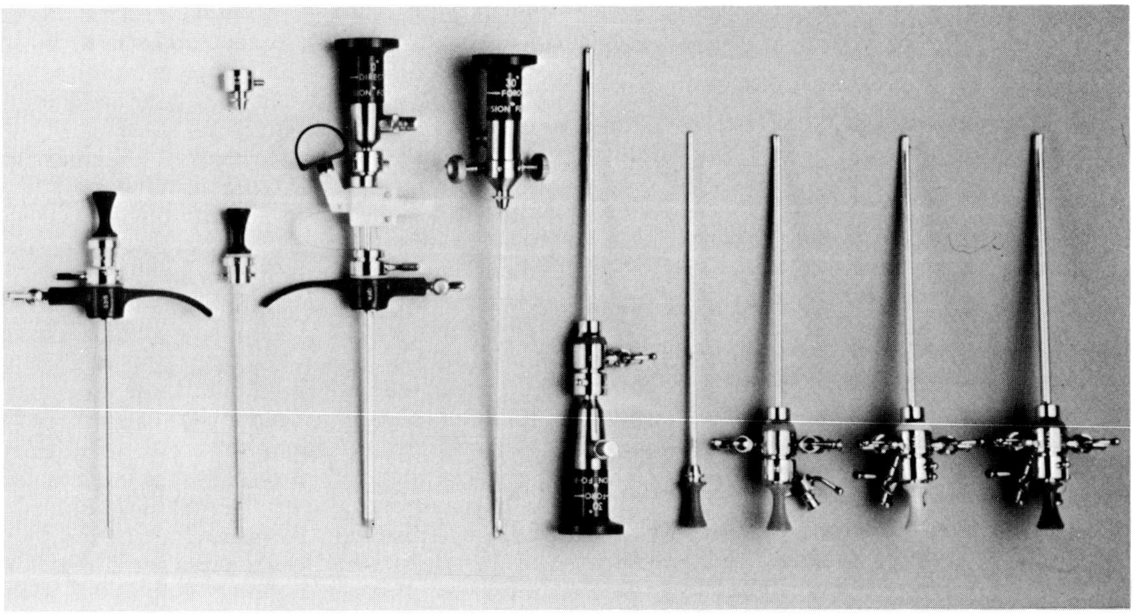

B

FIGURE 8–1. **A,** Standard adult and, **B,** pediatric cystoscopes. (Courtesy of Circon.)

A major development that gave flexible fiberoptic scopes a significant advantage was the incorporation into these devices of a directable steering mechanism. Some representative flexible ureteroscopes are shown in Figure 8–7.

The steerable mechanism permitted direct control in negotiating the normal ureteral curves and was even more advantageous in dealing with tortuous ureters. In addition, once the scope passed the ureteropelvic junction, this steerable mechanism allowed both intrarenal pyeloscopy and calycoscopy to be performed. The ability not only to look inside the kidney in a retrograde manner but to perform biopsies of intrarenal lesions has in-

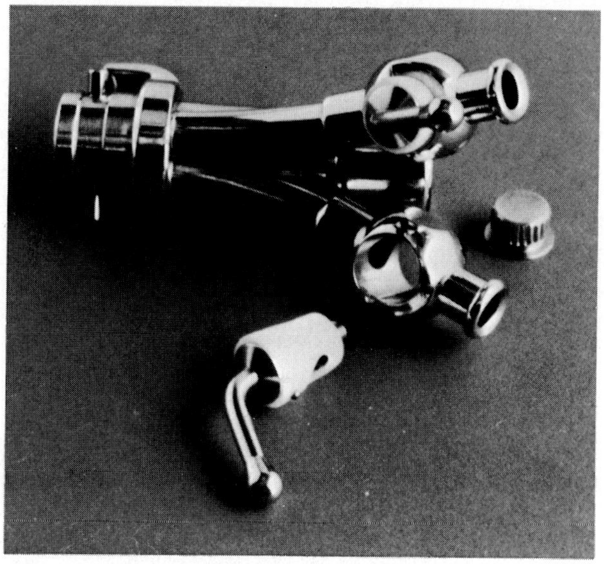

FIGURE 8–2. Working bridge supports both the viewing telescope and ports for working instruments. (Courtesy of Circon.)

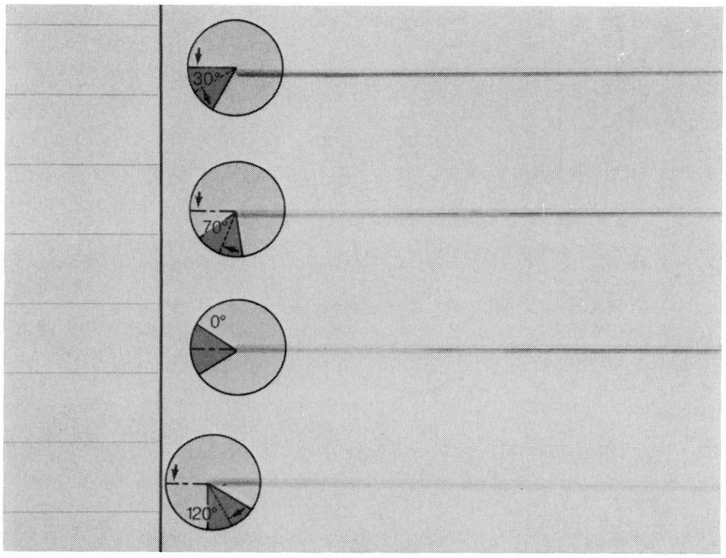

FIGURE 8–3. A variety of available viewing lenses for cystoscopy.

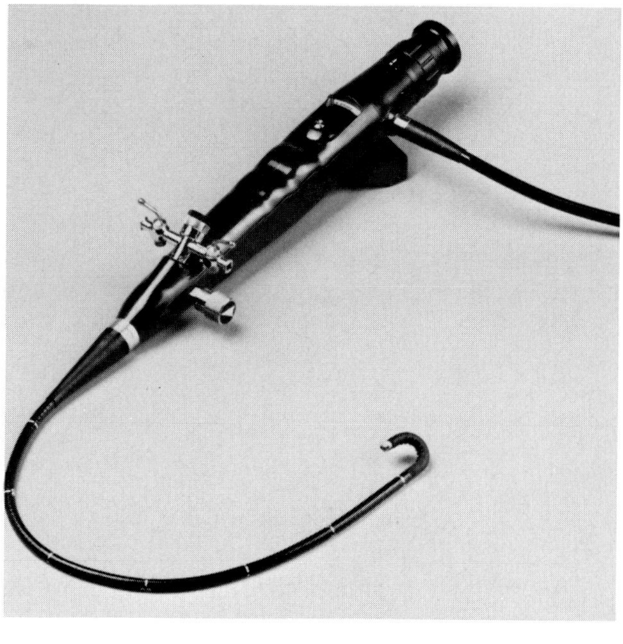

FIGURE 8–4. An 18F flexible fiberoptic cystoscope with steerable, deflectable tip. (Courtesy of Circon.)

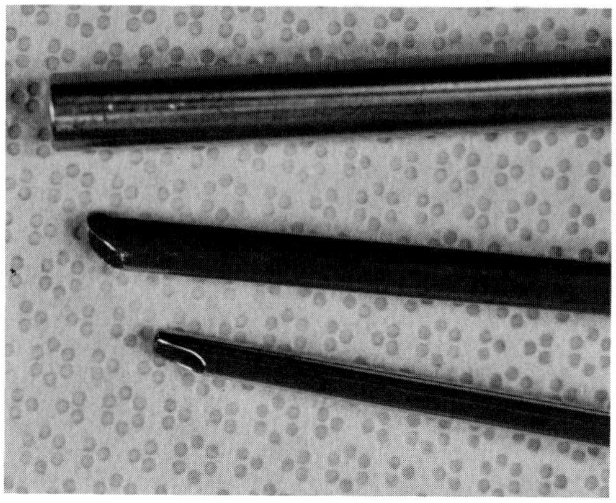

A

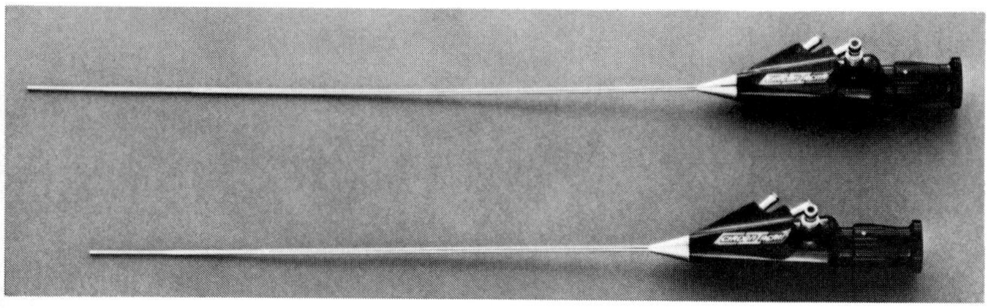

B

FIGURE 8–5. **A,** Miniaturization of ureteroscopes: 15F, 11.5F (courtesy of Karl Storz), and 8F (courtesy of Richard Wolf). **B,** Current miniureteroscope 6.2F. (Courtesy of Circon.)

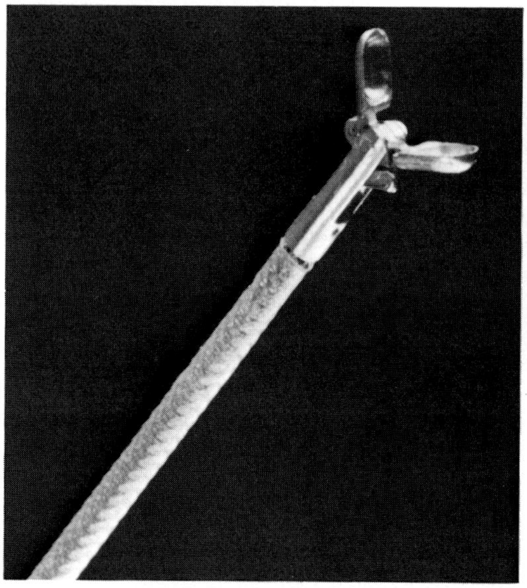

A

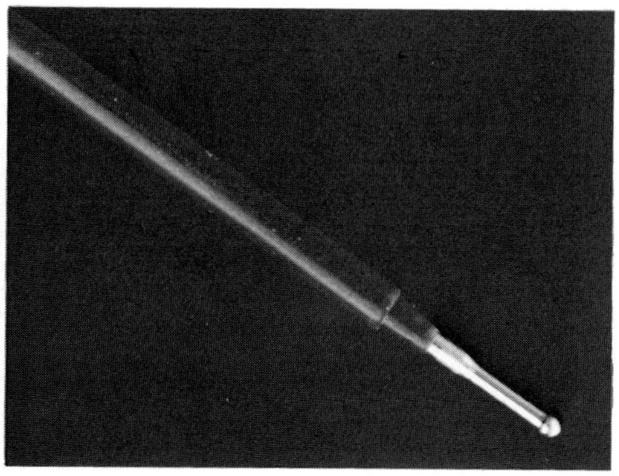

B

FIGURE 8–6. **A,** Ureteroscopic biopsy forceps. **B,** Electrocautery probe for hemostasis following biopsy. (**A** and **B** courtesy of Cook Urological.)

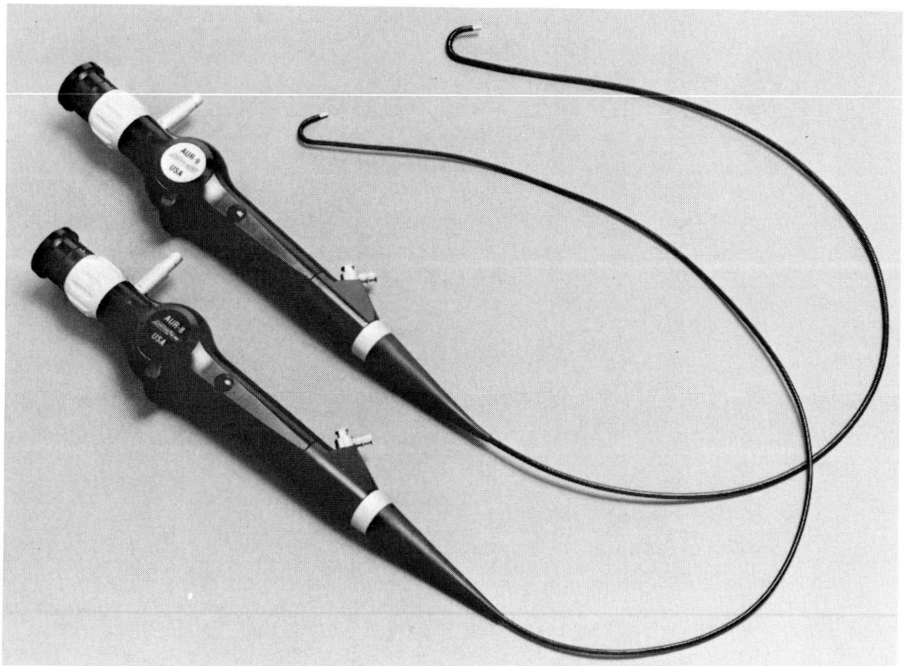

FIGURE 8–7. Flexible, steerable fiberoptic ureteroscopes, 8F and 9F. (Courtesy of Circon.)

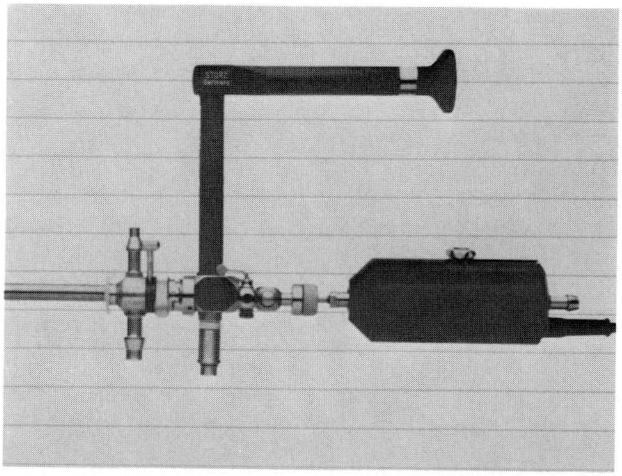

A

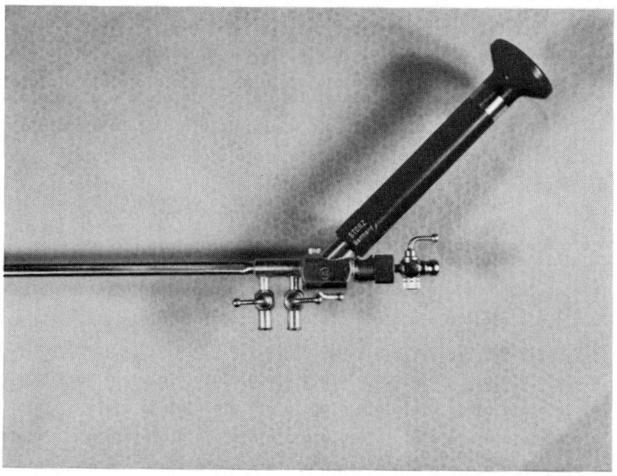

B

FIGURE 8–8. **A,** Offset viewing lens system for nephroscope. **B,** An 11.5F ureteroscope. The offset lens system allows use of the rigid ultrasonic lithotrite. (**A** and **B** courtesy of Karl Storz.)

creased diagnostic capabilities. Flexible ureteroscopes are sometimes useful for patients with upper tract calculi who are too obese to fit into conventional lithotripters. This vehicle has allowed fragmentation of stones with flexible intracorporeal lithotrites such as the pulsed dye laser and electrohydraulic probe. Often, markedly obese patients are unsuitable candidates for percutaneous nephrostolithotomy (PCNL) procedures because of the extremely long distance from their skin to the collecting system. Flexible ureteropyeloscopy has been successful in treating these stones.

PCNL itself has made unique demands on the endoscope (nephroscope).[2] Most stone surgeons have chosen to work through percutaneous tracts about 30F in diameter. Therefore a nephroscope of 28F has been the preferred design. The lens system had two specific requirements. First, of necessity, a straight-ahead or zero-degree lens system was required. Second, because of the nature of the large-diameter, rigid support instrumentation was required for stone removal (grasping forceps, ultrasonic, lithotrites), and an offset lens system was mandatory (Figure 8–8).

URETERAL ACCESS DEVICES

Before performing any urologic procedure within the ureter, the urologist must gain access and maintain that access. In practical terms, this means not only access at the level of the ureterovesical junction, but also access that allows controlled drainage of urine from the kidney into the bladder. The mainstays of ureteral access devices are the ureteric guidewires. As with most devices, they are produced in a variety of diameters and lengths and are composed of various materials. Two commonly used access devices are the floppy-tipped metal guidewire and the coated "glidewire" (Figure 8–9).

Floppy-tipped guidewires are flexible at the distal end to allow passive deflection around or by ureteric stones or ureteral kinks. Occcasionally a floppy-tipped guidewire is too flexible to bypass an obstruction. In response to limited options, the ability to add rigidity to the wire could mean the difference between ultimate failure or success. A "steerable" wire has a retractable stylet that allows its tip to be either rigid or floppy. As the stylet is advanced to the distal tip, the wire becomes rigid. As the stylet is retracted, the distal tip becomes floppy (Figure 8–10). This flexibility is valuable in preventing perforation of the ureteral wall, especially in areas resistant to passage of the wire.

In contrast, the glidewire has an outer coating that makes it slippery when wet, which aids in passage of the wire up the ureter. Both types of

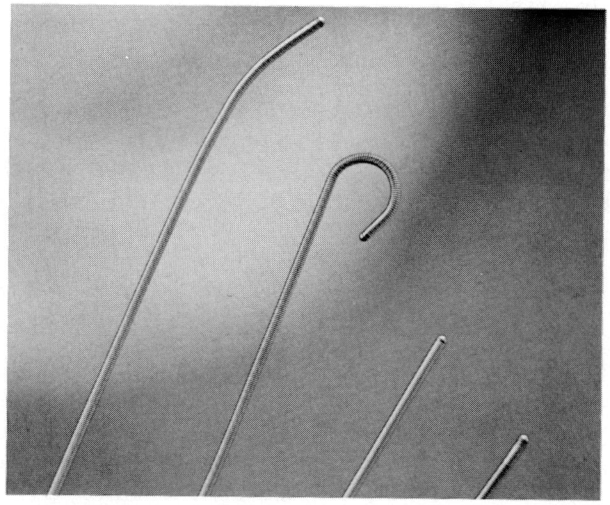

FIGURE 8–9. Various floppy-tip metal guidewires.

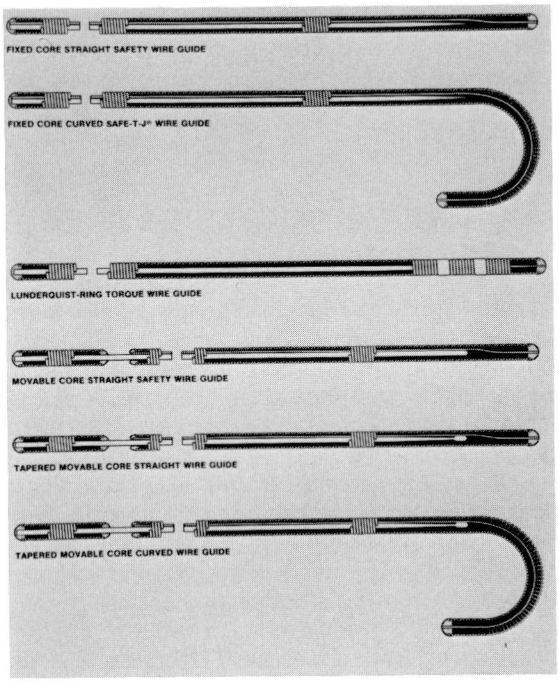

FIGURE 8–10. Diagrammatic sketch of the movable core (retractable stylet) guidewire.

wires are of diameters and lengths that can be used through standard working channels of most ureteroscopes. Furthermore, these diameters permit coaxial placement of most ureteral stent devices.

Guidewires can be placed into the ureter in a retrograde fashion under direct cystoscopic guidance. They can also be manipulated to the level of the renal pelvis, bypassing obstructions and rounding turns in the ureter. Once in place, they provide continuous access to the entire urinary tract. Thus they can be used as a visual guide for passing a ureteroscope up the ureter, either alongside or coaxially over the wire. More important, should a perforation occur during work in the ureter, a double J stent can be passed coaxially over the guidewire, the ureter adequately stented, and drainage secured to improve healing.

Skilled endourologists subscribe as a matter of course to the concept of "control of the urinary tract." Guidewires have provided urologists with the added measure of safety and flexibility to perform a variety of endoscopic manipulations in a controlled manner.

URETERAL BALLOON DILATORS

The normal ureter has three relatively narrow areas. One of these, the ureterovesical junction, often must be stretched or dilated to permit entry of a ureteroscope. Initially, urologists adapted dilation devices similar to those used for other structures (urethra, esophagus). Metal boule-a-bougie dilators were designed that could be passed into the

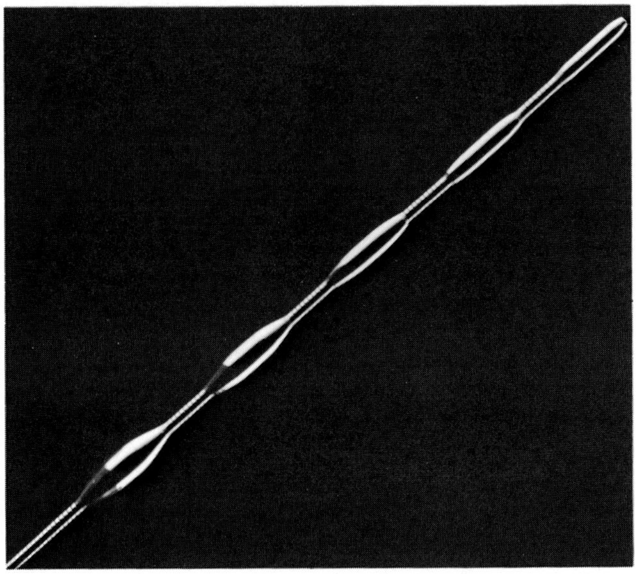

FIGURE 8–11. Progressively sized metal ureteral dilators, which are placed into the ureter coaxially over a guidewire. (Courtesy of Cook Urological.)

ureteral orifice under direct endoscopic vision via the cystoscope.[3] With the acceptance of the guidewire as a ureteral access device, these metal dilators were fashioned to be used coaxially over the guidewire (Figure 8–11). More recently, balloon dilation catheters have been devised to accomplish the same objective (Figure 8–12). Even with the continued miniaturization of ureteroscopes, dilating the ureteral orifice often has been necessary to gain endoscopic access. This maneuver not only facilitates passage of the ureteroscope, but also helps

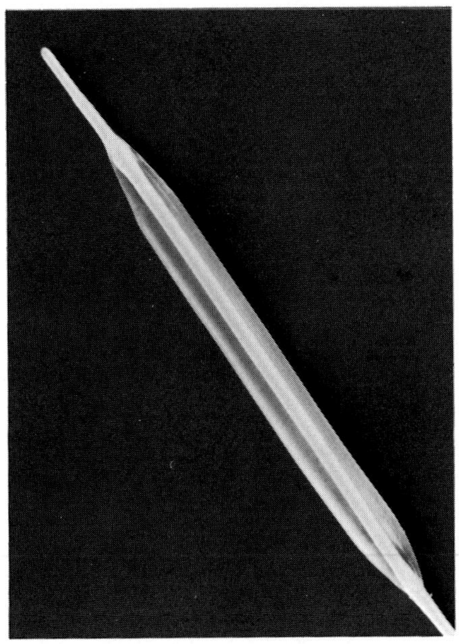

FIGURE 8–12. Inflatable balloon ureteral dilation catheter. (Courtesy of Cook Urological.)

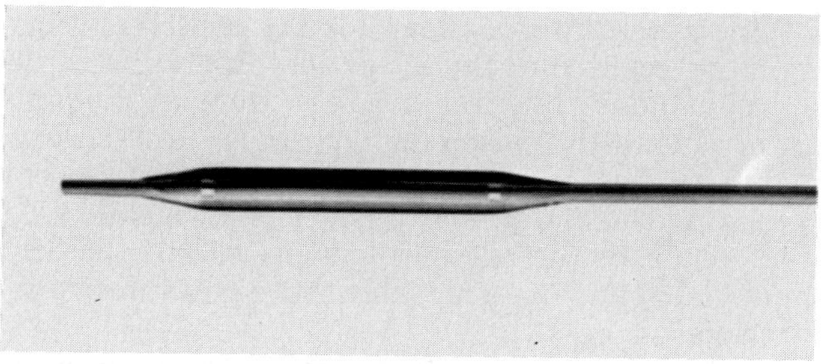

FIGURE 8–13. Ureteroscopic 5F balloon dilation catheter used through the ureteroscopic working port.

to prevent subsequent ureteral stricturing caused by pressure ischemia.

The technique of balloon dilation is straightforward. Once the guidewire is in place, the balloon dilation catheter can either be passed coaxially over the wire or be passed alongside the wire and inflated. Balloon dilation combines stretching and fatigue. Inflation of the balloon with either air or fluid stretches the ureteral walls. As with any muscular tube, prolonged and repeated stretching results in muscle fatigue. There is no commonly accepted method for routinely successful balloon dilation. Nevertheless, balloon inflation for 60 seconds repeated three times usually dilates the intramural ureter successfully and permits the easy passage of a 9.5F ureteroscope.

Balloon catheters have been manufactured to deal with the other narrow areas within the ureter. These catheters were, of necessity, smaller in diameter so that they could be delivered to the desired location through the working channel of the ureteroscope, which is usually 5F maximum (Figure 8–13). Thus, as the ureteroscope is passed retrograde and under direct vision up the ureter, thc balloon dilation catheter is passed through the working port of the ureteroscope and inflated when a narrow area is encountered. Common areas of use include the segment of the ureter that crosses the iliac vessels, the ureteropelvic junction, and the segment of the ureter just below a ureteral calculus. Two other balloon dilation catheters used in urologic practice are the percutaneous tract dilator for PCNL and the intraurethral prostatic balloon dilation catheter. These catheters are described in later sections.

CONDUIT DEVICES

Once the ureteral orifice has been adequately dilated, it is usually a simple task visually to direct a rigid ureteroscope into and up the ureter. Any passive resistance caused by anatomic constraints on the ureteroscope's passing from the urethra and into the ureteral orifice can usually be overcome. Men have anatomic undulations from the pendulous to the prostatic urethra, through the prostate and bladder, and into the ureteral orifice. The male anatomy often makes passage of flexible ureteroscopes difficult. As a result of the many curves in this path, leveraged advancement of the flexible ureteroscope is sometimes futile and the scope may buckle within the bladder. Rigid conduit devices have been fashioned to deal with this problem.

One of the earlier rigid conduit devices was a hollow sheath that was passed coaxially over a guidewire and placed into the ureteral orifice. The flexible ureteroscope was then passed into the lumen of the sheath and advanced up the ureter. The prototype of this conduit was the Finlayson ureteral peel-away sheath.[4] More recently developed cystoscopic assist devices provide slightly more visual control. With one such device the ureteroscope is inserted into a cystoscope and then passed directly into the ureter through the access port. This cystoscopic assist device allows minimal angulation of the ureteroscope and provides adequate leverage

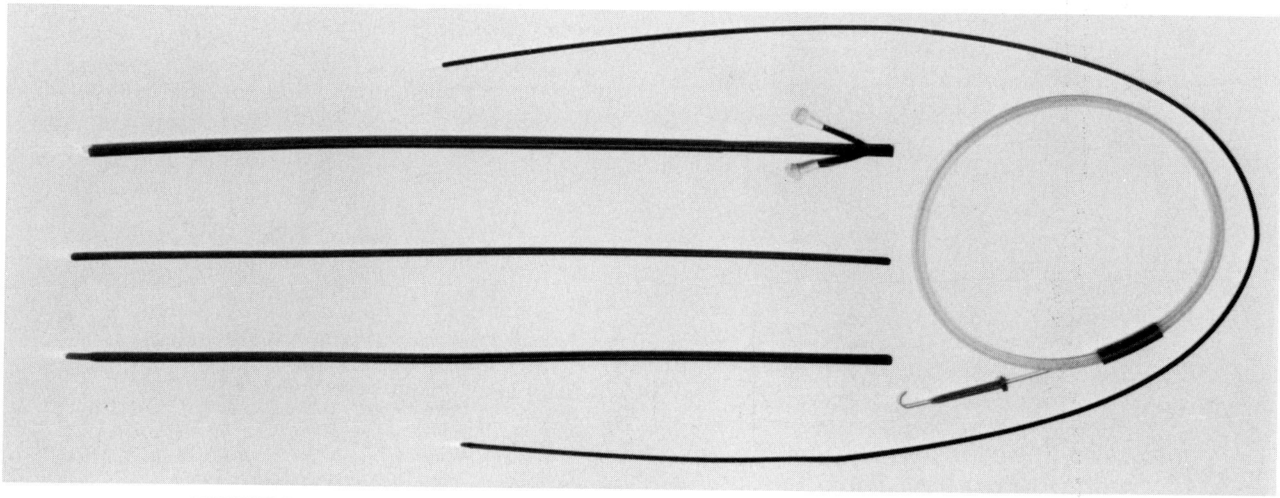

FIGURE 8–14. Finlayson ureteral peel-away dilation set. (Courtesy of Cook Urological.)

to pass the scope easily into the ureteral orifice. Once the ureteroscope is in place, the assist device is removed from around it (Figure 8–14).

IRRIGATION DEVICES

After the ureter has been accessed by guidewires and stretched by ureteral dilation catheters, the ureteroscope is put to work. Unfortunately, as ureteroscopes became miniaturized, so did their capacity to deliver irrigation fluid. Even hanging a large-volume bag of irrigation fluid at a substantial height may not provide adequate flow to perform the manipulations required within the ureter. This problem is not usually apparent during visual access and passage of the ureteroscope in a retrograde manner into the ureter. However, once the target (stone, tumor) is visualized, the working device (lithotrite, biopsy forceps) is passed into the working channel. This noticeably reduces the amount of irrigating fluid that can pass through the distal end of the ureteroscope. Consequently, equipment was developed that could overcome the limitations of passive irrigation pressure and allow adequate flow and good visualization.

The first of the irrigation devices was simple, practical, and inexpensive. It was basically a handheld instrument in which a one-way valve system allowed a syringe to self-fill and to infuse irrigation fluid through the ureteroscope (Figure 8–15). Not unexpectedly, a more sophisticated, less labor-intensive, and more expensive device has been developed that accomplishes the same end: adequate irrigation flow. The later device, the Ureteromat, not only provides an adequate flow rate for endoscopic visualization but also may accomplish ureteral dilation (Figure 8–16).[5]

One potential drawback for the ureteral irrigation devices is that the irrigation fluid must be delivered under high pressure to provide an adequate flow. Within the closed urinary tract (ureter, renal pelvis, and calyceal system), this high pressure can cause pyelotubular and pyelovenous backflow. In fact, at times the pressure generated may be high enough to cause a forniceal rupture and subsequent extravasation.

High-pressure irrigation rarely presents a problem if the system is stented postoperatively. However, if there is infection within the urinary tract at the time of irrigation, urinary sepsis may result. Consequently, anytime these manipulations are performed with the aforementioned irrigation devices, complete sterilization of the patient's urine is wise in case of prior urinary tract infection. If the urine is sterile, routinely employing prophylactic, broad-spectrum antibiotics is prudent.

STONE BASKETS

The pain of urinary colic is a result of obstruction within the urinary tract and not directly related to stone size. Similarly, successful stone removal does not depend solely on the size of the stone. The stone's hardness and the inflammatory response within the ureter are in many ways more predictive of ultimate success or failure in achieving stone removal. Nevertheless, there are realistic size limits that determine whether a stone can be physically extracted in one piece.

Before the advent of ureteroscopy, blind basket extraction of ureteral calculi was the standard method of management.[6] Initially a large-diameter, stiff metal basket was blindly passed up the ureter and past the offending calculus (Figure 8–17). The

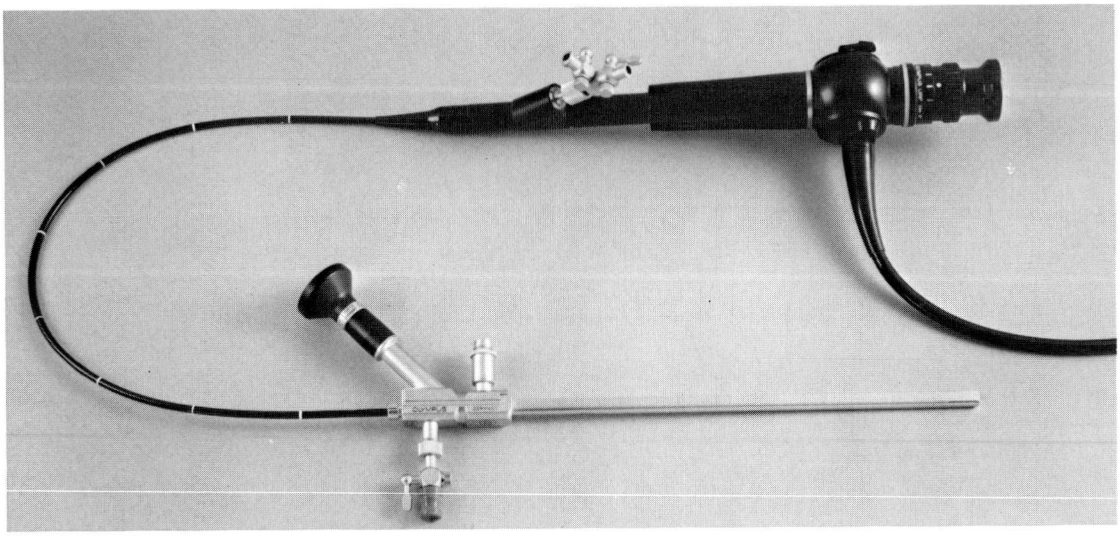

FIGURE 8–15. Direct viewing ureteroscopic assist device. (Courtesy of Olympus.)

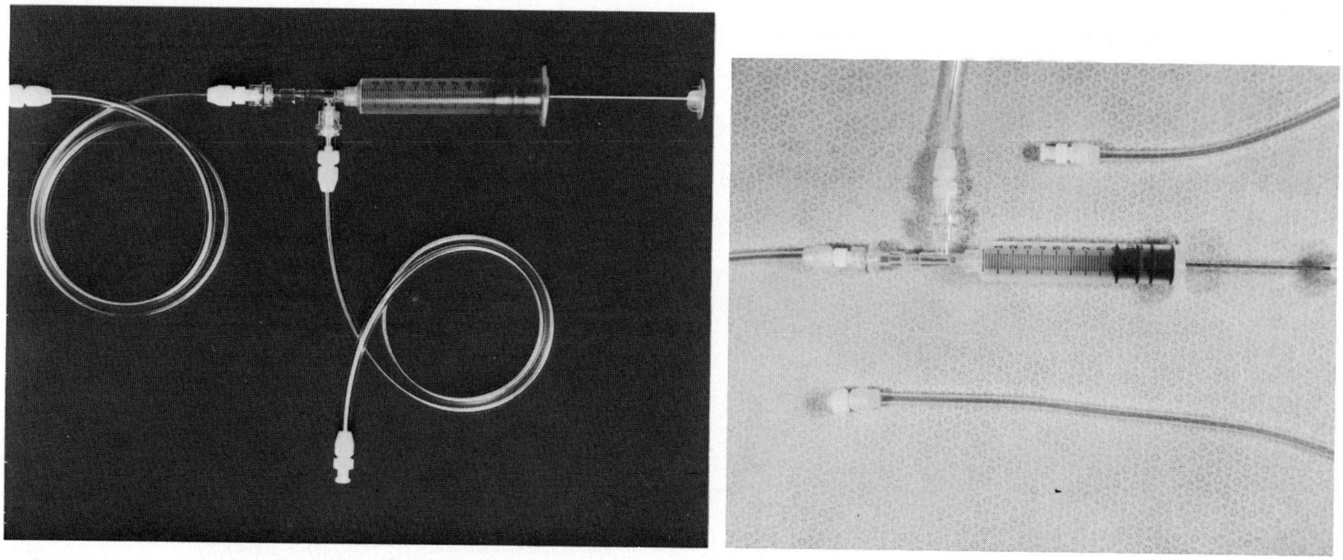

A B

FIGURE 8–16. **A,** Hand-held irrigation device with self-filling 10 ml syringe. (Courtesy of Vantec.) **B,** Close-up view showing one-way valve system.

basket was then slowly withdrawn and the stone engaged. If the stone was not removed at this first pass, passing the basket up beyond the stone again was often difficult. To help with this problem, filiform tips were placed on the distal end of the stone basket so that access above the stone could be maintained (Figure 8–18). Once the basket itself was drawn down below the stone, if it was not engaged with the stone inside of it, the filiform tip remained above the stone, allowing the basket to be passed again. However, the large, stiff metal stone baskets have many problems. First, they often cannot be passed by the stone because of their sheer size. More significantly, if the stone becomes engaged and resistance to extraction is encountered, serious damage could occur if excessive force is applied.

Despite the problems, baskets went through a process of refinement. As with most urologic instrumentation, they first were made smaller and more delicate. In addition, a variety of configurations emerged. The two most commonly employed were the flat wire and the helical stone baskets (Figure 8–19). Variations on this theme included the three-, four-, and five-wire baskets, filiform and nonfiliform tips, and sizes ranging from 5F to smaller than 2F (Figure 8–20).

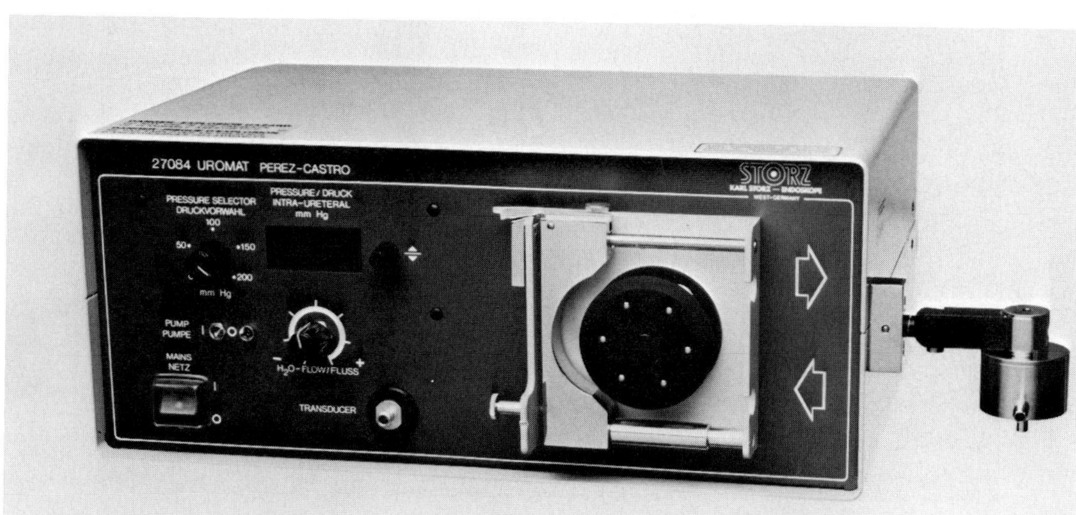

FIGURE 8–17. Ureteromat device for automated ureteroscopic irrigation. (Courtesy of Karl Storz.)

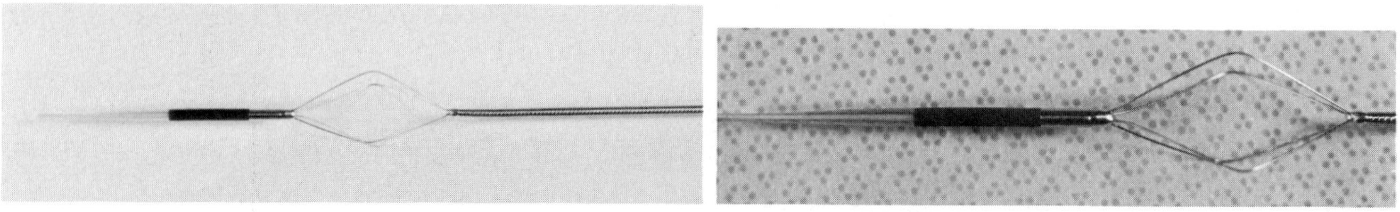

A B

FIGURE 8–18. **A,** Johnson stone basket. (Courtesy of Bard Urologic). **B,** Close-up view shows stiff, large-diameter metal wires.

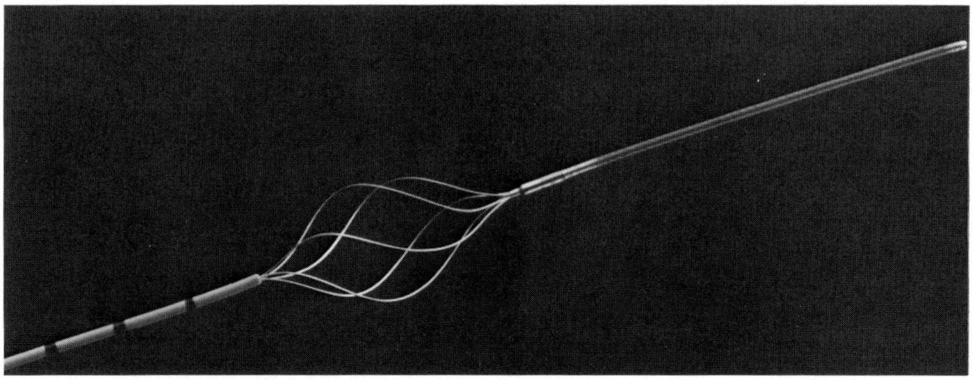

FIGURE 8–19. Filiform-tipped ureteral stone basket. (Courtesy of Cook Urological.)

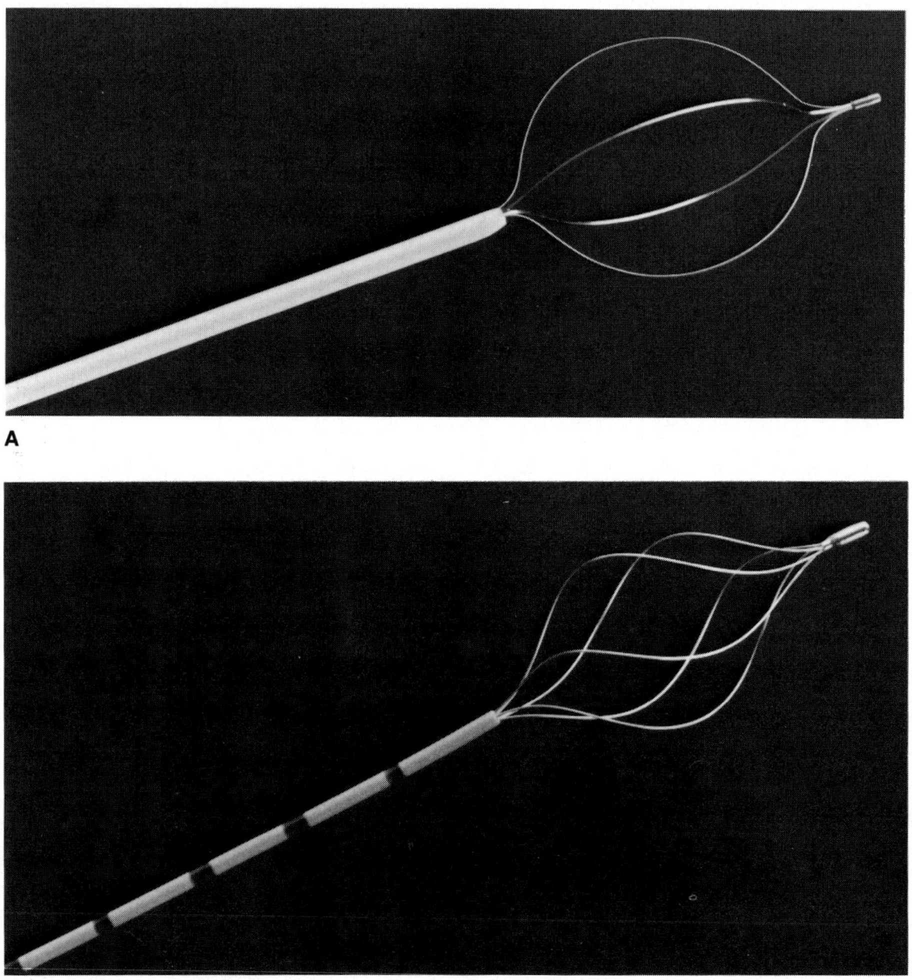

A

B

FIGURE 8–20. **A,** Flat wire stone basket. **B,** Helical stone basket. (**A** and **B** courtesy of Cook Urological.)

The art of stone basketing was greatly supported by the development of the ureteroscope. Direct vision basket extraction brought many things to light. The most obvious of these is that blind basket extraction is now rarely indicated.[7] Equally important is the realization that size limitations for the stones have been a significant consideration in the decision to use basket extraction. Despite visual guidance, the main drawback of stone basketing is that once the stone is engaged in the basket, it often cannot be disengaged. An entrapped stone basket is a significant problem. Occasionally open surgical removal is required. Technologic advances have made this problem rare.

GRASPING FORCEPS

In response to the basket's problems, mechanical grasping forceps were devised. These endoscopic forceps were already available for use in the bladder but required miniaturization for use in the ureter. Essentially two categories of grasping forceps are available. A two-prong metal forceps permits a firm grip on the stone and allows easy release if resistance is encountered during extraction (Figure 8–21). This device's major limitations are its 5F size, which precludes its use in ureteroscopes smaller than 9.5F, and its lack of flexibility, which restricts its application to rigid ureteroscopes.

The other device is a three-prong grasping forceps with a retractable sheath (Figure 8–22). This device ranges in size from 3F to 4.5F and comes in a variety of lengths, allowing use with both rigid and flexible ureteroscopes. This grasping forceps follows an old and accepted concept in endoscopic urology that the stone basket violated: that manipulation of the urinary tract should be *controlled.* The grasping forceps permits the urologist to both engage *and disengage* the stone, and thereby it clearly surpasses the ureteral stone basket.

INSTRUMENTS FOR STONE FRAGMENTATION

Ultrasonic Lithotrite

One of the first energy sources to be applied to the endoscopic fragmentation of calculi was the piezoceramic or ultrasonic shock wave generator.[8] This device incorporated high-frequency vibratory energy to generate acoustic sound waves that, when applied directly to calculi, could cause fragmentation. The device transmitted energy from the source (transducer) down a hollow metal tube (sonotrode) and achieved fragmentation when the sonotrode touched the calculus (Figure 8–23). This device was designed with a coaxial suction mechanism that enables removal of the stone fragments and resulting debris at the time of fragmentation. As a way to get rid of particles, this suction capability is obviously advantageous.

Originally designed as a large-diameter probe for percutaneous work within the renal collecting system, the ultrasonic lithotrite soon became miniaturized from approximately 10F to 5F for application within the ureter. Despite its ability not only to fragment calculi but also to remove small particles via suction, this device had one significant design limitation. Of necessity, the ultrasonic lithotrite was rigid and thus could be used only with an offset optical lens system within a rigid vehicle (nephroscope, ureteroscope). Offset lens systems do not present positional problems for intrarenal manipulation, but they are cumbersome for ureteral work. Moreover, the lithotrite can be used only within an offset ureteroscope with a minimum 5F working port. Most ureteroscopes having these requirements must be sized on the order of 11F to 12F. With the current popularity of miniaturized ureteroscopes that are 6F to 7F and flexible or semirigid, the ultrasonic lithotrite has fallen into disfavor. It nevertheless remains the preferred device for intrarenal lithotripsy because it is extremely safe, fragments stones efficiently, and removes small particles with its coaxial suction apparatus.

Electrohydraulic Lithotrite

Initially used within the confines of the bladder for fragmentation of vesical stones, the electrohydraulic lithotrite soon began to demonstrate its value compared with mechanical stone crushers (Figure 8–24).[9] This device generates a shock wave following the discharge of an electrical current across a coaxial spark gap. On contact with the surface of the stone, the expanding shock wave plasma bubble imparts its energy to break up the stone.

The electrohydraulic lithotrite fragments calculi less effectively than the ultrasonic lithotrite and also has other drawbacks. Rather than containing the debris and removing it simultaneously at the time of fragmentation as the ultrasonic lithotrite does, the electrohydraulic lithotrite disperses the fragments away from the calculus and throughout the surrounding area. Furthermore, fragment size following spark discharge of the electrohydraulic lithotrite is highly variable and unpredictable. Dispersion of fragments within the urinary bladder does not usually present a problem because these particles are often promptly discharged with voiding. However, within the confines of the renal collecting system, small particles that are retained, especially within dependent lower pole calyces, may remain there and ultimately lead to stone regrowth.

Probe size for use within the bladder and subsequently the kidney was initially designed to be

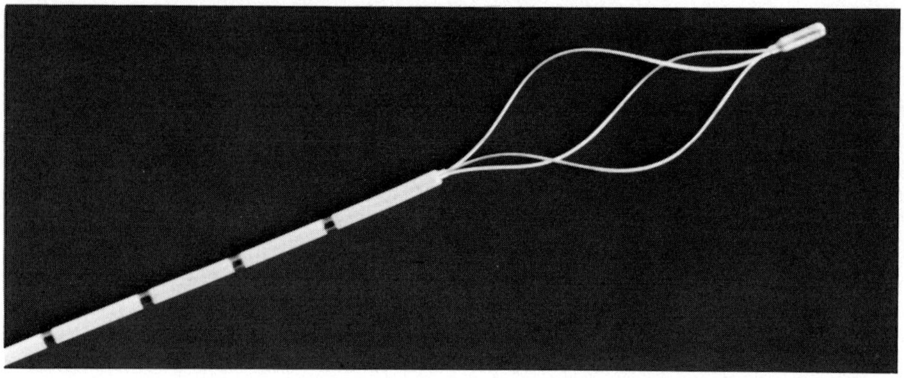

A

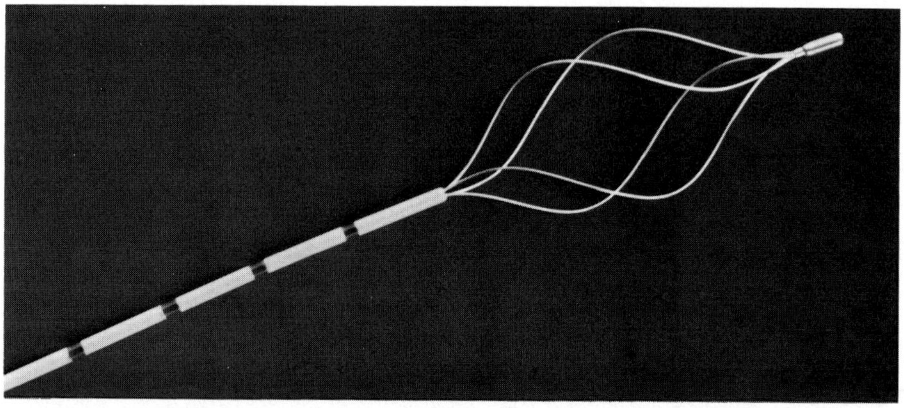

B

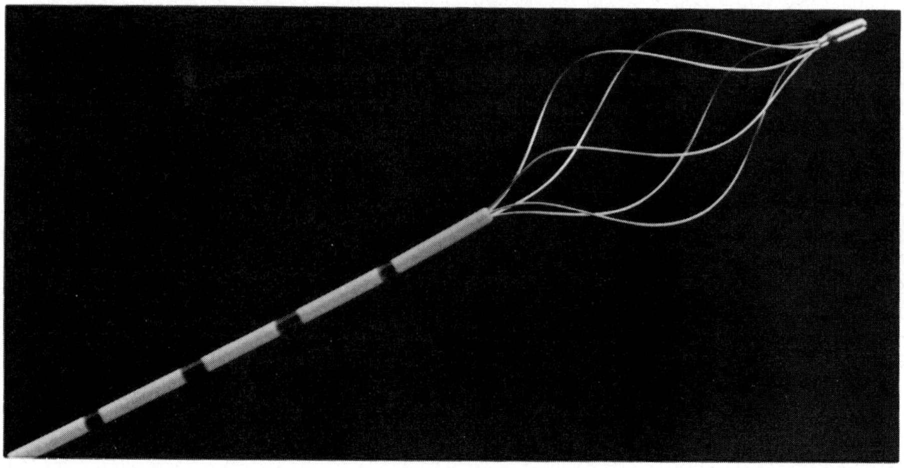

C

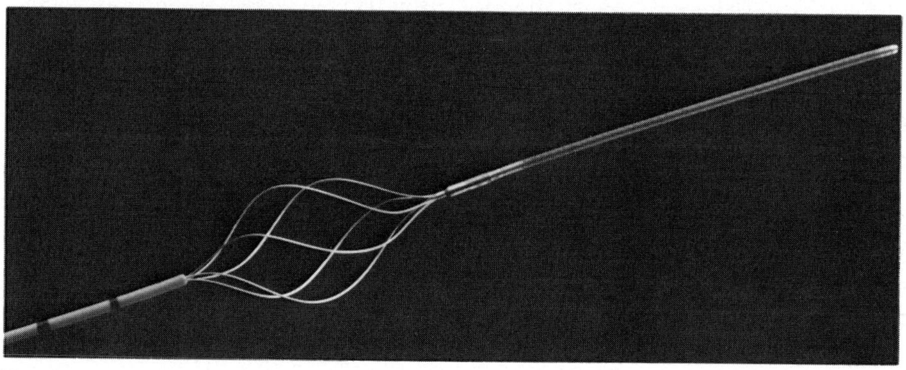

D

FIGURE 8–21. **A,** Three-wire basket. **B,** Four-wire basket. **C,** Five-wire basket, nonfiliform tip. **D,** Five-wire basket, filiform tip. (**A** to **D** courtesy of Cook Urological.)

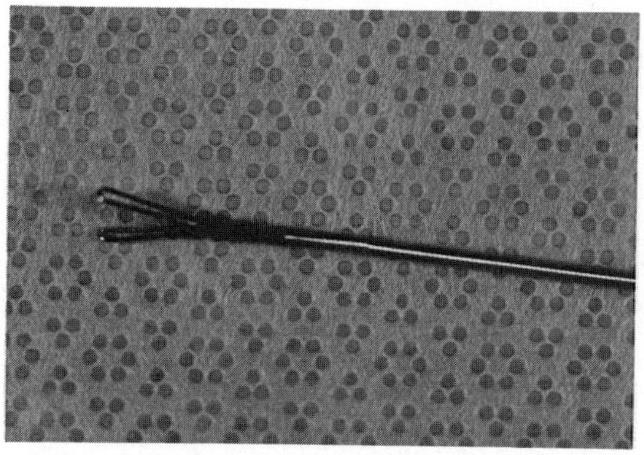

FIGURE 8–22. A 5F, two-prong metal grasping forceps. (Courtesy of Richard Wolf.)

9F (Figure 8–25). These probes were flexible and therefore did not require an offset lens delivery system. As with other devices, the 9F probe initially became downsized to 5F, which permitted its application to the treatment of ureteral calculi. Since the probe's flexibility makes it less cumbersome to manipulate than the ultrasonic lithotrite, the electrohydraulic lithotrite soon earned the cautious respect of most urologists.

The high energy output and minimally directed energy discharge of the electrohydraulic lithotrite quickly and easily caused ureteral damage. Because of the high energy discharge and heat generated within a small chamber such as the ureter, the lithotrite had to be placed precisely on the stone

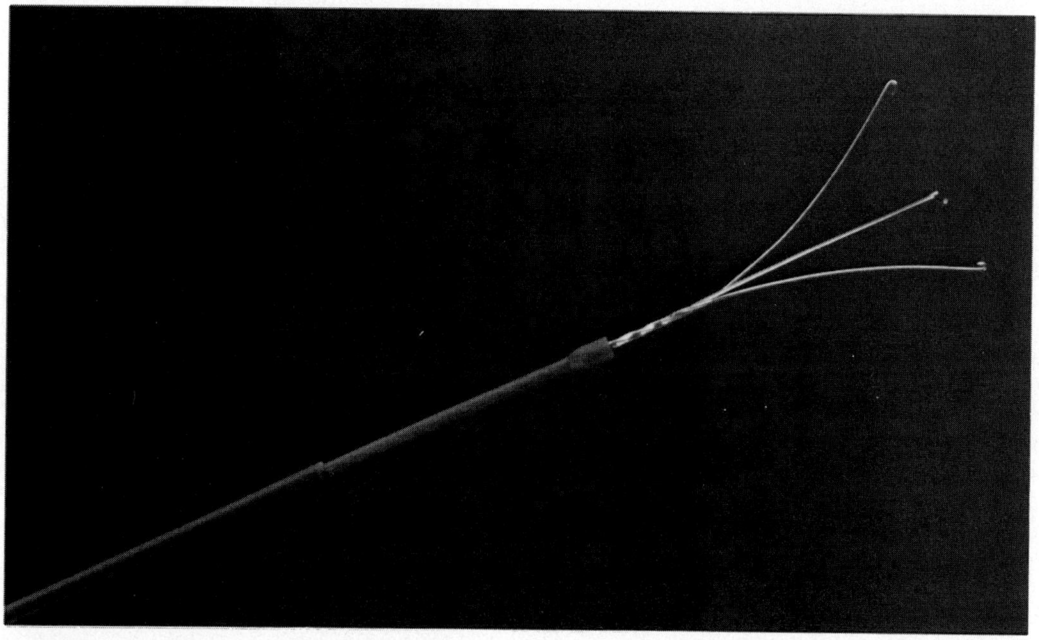

FIGURE 8–23. Three-prong, flexible, retractable sheath, wire grasping forceps. (Courtesy of Cook Urological.)

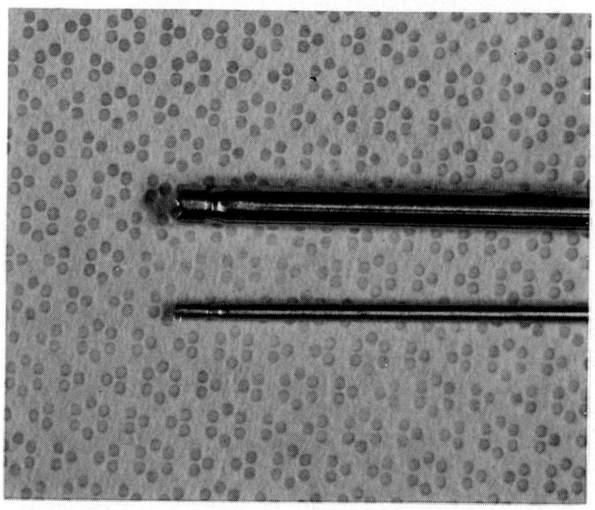

FIGURE 8–24. Ultrasonic lithotrites: 10F (nephroscopic) and 5F (ureteroscopic). (Courtesy of Karl Storz.)

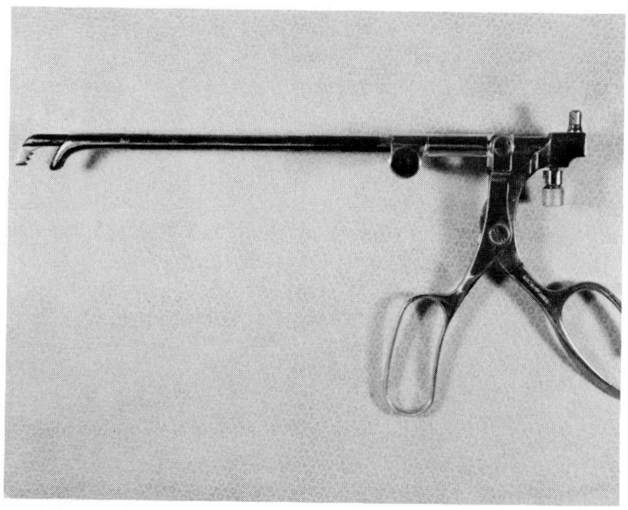

FIGURE 8–25. Direct viewing endoscopic mechanical lithotrite. (Courtesy of ACMI.)

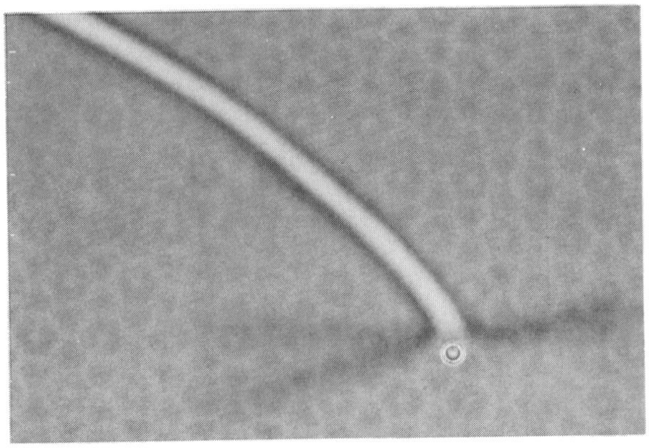

FIGURE 8–26. A 9F electrohydraulic lithotrite probe. (Courtesy of Northgate.) Note coaxial electrodes, which define the spark gap.

at the time of energy discharge. If the probe was in contact with the ureteral wall, it often resulted in ureteral perforation. Even under the best of circumstances, the shock wave energy, after being dissipated to the ureteral wall, resulted in epithelial hemorrhage from the already friable mucosa. This frequently compromised visibility within the ureter and led to premature termination of the stone removal procedure.

In an attempt to increase safety and broaden application for the potentially useful device, the probe was miniaturized further. Electrohydraulic lithotrite probes are now available in both 3F and 1.9F sizes (Figure 8–26). They appear to deliver energy comparable to that of larger probes and even demonstrate highly efficient stone fragmentation as a result of their concentrated energy density.[10] Perhaps more significant, they provide a wider margin of safety for intracorporeal lithotripsy. These smaller probes also are manufactured in a variety of lengths and thus can be used in both the rigid and the longer flexible ureterorenoscopes.

Laser Lithotrite

The most recent development in endourologically guided lithotripsy is the pulsed dye laser. This device generates a photoacoustic shock wave that safely and effectively fragments urinary tract calculi.[11] The shock wave generation modality and its delivery system demonstrate clear advantages over the previous lithotrites. The single obvious disadvantage is the cost. At approximately $250,000, the laser is as much as 50 times more expensive than other intracorporeal lithotrites. Despite this financial burden, the laser offers technologic developments that ultimately make it the safest device available for intracorporeal stone fragmentation.

The energy delivery system consists of a flexible quartz fiber that varies in size from 200 to 400 μm (Figure 8–27). This significant miniaturization in the energy delivery system has prompted further miniaturization in the vehicle delivery devices (ureteroscopes), and the laser is directly responsible for the development and manufacturing of the 6F and 7F "miniscopes." Naturally, a smaller ureteroscope means less chance for operative misadventure, ureteral perforation, and ureteral stricturing. In addition, this degree of endoscopic miniaturization has in most cases obviated the need for dilation of the ureteral orifice or the intramural ureter.

The wavelength of the laser energy is 504 nm. This wavelength is selectively absorbed by pigments in most ureteral calculi and permits an efficient absorption of the photoacoustic shock wave. Furthermore, the energy at this wavelength is minimally absorbed by the surrounding tissue, and thus this device is extremely safe for application within the ureter.

Stone fragmentation by laser energy at this wavelength usually results in minute (1 to 3 mm)

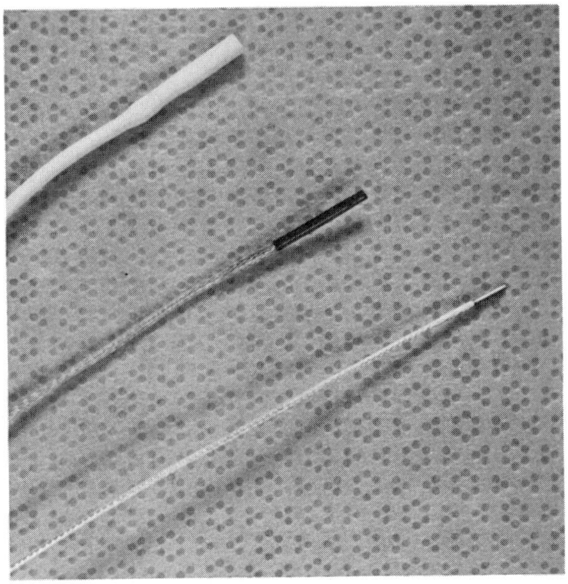

A

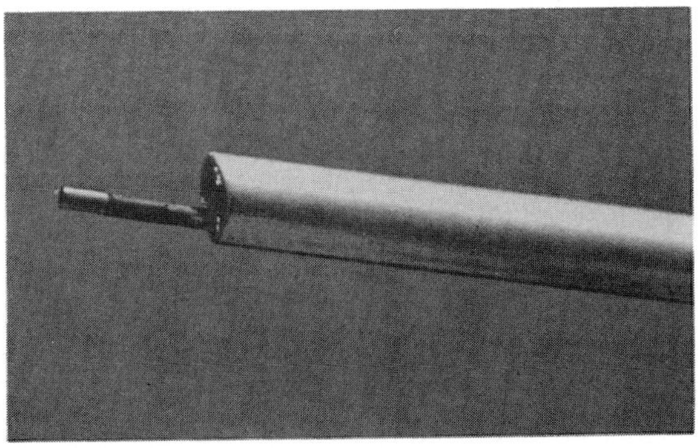

B

FIGURE 8–27. A, Electrohydraulic lithotrite probes: 9F, 5F, and 3F. (Courtesy of Circon.) B, New, 1.9F electrohydraulic probe (courtesy of Northgate), being used through a 6.2F ureteroscope (courtesy of Circon).

particles, and the fragments disperse from the main body of the stone at a low velocity. Obviously, such a small-diameter fiber (200 to 400 μm) is easily adapted for use in flexible ureteroscopes. Thus this device, in combination with the small-diameter flexible ureteroscopes, has permitted relatively safe venture into the proximal ureter.

Although in the United States the pulsed dye laser is the only laser approved for the treatment of urinary calculi, two other lasers are being investigated outside the United States. The neodymium:yttrium aluminum garnet (Nd:YAG) laser, a solid-state laser that for some time has been used in urology for the thermal destruction of tumors, has been Q-switched and thus adapted for pulsed application.[12] The other laser being investigated for treatment of urinary calculi is the alexandrite laser.[13] Whether either will provide any distinct advantage over the currently well accepted pulsed dye laser remains to be seen. Nevertheless, continued investigation into intracorporeal shock wave generation will ultimately define the most efficient wavelength for fragmentation of stones, the most effective level of energy density, and the safest delivery system.

STENTS

Although a number of devices theoretically allow access to a stone within the ureter, technical factors sometimes prevent access. Ureteral calculi usually elicit a caustic reaction within the ureter, which results in significant mucosal edema and ureteral spasm. As previously described, controlled access must be achieved before any endoscopic ureteral manipulation. If a guidewire can be passed by the calculus, the ureteroscope must be passed up to the stone. Although balloon dilation, minute-diameter rigid and flexible ureteroscopes, and a variety of lithotrites are now available, mucosal edema is often such that manipulation of the stone *should* not be attempted. Judgment dictates bypassing the stone (and relieving obstruction), allowing the mucosal edema and ureteral spasm to abate, and returning later to remove the stone.

Before the advent of ureteroscopes, urinary stones presented difficult problems. Endoscopy (cystoscopy) was performed for the purpose of basket extraction of stones. If the calculus could not be extracted or if the basket could not be passed up by the stone, the urologist at least wanted to unobstruct the kidney. To this end the urologist attempted to pass a ureteral catheter, which by its design was left in an externalized position. These catheters were originally designed for retrograde instillation of contrast material for pyelography. Nevertheless, their dual-purpose nature permitted their use for drainage of an obstructed kidney. The shortcoming of ureteral catheters was that they committed the urologist to intervention in the very short term and also committed the patient to both a Foley catheter and a hospital stay until further intervention (usually a ureterolithotomy) could be accomplished. Another significant drawback was that these catheters were subject to dislodgment by the careless patient, nurse, or x-ray technician.

Fortunately for all those involved, development of biocompatible materials allowed manufacturers to devise catheters that could safely remain inside patients for months.[14] This material was then fashioned to have a "positional memory." With the combination of these features, the double J or pigtail stent was manufactured. These relatively biocompatible, self-retaining, internalizable stents have revolutionized the management of both stone disease and ureteral obstruction. Over the past few years a wide variety of stents have been developed (Figure 8–28). The stents, like other technical devices, come in various lengths and French sizes and are made of different biocompatible materials. Stent selection is often a matter of the physician's preference and not a result of a specific difference in a stent's features. Thus, when lithotripsy or extraction of a ureteral stone is impossible or unsafe, a stent can be passed alongside the stone to unobstruct the kidney. The patient can subsequently be discharged and return when the edema and the ureteral spasm have resolved.

Many other clinical procedures have been either facilitated or made possible by the internalizable, self-retaining stent. These include the internalized drainage of an obstructed kidney resulting from malignancy, safe extracorporeal lithotripsy of large renal calculi (Steinstrasse prevention), difficult pyeloplasties, ureteral reimplantations, renal transplantation, and surgery on solitary kidneys, to name a few. The vast majority of stents employed

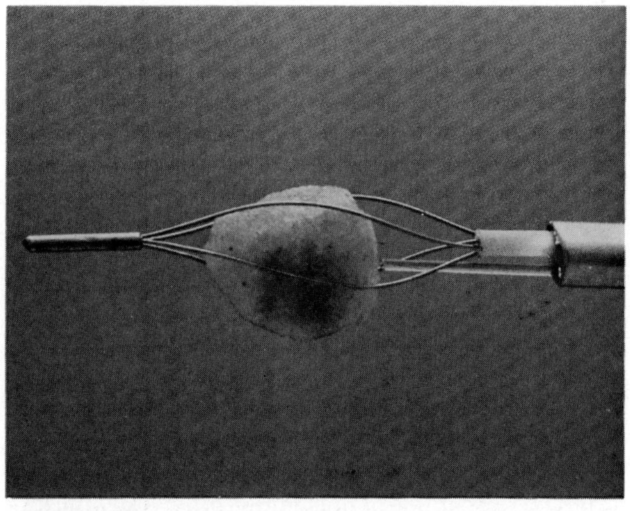

FIGURE 8–28. A 200 μm laser light guide (courtesy of Candela Laser) being used to fragment a stone within a four-prong wire basket, with a 6.2F ureteroscopic delivery vehicle (courtesy of Circon).

in urologic practice are put in place endoscopically. Of these, most are passed coaxially over a preplaced ureteral guidewire. If a guidewire cannot be passed up the ureter and into the renal collecting system, the stent cannot be positioned. In the case of ureteral obstruction from a stone or from a malignant process, the kidney must still be drained. Using similar biocompatible materials, direct drainage of the kidney can also be achieved.

NEPHROSTOMY TUBES

Before the revolution of the 1970s and 1980s in the management of stone disease, tubes placed within the urinary tract were considered an "evil." During the 1960s and early 1970s much of the material used for catheters, stents, and tubes was highly irritating and lithogenic. Long-term indwelling Foley catheters and suprapubic tubes have always been a "necessary evil" when indicated for patient management. During this time Foley and Malecot catheters were used to drain the kidney during the period surrounding open renal surgery. When used for temporary drainage, these nephrostomy tubes were seldom considered a problem. When left indwelling for longer periods, they quickly became a source of chronic infection, stricturing, and even stone formation. Furthermore, they required an open surgical approach to be placed properly.

As much of the equipment discussed in previous sections was developed, some of the access devices were applied to the placement of nephrostomy tubes. With the concurrent refinement in fluoroscopic and ultrasonic technology, imaging of the kidney (and the dilated collecting system) vastly improved. This ultimately increased confidence in direct needle puncture of the renal collecting system.[15] Fine, long needles could be placed percutaneously into the renal pelvis, the system opacified with contrast material, and selective calyceal puncture performed. Once inside the collecting system, a floppy-tipped guidewire served as a bridge between access to and therapeutic intervention in the kidney. With a guidewire passed through the hollow lumen of the needle, access to the kidney was secure and various manipulations became possible.

As biocompatible materials became more widespread, nephrostomy tubes were manufactured along design patterns similar to the self-retaining, internalized stents. These newly designed nephrostomy tubes, which were manufactured in a variety of French sizes, afforded distinct advantages over the prior generation of nephrostomy tubes (Figure 8–29). They could be placed percutaneously and thus did not require open surgery, and they were smaller, were made of biocompatible materials, and had self-retaining memory coils to prevent dislodgment. It was not difficult to predict that the concept

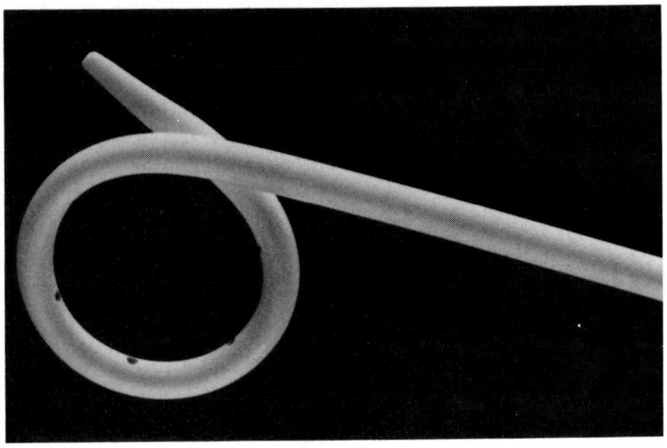

A

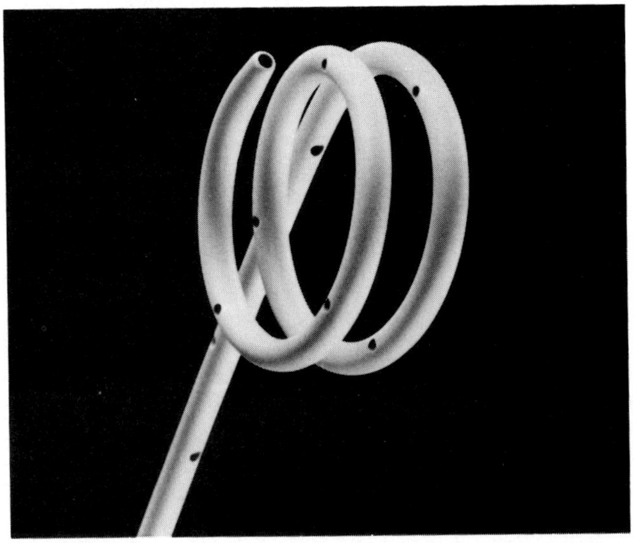

B

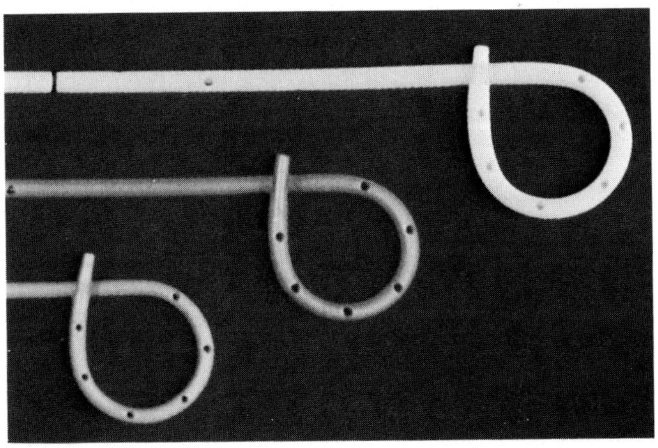

C

FIGURE 8–29. **A,** Single coil and **B,** multiple coil self-retaining indwelling ureteral stents (courtesy of Cook Urological). **C,** These are available in a variety of materials and French sizes.

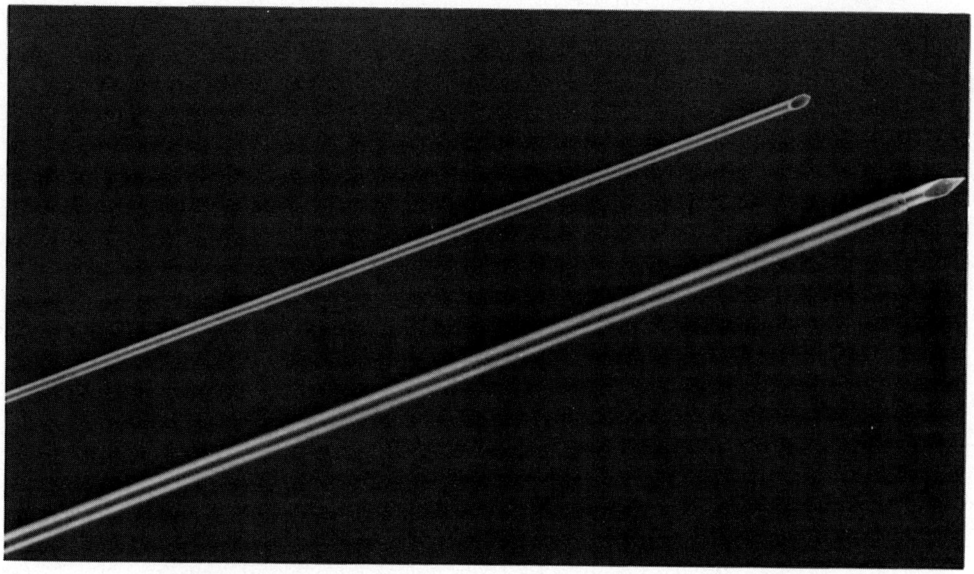

FIGURE 8–30. Percutaneous, hollow core needles for renal access.

of percutaneous renal access would blossom beyond that of simple nephrostomy tube placement. Clearly the establishment of "bigger access" to the kidney was required.

TRACT DILATORS

The development of percutaneous tract (skin to kidney) dilation closely paralleled that of ureteral dilation for endoscopic access. First were the coaxial metal facial dilators (Figure 8–30). Stout and effective, they earned physicians' wary respect. All percutaneous tract dilation should take place over a working guidewire, and caution dictates placement of a second guidewire, which can be used as a safety wire should the working wire become dislodged. The Amplatz dilation set quickly became the most common apparatus for tract dilation (Figure 8–31).[16] These tapered-end dilators come in sizes ranging from approximately 10F to 30F. They step up in size on the order of 2F per dilator. The sets come packaged with working sheaths (Figure 8–32) that fit coaxially over the dilator and are the conduits through which PCNL procedures are performed. Within the past few years a less labor-intensive and more rapid tract dilation system has been devised. It centers on a large, high-pressure balloon dilator (Figure 8–33). Placed coaxially over a working guidewire, this balloon can rapidly dilate the percutaneous tract up to approximately 30F. The balloon usually requires inflation with the Le-

FIGURE 8–31. Self-retaining percutaneous nephrostomy catheter *(center)* with accessory access and placement devices. (*Left to right:* Floppy-tipped guidewire, access needles, nephrostomy tube, drainage tube, dilation catheter.) (Courtesy of Cook Urological.)

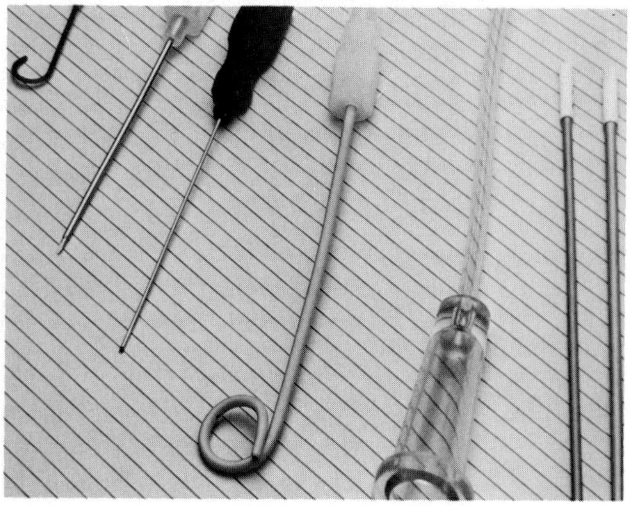

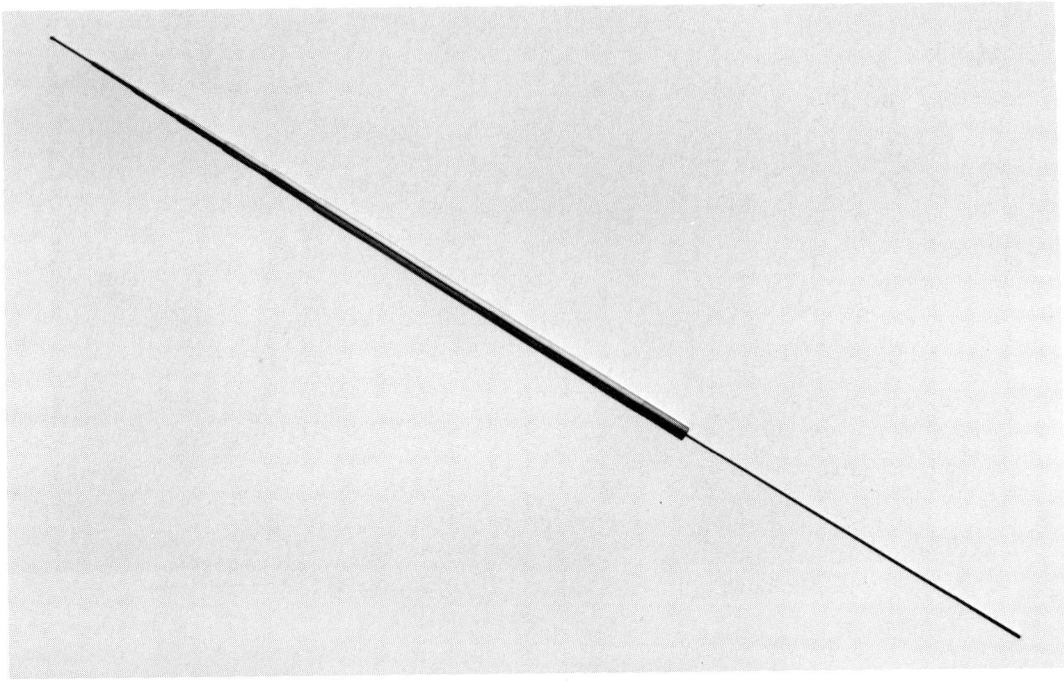

FIGURE 8–32. Coaxial metal fascial dilators. (Courtesy of Karl Storz.)

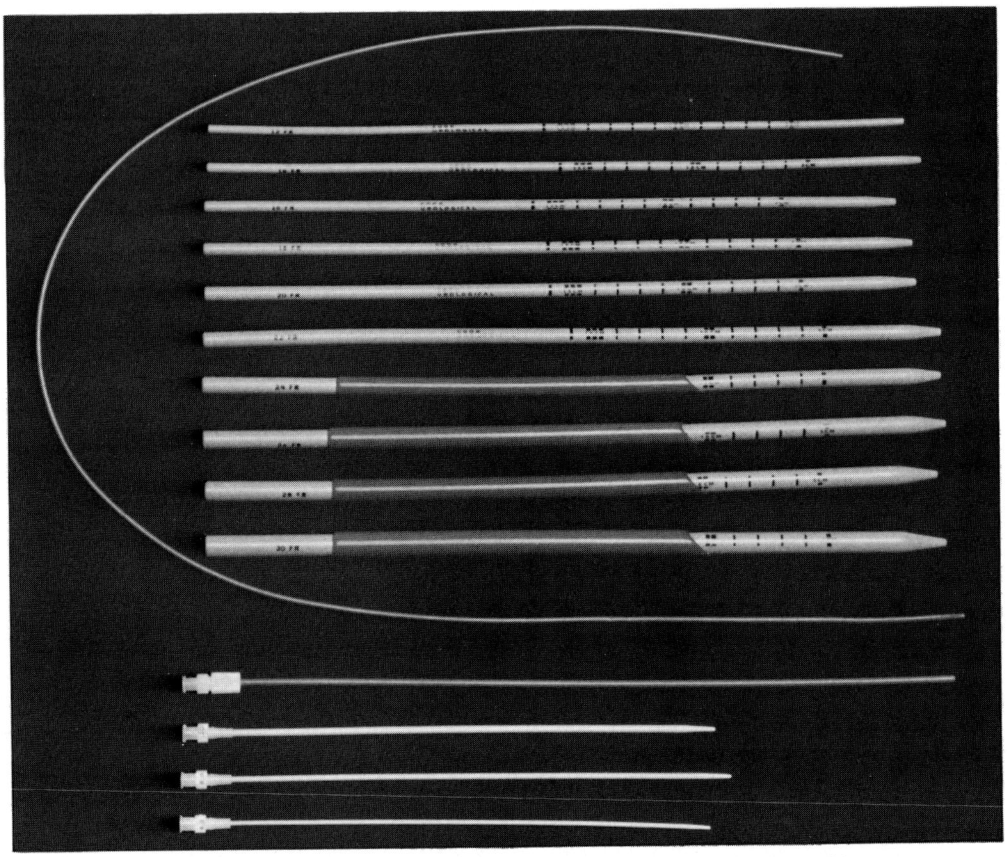

FIGURE 8–33. Amplatz dilation set. (Courtesy of Cook Urological.)

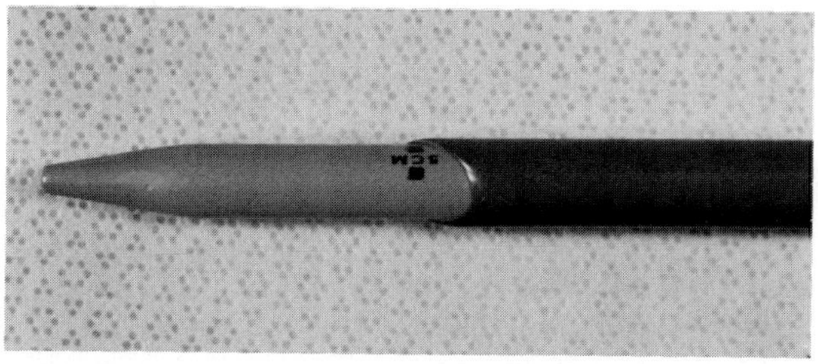

FIGURE 8–34. A 30F Amplatz dilator with coaxial outer working sheath.

vine-type syringe (Figure 8–34). Once the tract has been sufficiently dilated with the balloon, the final stages of dilation and sheath placement are performed, usually with the Amplatz system.

REFERENCES

1. Redman JF: Anatomy of the genitourinary system. In Gillenwater JT, Grayback JT, Howards SS, Duckett JW (eds): Adult and pediatric urology. Chicago: Mosby–Year Book, 1991, pp 30-33.
2. Segura JW, Patterson DE, LeRoy AJ, et al: Percutaneous lithotripsy. J Urol 130:1051-1054, 1983.
3. Bagley DH: Endoscopic diagnosis and treatment of urinary calculi with the ureteropyeloscope. In Harrison LH, Kandel LB, (eds): Techniques in urologic stone surgery. New York: Futura, 1986, Ch 3, pp 33-51.
4. Newman RC, Hunter PT, Hawkins IF, Finlayson, B: A general ureteral dilator sheathing system. Urology, March 1985, p 287.
5. Perez-Castro E: Ureteromat, method to facilitate ureterorenoscopy and avoid dilatation. In The urologic clinics of North America, update on endourology. Philadelphia: WB Saunders, 1988, pp 315-321.
6. Drach GW: Transurethral ureteral stone manipulation. In Harrison LH, Kandel LB (eds): Techniques in urologic stone surgery. New York: Futura, 1986, Ch 2, pp 17-31.
7. Abdelsayed M, Onal E, Wax SH: Avulsion of the ureter caused by stone basket manipulation. J Urol 117:868-870, 1977.
8. Marberger M: Physical dissolution of calculi. In Harrison LH, Kandel LB, (eds): Techniques in urologic stone surgery. New York: Futura, 1986, Ch 6, pp 121-151.
9. Mitchell ME, Kerr WS Jr: Experience with the electrohydraulic disintegrator. J Urol 117:159-160, 1977.
10. Murray SC, Dretler SP: An in-vitro comparison study of electrohydraulic (EHL) and laser lithotripsy [Abstract 404]. J Urol No. 4, Part 2. Presented at AUA Eighty-Third Annual Meeting, June 3-7, 1988.
11. Watson GM, Wickham JEA: Initial experience with a pulsed dye laser for ureteric calculi. Lancet 1:1357-1358, 1986.
12. Hofstetter A: The action of the pulsed Nd-YAG laserlithotripsy. Presented at the First International Workshop and Symposium on New Urological Technology, Sept 6-9, 1989, Leuven, Belgium.
13. Schildberg FW, Wenk H: Laser fragmentation. Presented at the Third International Symposium on Biliary Lithotripsy, Sept 13-15, 1909, Munich, West Germany.
14. Mardis HK, Kroeger RM: Ureteral stents. In The urologic clinics of North America, endourology update. Philadelphia: WB Saunders, 1988, pp 471-479.
15. Goodwin WE, Casey WC, Woolf W: Percutaneous trocar (needle) nephrostomy in hydronephrosis. JAMA 157:891-894, 1955.
16. Dyer RB: Percutaneous nephrostomy. In Harrison LH, Kandel LB (eds): Techniques in urologic stone surgery. New York: Futura, 1986, Ch 4, pp 53-104.
17. Lee LM, Goldenberg SL, Chan N: Mechanism of balloon dilatation of the prostate: pathologic study on organ donors [Abstract 378]. J Urol, vol 143, no 4, Presented at AUA Eighty-Fifth Annual Meeting, May 13-17, 1990.
18. Goldenberg SL, Perez-Marrero R, Lee LL, Emerson L: Endoscopic balloon dilatation of the prostate (EBDP) [Abstract 379]. J Urol, vol 143, no 4. Presented at AUA Eighty-Fifth Annual Meeting, May 13-17, 1990.
19. Denstedt JD, Chin JL, Grignon DJ, et al: Histopathologic study of changes induced by extensive balloon dilation of the prostate to 75F [Abstract 376]. J Urol vol 143, no 4. Presented at AUA Eighty-Fifth Annual Meeting, May 13-17, 1990.
20. Dowd JB, Smith JJ: Balloon dilation of the prostate without imaging: comparison with transuretheral resection of the prostate [Abstract 375]. J Urol vol 143, no 4. Presented at AUA Eighty-Fifth Annual Meeting, May 13-17, 1990.

CHAPTER 9

PERCUTANEOUS TECHNIQUES

JAY A. MOTOLA and ARTHUR D. SMITH

Over the last 20 years the approach to calculous disease of the kidney has undergone drastic change. Whereas most stones were once treated with a formal open procedure, nephrolithotomy and pyelolithotomy are rarely performed today. In the late 1970s endourologic procedures were developed for the treatment of renal calculi. This technology has since been refined, and endourologic techniques have been applied to pathologic entities of the genitourinary tract other than stone disease.

To some, the development of extracorporeal shock wave lithotripsy (ESWL) in the 1980s seemed to signal the end of the still new percutaneous stone procedures. However, percutaneous nephrolithotomy is still indicated for the management of a variety of conditions, including large cystine stones, large renal pelvic calculi, staghorn calculi, and stones that coexist with an underlying ureteropelvic junction obstruction, calyceal diverticulum, or infundibular stenosis.[1] Moreover, after the technique of accessing the kidney through a percutaneous nephrostomy has been mastered, numerous other endourologic procedures can be performed. Various diagnostic studies, including endoscopic examination and biopsy of lesions and filling defects and urodynamic studies, are possible. Endorenal surgery can now be performed safely to relieve ureteropelvic junction obstructions, resect transitional cell carcinomas of the renal pelvis, and treat other pathologic conditions of the kidney. The nephrostomy tract can also be used for chemolysis of various stones or for the administration of chemotherapeutic agents such as for the treatment of fungal infections or cancer.

This chapter reviews the applications of percutaneous manipulations of the kidney. After the principles of the creation of a percutaneous tract are established, the various percutaneous procedures are discussed.

PERFORMING A PERCUTANEOUS NEPHROSTOMY

> "The percutaneous nephrostomy tract must be regarded as a conduit to the upper urinary tract much the same way that the urethra is a conduit to the bladder."[2]

When first performed by Goodwin and associates in 1955, the percutaneous nephrostomy was intended simply for the decompression of a hydronephrotic kidney.[3] Since that time the technique has evolved into a crucial investigative tool and a method for diagnosing and treating renal pelvic and ureteral diseases. For these diagnostic or therapeutic procedures to be successful, however, a proper nephrostomy tract must first be created.

The patient should undergo preoperative evaluation that includes routine laboratory studies, a coagulation profile, a urinalysis, and a urine culture. An underlying coagulopathy represents the only absolute contraindication to this procedure and so must be corrected preoperatively.

Patients scheduled for percutaneous procedures should also have blood cross-matched. This is particularly important before a procedure on a pyelonephritic kidney that contains a stone, since such a kidney is more susceptible to bleeding because of the underlying inflammatory and infectious processes. At our institution patients are routinely cross-matched for 2 units of packed red blood cells. In our experience of more than 2000 percutaneous stone extractions, the transfusion rate has been nearly 10%. The use of autologous transfusions and designated donor blood units is preferred by patients today, and most patients with large stones routinely make arrangements with the blood bank. We have found intraoperative blood salvage and retransfusion (Cell Saver, Haemonetics, Corp.,

Braintree, Mass.) during endourologic procedures to be safe and useful, and it decreases the postoperative transfusion needs of the patients.

A positive urine culture represents only a relative contraindication to the procedure. Certainly, emergency percutaneous nephrostomies should be performed in patients manifesting severe systemic signs or infected stones, since the procedure may be lifesaving. However, elective therapies such as stone removal should be deferred until the appropriate antibiotics have been administered.

Preoperative intravenous urograms should be available at the time of the procedure so that the surgeon can select the appropriate nephrostomy site and assess the extent of obstruction. An abdominal film should be obtained the day of surgery or before the day of surgery to avoid inappropriate procedures in cases of stone passage or stone migration. Before the procedure, broad-spectrum parenteral antibiotics are always administered. The results of the urine culture must be considered when selecting these drugs. Aminoglycoside coverage is administered to patients with staghorn calculi.

Anatomic Considerations

Renal Relations

The surgeon must understand the three-dimensional anatomy of the retroperitoneum before performing any percutaneous procedures on the kidney. The kidneys are lateral to the twelfth thoracic vertebra superiorly and the second or third lumbar vertebra inferiorly. The right kidney is approximately 2 cm lower than the left kidney because of the caudal displacement of the right kidney by the right lobe of the liver. The kidneys are not fixed in location: they move during breathing and may descend as much as 2.5 cm with a change from the supine to the erect position.[4] Body habitus also has some bearing on location, with tall, thin individuals tending to have their kidneys lower lying than short, stout individuals.

The axes of the kidneys are 13 degrees off the sagittal plane, with the upper poles tilted slightly toward each other. The medial borders of the kidneys are tilted slightly forward on the edges of the psoas muscles. The renal hilum is in the middle of the medial surface of each kidney. The renal vein, renal artery, renal pelvis, nerves, and lymphatics pass through the hilum.

When a transparenchymal puncture is performed, the surrounding structures of the kidney should be considered, since inappropriate needle passage may result in a puncture of any of these structures (Figure 9–1). The anterior relations of the left kidney include the left adrenal gland, spleen, stomach, and left side of the colon. The jejunum and tail of the pancreas are located medially. The right kidney is related to the right adrenal gland, the right side of the colon, and the liver. The duodenum is situated medially.

The posterior anatomic relations are similar for both kidneys and are not vital structures such as those located anteriorly. The quadratus lumborum muscle is medial to both kidneys, and the psoas muscle provides support to the lower aspects. The erector spinae muscles are located posteriorly. The internal and external oblique and transversus abdominis muscles are located laterally. The postero-inferior serratus and latissimus dorsi muscles are located posterolaterally.

To avoid causing the complications of pneumothorax or hydrothorax when performing a percutaneous nephrostomy, the surgeon must consider the close proximity of the kidneys to the contents of the thoracic cavity. Both kidneys have a superior relation to the diaphragm; that of the right kidney is less significant because of its lower position. One half of the right kidney and two thirds of the left kidney lie above the twelfth rib. The kidneys are separated from the lungs by the diaphragm, which

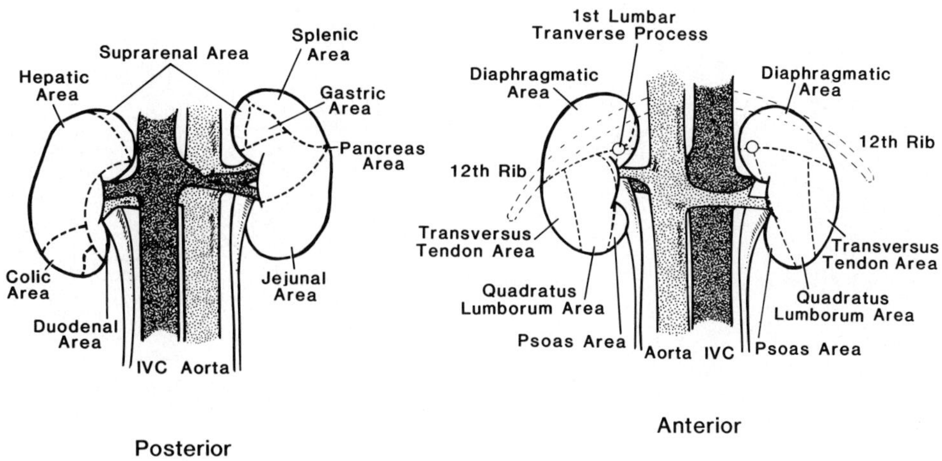

FIGURE 9–1. Anterior and posterior renal anatomic relations.

attaches to the inner aspect of the twelfth rib. The pleural reflection is located posteriorly at the level of the twelfth rib and in the midaxillary line at the level of the tenth rib. The inferior aspect of the lung parenchyma is located posteromedially at the eleventh costovertebral joint, at the tenth rib in the scapular line, and at the eighth rib in the midaxillary line.

These anatomic relations have great clinical relevance. The ideal percutaneous puncture is performed beneath the twelfth rib because a puncture over the twelfth rib may violate the pleura and the diaphragm. Stones often are in upper pole calyces, which are above the twelfth rib. The placement of an intercostal nephrostomy tract facilitates treatment of upper pole stones, but this access is associated with a higher morbidity rate. An approximately 12% serious complication rate has been reported with an intercostal approach, with most of the problems related to crossing the pleural space.[5,6]

The superior calyces can be approached safely by a recently described endourologic technique.[7] An Amplatz sheath placed through a central or lower pole calyx can be pushed caudally while the descent of the kidney is monitored fluoroscopically. After this maneuver has been performed, an 18-gauge TLA (translumbar angiography) needle is passed through the initial skin puncture, and a Y tract is created with the original nephrostomy tract for safe access to the upper pole (Figure 9–2). We have used this technique in 25 patients and have had no com-

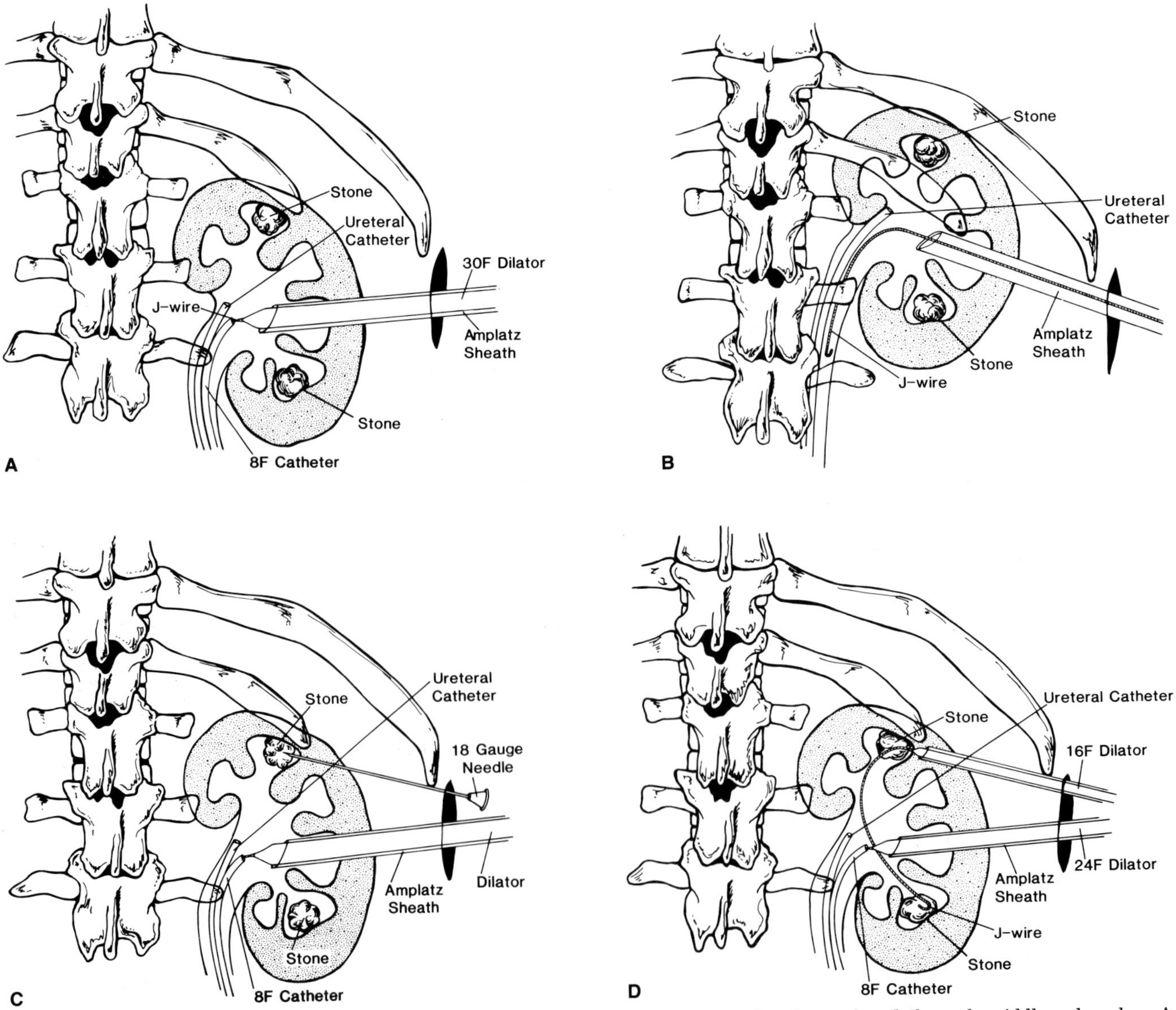

FIGURE 9–2. **A,** Superior calyx stone and lower calyx stone. Nephrostomy tract has been placed through middle pole calyx. A ureteral catheter and guidewire are in position across the ureteropelvic junction. **B,** Amplatz sheath and dilator being pushed caudally to cause the descent of upper pole calyx beneath the twelfth rib. **C,** Y tract being created with a TLA needle to access the superior calyx. **D,** Superior calyx nephrostomy tract being dilated beneath the level of the twelfth rib as a 24F Amplatz sheath and dilator provides caudal displacement of the kidney. (From Karlin GS, Smith AD: J Urol 142:774, 1989. Used by permission.)

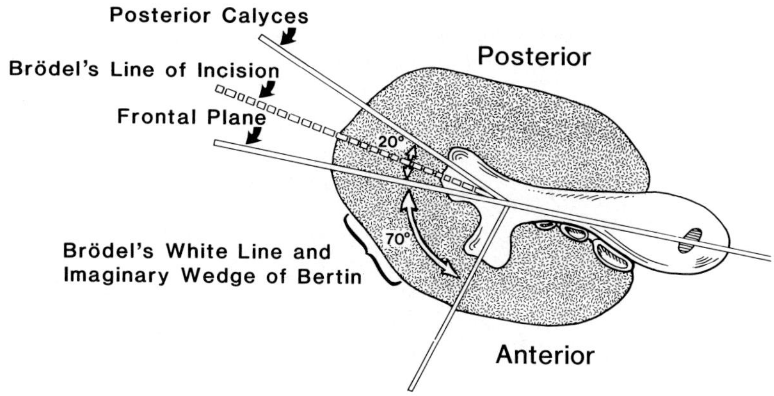

FIGURE 9–3. Angulation of anterior and posterior calyces and Brödel's avascular line of incision.

plications. It is ideal when percutaneous stone extraction requires access from a middle and an upper pole calyx.

Intrarenal Anatomy

The most vital anatomic concept for successful endourologic instrumentation is that of the intrarenal anatomy. Marked interindividual variation is encountered. The kidney has 4 to 28 fused but anatomically separate lobes, each composed of a central cone-shaped mass of medullary tissue surrounded by cortical tissue except at the apex.[8] The apex of this conical tissue is the papilla, and each invaginates a cup-shaped minor calyx. The minor calyces join to form two or three major divisions of the renal pelvis, the major calyces, which then join to form the renal pelvis.

The configuration of the calyceal system and renal pelvis also exhibits great variability, and several models have been proposed to help explain it. Between 4 and 12 calyces (average 8) are found in the classic renal pelvis. In a description of calyceal anatomy it is best to regard the anterior calyces as being seen end-on radiographically and the posterior calyces side-on. A computerized tomographic (CT) study of the calyceal position has revealed that the anterior calyces tend to be located more laterally than the posterior calyces (Hodson model).[9] These findings place the anterior calyces 70 degrees and the posterior calyces 20 degrees from the coronal plane. Proper positioning of the patient in a prone semioblique position with the patient's body rotated 30 degrees from the table surface (or rotating the C-arm 30 degrees) places the posterior calyces, especially the lowest one, to lie tangentially with the surgeon's view.

Blood Supply

One last anatomic consideration is the blood supply to the kidney. The main renal artery splits into a large anterior branch and a smaller posterior branch. This smaller branch passes posterior to the renal pelvis and has only one segmental artery. The anterior branch splits into four segmental arteries: an apical, two anterior, and a basilar vessel. The anterior vessels supply the anterior aspect, the apical vessel the superior aspect, and the basilar vessel the inferior segment of the kidney. These segmental vessels divide into interlobar arteries, the second-order branches of the renal artery, which may be paired. The pairs develop at the base of each major calyx, then separate and course toward the papilla along opposite margins of the major calyx. These vessels divide once again into transmedullary vessels, the third-order branches of the renal artery, and then enter the parenchyma. The transmedullary vessels are also paired. They traverse the medulla and form the arcuate vessels at the renal cortex.

Brodel first described the white line on the anterolateral surface of the kidney that overlies the column of Bertin separating the lobes in the middle of the kidney into anterior and posterior regions. This white line is hypervascular and must be avoided during a percutaneous nephrostomy.[10] In 70% of patients, Brodel's avascular plane (a bloodless line of incision) is located approximately 1 to 2 cm posterior to the lateral margin of the kidney (Figure 9–3). Proper patient positioning and manipulation of the fluoroscopic C-arm bring the posterior calyces into the proper position to allow a safe puncture lateral to the thick paraspinal muscles at a 20- to 30-degree angle through Brodel's avascular plane.

Antegrade Creation of the Nephrostomy Tract

Ureteral Catheter Use

Although its use is optional, the placement of an open-ended ureteral catheter retrograde under fluoroscopic guidance on the affected side facilitates the creation of the nephrostomy tract. Contrast medium can be injected through the catheter to opacify and distend the renal collecting system. The catheter also has other advantages. For example, it is easily seen fluoroscopically, allowing easy confirmation of the site of the problem before insertion of the needle. The catheter also can be used to push

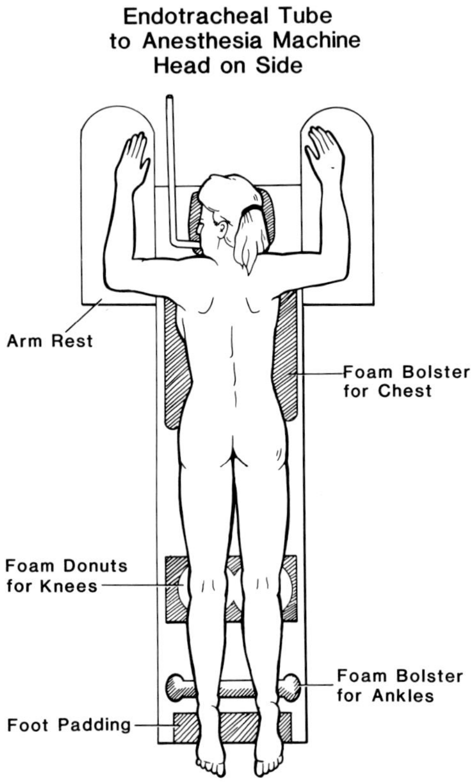

FIGURE 9–4. Patient positioning for percutaneous renal procedures.

a stone toward the renal pelvis and to block the antegrade migration of other stones. The passage of a guidewire through the external meatus, which is needed to position some nephrostomy tubes or stents, is more easily accomplished with a ureteral catheter in place.

Positioning and Draping

After completion of the cystoscopic procedure, intravenous extension tubing should be attached to the ureteral catheter to allow injection of contrast medium during the procedure. The patient is then taken out of the dorsal lithotomy position and placed prone on the operating table, which should have a radiolucent middle section to allow the use of a C-arm with fluoroscopy (Figure 9–4). Foam bolsters should be placed beneath the patient bilaterally from the shoulders to the iliac crest to elevate the chest wall off the operating table and so permit its free movement for ventilation. Foam pads also are needed to protect potential sites of pressure sores during the procedure, such as the knees and anterior aspects of the ankles. The skin of the flank is then prepared. Cleansing the skin with alcohol after it has been prepared with povidone solution is useful because this helps the surgical drapes adhere to the patient. We use an endourology drape (Surgikos) with a side pouch that collects the overflow of the irrigating solution. The pouch has a valve on the bottom that is attached to suction, which helps to keep the patient and operating room dry. The outlet valve also permits the connection of an autologous blood recovery system. Alternatively, a craniotomy sheet can be used to drape the patient.

Puncture

A variety of techniques are used to localize the collecting system. In the operating room, fluoroscopic guidance is preferable. CT scanning, ultrasonography, intravenous administration of contrast medium, and blind puncture of the collecting system are alternative methods.

In our procedures contrast medium is injected through the ureteral catheter to opacify the collecting system for fluoroscopy. The fluoroscope C-arm is rotated 20 to 30 degrees toward the operator (Figure 9–5). This places the angle of the C-arm in the same central posterior plane of the kidney and allows "down the barrel imaging." A posterolateral percutaneous approach with an 18-gauge TLA needle is used to puncture the chosen calyx; this approach along the margin of the kidney approximates the avascular line of Brodel, encroaching on the infundibulum as laterally as possible. Ideally a posterior calyx of the lower pole or middle region is punctured, since this approach minimizes bleeding. Direct punctures of the renal pelvis or upper pole should be avoided because the incidence of vascular injury is greatest when this approach is used.[11] Puncture of anteriorly located calyces is undesirable because of their proximity to the spleen and liver, a sharper angle of entry onto the pelvis, and a greater intraparenchymal distance that must be spanned.

With the C-arm in position the TLA needle is advanced approximately 5 to 8 cm into the desired

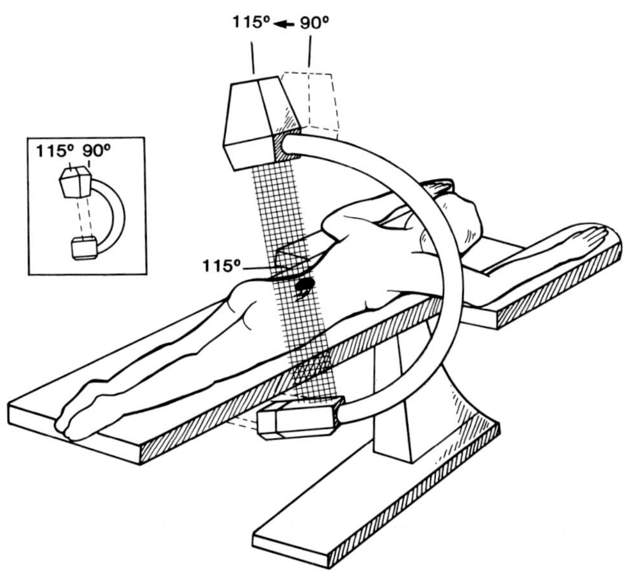

FIGURE 9–5. C-arm positioned so that the axis of the fluoroscope approximates the avascular line of Brodel.

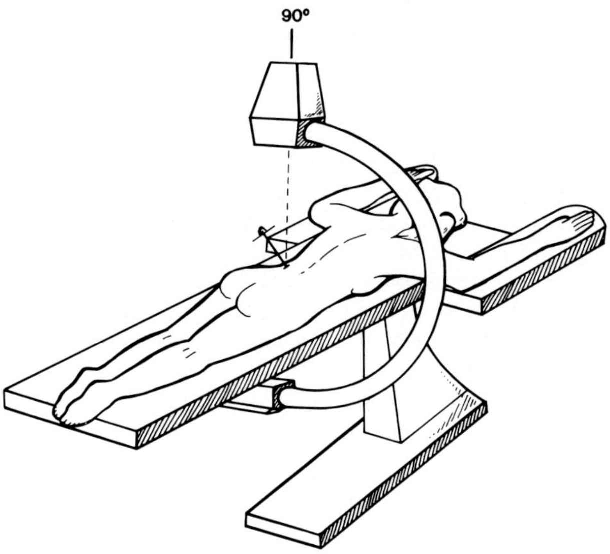

FIGURE 9–6. C-arm positioning after the collecting system is accessed to assess depth of penetration.

calyx. The fluoroscopic image reveals an end-on view of the collecting system. The depth of penetration is assessed by rotation of the C-arm back to 90 degrees, providing a parallax image (Figure 9–6). The needle is inserted further until it enters the renal collecting system. As it is advanced, resistance to the needle changes twice. The first change represents the needle passing through the renal capsule, and the second is the needle entering the collecting system. The stylet of the needle is removed, and aspiration of urine through the TLA needle confirms proper placement within the collecting system (Figure 9–7).

A 0.038-inch floppy-tip J guidewire is inserted into the needle and either advanced across the ureteropelvic junction or coiled within the renal pelvis if it will not pass into the ureter (Figure 9–8). The needle is then removed. If further endourologic manipulation is not warranted, as may be the case with ureteral obstruction arising from advanced cervical or prostatic carcinoma, it is possible to dilate the tract over this guidewire and insert one of the many available nephrostomy tubes. The tract needs to be dilated only 1F to 2F beyond the diameter of the intended tube, which usually is 12F.

Tract Dilation

For stone removal or intrarenal surgery the nephrostomy tract must be large enough to accept a working sheath that will hold the nephroscope. After the skin puncture is elongated with a scalpel, gradual dilation of the tract can begin. A variety of methods are used; however, we find the Amplatz Renal Dilating Set (Cook, Bloomington, Ind.) to be quicker and more reliable than metal coaxial or balloon dilators. This system consists of Teflon sheaths that fit over fascial dilators ranging in size from 6F to 30F. Over the floppy-tip J wire, the nephrostomy tract is dilated beginning at 6F and proceeding sequentially to 10F (Figure 9–9). This is done under fluoroscopy to avoid kinking of the guidewire and unnecessary perforations of the renal capsule. The dilators should be inserted with a slight twisting motion. Once the 10F sheath has been inserted, a stiffer torque guidewire is advanced into the renal pelvis. This torque wire acts as a safety wire in case of the inadvertent dislodgment of the initial guidewire. Ideally, one of the two guidewires is advanced beyond the ureteropelvic junction; however, this may not be possible, especially if the junction is obstructed. If a wire cannot be advanced down the ureter, an opportunity to advance it under direct vision will exist once the nephroscope is in place. A guidewire that bridges the ureteropelvic junction provides maximum sta-

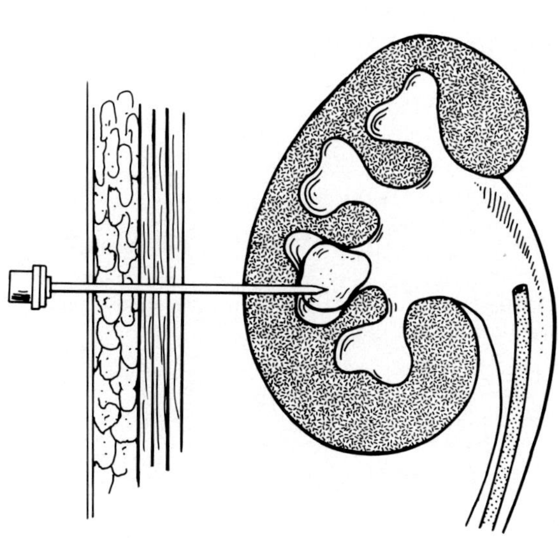

FIGURE 9–7. TLA needle in chosen calyx.

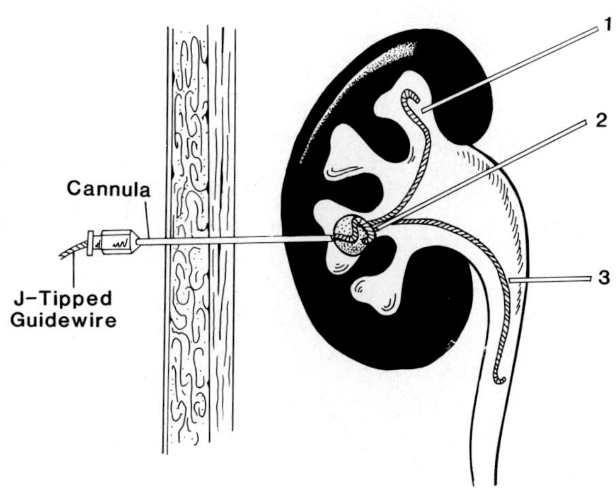

FIGURE 9–8. Floppy-tipped guidewire advanced through TLA needle.

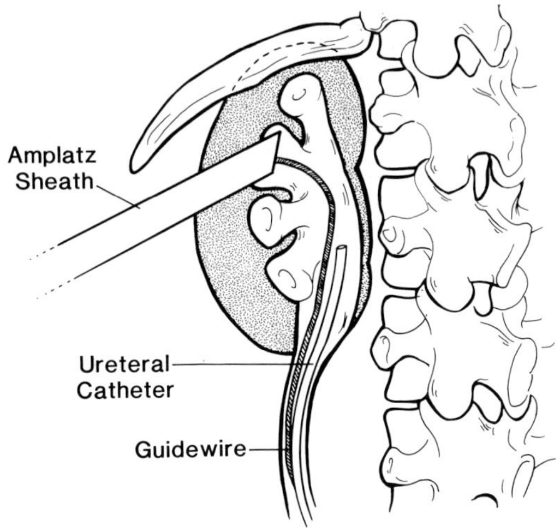

FIGURE 9–9. Amplatz sheath placed over floppy-tipped guidewire.

bility during the procedure and also provides access to the entire genitourinary system.

Once the second guidewire has been positioned, the tract is dilated to 34F (Figure 9–10). The 34F Amplatz sheath is left in position and used as the working sheath. A 26F rigid nephroscope fits easily into this sheath. The difference in size between the sheath and the nephroscope is advantageous, since providing an outlet for irrigation fluid minimizes intrapelvic pressure. Maintaining this pressure below 15 cm H_2O reduces the problems of pyelovenous and pyelosinus backflow and the associated risks of sepsis, as well as the absorption of irrigating fluid.[12]

Concern about parenchymal damage attributable to dilation to 34F has been allayed. The absence of persistent elevation of urinary brush border enzymes such as lysozyme in the postoperative period[13] is evidence of the kidney's tolerance for nephrostomy puncture, tract dilation, and percutaneous manipulation.

Retrograde Percutaneous Nephrostomy

Occasionally a percutaneous nephrostomy cannot be performed antegrade and must be performed in a retrograde manner (Table 9–1). Retrograde percutaneous puncture has several advantages. For example, this technique is ideal for the puncture of a nondilated collecting system with the puncture occurring away from the hilar vessels. The guidewire, which is passed out the flank from the urethra, makes loss of access virtually impossible. Most important, urologists are well trained in passing instruments in a retrograde manner.

Technique

The puncture is performed with the patient in the dorsal lithotomy position with a roll placed under the hips. Cystoscopic examination is performed. A 5F 100 cm straight Teflon catheter with a bevel tip is inserted into a 9F 90 cm Teflon catheter with a distal curve, and the two are locked together with an O ring. A 120 cm long 0.035-inch floppy-tip J guidewire passed through the catheter completes the assembly. The catheter assembly is passed transurethrally through the cystoscope, and the floppy-tip wire is advanced into the ureteral orifice. At that time the floppy guidewire should be replaced by a torque or tip-deflecting guidewire and the entire assembly passed retrograde up the ureter. The collecting system is then opacified. The wire is then manipulated into the chosen calyx and proper positioning confirmed with radiographs taken in both the supine and oblique positions. Posterolateral positioning of the wire is ideal, as is true for an antegrade nephrostomy. The Teflon catheters are advanced into the calyx, and the guidewire can then be removed. A 120 cm long 20- or 21-gauge hypodermic needle is passed through the ureteral catheter and advanced transparenchymally out through the skin. A "rocket" wire, a 0.021-inch 260 cm wire stylet with a sharpened tip, can be advanced through the hypodermic needle to facilitate

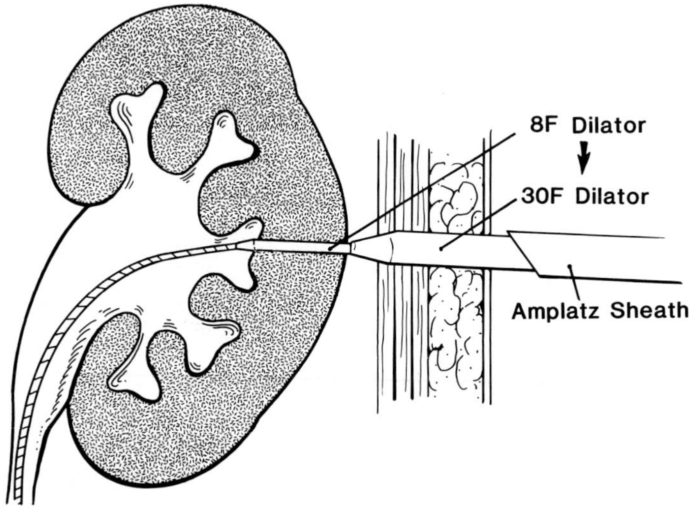

FIGURE 9–10. Dilation of the nephrostomy tract with the Amplatz sheath in position.

TABLE 9–1. Indications for Retrograde Percutaneous Nephrostomy

Malrotated kidney
Abnormally positioned kidney
Horseshoe kidney
Kidney with nondistensible collecting system
Hypermobile kidney

passage of the needle through the flank. After the needle has been passed out the flank, the nephrostomy tract can be dilated as described previously.

Applications

We have found the retrograde nephrostomy to be extremely useful with congenital ectopic kidneys.[14] These kidneys generally are nonpalpable, and the abdominal contents that overlie them anteriorly make them poorly suited for antegrade nephrostomy. Such kidneys differ from transplanted pelvic kidneys, which are palpable and therefore amenable to direct puncture. After a retrograde transparenchymal puncture of an ectopic kidney has been created, laparoscopic examination is performed to displace the bowel. Laparoscopic forceps can then be used to advance the needle from the anterior renal surface through the abdominal wall. Once the needle is passed through the abdominal wall, the nephrostomy tract can be dilated in the usual fashion. Because of the posterior direction of their calyces, horseshoe kidneys are also well suited to antegrade nephrostomy because this technique minimizes the risk of inadvertent bowel puncture. Malrotated kidneys are also candidates for retrograde nephrostomy because the location of the renal arteries is not always obvious. A retrograde nephrostomy in these cases minimizes the risk of hemorrhage from an inadvertent puncture of the renal vessels.

Retrograde nephrostomy has additional advantages. For example, it can be performed easily in obese patients and in those who have kidneys scarred by previous procedures or recurrent infections.

Disadvantages and Contraindications

Calyx selection is a vital part of the technique, and complications are more common with upper calyceal punctures. One of the few disadvantages encountered with this procedure is that after a successful puncture the patient must be repositioned prone to permit access to the tract.

The contraindications are similar to those for an antegrade procedure, but additional constraints exist. Patients with complete staghorn calculi or other large stones are not well suited to a retrograde puncture, since manipulating the needle into the appropriate calyx is difficult. Also, retrograde techniques may not be possible in patients with lower tract abnormalities that preclude cystoscopic examination or ureteral catheterization, such as advanced pelvic malignancies or a markedly enlarged prostate gland. Patients with ureteral obstruction that cannot be bypassed with a catheter also are not candidates for this procedure.

Nephrostomy Complications

The complications of retrograde and antegrade nephrostomy are similar and may occur early or late (Table 9–2). Excessive bleeding, pleural effusion, pneumothorax, hydrothorax, and puncture of adjacent organs have all been reported. The exit of the needle through the upper ureter and back into the renal pelvis has also occurred.

Endourologists are most fearful of vascular complications. Most complications resolve with conservative management, including bed rest, controlled pressure dressing, clamping of the nephrostomy tube, and transfusion. Fortunately, less than 10% of patients require transfusion. More serious vascular complications, including pseudoaneurysm, arteriovenous fistula, and retroperitoneal hematoma formation, usually require angiographic embolization of the bleeding site. If this approach fails, surgical repair of the injured vessel should be attempted. The nephrectomy rate attributable to severe vascular injury is less than 1 in 1000. The lowest incidence of complications is obtained by surgeons who are extremely familiar with these instruments and techniques. Careful selection of the appropriate calyx helps to ensure a safe puncture.

Management of the Stone

Once the nephrostomy tract has been created, direct visualization of the stone is easily accom-

TABLE 9–2. Complications of Percutaneous Nephrostomy

EARLY
Bleeding
Pseudoaneurysm
Arteriovenous fistula
Retroperitoneal hematoma
Injury to adjacent organs
Hydrothorax or hemothorax
Perforation
Extravasation
Infection or bacteremia
Urinoma
LATE
Stricture of ureter
Ureteropelvic junction obstruction
Retroperitoneal fibrosis
Failed procedure: incomplete stone or tumor removal

plished (Figure 9–11). Since the advent of shock wave lithotripsy, a surgeon would rarely perform a percutaneous puncture primarily to remove a stone small enough to be extracted without intrarenal lithotripsy. Exceptions to this are stones resistant to lithotripsy (cystine or some calcium oxalate monohydrate stones) or failure of the fragments to clear, such as when they are within a calyceal diverticulum, behind a stenotic infundibulum, or in a lower pole calyx. Patients whose body habitus precludes shock wave lithotripsy are also in this group. For these instances a variety of baskets and forceps can be used to grasp the fragments or the entire stone.[15] These instruments may also be used to extract fragments resulting from lithotripsy that are not cleared.

Baskets can be introduced through the Teflon sheath of the Amplatz system and manipulated to snare the stone under fluoroscopic guidance. Examples are the Hawkins, Dormia, Pfister-Schwartz, and Segura stone baskets. These are used mainly through a flexible nephroscope to grasp stones that are in the proximal ureter or in a calyx inaccessible to the rigid nephroscope. Their use helps to avoid additional percutaneous punctures. Stones or fragments smaller than 7 mm are best grasped with alligator forceps which, because of their small teeth, are unlikely to grab any adjacent tissue. Foreign body forceps are best for removing fragments between 7 mm and 1 cm, and 1 cm stones are most easily manipulated with three-pronged grasping forceps. When a second (safety) guidewire is in place and the nephrostomy tract has been dilated to 34F, stones as large as 1.2 cm may be extracted by pulling them against the working sheath and removing the stone and sheath together. Randall or Mazzariello-Caprini forceps modified to permit passage over a guidewire can also be used for extracting large stones.

Today, the most common indication for performing a percutaneous nephrostomy for stone removal is a large stone burden. These stones require fragmentation before their removal. Three modalities—electrohydraulic, ultrasonic, and laser—are now available for intrarenal lithotripsy, and they are discussed here in order of decreasing strength. Removal of stones or fragments often necessitates placement of instruments in various parts of the collecting system and sometimes requires the creation of multiple nephrostomy tracts or the use of a Y tract (Figure 9–12). The Y tract involves creating a branch off the established tract through a common skin puncture; this offers access to many parts of the collecting system and permits more efficient removal of the stone.

Electrohydraulic Lithotripsy

The electrohydraulic lithotripsy (EHL) probe is a bipolar electrode that creates a spark gap between its inner and outer layers. This spark forms an electrical discharge that vaporizes the irrigating liquid, creating a cavitation bubble whose expansion and collapse generate a series of shock waves. These shock waves cause fragmentation of the stone because most of their energy is dissipated at the fluid-stone interface. This technology is similar to shock wave lithotripsy except that the energy is not focused. The EHL probes are flexible, range in diameter from 3F to 9F, and can be used with both flexible or rigid nephroscopes. The frequency and duration of the electrical discharge, as well as the energy it releases, can be adjusted.

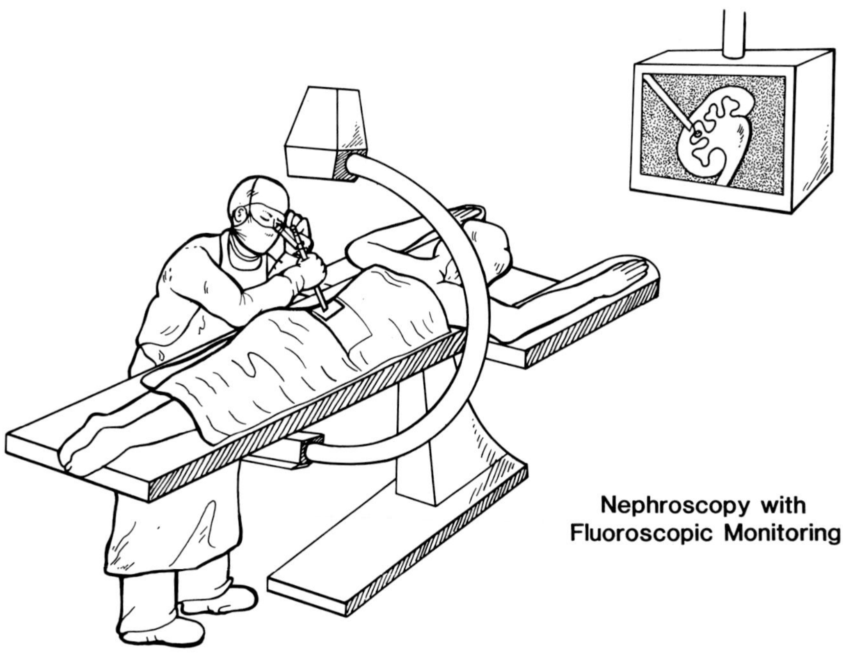

FIGURE 9–11. Nephroscopy after successful creation of nephrostomy tract.

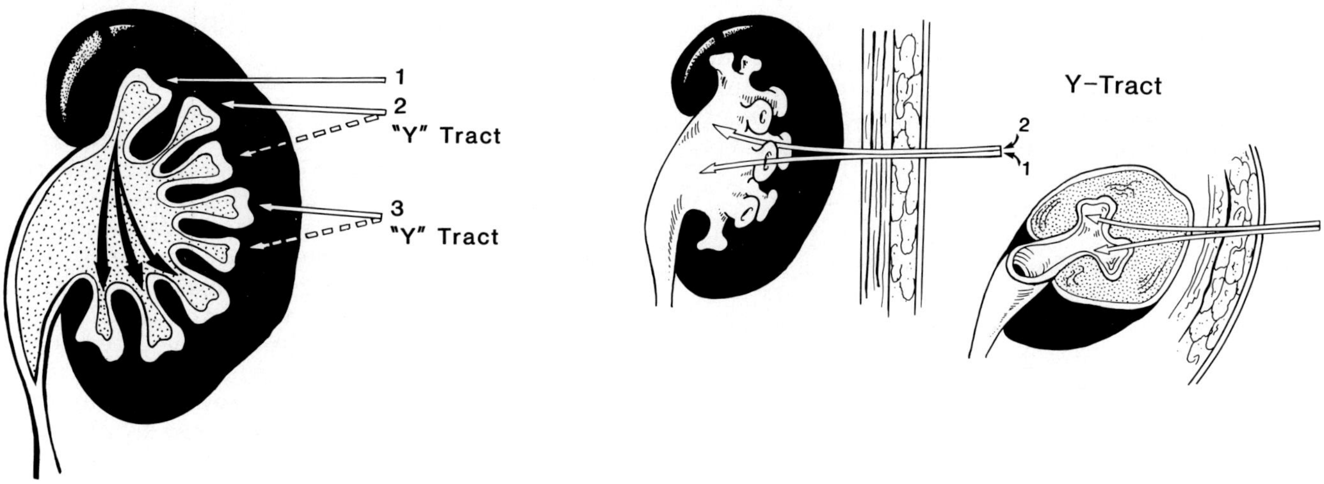

FIGURE 9–12. Y tracts providing access to all portions of the collecting system.

The EHL technique is easy to use in the kidney, but several points must be kept in mind for maximum effectiveness. First, the life span of an individual probe is 15 to 50 seconds, depending on the voltage and pulse frequency of each discharge. The efficiency of these probes is reduced as their edges erode, and therefore the tips must be inspected periodically. Second, these probes are most efficient when ⅙ normal saline solution is the irrigating fluid (500 ml of normal saline + 3000 ml of distilled H_2O = ⅙ normal saline). Third, the energy discharge may damage the lens of the nephroscope. Keeping the tip of the probe at least 3 mm from the end of the nephroscope minimizes this risk. Moreover, discharge from the probe can cause local tissue damage if the probe contacts the epithelium. Fourth, the tip of the electrode need not come in contact with the stone for fragmentation to occur. Positioning the electrode tip near the roughest or most irregular surface of the stone also increases the efficiency of this technique. The ability to use this probe through a flexible nephroscope allows precise positioning of the tip around corners.

Safety is of special concern with EHL. The probe should always be controlled because it may cause perforation by direct pressure with or without discharge. Fragmentation should be performed with the lowest energy level that disrupts the stone. Although safety should remain a concern, the new 3F probes that can be passed through the working port of all flexible nephroscopes are safer than the larger probes used in the past.

The low cost of EHL makes it extremely attractive; however, it cannot be used universally. Its principal use intrarenally is for very hard stones such as those of calcium oxalate monohydrate, uric acid, or cystine. It is less effective for calcium oxalate dihydrate and struvite stones. The major drawback of EHL is the necessity to extract mechanically fragments that are not flushed out through the nephrostomy tract and the need to use several probes to destroy large stones.

Ultrasonic Lithotripsy

Ultrasonic lithotripsy exploits mechanical vibrations at frequencies above the normal limit of audibility (>17 kHz) to fragment calculi. Alternating current applied to a ceramic crystal causes its expansion and contraction. The resulting vibration transmitted to the tip of the probe creates a drilling effect. Cavitation, the formation of bubbles and their contraction, also occurs at the tip. Contraction of the bubbles releases a large amount of energy that is effective over a small area, and this energy also contributes to stone fracture. Ultrasonic lithotripsy has a thermal effect and causes ultrasonic irradiation, but these effects probably play no clinical role in fragmentation.

Ultrasonic lithotripsy probes range in size from 3F to 9F. The smaller probes are solid and therefore cannot be used to aspirate the fragments, unlike the larger probes, which have a hollow core. Contact of the probe with the collecting system is not deleterious provided the suction core is not obstructed with stone debris. When obstruction occurs, irrigation is less efficient, the tip of the probe heats up, and focal thermal injury may occur. Although the tip of the probe must be in contact with the stone, excessive force may cause a perforation of the renal pelvis with migration of stone fragments into the retroperitoneum. If a perforation does occur, efforts should be directed at stone extraction with forceps because further lithotripsy will result in further spillage of fragments into the retroperitoneum and increase the size of the perforation.

The major disadvantage of ultrasonic lithotripsy is that the probe is not flexible. Therefore the nephrostomy tract must be carefully positioned to create a straight path between the lithotripter and the stone so that the tip of the probe can contact the stone. Stones with a shell or central core of uric acid are the most resistant to ultrasonic lithotripsy, whereas calcium oxalate and struvite stones are the easiest to fragment.

Laser Lithotripsy

Laser lithotripters can fragment calculi as successfully as electrohydraulic or ultrasonic lithotripters while using less energy than either of the other modalities. Most clinical experience with the laser has been obtained in the ureter; however, intrarenal stone fragmentation is easily performed. The principal advantage of laser lithotripsy is that it preserves the surrounding tissues because the wavelengths employed are absorbed by stones but not by tissues. The energy available for fragmenting a stone with a laser is a function of several factors, including wavelength, fragmentation threshold, length of time the laser is fired, pulse duration, and cross-sectional area of the laser fiber.[16]

Laser lithotripsy works on the principle of the formation of a plasma at the surface of the calculus. This plasma is a rapidly expanding and contracting cavity of electrons and ions. The collapse of the plasma after the laser pulse produces a mechanical shock wave, which is confined locally by the irrigating solution. The mechanical shock wave subjects the stone to high pressures that cause fragmentation in a manner similar to EHL.

Early attempts with laser lithotripsy were impractical because of the great amounts of energy required to cause fragmentation, the poor absorption of energy by the stone, and the lack of an adequate delivery system.[17,18] The lasers commonly used today (Pulsolith, Technomed Corp., Danvers, Mass.; MDL 2000 Laser Tripter, Candela Corp., Wayland, Mass.) are tunable pulsed dye lasers that use coumarin green. The wavelength emitted is 504 nm, which lies between the major absorption bands of the hemoglobin molecule and therefore results in selective absorption of the energy by the stone pigment instead of the surrounding tissues.

The laser fibers range in size from 200 to 320 μm, feature a helium-neon aiming beam, and have a pulse duration of 1 μsec. The laser fiber is easier to manipulate when passed through a small-caliber ureteral catheter, which can then be passed into the working channel of the nephroscope (flexible or rigid). The fiber must be in contact with the stone for fragmentation to occur.

The principal advantage of laser lithotripsy is the absence of local tissue damage. The cost of these units (nearly $250,000) remains the major drawback. Also, fragments have to be extracted manually unless they can be flushed out through the nephrostomy tract.

Postoperative Drainage

Once the stone has been removed, postoperative drainage of the collecting system must be established. A large-bore nephrostomy tube is required. Our tube of choice is a 24F Re-entry tube (Microvasive, Watertown, Mass.), which consists of a ureteral segment attached to a Malecot catheter whose wings open in the renal pelvis (Figure 9–13). The tube is positioned over a guidewire and advanced into position under fluoroscopic guidance. A nephrostogram is performed through the tube to confirm its proper position, and the tube is then secured to the patient's flank with a heavy silk suture.

The nephrostomy tube has several advantages. For example, 48 hours postoperatively, a nephrostogram is easily obtained. If no radiographic evidence of obstruction, extravasation, or residual fragments is found, the tube is removed. The patient is discharged after the tract to the skin becomes obliterated and the patient no longer has any flank drainage. When residual fragments, obstruction, or extravasation exists postoperatively, other advantages of this tube become apparent. The Re-entry tube allows easy extraction for the fragments and provides adequate drainage above the ureteropelvic junction if edema persists. Any necessary chemolysis can also be performed through this tube.

Chemolysis

Even though chemolysis of renal calculi is not so important as it once was in the management of retained fragments after a percutaneous procedure, it can be valuable for inaccessible parts of the stone. It also is helpful for fragments resistant to shock wave lithotripsy. For example, residual stone rates as high as 34% at 3 months after shock wave lithotripsy have been reported.[19] If these fragments are of appropriate composition, chemolysis may be preferable to repeat lithotripsy, particularly if the frag-

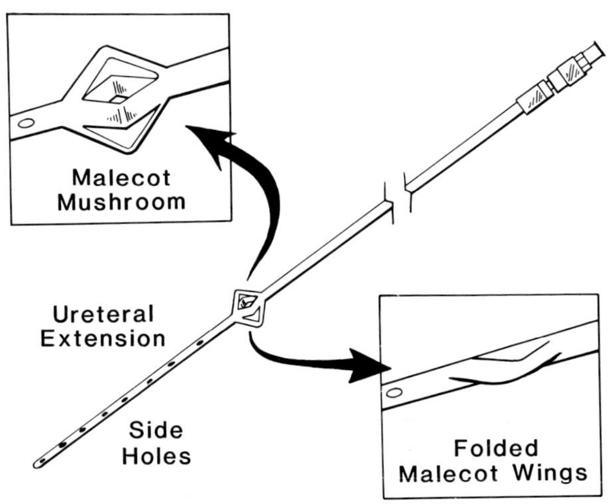

FIGURE 9–13. A 24F Re-entry tube.

ments are small and difficult to localize for external management. In selected patients with nonobstructing cystine, uric acid, or struvite stones, chemolysis may be used as a primary treatment for stone disease. Patients who are poor surgical candidates may also undergo primary chemolysis.

The ultimate goal of shock wave lithotripsy should not be fragmentation, but rather removal of all stones. Similarly, fragments retained after percutaneous stone extractions should be removed. Residual fragments, regardless of size, can act as a nidus for regrowth, can cause obstruction or sepsis, or can be the source of persistent pain. Retained struvite fragments contain bacteria in the interstices. Therefore, as long as residual fragments exist, the patient's infection will not be cured, nor will the potential for forming additional stones be eliminated. The value of total stone removal is shown by the finding that the routine use of hemiacidrin irrigation after shock wave lithotripsy or percutaneous stone extraction of struvite stones has been associated with a decreased incidence of recurrent stone formation.[20]

Various pharmacologic agents are available for the dissolution of renal calculi. The stone composition and location determine which of these agents is appropriate. In addition, multiple routes of administration (oral, intravenous, or direct percutaneous) are possible. Stone burden, location, and composition play a role in determining which route should be used.

Before chemolysis therefore the composition of the stone must be determined. Fragments removed percutaneously may be analyzed. Radiographic appearance and laboratory evaluation may also be helpful. For example, laminations, a central nucleus, and radiolucency are characteristic of uric acid stones. Cystine stones are faintly radiopaque with a homogeneous or ground-glass appearance and an irregular surface and shape. Urinalysis reveals a characteristic microscopic appearance of hexagonally shaped crystals in cystine stones. Struvite stones, with their typical staghorn appearance filling the renal pelvis, are also easily identified radiographically. Various epidemiologic[21] and genetic factors, as well as some postoperative states, contribute to stone formation. Drugs the patient is taking may also be a factor. The knowledge of these factors can add insight into the most likely stone composition.

SPECIAL CONSIDERATIONS FOR PARTICULAR STONES

Cystine Stones

Cystine calculi are uncommon, accounting for 1% to 3% of all renal calculi. They develop almost exclusively in patients homozygous for the hereditary disorder familial cystinuria.[22] The poor solubility of cystine in urine (300 mg/L at pH 6) leads to the formation of stones.

General Measures

The goal of dissolution therapy and prophylaxis is to increase the solubility and decrease the concentration of cystine in urine. Copious fluid intake, including overnight fluid ingestion, to obtain a urine output of 3 to 4 L/day is vital. A low-methionine diet with restrictions of milk, eggs, cheese, and fish is also part of the treatment regimen. The solubility of cystine increases sharply with alkalinization of the urine. For example, increasing the urinary pH from 6 to 8 triples the solubility of cystine, with 1 g being soluble in 1 L of urine at the higher pH. Despite this change in solubility, medical dissolution of cystine calculi is effective in only 30% to 40% of patients after long-term therapy,[23] and therefore conservative management with fluids and diet can be attempted only in patients with nonobstructive stones.

Alkalinization should be directed at maintaining the urinary pH between 7.5 to 8.5. Adequate alkalinization can be provided with intake of 13.5 to 22.7 g of sodium bicarbonate every 24 hours in equally divided doses. Alternatively, potassium citrate solutions (80 to 135 ml) may be used. These agents are available in both liquid (Polycitra) and tablet forms (UrocitK). Diamox administered at bedtime can help to keep the urine alkalinized overnight. This carbonic anhydrase inhibitor increases the excretion of bicarbonate and accelerates urinary acidification. The use of this agent during the daytime hours has also been advocated.[24] Because of the underlying metabolic disorder in patients with cystine stones, lifelong prophylactic alkalinization is required, and compliance can be a problem.

Sodium overload is a complication of therapy, and caution is needed with patients who have hypertension, renal insufficiency, or cardiovascular disease. Gastrointestinal side effects are common with alkalinizing agents, especially when larger doses are administered.

Chemolysis

When alkalinization and increased fluid intake fail, which is often the case, thiol solutions can be attempted. D-Penicillamine (Cuprimine; Merck, Sharp & Dohme, West Point, Penn.) and Tiopronin (alpha-mercaptoproprionylglycine, Thiola; Mission Pharmacal, San Antonio, Tex.) are thiol disulfide exchange substances. Penicillamine, a chelating agent, forms a water-soluble mixed disulfide with cystine. This action may prevent the formation of further stones and helps to dissolve previously formed stones. The complex is 50 times more soluble than cystine. The average adult dosage is 500 mg three or four times daily. Side effects are common and some reactions are potentially fatal. Sensitivity rashes (erythematous, maculopapular, or morbilliform) may be diminished by concomitant administration of antihistamines or steroids. A reduction in dosage or discontinuing the agent causes a resolution of symptoms. Restarting the drug at a smaller dosage and gradually increasing the dosage rarely causes a recurrent rash. More serious toxic effects include bone marrow suppression and the development of immune disorders. Abnormal urine findings, including proteinuria (protein level >2 g/24 hr), nephrotic syndrome, and glomerulonephritis necessitate immediate discontinuation of drug therapy.

Tiopronin forms a water-soluble mixed disulfide with cystine. This agent may be more effective than penicillamine, and its toxicity has been reported to be less.[25] Side effects include a dose-related nephrotic syndrome, urticaria, and lymphadenopathy. The dose for stone dissolution is between 60 and 1800 mg/day but less than 50 mg/kg per day.

Cystine stones that do not respond to conservative management, those that are large and obstructing, or large residual fragments after shock wave lithotripsy may be treated by direct dissolution through a nephrostomy tube. Alkalinizing agents such as sodium bicarbonate or tromethamine-E (THAM-E; Abbott Laboratories, N. Chicago, Ill.) may be used. The goal is to create an alkaline urine (pH >7.5) to foster stone dissolution. The duration of therapy with THAM-E, an organic amine buffer of pH 10.2, ranges from 5 to 37 days; this agent is reported to be more effective than sodium bicarbonate irrigations.[26]

Disulfide and thiol compounds such as *N*-acetylcystine (Mucomyst; Meade Johnson Laboratories, Evansville, Ill.) or D-penicillamine can also be administered through the nephrostomy tube. Acetylcysteine is superior to THAM-E for the dissolution of cystine stones.[27,28] The addition of the strong alkalinizing agent sodium hydroxide increases the effectiveness of this therapy[28] because of a synergistic effect of the pH-dependent increase in the solubility of cystine and a thiol-disulfide interchange. The low cost of Mucomyst also makes it an attractive agent.

Struvite (Magnesium Ammonium Phosphate) Stones

Magnesium ammonium phosphate stones are associated with urinary tract infection with urease-producing organisms such as *Proteus, Staphylococcus, Pseudomonas,* and *Klebsiella.* Infection with *Proteus* is most common. The splitting of urea by urease produces ammonia and carbon dioxide, which are further hydrolyzed into ammonium, hydroxyl, and carbonate ions. The alkalinization of the urine by the negatively charged ions (hydroxyl and carbonate) permits its supersaturation with magnesium, ammonium phosphate, calcium phosphate, and carbonate apatite crystals. Stones, often of a staghorn configuration, subsequently form. *Proteus* organisms themselves may contribute to stone formation by the production of a matrix substance.[29]

Bacteria are often located within the interstices of struvite stones, and therefore the only successful therapy is removal of all stones. Because percutaneous nephrostolithotomy and shock wave lithotripsy often leave residual fragments, dissolution is a useful adjunct. Therapy should inhibit the urease enzyme and eradicate the bacterial infection.

Oral dissolution therapy of struvite stones is directed at inhibiting urease. Acetohydroxamic acid (Lithostat; Mission Pharmacol Co., San Antonio, Tex.) can prevent the growth of struvite stones,[30] but it is not used extensively because many patients cannot tolerate it. Its principal use is in prophylaxis and not dissolution, since no more than 50% of patients receiving acetohydroxamic acid exhibit significant stone dissolution.[31] Hydroxyurea also inhibits urease, but its side effects, cytotoxicity, and lesser effectiveness compared with acetohydroxamic acid have prevented its common use.[32]

The direct dissolution of struvite stones with irrigation through a nephrostomy tract is far more effective than oral therapy. Magnesium citrate solutions are most useful for accomplishing this. Suby's Solution G (Travenol, Deerfield, Ill.) and hemiacidrin (Renacidin; Guardian Chemical Co., Hauppauge, N.Y.) are commonly used. Suby's Solution G contains the sodium salt of carbonic acid. Hemiacidrin contains four times as much magnesium as Suby's and also the calcium salt of carbonic acid. The initial use of organic acid solutions for irrigation was complicated by severe irritation of the bladder mucosa. The addition of magnesium to these solutions by Suby decreased the irritative effects and made the use of these substances possible.[33] Magnesium also has the beneficial effect of enhancing chemolysis by an ion exchange mechanism with calcium.[34] The success of these agents is related to several factors. Both solutions have a pH of 4, and because of this acidity they dissolve struvite calculi. In addition, calcium citrate complexes are formed, which promote dissolution.

Death has been associated with the use of Suby's Solution G and Renacidin. Reevaluation of the safety profile of these organic acid solutions did not show inherent toxicity but rather revealed sepsis during the infusion as the cause of death.[35,36] This sepsis was the result of high infusion pressures generated through the nephrostomy tract in a kidney containing bacteria.

One other significant side effect is hypermagnesemia, which can be fatal. Possible signs are nausea, vomiting, drowsiness, hypotension, and hyporeflexia. Peripheral vasodilation and respiratory depression resulting from the curare-like action of magnesium at the neural end-plates are seen later. If signs and symptoms of hypermagnesemia appear or the serum magnesium level exceeds 2.4 mg/dl, the irrigation should be stopped immediately and intravenous fluid and furosemide administered to facilitate diuresis. Other complications are renal and perirenal abscesses, fungal infections, flank pain, thrombophlebitis, pulmonary emboli, and ulcerations of the urothelium.

Despite the sometimes serious problems, several series have confirmed the safety of using these substances for irrigation.[37,38] Guidelines have been established to prevent the septic or metabolic complications previously encountered (Table 9–3).

Uric Acid Stones

Approximately 10% of urinary calculi are composed of uric acid. In some cases the patient has abnormally high production of this organic acid. Inherited metabolic diseases such as Lesch-Nyhan syndrome can be responsible, in which case patients also have hyperuricemia. Overproduction of uric acid can be seen in myeloproliferative disorders, obesity, or excessive alcohol ingestion. The abnormal excretion of uric acid also causes stone formation, such as that seen with a high-purine and high-protein diet or with the use of uricosuric drugs such as thiazides or salicylates. Uric acid lithiasis can develop because of excessive loss of water to the environment, as occurs with ileitis and colitis. Finally, idiopathic uric acid lithiasis is encountered. These patients excrete a normal amount of uric acid daily and do not have elevated serum uric acid levels but do have a constantly low urinary pH.

Urine pH is the most important factor to consider when treating patients with uric acid stones. The pK of uric acid is 5.75, and raising the urinary pH from 5 to 7 results in a greater than 200-fold increase in its solubility. Therefore increased fluid intake may be begun for confirmed uric acid stones that are not obstructive, provided the patient can tolerate the regimen. The goals are to increase the urinary volume, reduce uric acid excretion, and alkalinize the urine. An output between 2 and 3 L/day should be maintained, with patients monitoring their fluid status. Also, 300 mg of allopurinol daily and a low-purine diet should be instituted to reduce urinary uric acid. By inhibiting xanthine oxidase, allopurinol blocks the enzymatic conversion of hypoxanthine to xanthine and of xanthine to uric acid. The side effects of allopurinol are few, but gout may be precipitated in patients with hyperuricemia.

Alkalinization should be directed at maintaining a urinary pH between 6.5 and 7.0. The pH should not be allowed to rise over 7, since this could precipitate calcium phosphate (brushite). Administration of potassium citrate 60 mEq/day provides effective alkalinization and also increases the excretion of citrate, an inhibitor of calcium oxalate and calcium phosphate precipitation.[39]

Potassium salts generally are preferable to sodium salts such as sodium bicarbonate or sodium citrate for several reasons. In patients with hypertension or congestive heart failure, the sodium load of an effective alkalinization regimen may be excessive. The by-products of dissolution must also be taken into consideration. Alkalinization with sodium citrate increases urinary concentration of calcium phosphate (brushite)[40] and monosodium urate,[41] possibly supersaturating the urine with two crystals (monosodium urate and brushite) that predispose to secondary calcium stone formation. Hyperkalemia is one side effect of potassium citrate.

Because it provides steady urinary alkalinization, intravenous therapy can be used for a more rapid and sustained urinary alkalinization. One-sixth molar lactate is effective for systemic alkalinization,[42] but its use requires hospitalization, because congestive heart failure, hypertension, and hypernatremia may develop.

Because of the great effectiveness of alkalinization in dissolving calculi, urinary diversion is required only in patients with high-grade obstruction, unremitting colic, or sepsis. Once some form of diversion (ureteral catheter or nephrostomy tube) has been placed, dissolution may be facilitated with direct irrigation through this tube. Chemolysis can be used as a primary mode of treatment in patients unable to tolerate oral alkalinization, since little systemic absorption of the irrigant occurs.

Sodium bicarbonate can be infused through either a ureteral catheter or a nephrostomy tube. Four ampules of sodium bicarbonate added to 1 L of normal saline solution creates a final concentration of 178 mEq/L. This easily prepared, inexpensive solution has a pH of approximately 7.6. Tromethamine-E has also been used and dissolves stones more rapidly than sodium bicarbonate.[43]

TABLE 9–3. Guidelines for Safe Irrigation with Suby's Solution G or Hemiacidrin

1. Nephrostogram before irrigation to rule out extravasation or obstruction
2. Sterile urine confirmed by daily cultures
3. Careful monitoring of vital signs
4. Intravenous administration of antibiotics during the infusion
5. Continuous monitoring to maintain intrarenal pressures of less than 25 to 30 cm H_2O (i.e., that pressure below which pyelovenous backflow occurs)
6. Monitoring of serum magnesium levels
7. Monitoring of progress of dissolution radiographically to minimize treatment time
8. Discontinuation of irrigation with development of pain or fever

Calcium Stones

Unfortunately, greater than 80% of renal calculi contain calcium, and no reliable agent for dissolving these stones is available. Stone formation as a result of idiopathic hypercalcuria may be controlled with a regimen of copious fluid intake, thiazide administration, and sodium restriction.[44] Patients who have underlying hypocitraturia may demonstrate a reduction in stone recurrence and formation rates with the administration of potassium citrate.[45] Any identifiable underlying cause should be corrected (e.g., alkalinization in renal tubular acidosis; parathyroidectomy for hyperparathyroidism).

Several reasons exist for the absence of an adequate dissolution agent for calcium stones. First, simple acidic or basic solutions are ineffective because the solubility of calcium oxalate remains relatively constant over the pH range from 3 to 8. In addition, calcium oxalate stones are often complex, with various combinations of calcium oxalate and calcium phosphate arranged in various configurations. Each layer of one of these stones can require a different agent, making dissolution unfeasible.

Chelation with ethylenediaminetetraacetate (EDTA) has been attempted for calcium oxalate stones. However, in these stones EDTA elicits only a slight response that is somewhat enhanced by an alkaline environment.[46] Given its minimal effect on stone dissolution and the marked urothelial irritation it produces, little role exists for EDTA in the management of calcium stones.

ENDOPYELOTOMY

Once intrarenal stone removal had been mastered, intrarenal surgery seemed to be the next logical outgrowth of endourology. Several experimentally derived principles led to investigation of the possibility of relieving ureteropelvic junction (UPJ) obstructions percutaneously.

The procedure endopyelotomy is essentially a percutaneous pyeloplasty. Previously it had been shown that the muscularis and mucosa of the ureter healed after a narrowed segment was excised and stented.[47] These healed ureters exhibited peristalsis without adynamic dilation. In addition, provided the defect was no greater than 2 cm and the ureter was stented for at least 6 weeks, the ureter was regenerated by muscle hyperplasia without muscle contraction.[48] Endopyelotomy is based on these findings.

Diagnosis of Obstruction

Common symptoms of UPJ obstruction include gross hematuria after minimal trauma, intermittent flank pain with nausea and fever, persistent urinary tract infections, and in young patients abdominal pain associated with increased fluid intake. Preoperative evaluation is needed to confirm the obstruction and may include intravenous urography, diuretic renography, retrograde pyelography, and, in children, voiding cystourethrography. Ideally the patient has a minimum of 20% of total renal function on the affected side. Approximately 5% of our patients have had an equivocal diagnostic evaluation, and these patients undergo a Whittaker test to confirm the diagnosis of obstruction. Patients with severe obstruction and poor function may benefit from a trial of decompression of the hydronephrotic system with either a ureteral stent or a percutaneous nephrostomy tube. If renal function improves when the obstruction is temporarily relieved, these patients become surgical candidates.

Technique

After obstruction is confirmed, an endopyelotomy may be performed. The placement of a ureteral catheter transurethrally is extremely important, especially in the case of dense strictures that will not allow the passage of a floppy-tip or Bentsen guidewire across the narrowed area. In this case the ureteral catheter should be left in place just beneath the strictured area so it will serve as a landmark during the procedure.

A percutaneous nephrostomy should then be performed as described previously. Careful selection of the puncture site is vital to a successful endopyelotomy. The ideal approach to the narrowed area is along the straightest possible path. A tangential approach provides maximum maneuverability and visibility down the stenotic segment. Creating the nephrostomy through a posterior middle or upper pole calyx best accomplishes this. Lower pole tracts are not in the proper anatomic orientation for this procedure.

After the nephrostomy tract has been created, controlling the UPJ becomes important. The 26F nephroscope is inserted into the working sheath for visual inspection of the renal pelvis and the ureteropelvic junction. If the ureteral catheter was passed across the stenotic segment, it is now seen. A two-prong grasping forceps is inserted through the working channel, and the ureteral catheter is withdrawn through the nephrostomy tract. A 0.038-inch floppy-tip Teflon-coated wire is fed through the catheter and advanced antegrade. Once it emerges from the urethral meatus, a circulating nurse can withdraw the ureteral catheter.

The narrowed region and the redundant renal pelvis can be obstacles to gaining control of the UPJ. If the ureteral catheter was not passed retrograde, additional manipulation is required to negotiate a guidewire across the segment. Flexible nephroscopy may be of some use with the redundant renal pelvis. A Hunter-Hawkins retrograde nephrostomy may also be used. Alternatively, with the ureteral catheter advanced as far as possible retrograde while the area of the narrowed segment is observed with the nephroscope, a two-pronged forceps can be used to dissect bluntly over the catheter until the catheter appears in the visual field. Methylene blue can also be injected via the ureteral catheter, and the jet of blue can be followed nephroscopically. The area can then be incised with a cold knife until the catheter appears. This technique with the cold knife offers little room for error and should be attempted only as a last resort because total dismemberment of the ureter may occur.

At times recovering the catheter is tedious, and the surgeon may be tempted to bypass this step. However, replacing the catheter with a guidewire has some advantages. Not only does the wire act as a guide, but also it readily identifies the ureter when the UPJ is being incised. In addition, the guidewire will be used to place the stent in proper position at the completion of the procedure.

Any stones should be removed before the endopyelotomy. Occasionally a stone is impacted in the UPJ and leads to a reactive obstruction. In such cases the stone should be removed and the UPJ should not be incised. Instead the nephrostomy tube is left in place until the edema resolves. Patients who do not have a resolution of this obstruction after several weeks are candidates for an endopyelotomy.

After control of the UPJ has been obtained, the nephroscope is exchanged for a direct-vision endopyelotome. We believe that this instrument provides the best configuration for performing the incision. A hook-shaped, cold-knife cutting blade is used. The hook on the distal end of this blade lifts the tissue up before it is incised, permitting visual inspection of the mucosa to assess its viability and

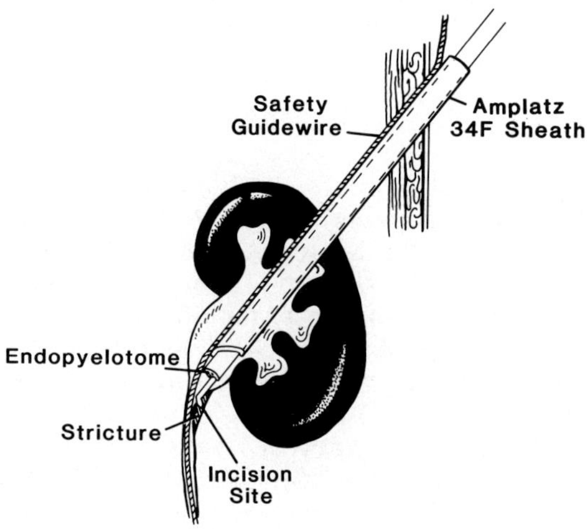

FIGURE 9–14. Endopyelotome in position across ureteropelvic junction obstruction.

TABLE 9–4. Types of Postprocedure Stenting Used in Endopyelotomy, October 1983–November 1991

Stent Type	No. of Patients
8F universal	42
12F universal	32
12F/7F endopyelotomy	14
14F/8.2F endopyelotomy	98
Re-entry tube	3
TOTAL	189

locate any arterial pulsations. Early in our series attempts were made with the urethrotome, hot-knife incision, and balloon dilation of the UPJ; however, our success with these techniques was not equal to the rate we are achieving with our present technique. Other groups have also had poor success with balloon dilation, finding it useful only in the immediate postoperative period, not for long-standing obstructions.[49]

The hook knife is advanced alongside the guidewire, and an incision is made in the strictured region (Figure 9–14). This incision should be made through the full thickness of the mucosa and smooth muscle until the periureteral fat is visible. The hook knife is advanced down the UPJ; when the knife is retracted into the endopyelotome, the segment is cut. As subsequent cuts are made, the UPJ begins to open up. The incision should be extended inferiorly until the ureter takes on a funneled appearance, with healthy pink mucosa visible through the endopyelotome. The incised area is then enlarged with an 18F Amplatz dilator.

The location of the incision should be chosen with special regard for the blood supply of the upper ureter. Basilar segmental renal arteries, which arise anteromedially, supply this segment of ureter. The full-thickness endopyelotomy incision should be made in such a manner as to avoid these vessels. A posterolateral incision is ideal. Any vessels that were transposed posteriorly during a previous pyeloplasty, as well as aberrantly located vessels, which are found in 20% to 30% of the general population, are also avoided with a posterolateral incision.

Once the endopyelotome has been withdrawn, a stent is positioned across the repaired area. The ideal stent is large enough to maintain urinary diversion and to ensure an adequate lumen size after healing has been completed, but narrow enough to avoid ischemia or pressure necrosis of the ureter, which would interfere with the healing process. Our method of stenting the UPJ has been evolving over the last several years (Table 9–4). Initially we used an 8F universal (Smith) stent. The drawback to this multipurpose stent was that the entire length of ureter was not being stented, and ureterovesical junction stenosis occurred in a small percentage of cases. Similarly, the 12F universal (Smith) stent proved unsatisfactory because its insertion required the concomitant use of a 14F or 16F peel-away introducer, and difficulty was encountered. A tapered stent with multiple distal coils was designed for this procedure, but its use was associated with irritative bladder symptoms or migration down the urethra while it was being positioned.

Although the success rates are similar with all the stents we have used, we have come to rely on an endopyelotomy stent manufactured by Cook Urological (Bloomington, Ind.). This stent is tapered and easily positioned. The proximal portion, the part that lies in the renal pelvis, measures 14F. The stent has multiple side holes and a proximal radiopaque marker. The intravesical portion measures 8.2F to reduce the risk of pressure necrosis and has a single coil (Figure 9–15). This stent is easily positioned by passage over the guidewire previously put into position across the UPJ. Also available is a pediatric stent, which is 10F proximally and tapers to 5F distally. In males the distal coil may migrate during stent placement. A pusher, such as a cystoscope sheath or ureteral catheter, may be placed in the urethra to position the coil properly within the bladder lumen. Proper positioning of the stent is crucial because inadequate proximal diversion of urine leads to extravasation at the site of incision, which is thought to contribute to fibrosis and subsequent failure of the UPJ procedure.

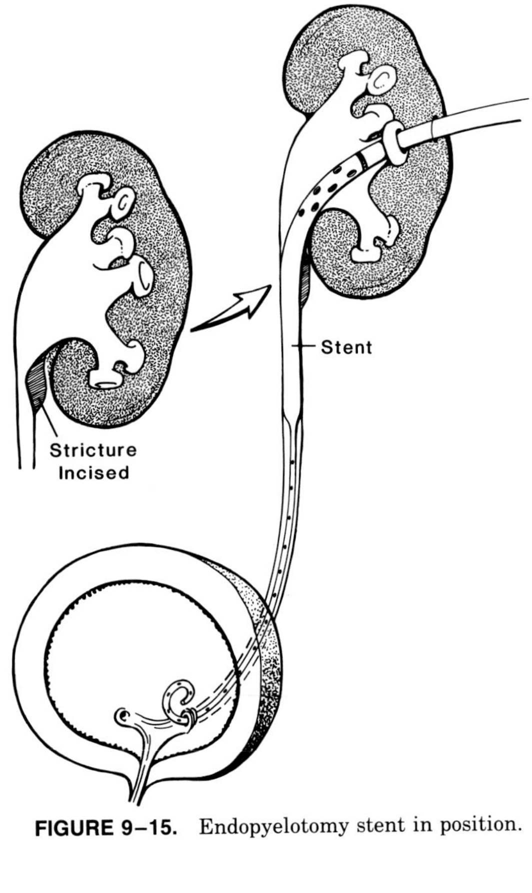

FIGURE 9–15. Endopyelotomy stent in position.

The guidewire and working nephrostomy sheath can be removed after the stent extends into the bladder and its correct position has been confirmed fluoroscopically. The stent should be secured to the patient's flank with a heavy silk suture and attached to a urinary drainage bag. The stitches must be carefully placed, avoiding perforation of the stent. The stent is left to gravity drainage for 48 hours.

On the second postoperative day a nephrostogram is obtained. Good stent position, adequate urinary drainage, and absence of significant extravasation should be identified. If these criteria are met, the stent is clamped overnight. If the patient has a spiking fever or discomfort, drainage is continued for an additional 48 hours, after which a repeat nephrostogram is obtained. Patients who do not tolerate the clamping often need repositioning of the tube, which may be accomplished with fluoroscopic guidance. The patient is discharged from the hospital with the external portion of the stent coiled under a sterile dressing.

The endopyelotomy stent is left in place for 6 weeks. This duration of stenting was determined on the basis of experimental work performed by others.[47,48] Despite reports of success with shorter periods of stent placement,[50] we have obtained good results with 6 weeks of stenting and do not plan to alter our management protocol.

Patients return at 6 weeks for a repeat stentogram. The stent is removed via the flank based on the results of this examination. Three months later, patients undergo repeat intravenous urography or radionuclide scanning. Radiographic studies are evaluated for gross architecture and adequacy of pelvic emptying. The urologist must remember that unchanged radiographs may not be the result of a surgical failure but rather of irreversible damage to the collecting system caused by long-standing obstruction. Therefore patients not exhibiting improvement on intravenous urograms should undergo diuretic renal scanning. Our minimal criteria for success are the relief of symptoms and stabilization of the radiographic appearance.

Results

Over the last 7 years we have performed 189 endopyelotomies on both primary (93 patients) and secondary (96 patients) obstructions of the ureteropelvic junction. In this time treatment has been successful in 162 patients, for an overall success rate of 85.7% (162/189).[51] Among the successful outcomes, the average follow-up time has been 44.5 months (range 2 to 97 months): 92% (150/162) have been followed a minimum of 1 year, 70% (123/162) a minimum of 2 years, and 63% (102/162) at least 3 years. Therefore we can say that good results appear to be long lasting. The success rate is approximately 85% for both primary and secon-

TABLE 9–5. Findings at Exploration in Failed Endopyelotomies

Tortuous ureter
Massively redundant renal pelvis
Fibrotic ureteropelvic junction
Impacted intramural crystals and fibrosis
Unsuspected transitional cell carcinoma

dary obstructions of the ureteropelvic junction. Patients in this series ranged in age from 2¾ to 80 years.

A learning curve does not appear to exist for this procedure. In each group of 20 successive endopyelotomies we have performed, the success rate is similar to that for the overall series.

When endopyelotomy failed and subsequent open repair was performed, the excised narrowed segments were examined histologically. Some degree of fibrosis of the excised UPJ was universally encountered. In a few cases anatomic anomalies probably contributed to the failure (Table 9–5). In other instances the condition of the tissue was not conducive to healing. For example, in some cases crystals were probably interfering with the normal healing process and serving as a nidus for further fibrosis. Foreign body granulomas were detected in the specimens excised from these patients.

It appears that endopyelotomy can be offered to most patients with UPJ obstructions, regardless of previous surgery. However, a long (>2 cm) stricture of the UPJ poses a limitation to the procedure. In addition, the procedure is not well suited to strictures below the level of the UPJ. In our experience, patients who had undergone endopyelotomy for a stricture of the upper third of the ureter inevitably required an open procedure to relieve the obstruction.

The majority of complications we have encountered are minor (Table 9–6). Stent-related complications are most common, but stenosis of the ureterovesical junction is also seen. Serious hemorrhage in two patients and ureteral avulsion in one were the only major complications; fortunately, these are rare occurrences.

Comment

The failures we have had were not intraoperative failures, and technical difficulty has never precluded endopyelotomy. Symptoms of failure usually appear within 2 weeks after removal of the endopyelotomy stent and are consistent with a recurrent stricture. Subsequent open pyeloplasties performed in this group of patients were not complicated by the previous endopyeloplasty.

Compared with an open pyeloplasty, endopyelotomy causes less morbidity and has a shorter operating time and hospital stay. These factors, as well as the lesser postoperative pain, the faster return to work, and a success rate comparable to that of open pyeloplasty, make endopyelotomy attractive to patients. Moreover, because the blood supply to the ureter is kept intact, less scar tissue should form at the surgical site, which lessens the likelihood of postoperative restenosis. Our long-term follow-up of these patients indicates that this procedure is a cure for both primary and secondary UPJ obstructions.

ENDOPYELOPYELOTOMY

Endopyelopyelotomy is an extension of the endopyelotomy procedure. It is used in the small group of patients who have a bifid renal pelvis with obstruction of one segment at the level of its UPJ. When the stenotic segment is too long for an endopyelotomy, endopyelopyelotomy is a valid percutaneous option.[52]

The procedure is an endourologic creation of a controlled fistula between the obstructed and nonobstructed segments of the bifid system (Figure 9–16). A percutaneous nephrostomy into the obstructed collecting system should first be created as described previously. After nephroscopic examination is performed and the determination made that the obstructed segment cannot be relieved by an endopyelotomy, a second percutaneous nephrostomy tract is created in the nonobstructed segment. This tract is dilated to 28F, and the 28F sheath is left in place. A Fogarty catheter is positioned over a guidewire placed during creation of the tract. This catheter is then positioned alongside the UPJ within the lumen of the ureter belonging to the nonobstructed segment. The Fogarty balloon is inflated with contrast material, which allows fluoroscopic monitoring.

An endopyelotome is inserted through the obstructed nephrostomy tract, and the extrinsic indentation of the inflated Fogarty balloon, which is abutting the obstructed system, is identified. If this bulge cannot be located directly, the endopyelotome may be viewed in various positions with fluoroscopy until it is next to the balloon. The endopyelotome is then used to incise any tissue that lies between the obstructed segment and the Fogarty catheter in the nonobstructed moiety. The incision is continued until the Fogarty balloon ruptures and the

TABLE 9–6. Complications of Endopyelotomy in 189 Cases

MAJOR
Serious hemorrhage (2)
Ureteral avulsion (1)
MINOR
Stent related (29)
Ureterovesical junction stenosis (2)

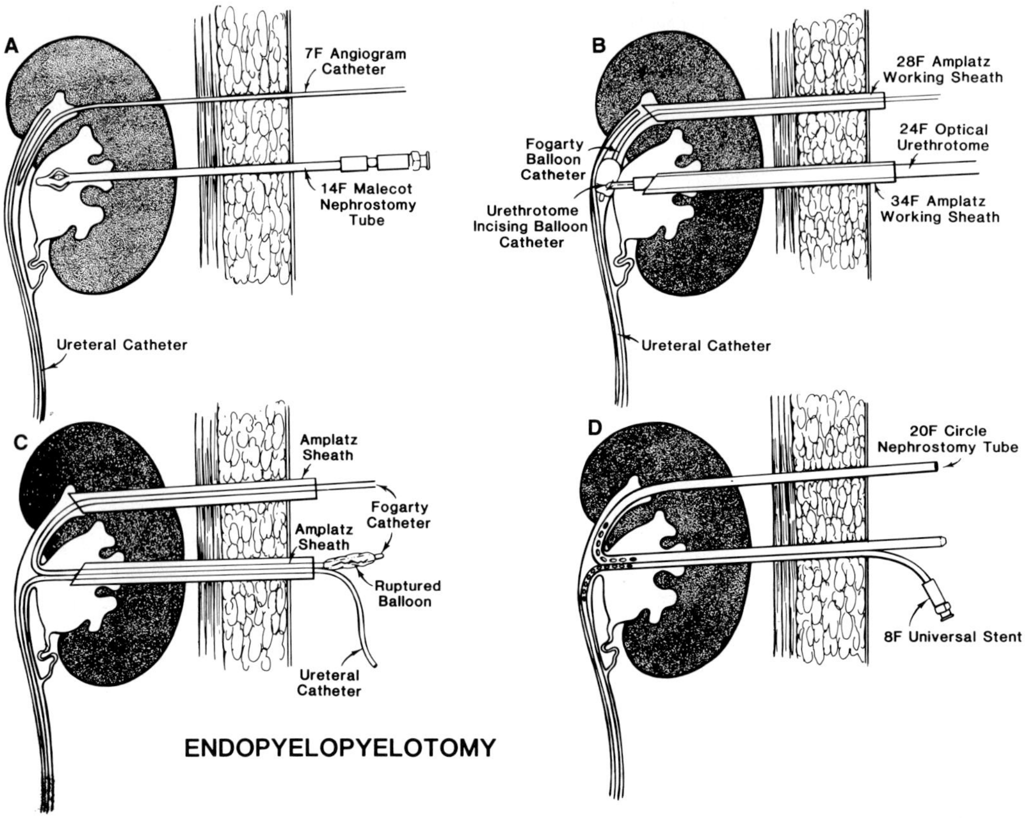

FIGURE 9–16. **A,** Access of upper and lower pole moieties. **B,** Dilation of both tracts with Fogarty balloon in position. **C,** Ruptured Fogarty balloon withdrawn through lower tract. **D,** A 20F circle tube and 8F universal stent in position. (From Saltzman B, Smith AD: Semin Urol 4:153, 1986. Used by permission.)

passage is wide enough to identify and extract the Fogarty catheter.

A grasping forceps is passed through the working channel of a nephroscope inserted through the tract of the obstructed segment. The Fogarty catheter and its guidewire are extracted through this tract and exteriorized. Once both the Fogarty catheter and the guidewire are in position, the catheter may be removed. The guidewire, which remains in place, now extends through the upper segment, traverses the newly created gap created between the two renal pelves, and passes out the lower pole. This wire is in the proper position for placement of the stent, a 20F silicone circle tube. Radiopaque markers on both sides of the drainage holes help in the proper positioning of this tube. In addition, an endopyelotomy stent is put into position across the patent UPJ. Last, a small Malecot catheter is introduced into this common renal pelvis to ensure adequate drainage of the renal pelvis during the first 48 hours postoperatively.

The patient is discharged from the hospital with the circle tube and endopyelotomy stent in place after their positions are confirmed with a nephrostogram obtained on the second postoperative day. An additional nephrostogram is obtained 6 weeks later, and if the new fistula is patent, both nephrostomy tubes are removed. A 6-month follow-up examination, including intravenous urography, is performed.

PERCUTANEOUS MANAGEMENT OF CALYCEAL DIVERTICULA AND STENOTIC INFUNDIBULA

Like UPJ obstructions, calyceal diverticula and infundibular stenosis are correctable anatomic abnormalities that predispose the patient to urinary stasis and concomitant stone formation. As is true for UPJ obstructions, these entities may be successfully managed with endourologic techniques.

Stones within a calyceal diverticulum are fairly common. Routine intravenous urography reveals an incidence of diverticula of 0.21% to 0.45%, with nearly 40% of these patients having a stone.[53] The narrow neck of the diverticulum precludes the spontaneous passage of these stones. Although obstruction of calyceal diverticula can lead to serious complications, only with the recent technologic advances in percutaneous procedures is an aggressive approach to these stones being undertaken.[54] Extracorporeal shock wave lithotripsy (ESWL) of stones in a diverticulum or proximal to an infundibular stenosis is contraindicated because the narrow neck of the diverticulum or the stenotic region

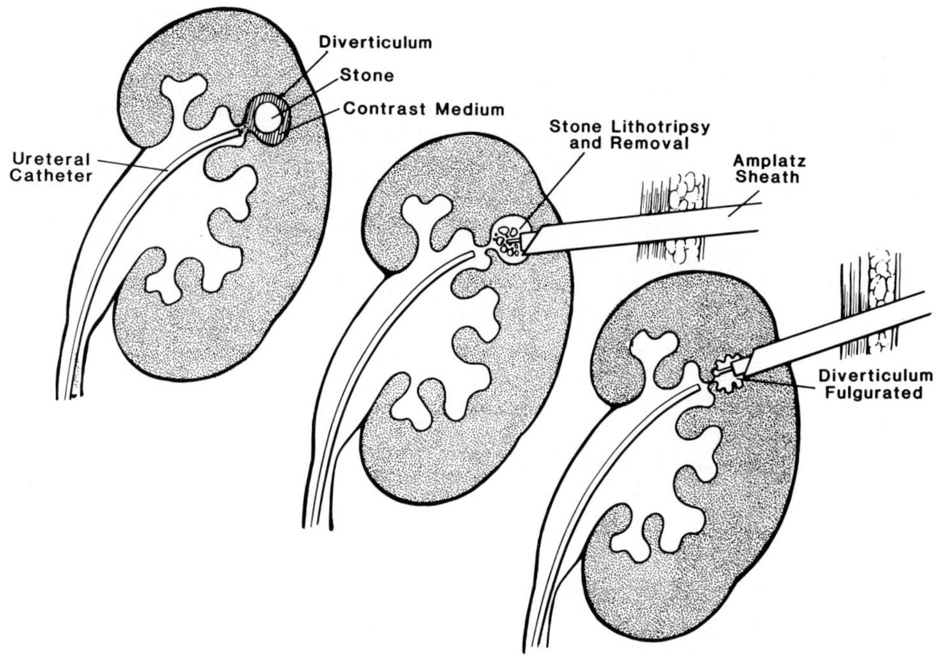

FIGURE 9–17. Management of stones within a calyceal diverticulum.

of the infundibulum is a form of distal obstruction, and the fragments will not clear. For example, in one series ESWL of stones contained within calyceal diverticula resulted in only a 50% stone-free rate and a 45% retreatment rate, with 62% of the patients remaining symptomatic.[55] In contrast, a 95% stone-free rate occurs after percutaneous procedures for such stones. More important, the percutaneous route corrects the underlying disorder, whereas ESWL does nothing for the anatomic abnormality and therefore patients are likely to form recurrent stones.

The percutaneous nephrostomy should be performed directly into the affected calyces provided they are posterior and located below the twelfth rib (Figure 9–17). A guidewire is passed through the stenotic region (i.e., stenotic infundibulum or neck of the diverticulum). Depending on the degree of obstruction, passage of a guidewire may not be a simple feat. When the area is extremely stenotic, the passageway into the collecting system may not be visible at all. The injection of methylene blue retrograde through a ureteral catheter may help identify this opening.

If the calyx in question is above the twelfth rib, two options are available. An indirect approach may be used (Figure 9–18, *A*), with the nephrostomy performed through a lower pole calyx. A flexible nephroscope may then be manipulated to the stenotic upper infundibulum or neck of the diverticulum and a guidewire passed through the narrowing. This indirect technique is also useful for anterior calyces, which are technically more challenging because they are harder to reach.[56] Direct approaches may also be used, but the incidence of complications is increased with high nephrostomies. High nephrostomies require special care to minimize complications.

When the direct approach is used (Figure 9–18, *B*), with the guidewire in place, the tract can be dilated. The stone should be extracted as soon as it is visible because further manipulation would widen the anatomic obstruction. If this occurs, the

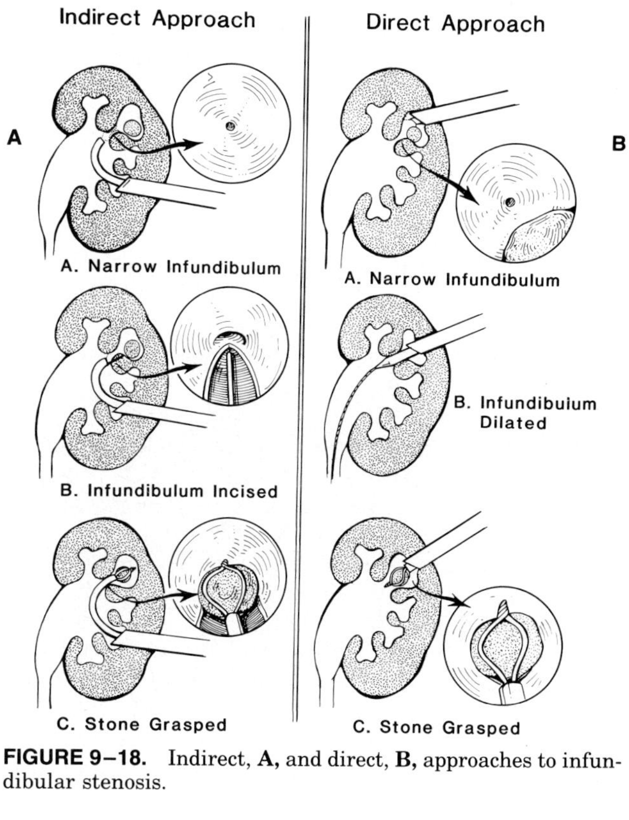

FIGURE 9–18. Indirect, **A**, and direct, **B**, approaches to infundibular stenosis.

stone could easily be displayed distally, resulting in a more difficult extraction. After the stone has been removed, balloon dilation of the diverticular neck or stenotic infundibulum is performed. A cold-knife infundibulotomy can be performed in selected patients. The indirect approach requires relieving the obstruction before extracting the stone.

Any incision of the stenotic region should be done with a cold knife. A cutting current can injure the segmental arteries, which are adjacent to the area being incised,[57] and a full-thickness incision of the infundibulum should be avoided. In treatment of a diverticulum, after dilation has been performed, the wall should be fulgurated. This traumatization of the epithelial lining ensures granulation and ablation of the diverticulum.[58]

Regardless of the approach, a large nephrostomy tube (24F reentry) is used to drain the kidney postoperatively.

PERCUTANEOUS MANAGEMENT OF UPPER TRACT TRANSITIONAL CELL CARCINOMA

Another use for intrarenal (endorenal) surgery is the percutaneous management of upper tract transitional cell carcinoma. Renal pelvic transitional cell carcinoma has traditionally been managed by nephroureterectomy with the additional removal of a bladder cuff.[59,60] Conservative (nephron-sparing) approaches to lesions of the renal pelvis have been advocated for many years,[61,62] but because this disease is commonly multifocal, few urologists have been willing to treat it with less than radical surgery. However, advances in endourologic technique and instrumentation and the successes being achieved by various groups[63-65] have increased the popularity of the nephron-sparing approach for selected patients.

Patient Selection

When a conservative approach is considered, careful patient selection is important. The grade and stage of the tumor should be determined by a combination of endoscopic, radiographic, and selective cytologic and histologic analyses. The ideal lesion for endorenal management is small (<2 cm), unifocal, papillary, low grade, and superficial. The need for deep resection of the thin renal pelvis and the tendency of these cancers to multifocality limits the usefulness of the percutaneous approach in patients with high-grade lesions and a normal contralateral kidney.[66,67] However, the presence of a high-grade lesion does not preclude this approach if the patient would require dialysis when treated with traditional means. Thus percutaneous management is appropriate for high-grade lesions in patients with functionally or anatomically solitary kidneys or bilateral synchronous disease, since this approach may be the only means of avoiding dialysis of these patients. Patients who are poor surgical risks for nephroureterectomy also benefit. In addition, patients with an increased risk for contralateral recurrences, such as those with Balkan or analgesic nephropathy, benefit from the percutaneous approach.

The possibility of seeding a nephrostomy tract with spilled tumor cells is real, but we have not encountered this in any of the patients we have treated percutaneously. A ureteroscopic resection is the treatment of choice for these lesions if adequate resection can be performed, since this eliminates any potential for nephrostomy tract seeding. However, when ureteroscopy is not possible, which is often the case, the percutaneous route is preferred because of the greater access it provides to the renal pelvis. An iridium (^{192}Ir) wire has been left in the nephrostomy tube for several days postoperatively to kill any tumor cells that have been spilled.[65]

Technique

A percutaneous nephrostomy is performed as described previously. After access has been established, the entire collecting system is examined with a rigid or flexible nephroscope. Endoscopic examination should include the proximal ureter.

Before resection of the lesion, random cold cup biopsies of the renal pelvis are performed. During this step, polyethylene catheters are placed over any guidewires to prevent the tissue damage that would be associated with passage of electrical current down the guidewire. A combination of a resectoscope and cold cup biopsy forceps is used to resect the lesions completely (Figure 9–19). Because of the small capacity of the renal pelvis and the free flow of irrigating solution, each loop of tissue must be removed manually. The resection should include deep tissue layers, both to remove all of the tumor and to provide the pathologist with adequate architecture to determine the level of invasion.

Once the lesion appears to have been fully resected, the base of the tumor and any suspect regions should be fulgurated with either an Nd:YAG laser or a Bugbee electrode. The kidney should be drained postoperatively with a 24F reentry nephrostomy tube. This tube can easily be positioned over the previously placed guidewires after the polyethylene shields have been removed.

Nephrostograms are obtained 48 hours postoperatively. If the nephrostogram does not reveal any evidence of extravasation, the nephrostomy tube is clamped. If the patient tolerates this (pain free, no elevation of fever), he or she may be discharged home.

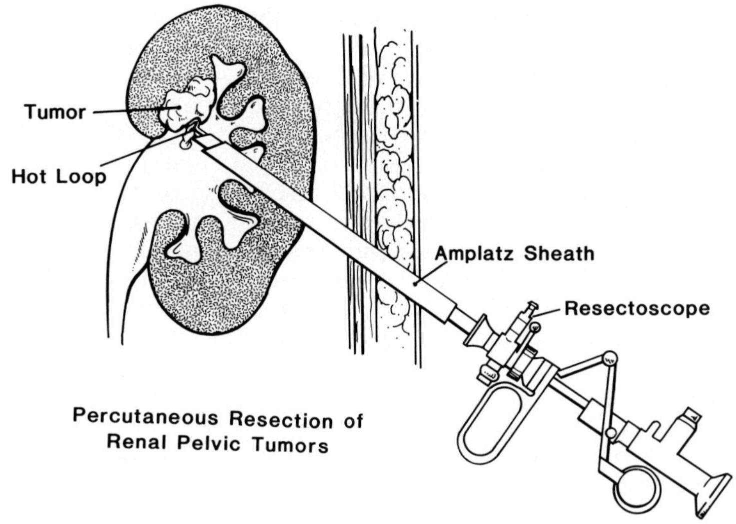

FIGURE 9–19. Percutaneous resection of upper tract transitional cell carcinoma.

Adjunctive Treatment

Even when the entire tumor is thought to have been resected, further management is required. Our current treatment protocol is reviewed in Table 9–7. Approximately 2 weeks postoperatively patients undergo a second-look nephroscopic examination. We consider 2 weeks to be long enough for most of the significant edema and erythema associated with the first procedure to resolve. Second-look procedures may be performed with intravenous sedation. If nephroscopy reveals suspect lesions, further biopsies, resection, and fulguration of these areas are performed. The patients then are treated with intracavitary bacille Calmette-Quérin (BCG) through the nephrostomy tube, which is left in place. Patients without evidence of disease have the nephrostomy tube removed. These patients require intravenous urograms, cystoscopy, and selective cytologic studies at 3-month intervals. Endoscopic intervention is indicated when recurrent disease is suspected.

Intracavitary BCG is administered weekly for 8 weeks on an inpatient basis. An adequately draining nephrostomy tube is required for these treatments. The patency and placement of the tube should be confirmed with a nephrostogram before the treatment begins. In addition, a nephrostogram should be obtained halfway through the course of therapy. The renal pelvis is irrigated with 300 ml of normal saline solution with an infusion pump at a rate of 100 ml/hr. A manometer should be attached in line with the pump, and the nephrostomy tube and renal pelvic pressures should be main-

TABLE 9–7. Treatment Protocol for Percutaneously Resected Upper Tract Transitional Cell Carcinoma

Creation of nephrostomy tract
Tumor biopsy → High-grade or invasive tumor → Nephroureterectomy
Tumor resection
Fulguration of tumor base

↓

Second look → High-grade or invasive tumor → Nephroureterectomy
Second look → Residual low-grade disease → Nd:YAG laser + BCG → Third look
↓ (Third look) → No evidence of disease

↓

No evidence disease

↓

Intracavitary BCG ← No evidence of disease

↓

Every 3 months

Intravenous urography
Cystoscopy
Selective cytology
+/− Endoscopy

BCG, Bacille Calmette-Guérin.

tained at less than 15 cm H_2O. For each treatment, 1 vial of BCG (Tice strain: 1 to 8 × 10^8 colony-forming units) is administered. The BCG is mixed with 50 ml of sterile water and infused over 1 hour. The patient is observed overnight and discharged the following morning.

During the course of therapy, chest radiography is performed on alternate weeks. In addition, complete blood cell counts, serum chemistry evaluations, and urine cultures for acid-fast bacilli are obtained. The dosage of BCG is reduced if the patient shows a systemic toxic effect during the infusion. After the intracavitary therapy has been completed, additional nephroscopic examination is performed. Chronic and acute inflammatory reactions may be seen at this time. Granulomas may be present in biopsy specimens.

Results

We recently reviewed our experience with the percutaneous management of upper tract transitional cell carcinoma.[68] Over the past 6 years 20 patients have been treated with these techniques. Five patients have died, four of them from transitional cell carcinoma. Thirteen (65%) of the patients are alive with no evidence of disease after a mean follow-up of 31 months. Recurrence rates between zero and 14% have been identified in patients with low-grade (grade I) single lesions or superficial (noninvasive) disease. Lesions that were multifocal, high grade (grade II or III), or invasive had recurrence rates between 66% and 100%. A second-look procedure, the use of the Nd:YAG laser to fulgurate the tumor base, and the instillation of BCG have all been associated with lower recurrence rates. These findings have led us to restructure our management plan so that all patients now get a second-look procedure, fulguration of the tumor base, and BCG therapy for 8 consecutive weeks. During the course of BCG treatment, renal function remained unchanged. No evidence of extrarenal BCG toxicity such as abnormal results of liver function tests or distant granulomas have been found. The only complications encountered have been the development of a UPJ obstruction, easily relieved by an endopyelotomy, and significant bleeding through the nephrostomy tube that necessitated transfusion in one other patient.

The nephron-sparing approach to upper tract transitional cell carcinoma can be successfully accomplished percutaneously. Small low-grade unifocal lesions are best suited to treatment with this approach. Patient compliance is another factor that should be considered, since a rigorous postoperative examination is required every 3 months. Additional use of this technique may be feasible for palliation in patients with metastatic disease who have bleeding or obstruction.

PERCUTANEOUS MANAGEMENT OF SIMPLE RENAL CYSTS

Simple renal cysts (retention cysts) are the most common cystic abnormality of the kidney and are common incidental radiographic and postmortem findings.[69] Except in the event of rupture, these masses do not communicate with the collecting system. The vast majority are asymptomatic. However, they may occur as abdominal masses. Acute bleeding into the cyst is associated with abdominal pain. Other findings may include polycythemia or the development of hypertension if significant compression of the renal vasculature or parenchyma occurs. Large size, recurrent pain, bleeding, and hypertension have been indications for resection or decompression in selected patients. Obstruction leading to parenchymal atrophy is another indication for intervention.

The percutaneous decompression of renal cysts under ultrasound guidance is a well-accepted technique.[70] However, even when the cyst cavity is treated with sclerosing agents, the cyst may recur. Also, the use of these sclerosing agents has been associated with serious complications, including severe inflammatory reactions that have even necessitated nephrectomy.[71] With this in mind, various investigators have attempted more elaborate percutaneous management of cysts that require treatment.

The percutaneous resection of renal cysts with standard urologic equipment has been described.[72,73] Cyst puncture is performed, and provided that the cyst fluid is clear and nonhemorrhagic and that cytologic and biochemical findings are normal, percutaneous resection of the cyst can be undertaken. The cysts may be approached through the renal parenchyma. After a guidewire is introduced through the needle into the cyst cavity, the nephrostomy tract and cyst wall can be dilated as described previously.

The cyst wall is then visualized through the nephroscope. The cyst at this point is decompressed, and the peripheral cyst wall can be identified. An intentional perforation is created through the cyst wall into the perirenal fat with a grasping forceps. The nephroscope is withdrawn and the resectoscope inserted. A standard transurethral resectoscope can be used in place of the endopyelotome (Figure 9–20). Hot current is used. Under direct vision, beginning at the site of the perforation, the cyst wall is electrocauterized. Before the procedure is completed, perirenal fat is pulled into the previous cyst cavity to help prevent recurrence.

The intrarenal marsupialization of a simple cyst has also been described.[74] Much as an endopyelopyelotomy relies on the creation of a controlled fistula between the upper and lower pole segments, this technique creates a short-term controlled fistula between the renal cyst and the collecting sys-

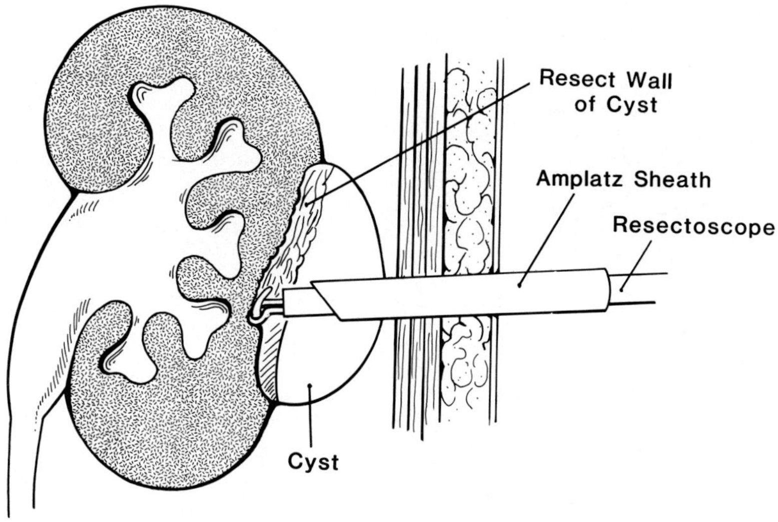

FIGURE 9–20. Percutaneous management of simple renal cyst.

tem. A direct puncture into the cyst cavity is performed, and the cyst wall is then electrocauterized or photocoagulated with an Nd:YAG laser to effect obliteration (Figure 9–20). The cyst cavity is marsupialized internally by endourologic creation of a puncture from within the cyst cavity into the adjacent aspect of the collecting system. A stent is placed from the cyst cavity down into the bladder. This technique has provided the long-term resolution of symptoms in patients whose lesions were resistant to conventional procedures.[74]

Although the reports are of preliminary investigations, these innovative percutaneous techniques seem to be successful. Further investigation will probably prove this to be a valuable alternative to traditional surgery in patients whose renal cysts require intervention. The long-term resolution of these cysts appears to be more likely than with standard techniques, and the need for subsequent procedures appears to be lower.

SUMMARY

Although ESWL has supplanted percutaneous stone extraction as the most common procedure for the treatment of renal calculi, percutaneous procedures will continue to have a well-defined role in renal stone management. Percutaneous operations should be the procedure of choice for staghorn calculi and other large stone burdens. Large cystine stones also are more efficiently treated via a percutaneous route, as are stones associated with an underlying anatomic obstruction or stones resistant to ESWL.

The technologic advances that have been made with the percutaneous renal approach are beginning to be applied in other surgical disciplines. Whereas urologists have used the percutaneous approach for many years, it is only recently that general surgeons have begun to do so. Much of the technology required to treat gallbladders percutaneously was developed by urologic surgeons. Lymph node surgery via a percutaneous route (laparoscopic lymphadenopathy) is now common in most major medical centers.

Percutaneous renal surgery is progressing and will have a definitive role in the future. The relief of UPJ obstructions with an endopyelotomy is clearly an alternative that should be offered to patients. Similarly, calyceal diverticula, infundibular stenoses, and renal cysts may be successfully managed percutaneously. Percutaneous nephrectomy is also a reality.[75] The percutaneous approach to cystotomy, bladder repair, and ureteral isolation with ligation is undergoing laboratory trials.[76] Continued investigation by creative individuals will widen the range of indications for percutaneous procedures.

REFERENCES

1. Motola JA, Smith AD: Therapeutic options for the management of upper tract calculi. Urol Clin North Am 17:191, 1990.
2. Smith AD, Lange PH, Fraley EE: Applications of percutaneous nephrostomy: new challenges and opportunities in endo-urology [letter]. J Urol 121:382, 1979.
3. Goodwin WB, Casey WC, Woolf W: Percutaneous trocar (needle) nephrostomy in hydronephrosis. JAMA 157:891, 1955.
4. Kaye KW, Goldberg ME: Applied anatomy of the kidney and ureter. Urol Clin North Am 9:3, 1982.
5. Young AT, Hunter DW, Castaneda-Zuniga WR, et al: Percutaneous stone extraction: use of the intercostal approach. Radiology 154:633, 1985.
6. Picus D, Weyman PJ, Clayman RV, McClennan BL: Intercostal space nephrostomy for percutaneous stone removal. AJR 147:393, 1986.
7. Karlin GS, Smith AD: Access to supracostal calices: renal displacement technique and review of options. J Urol 142:774, 1989.
8. Hodson CJ: The lobar structure of the kidney. Br J Urol 44:246, 1972.
9. Kaye KW, Reinke DB: Detailed caliceal anatomy for endourology. J Urol 143:1085, 1984.

10. Brodel M: The intrinsic blood vessels of the kidney and their significance in nephrotomy. John Hopkins Hosp Bull 12:10, 1901.
11. Thornbury JR: Perirenal anatomy: normal and abnormal. Radiol Clin North Am 27:321, 1979.
12. Saltzman B, Khasidy LR, Smith AD: Measurement of renal pelvic pressures during endourologic procedures. Urology 30:472, 1987.
13. Urivetsky M, Motola JA, King L, Smith AD: Impact of percutaneous renal stone removal on renal function: assessment by urinary lysozyme activity. Urology 33:305, 1989.
14. Eshghi AM, Roth JS, Smith AD: Percutaneous transperitoneal approach to a pelvic kidney for endourological removal of a staghorn calculus. J Urol 134:525, 1985.
15. Smith AD, Castaneda-Zuniga WR: Technique for removal of kidney stones intact. In Smith AD, Castaneda-Zuniga WR, Bronson JG (eds): Endourology: principles and practice. New York: Thieme, 1986, p 152.
16. Watson G, Dretler SP, Parrish J: The pulsed dye laser for fragmenting urinary calculi. J Urol 138:195, 1987.
17. Mulvaney WP, Beck CW: The laser beam in urology. J Urol 99:112, 1968.
18. Tanahashi Y, Orikasa S, Ciba R, et al: Disintegration of urinary calculi by laser beam: drilling experiment in extracted urinary stones. Tohuko J Exp Med 128:189, 1979.
19. Drach GW, Dretler SP, Fair W, et al: Report of the United States Cooperative Study of Extracorporeal Shock Wave Lithotripsy. J Urol 135:1134, 1986.
20. Silverman DE, Stamey TA: Management of infection stones: the Stanford experience. Medicine 60:44, 1983.
21. Gill WB: Renal calculous disease: classification, demographics and etiological considerations. Semin Urol 2:1, 1984.
22. Prien EL: Crystallographic analysis of urinary calculi: a 23 year study. J Urol 89:917, 1963.
23. Dahlberg PJ, Van Den Berg CJ, Kurtz SB, et al: Clinical features and management of cystinuria. Mayo Clin Proc 52:533, 1977.
24. Freed SZ: The alternative use of an alkalinizing salt and acetazolimide in the management of cystine and uric acid stones. J Urol 113:96, 1975.
25. Koide T, Kinoshita K, Takemoto M, et al: Conservative treatment of cystine calculi: effect of alpha-mercaptoproprionylglycine on cystine stone dissolution and on prevention of stone recurrence. J Urol 128:513, 1982.
26. Crissey MM, Gittes RF: Dissolution of cystine ureteral calculus by irrigation with tromethamine. J Urol 121:811, 1979.
27. Schmeller NT, Kersting H, Schuller J, et al: Combination of chemolysis and shock wave lithotripsy in the treatment of cystine renal calculi. J Urol 131:433, 1984.
28. Saltzman N, Gittes RF: Chemolysis of cystine calculi. J Urol 136:846, 1986.
29. Rosenstein IJM, Hami Hon-Miller JMT: Inhibitors of urease as chemotherapeutic agents. CRC Crit Rev Microbiol 11:1, 1984.
30. Griffith DP, Gibson JR, Clinton C, et al: Acetohydroxamic acid: clinical studies of a urease inhibitor in patients with staghorn calculi. J Urol 119:9, 1978.
31. Williams JJ, Radman JS, Peterson CM: A randomized double-blind study of acetohydroxamic acid in struvite nephrolithiasis. N Engl J Med 311:760, 1984.
32. Stegmayr B, Stegmayr B: Crystal formation induced by uropathogenic bacteria. Scand J Urol Nephrol 17:197, 1983.
33. Suby HI, Suby RM, Albright F: Properties of organic acid solutions which determine their irritability to the bladder mucous membrane and the effect of magnesium in overcoming this irritability. J Urol 48:549, 1942.
34. Dretler SP, Pfister RC: Primary dissolution of struvite calculi. J Urol 131:861, 1984.
35. Rosen DI, Nemoy NJ, Wolf PL, et al: Intravenous infusion of Renacidin in dogs. Invest Urol 9:31, 1971.
36. Nemoy NJ, Stamey TA: Surgical, bacteriological and biochemical management of infection stones. JAMA 215:1470, 1971.
37. Dretler SP, Pfister RC, Newhouse JH: Renal stone dissolution via percutaneous nephrostomy. N Engl J Med 300:341, 1979.
38. Fam B, Rossier AB, Yalla SB, et al: The role of hemiacidrin in the management of renal stones in spinal cord injury patients. J Urol 116:696, 1976.
39. Pak CYC, Fuller C, Sakjaee K, et al: Long term treatment of calcium nephrolithiasis with potassium citrate. J Urol 134:11, 1985.
40. Pak CYC, Diller EC, Smith GW, et al: Renal stones of calcium phosphate: physiochemical basis for their formation. Proc Soc Exp Biol Med 130:753, 1969.
41. Pak CYC, Watters O, Arnold L, et al: Mechanism for calcium urolithiasis among patients with hyperuricosuria: supersaturation with respect to monosodium urate. J Clin Invest 59:426, 1977.
42. Kursh ED, Resnick MI: Dissolution of uric acid calculi with systemic alkalinization. J Urol 132:286, 1984.
43. Sadi MV, Saltzman N, Feria G, Gittes RF: Experimental observations on dissolution of uric acid calculi. J Urol 134:575, 1985.
44. Smith C, Linner J: Dissolution of calcium oxalate calculi. Urology 19:21, 1982.
45. Pak CYC, Fuller C: Idiopathic hypocitraturia calcium oxalate nephrolithiasis successfully treated with potassium citrate. Ann Intern Med 104:33, 1986.
46. Kallistratos G: Litholytic agents: preventative and curative drugs for nephrolithiasis. Drug Design 4:237, 1973.
47. Davis DM, Strong GH, Drake WM: Intubated ureterotomy: experimental work and clinical results. J Urol 59:851, 1948.
48. Oppenheimer R, Hinman F Jr: Ureteral regeneration: contracture vs. hyperplasia of smooth muscle. J Urol 74:476, 1955.
49. King LR, Coughlin PW, Ford KK, et al: Initial experience with percutaneous and transurethral ablation of postoperative ureteral strictures in children. J Urol 131:1167, 1984.
50. Amer M, Abdel H: Endopyelotomy for ureteropelvic junction obstruction: is long term stenting mandatory? J Endourol 1:265, 1987.
51. Motola JA, Badlani GH, Smith AD: 210 consecutive endopyelotomies: An 8 year follow-up (submitted for publication).
52. Badlani GH, Smith AD: Percutaneous endopyelopyelotomy: endourological management of a bifid pelvis with ureteropelvic junction obstruction. J Urol 134:327, 1985.
53. Timmons JW Jr, Malch RS, Malek RS, et al: Caliceal diverticulum. J Urol 114:6, 1975.
54. Hulbert JC, Reddy PK, Hunter DW, et al: Percutaneous techniques for the management of caliceal diverticula containing calculi. J Urol 135:225, 1986.
55. Van Cangh PJ, Aad AA, Lorge F, et al: Management of symptomatic calculi located in caliceal diverticula: a review of 38 patients. Presented at the 84th Annual Meeting of the American Urological Association, Dallas, May 1989.
56. Saltzman B, Smith AD: Percutaneous renal surgery. Semin Urol 4:153, 1986.
57. Clayman RV, Hunter D, Surya V, et al: Percutaneous intrarenal electrosurgery. J Urol 131:864, 1984.
58. Motola JA, Smith AD: Management of upper tract calculi. Urol Clin North Am 17:191, 1990.
59. Johansson S, Wohlquist L: A prognostic study of urothelial renal pelvic tumors: comparison between the prognosis of patients treated with intrafascial nephrectomy and perifascial nephroureterectomy. Cancer 43:2525, 1979.
60. McCarron JP, Mills C, Vaughan ED Jr: Tumors of the renal pelvis and ureter: current concepts and management. Semin Urol 1:75, 1983.
61. Ferris DO, Daut RV: Epithelioma of the pelvis of a solitary kidney treated by electrocoagulation. J Urol 59:577, 1948.

62. Carrol G: Bilateral transitional cell carcinoma of the renal pelvis. J Urol 93:135, 1965.
63. Smith AD, Orihuela E, Crowley AR: Percutaneous management of renal pelvic tumors: a treatment option in selected cases. J Urol 137:852, 1987.
64. Streem SB, Pontes JE: Percutaneous management of upper tract transitional cell carcinoma. J Urol 135:773, 1986.
65. Woodhouse CRJ, Kellett MJ, Bloom HJG: Percutaneous renal surgery and local radiotherapy in the management of renal pelvic transitional cell carcinoma. Br J Urol 58:245, 1986.
66. Murphy DM, Zincke H, Furlow WL: Management of high grade transitional cell cancer of the upper urinary tract. J Urol 125:25, 1981.
67. Zincke H, Neves RJ: Feasibility of conservative surgery for transitional cell cancer of the upper urinary tract. Urol Clin North Am 11:717, 1984.
68. Moldwin RM, Smith AD: Update on percutaneous treatment of upper tract urothelial tumors. Presented at the 8th World Congress on Endourology and ESWL, Washington, DC, August 29–Sept 2, 1990.
69. Laucks SP Jr, McLachlan MSF: Aging and simple cysts of the kidney. Br J Radiol 54:12, 1981.
70. Bach D, Weissbach L, Granthoff H, Lachner KJ: Percutaneous puncture of renal cysts for diagnostic and therapeutic purpose. Urol Int 35:281, 1980.
71. Beyer D, Fiedler V: Is renal cyst puncture an available diagnostic procedure for differentiation of avascular space-occupying lesions? Urologe (A) 16:339, 1977.
72. Hubner W, Pfab R, Porpaczy P, Hartung R: Renal cysts: percutaneous resection with standard urologic instruments. J Endourol 4:61, 1990.
73. Meyer WM, Jonas D: Endoscopic percutaneous resection of renal cysts. Presented at the 8th World Congress on Endourology and ESWL, Washington DC, August 29–Sept 2, 1990.
74. Hulbert JC, Hunter D: Percutaneous techniques for intrarenal marsupialization of difficult symptomatic renal cysts. Presented at the 85th Annual Meeting of the American Urological Association, New Orleans, May 1990.
75. Clayman RV, Soper N, Kavoussi LR, et al: Laparoscopic nephrectomy: initial report of pelviscopic total organ ablation. Presented at the 8th World Congress on Endourology and ESWL, Washington, DC, August 29–Sept 2, 1990.
76. Winfield HN, Ryan KJ: Experimental laparoscopic surgery: potential clinical applications in urology. J Endourol 4:37, 1990.

CHAPTER 10

FLOW CYTOMETRY IN UROLOGY

IHN SEONG WHANG and MITCHELL C. BENSON

In 1941 Papanicolaou and Traut established the clinical relevance of nuclear morphology and cytochemistry for diagnosis of cervical cancer from exfoliative cytologic specimens.[1] This provided a rationale for the development of automated apparatus to perform clinical cytologic tests, leading to the construction of the first cell sorter in 1965 by Fulwyler.[2] In 1967 Kamentsky and Melamed established that nucleic acid content and cell size were useful parameters for cytologic classification of cervical cells and proceeded to build a flow cytometer that measured nucleic acid content and cell size.[3]

When it became evident that measurements of DNA ploidy could be used to detect and diagnose cancer and predict patient prognosis, the application of flow cytometry to the assessment of a wide range of human tumors proliferated rapidly. Flow cytometry can now be used to analyze total DNA content, individual chromosomes, RNA content, cell surface antigens, cell size, and numerous functional characteristics of individual cells. Samples can be further analyzed by computer determination of cell cycle and by cell sorting for assessment of specific populations.[4]

Flow cytometry has been extensively employed in the evaluation of tumors in the genitourinary tract. This chapter discusses the knowledge obtained from these flow cytometric evaluations, as well as the basic methods necessary to use and understand flow cytometric determinations.

METHODS

Numerous flow cytometry instruments are available commercially. Regardless of which instrument is employed, the basic tenets are the same.[4,5] These automated cell analysis and cell sorting instruments combine optical and electrical sensing techniques that, with the aid of computer data storage, permit several simultaneous measurements on the same cell. Typical measurements are cell volume, multicolor fluorescence from stains bound to cellular constituents, and light scatter with which cell size and intracellular structure can be assessed. Figure 10–1 is a schematic drawing of a typical flow cytometer. Before a discussion of how a flow cytometer operates, a brief explanation of sample preparation is appropriate because the data obtained from analysis of a sample can be no better than the sample itself.

Proper sample preparation is crucial if meaningful conclusions are to be drawn from the analysis of a specimen. An in-depth discussion of sample preparation can be found in a text by Pretlow and Pretlow.[6] For routine analysis of DNA ploidy, we use a technique developed at our institution by Dietch, Law, and DeVere White.[7]

Once a single cell suspension derived from a viable tumor sample has been prepared, cell integrity should be assessed by trypan blue exclusion. This is necessary for all cytometric studies, even if living cells are not required. Suspensions with less than 70% viability may lead to spurious results owing to leakage of cellular components or DNA into the media and analysis of incomplete cells. To allow retrospective analysis of archival material, Hedley and associates developed a method to extract nuclei from formalin-fixed, paraffin-embedded tissue blocks.[8] This major advance opened the way for numerous studies of patient prognosis by flow cytometric DNA analysis of pathologic tissue. Tissues fixed in Bouin's solution are generally not amenable to retrospective analysis, since the picric acid in the fixative causes an ongoing degradation of DNA even in the paraffin block. Attempts to analyze such samples either are unsuccessful or result in histograms with large standard deviations.

Flow cytometric analysis begins by introduction of the cell sample into the flow chamber. Smooth nonturbulent flow is ensured by the introduction of the sample into the center of a faster moving

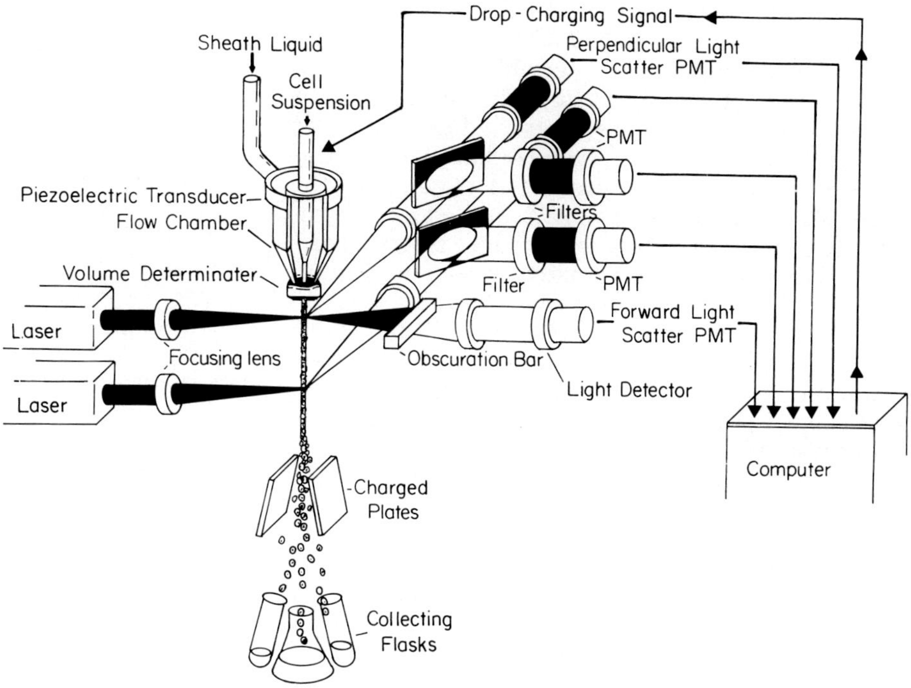

FIGURE 10–1. A schematic drawing of a dual laser flow cytometer. The flow cytometer shown is capable of cell sorting.

stream of sheath fluid as described by Reynolds' formulation of fluid flow. The proximity of the cells to one another can be controlled by the rate at which sample fluid enters the flow chamber. The speed at which fluid exits the flow chamber is held constant, and this principle allows the measurement of multiple parameters at distinct sensing stations along the course of the fluid stream. The distance between the excitation lasers is governed by the configuration of the flow system. Since the rate at which a cell is traveling is constant, data can be correlated as having originated from a single source by the time elapsed between readings. For example, a cell enters the flow chamber and passes through an electronic cell volume detector at time 0 (Figure 10–1). At time 0 + W, that cell is illuminated by light source 1 and bound stains fluoresce accordingly. At time 0 + W + X, that cell is illuminated by light source 2 and stains similarly fluoresce. Since these events are separated in time, the dedicated computer can record all readings as having originated from a single cell and store the data accordingly. This type of data collection is called list mode data acquisition. Later the experiment can be repeated with the data signals arising from computer storage. This type of data analysis is called list mode data analysis and is useful for analyzing complex populations.[5]

Cell sorting is accomplished by carrying these concepts one step further. A piezoelectric transducer (which converts electrical energy to mechanical energy) is activated and causes the fluid stream to vibrate. These vibrations eventually disrupt the stream and at a definable point cause it to break into droplets. Some of these droplets contain the desired cells. Since the stream is traveling at a constant rate, the distance between the sensors and the deflection plates defines the time at which a droplet containing a desired cell will be at the deflection plates. By knowing the distance between the sensors and the point at which droplets are forming, the urologist can determine the times at which to charge the stream and activate the deflectors. For example, a prostate cancer cell has its volume determined at time 0. At times 0 + W and 0 + W + X, various determinations are made and this cell type is found to be of interest. The cell continues to move down the intact sample stream and at time 0 + W + X + Y, just before disruption of the stream begins, the stream is given a positive (+) charge. The stream is then disrupted, and the droplet continues to carry this (+) charge. The intact stream is then neutralized so that future droplets are not charged and inadvertently deflected. At time 0 + W + X + Y + Z, the charged droplet containing the desired cell passes through the charged deflector plates and reacts according to the charge placed on the droplet. This process, called cell sorting, allows populations of interest to be captured and further analyzed.[5]

Cells can be sorted directly onto microscope slides for visual identification or sorted into wells containing growth media and subsequently placed in cell culture. Researchers are also collecting cells for further evaluation employing polymerase chain reaction (PCR).[9] We believe that cell sorting should be a part of any new experiment to ensure that the researcher is dealing with a true population and not an artifact.

Most flow cytometers are equipped with laser light sources. The most commonly employed is the 5 W argon laser, since it has substantial power output in both the ultraviolet and visual ranges. When a flow cytometer is equipped with two argon lasers, one is often used to drive a secondary compound in the form of a tunable dyer laser. This allows a wider range of excitation wavelengths and the ability to employ more fluorescent labels. The main drawback to laser light sources is the expense of the laser. Mercury arc lamps are a less expensive alternative and are available on some instruments. The schematic flow cytometer shown in Figure 10–1 would have laser light sources.

Once a cell or cellular component is illuminated, it emits a wavelength of light specific for the fluorochrome with which it is labeled. Optical filters are used to collect only the spectrum of fluorescence being studied. Two types of detectors are available: the photovoltaic photodiode detector, which collects forward light scatter, and photomultiplier tubes, which detect fluorescence. Both generate a current in response to a photon strike.[4]

Those wishing additional information on the techniques of flow cytometry are referred to the textbooks and articles in references 4, 10 and 11.

QUALITY CONTROL

Variability can occur from numerous sources. As mentioned previously, sample preparation is an important first step in flow analysis. Second is the process of staining the sample with a given dye or fluorochrome. Errors produced by inappropriate dye concentration can result in an increased standard error. The flow cytometer itself can also be the source of error. The machine must be calibrated and well maintained, and the optics must be in proper alignment.

When performing DNA analysis, we always include an internal control. Either chicken or trout erythrocytes (red blood cells [RBCs]) are excellent for this, since they have a total DNA content approximately one-third that of humans. Therefore the animal RBCs can be added directly to a sample without perturbing the human portion of the histogram (Figure 10–2).

Others have recognized the importance of quality control. To assess different laboratories, the National Cancer Institute established a Bladder Cancer Flow Cytometry Network.[12] This network involved five laboratories, Memorial Sloan-Kettering Cancer Center, Montefiore Medical Center, Rush-Presbyterian Medical Center, University of California at Davis, and University of Rochester. The investigators performed studies using "cocktail" samples to assess the reproducibility of flow cytometry results among the five laboratories. They found two types of variation among the laboratories. First were variations that were constant across runs. This constant variability is due to differences in instrumentation, instrument setup, and laboratory techniques, as well as consistent differences in the number of cells analyzed. Second, the investigators found differences among the laboratories that were not constant across runs. The source of these errors appeared to be inconsistency in sample preparation, staining, and analysis. The elimination of this latter type of variation is necessary for meaningful comparison of data within and among laboratories and for the creation of universal laboratory data bases.

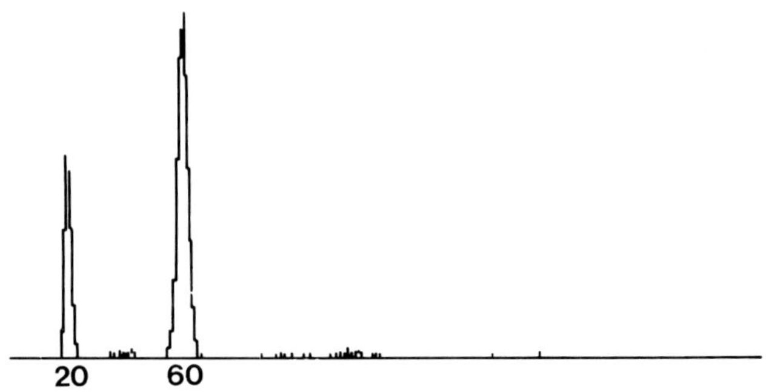

FIGURE 10–2. A sample histogram demonstrating the chicken red blood cell DNA peak in channel 20 and a human diploid population in channel 60.

CYTOCHEMICAL STAINS

Quantitative cytochemical stains provide a rapid, accurate, reproducible means of assaying genetic, cytologic, biochemical, and functional properties of normal cells and benign and malignant tumor cells. Quantitative measurement of fluorescent dyes that bind to particular cellular constituents has received the most attention in flow cytometry. In addition, fluorescent dyes can be combined with antibodies and lectins for the study of cell surface moieties.[13,14]

The measurement of fluorescence has three major advantages in flow cytometry: (1) fluorescence intensity is directly proportional to the quantity of the dye present and, by inference, the amount of the material being bound; (2) low concentrations of dye per cell can be detected; and (3) nonfluorescent substrates can be activated to a fluorescent state by cellular enzymes and used to quantitate cellular function.[15]

CELL CYCLE

Based on the early work of Howard and Pelc, cell growth and division have been described in terms of specific phases through which a cell cycles.[16] Cells not proliferating and not part of the cell cycle are labeled G-0. The four phases of cell proliferation are designated G-1, S, G-2, and M. After a cell leaves the quiescent state, G-0, it enters a phase during which no DNA synthesis takes place. This is called the G-1 (Gap 1) phase. No difference in DNA content between G-0 and G-1 cells has been identified but differences in RNA content have been found.[17] The next phase is the synthesis phase, or S phase. In the S phase the DNA content of the cell increases until the genome is duplicated. The S phase is followed by a premitotic nonsynthetic phase called G-2 (Gap 2). The G-2 phase ends when mitosis (M phase) begins. Mitotic division takes up only a small part of the cell cycle. Following mitosis, cells can return to G-1 and recycle or enter G-0 and become quiescent. Cells in G-0 and G-1 phase have unit DNA content, whereas cells in G-2 and M phases have twice the G-0 and G-1 phase DNA content.[17] The percentage of cells in the S, G-2, and M phases is called the proliferative fraction.[18] In general, the proportion of cells in S phase increases with decreasing degree of differentiation and with increasing invasiveness of tumors.

DNA PLOIDY

To date, the assessment of DNA ploidy and proliferative fraction has received the most attention in flow cytometric tumor analysis. In some studies the incidence of tumors with abnormal DNA content was found to be low, whereas in others the incidence of aneuploid abnormalities has been as high as 90%.[19] This discrepancy is due in part to experimental technique and in part to the definition of abnormal ploidy employed in different studies.[20] DNA distributions invariably contain pulses resulting from cellular debris that produces nonspecific background fluorescence. These background pulses overlie all parts of the histogram. The percentage of cells in the cycling compartment is usually much smaller than the percentage of cells in the main population of the tumor. Thus the inadvertent addition of spurious pulses to the smaller cycling compartment can have a significant effect on the analysis of that compartment while having little or no effect on the analysis of the main population. This can lead to an overestimation of the cycling cell fraction or the erroneous labeling of a tumor as aneuploid. Therefore correction procedures for nonspecific background fluorescence are important for correct calculations of cell cycle phases.[21] In addition, admixtures of different cell populations, especially lymphocytes in samples from complex tumors, can occur. This problem can be handled in two ways: (1) isolation of epithelial cells using monoclonal antibodies directed against epithelial cell membranes or cytokeratins and (2) separation of lymphocytes by centrifugation on a lymphocyte separation medium or subtraction of lymphocytes using panleukocyte monoclonal antibodies.[21] No definition of abnormal proliferation is universally accepted. Some consider less than 10% proliferative fraction normal, 10% to 15% suspicious, and greater than 15% abnormal. Others seem to have varied these percentages to fit their results.

BLADDER CANCER

Flow cytometry is a useful adjunctive method for examination of bladder cancer. In 1980 Collste and colleagues reported on a series of patients studied by flow cytometry using bladder irrigation specimens collected at the time of cystoscopy.[22] Since then, transitional cell carcinoma (TCC) of the bladder has been the urological tumor most extensively studied by flow cytometry.[23] TCC of the bladder is often multicentric, and since carcinoma in situ is not always easily detectable at cystoscopy, flow cytometry has been valuable in detecting these changes in the urothelium. In addition, because studies of cells in voided urine or bladder washings can easily be repeated, the method is valuable for studying the effects of different treatment regimens.[24]

DNA ploidy studies in bladder cancer have shown that the degree of ploidy is generally related to grade and stage of the tumor; diploid tumors are generally of low grade and aneuploid tumors of high grade. In a study of 383 newly detected bladder tumors, all grade I tumors were found to be diploid and all grade III tumors were aneuploid.[18] Grade II tumors were half diploid and half aneuploid. This is in agreement with the findings of a majority of studies, in which the degree of differentiation correlated with ploidy. DNA ploidy determinations have also been employed to detect the presence of TCC, predict the recurrence rate and progression of superficial tumors, and determine the malignant potential of high-grade tumors.[25]

Detection of Bladder Cancer

The bladder is particularly amenable to examination with flow cytometry, since specimens can be easily and noninvasively obtained. One of the most important applications of flow cytometry may be in follow-up of patients who have undergone local transurethral resection of their first superficial tumor. This is because flow cytometric measurements are objective, are reproducible, and can predict and detect tumor recurrence.[26] The sensitivity of flow cytometry is at least equal to that of conventional cytology.[27-30] Using flow cytometry of bladder washing specimens, Klein and associates correctly identified 69 of 71 patients with bladder cancer.[30] Devonec and co-workers in a study of 84 patients found that flow cytometry had higher sensitivity than conventional cytology.[28] This was further supported by Badalament and colleagues, who compared sensitivities among bladder washing flow cytometry, bladder washing cytology, and cytology of three voided urine specimens.[27] They found sensitivities of 83% with bladder washing flow cytometry, 61% with bladder washing cytology, and 60% with cytology of three voided specimens. The sensitivities of all modalities decreased when only women were studied owing to the frequent presence of pyuria in women with bladder tumors. Hermansen and associates found a sensitivity of 64% for bladder washing flow cytometry, 31% for urine cytology performed at cytoscopy, and 32% for cytology of three voided urine specimens in women with bladder tumors.[29] These studies show that flow cytometry is as sensitive a test as conventional cytology.

A technique for simultaneous analysis of DNA, RNA, and nuclear size by flow cytometry has been described by Collste and co-workers.[22] This was performed in an attempt to increase sensitivity and specificity of cytometry. To quantitate RNA and DNA, the authors used acridine orange, which binds to single-stranded RNA and double-stranded DNA via different mechanisms. The method of binding results in unique wavelength fluorescence and permits discrimination between granulocytes and epithelial cells based on differences in RNA content and size. Collste and associates were able to detect 11/13 papillary cancers, 12/13 invasive cancers, and 24/28 carcinomas in situ. Thus the simultaneous analysis of DNA and RNA in flow cytometry can increase sensitivity and specificity.

To determine the predictive value of flow cytometric DNA ploidy and urine cytology in patients with superficial TCC of the bladder, we conducted a retrospective analysis of 181 patients who underwent cystoscopy, flow cytometric DNA ploidy, and cytology from 1984 until 1989.[31] Ninety-nine patients continued to be followed serially for superficial TCC and underwent 637 separate examinations, a mean of 6.5 per patient. At initial evaluation, flow cytometric DNA ploidy had 75% sensitivity and 57% specificity; cytology was 72% sensitive and 94% specific. During the course of follow-up, flow cytometric ploidy was 76% sensitive and 36% specific. Cytology was less sensitive (40%) but more specific (81%) than flow cytometric DNA ploidy in follow-up evaluation. These results were similar whether or not intravesical chemotherapy or bacillus Calmette Guerin (BCG) was administered. Patients with flow cytometric DNA ploidy and cytology positive for TCC were followed up longitudinally to ascertain whether a false positive flow cytometric DNA ploidy represented early detection of recurrent TCC not apparent at cystoscopy. "False positive" flow cytometric DNA ploidy and cytology were equally predictive of recurrent TCC progressively with time, but for any given examination flow cytometry was more likely to detect and predict TCC recurrence. At 4 years the incidence of TCC for false positive flow cytometric DNA ploidy and for cytology was 87% and 84%, respectively.[31]

The sensitivity of flow cytometric DNA ploidy in detection can be enhanced by the use of secondary cell surface markers. Unfortunately, many markers are too specific and do not label all TCC. For this reason we have developed a technique using a surface marker, epithelial membrane antigen (EMA; Dako Corp.) that is specific for epithelial cells. EMA reacts with normal epithelium from a variety of tissues, as well as a number of neoplasms, including adenocarcinoma, TCC, and squamous cell cancer. Using this technique on alcohol-fixed cells from bladder washings, we have enhanced our detection of abnormal cell populations and reduced artifacts caused by lymphocyte contamination.[32]

Flow cytometry has some disadvantages as a means to detect recurrence in patients with a history of bladder cancer. First is the cost of instrumentation, although this must be weighed against the cost of other means of detection. Second is that for best results the test requires a sample obtained by bladder irrigation rather than one obtained from a voided specimen.[26] However, bladder catheterization is not highly invasive and has low morbidity. If the detection rate by flow cytometry was sufficient and cystoscopy could be avoided, the arguments against expense and catheterization would be moot.

DNA Patterns in Macroscopically Normal Bladder

In extensive studies using flow cytometry, Farsund, Hoestmark, and Laerum[33] found that macroscopically normal-appearing bladder mucosa in patients with bladder cancer had abnormal DNA content that was a function of the grade of the primary tumor. In their study all grade I tumors were diploid, whereas 43% of grade II and 91% of grade III tumors demonstrated aneuploidy. Among patients with aneuploid grade II and III tumors, 44% demonstrated aneuploidy in macroscopically and histologically normal-appearing mucosa away from the tumor. The frequency of occurrence of aneuploidy in the macroscopically normal mucosa increased from 25% in patients with tetraploid tumors to 86% in those with nontetraploid aneuploid tumors.

DNA Patterns in Carcinoma in Situ

Carcinoma in situ of the bladder was first described by Melicow and Hollowell in 1952.[34] Primary carcinoma in situ may progress to a noninvasive papillary tumor or an invasive sessile or papillary cancer. The interval between diagnosis and progression varies from a few months to many years.[35] The DNA ploidy pattern of carcinoma in situ does not differ from the pattern found in other grade III tumors; that is, most are aneuploid. In one prospective study of 20 patients with carcinoma in situ, all 20 tumors were aneuploid.[35] Among the 20, 7 had multiple aneuploid lines and all 7 became invasive within 2 years. The percentage of S phase DNA was noted to be highest in those tumors that progressed.[18,35] Thus the combination of more than one aneuploid cell line and a high proliferative fraction (percentage of S phase) portended a particularly unfavorable prognosis in primary carcinoma in situ.

DNA Patterns in Superficial Bladder Tumors

The natural history of superficial bladder tumors has been well characterized by the National Bladder Cancer Collaborative Group A.[36] They reported on 249 patients with superficial bladder cancer (stages Ta and T1) with a median follow-up of 39 months. Progression correlated with the grade and stage of the tumor. Only 2% of grade I tumors progressed, whereas 4% of grade II and 45% of grade III tumors did. The majority of progression occurred within 24 months of diagnosis. Similar correlations could be made with stage. Only 4% of Ta tumors, but 30% of T1 tumors, progressed. When the tumor size was examined as an independent variable, a significant difference in progression rate was observed only with tumors larger than 5 cm. DNA ploidy studies have been performed to better stratify patients within stage and grade categories.

Gustafson, Tribukait, and Esposti studied 229 patients with superficial (stage Ta and T1, grade I and II) tumors.[37] None of the 175 diploid tumors progressed during 30 months of follow-up, but 19 of the 54 aneuploid tumors did. This progression led to a cancer-related death in 11 patients. Among the patients with aneuploid tumors, only 10% of tetraploid tumors progressed whereas 51% of nontetraploid tumors did. Thus, even among aneuploid tumors, triploid tumors are more aggressive. As expected, most of the progressive tumors had a high proliferative fraction (percentage of S phase). The recurrence rate of these superficial low-grade tumors was also related to their ploidy. The mean annual recurrence rate of a diploid grade I tumor was 0.28 recurrence per year, and that of diploid grade II tumor was 0.52 recurrence per year. The risk of recurrence for an aneuploid grade II tumor was 1.54 recurrences per year.[37]

DeVere White and colleagues in a retrospective analysis studied deparaffinized archival material from patients with stage Ta bladder cancer (grade I or II).[38] They found that all patients with aneuploid tumors had recurrences but only 29% of patients with diploid tumors did. In 20 of the 28 patients with recurrences, the ploidy had changed at the time of recurrence from the ploidy noted at initial diagnosis; that is, diploid tumors became aneuploid. In addition, when patients with aneuploid tumors had recurrence with an aneuploid tumor, two thirds were invasive, whereas only one third were invasive when the recurrence was nonaneuploid.

In a subsequent study of 477 patients with superficial bladder tumors, Gustafson, Tribukait, and Esposti found that recurrences developed in 60% of patients with single tumors and 89% of patients with multiple tumors.[39] Similarily, only 63% of grade I tumors recurred, but 79% of grade II tumors did. These data could be further stratified by DNA ploidy. The recurrence rate among patients with aneuploid tumors was 94%, whereas 71% of diploid tumors recurred.

The ability to predict the natural history of superficial TCC can be enhanced by the use of monoclonal antibodies to cell surface glycoproteins. Fradet and associates analyzed bladder tumor specimens simultaneously for DNA content and for expression of certain surface glycoproteins.[40] They found that the expression of surface glycoprotein T138 and the degree of ploidy gave the best prognostic correlation for bladder cancer. Among patients with diploid tumors, 26 did not have expression of the T138 antigen and none of these patients died of cancer, whereas 5 of 15 (33%) who had expression of T138 antigen died of cancer ($p < 0.01$). Among the 10 patients with aneuploid tumors in whom T138 was not expressed, only 2 cancer deaths occurred. T138 was expressed on an aneuploid tumor in 19 patients, 12 of whom died of cancer. Fradet and associates concluded that the use of multiparameter flow cytometry to analyze both DNA content and surface antigen yielded more prognostic information about human bladder cancer than either modality alone.

DNA Patterns in Invasive Bladder Tumors

Approximately one third of bladder tumors are invasive when diagnosed, and studies have shown that almost all invasive tumors are aneuploid.[38,41] Surprisingly little attention has been focused on the relationship between DNA ploidy and survival after cystectomy. Patients with invasive bladder cancers treated with radiation therapy or chemotherapy in addition to cystectomy have been the subject of numerous analyses that have tried to use DNA ploidy to select appropriate candidates for these alternative and adjuvant therapies.

In an older study with Feulgen-stained material, Fossa, Kaalhus, and Scott-Knudsen examined 123 patients with bladder cancer in all stages followed up for 2 years.[42] The relative frequency of nondiploid tumors increased with increasing clinical stage and decreasing histologic differentiation. Among what they called stage I (stage Ta and T1) tumors, 43 were diploid and 20 were nondiploid. Among more deeply invasive, stage II and III (stage T2 and T3) tumors, 8 were diploid and 18 were nondiploid. For stage IV (stage T4) tumors, 12 were diploid and 22 were nondiploid. Patients with advanced diploid tumors (stages II to IV) had better actuarial survival at 18 months than those with nondiploid tumors. However, this survival advantage was no longer present at 24 months, which may reflect the absence of effective adjuvant therapy in the 1970s.

Lymph Node Metastases

The DNA pattern in lymph node metastases has been studied by Ghoneim.[18] Lymph node metastases were found in 43 of 136 patients who underwent cystectomy for bladder cancer. All except 2 were muscle invasive tumors (≥T2). Thirty tumors were diploid and 106 were aneuploid. Only 2 of 30 diploid tumors had lymph node metastasis, whereas 41 (39%) of aneuploid tumors had metastasized to the lymph nodes. In 54% of 43 patients with lymph node metastasis the degrees of ploidy in the primary tumor and the metastatic lymph nodes were the same, whereas in 30% the degrees of ploidy in the primary tumor and the metastatic lymph nodes were completely different. This may have been due to a change in ploidy during evolution of the tumor or to the existence of undetected additional cell populations in the primary tumor. Furthermore, all tumors with an S phase greater than 20% had lymph node metastases, whereas 50% of tumors with an S phase between 10% and 20% had lymph node metastases. Of the tumors with an S phase less than 10%, 33% had lymph node involvement.[18] This provides further support for the idea that DNA ploidy as well as the proliferation fraction affects the incidence of metastatic disease and thereby affects overall prognosis in bladder cancer.

DNA Patterns and Response to External Radiation Therapy

Although external radiation therapy has the potential of preserving a functioning bladder, not all patients have tumor control after a full course of radiation therapy. In an attempt to select patients whose tumors may be more radiosensitive, flow cytometric DNA ploidy has been used. Wijkstrom and co-workers used external beam radiation to treat 73 patients with advanced bladder cancer and studied whether pretreatment flow cytometric DNA characteristics affected the outcome over a 5.6-year period.[18] They found that tumor grade, tumor stage, and endoscopic findings were not useful in predicting the likelihood of radiation response. However, flow cytometric DNA ploidy identified some patients who would have a low likelihood of responding to external radiation therapy. In their series 50% of patients had residual tumors following radiation therapy and all died of disease. Twenty-seven of the 73 patients had tumors with several aneuploid cell lines, and 85% of these patients failed to respond to radiation therapy.

Radiation therapy employed before cystectomy can result in clinical downstaging. In a study by Klein and associates, clinical downstaging was documented by flow cytometric DNA ploidy in 43% of patients.[43] They studied 28 patients with grade II and III muscle invasive TCC of the bladder treated with 2000 rads to the pelvis over 5 days. A barbotage specimen of the bladder was obtained before and after radiation therapy. All 28 patients had aneuploidy before radiation therapy. Despite only 5 days of therapy, 12 patients no longer demonstrated aneuploidy at the end of treatment. This was interpreted as downstaging of the tumor and was considered a favorable prognostic sign.

DNA Patterns and Survival in Bladder Cancer

Flow cytometric DNA ploidy is an independent prognostic variable. An overall (all stages and grades) 5-year survival of 91% has been reported for patients with diploid bladder tumors, whereas 5-year survival of patients with tetraploid bladder tumors was 83%. In patients with aneuploid tumors the overall 5-year survival decreased to 59% if only one aneuploid stem line was found and 30% if multiple aneuploid stem lines existed.[18] In addition to correlating with DNA ploidy, survival is a function of a tumor's proliferative index. Survival is inversely proportional to percentge of S phase. In patients with grade II bladder tumors in whom the S phase percentage was less than 10%, the 5-year survival rate was 92%. Survival decreased to 48% when the S phase was 10% to 14% and to only 14% when the S phase was greater than 15%.[18] These data strongly support the classification of bladder tumors by both DNA ploidy and proliferative fraction.

Not all investigations have demonstrated an independent correlation between DNA ploidy and survival. Murphy, Chandler, and Trafford found that DNA ploidy did not offer prognostic information that was not already available with histologic grade alone.[44] They studied deparaffinized specimens from 64 patients with grade I to III TCC. A significant correlation existed between DNA ploidy and survival. However, the authors noted that DNA ploidy did not provide important new prognostic information about grade II neoplasms and believed that DNA ploidy did not add to the information available by histologic grading alone.

Most experts agree that flow cytometric determinations of DNA ploidy are useful in the study of bladder tumors. Generally these studies offer unique information about the risk of recurrence and progression for superficial disease. In addition, DNA ploidy appears useful in predicting clinical outcome in patients with invasive and metastatic disease. The utility of this and similar technologies as a replacement for cystoscopy in the monitoring of patients remains to be determined. DNA ploidy measurements and determinations of proliferative fraction do appear to increase the ability to predict the malignant potential of a given tumor.

TRANSITIONAL CELL CANCER OF THE RENAL PELVIS AND URETER

DNA ploidy analysis of TCC of the upper urinary tract mirrors the findings concerning bladder TCC. Oldbring and co-workers prospectively studied 11 patients with TCC of the renal pelvis and the ureter.[45] They found DNA ploidy to correlate well with histologic findings. Aneuploidy was found in half of grade II tumors and all grade III tumors. In addition, they demonstrated aneuploidy in histologically normal urothelium. This has also been demonstrated in the bladder.[33] Aneuploidy was also associated with an increased risk of carcinoma in situ in areas away from the primary tumor.

RENAL CELL CARCINOMA

Renal cell carcinoma can be a highly unpredictable neoplasm with a tendency to recur and cause death many years after initial therapy. The best available predictor of outcome is tumor stage at diagnosis.[18,46-49] Cell differentiation (grade) and histologic pattern have also been shown to affect prognosis.[18,49] The presence of either sarcomatous elements or poor differentiation indicates a less favorable prognosis. However, the majority of renal cell carcinomas are moderately differentiated, and these tumors behave in an unpredictable fashion.[18] DNA ploidy has been used in attempts to stratify patients. These studies have been aided by the use of archival material, which has enabled retrospective study of cases with long-term follow-up. Retrospective analysis has been important in evaluating the role of DNA ploidy in renal cell cancer because of the tumor's ability to recur or metastasize many years after initial therapy.

Numerous studies have examined the role of DNA ploidy in predicting the malignant potential and ultimate behavior of renal cell carcinoma. As with the bladder cancer, most studies have shown that ploidy correlates well with stage and prognosis.[18,46,48-51] However, some have found no correlation.[47,52]

DNA Patterns in Localized Renal Cell Carcinoma

Grignon and colleagues studied DNA ploidy in 103 patients with renal cell carcinoma.[46] Fifty-two patients had Robson stage I, 21 had Robson stage II, and 30 had Robson stage III tumors. The Robson stage, tumor ploidy, and mitotic rate were all statistically significant and independent predictors of outcome. Based on stage, 10-year survivals of 88%, 38%, and 39% were observed for stage I, II, and III renal cell carcinomas, respectively. DNA ploidy analysis revealed the tumors to be diploid in 52 cases, aneuploid in 49 cases, and tetraploid in 2 cases. Regardless of stage, the 10-year survival was 79% for diploid tumors and 49% for nondiploid tumors. The 10-year survival was 73% for tumors with a low mitotic index and 16% for tumors with a high mitotic rate.

In 1982 Baisch and colleagues studied 46 patients with renal cell carcinoma and found a significant correlation between the presence of aneuploidy and poor outcome.[20] However, this study did not stratify patients according to their pathologic stage. Later, Baisch, Otto, and Kloppel expanded the study and found that DNA ploidy was a significant predictor of outcome independent of stage and nuclear grade.[50]

Otto and associates studied 68 patients with renal cell carcinoma.[48] Metastatic disease developed within 1 to 4 years in 21% of patients with diploid tumors and in 89% of patients with aneuploid tumors. Furthermore, the proliferative activity of aneuploid tumors was greater than that of diploid tumors (12% versus 5%), and the proliferative activity in aneuploid patients with metastatic disease was higher (12%) than in those without metastatic disease (5%).

Ljungberg, Stenling, and Roos found a 48% incidence of diploidy, an 8% incidence of polyploidy, and a 44% incidence of aneuploidy in a series of patients treated for renal cell carcinoma.[53] No correlation between tumor size and DNA content was found, but aneuploid renal cell carcinomas had higher percentages of S phase cells than either diploid renal cell tumors or normal kidney parenchyma. Survival was not assessed in this study.

DNA Patterns in Metastatic Renal Cell Carcinoma

Unfortunately, about one third of patients with renal cell carcinoma have metastatic disease at the time of diagnosis. The survival rate for these patients has been reported to be 30% at 1 year, 7% at 2 years, and 5% at 5 years.[51] Stratification of patients with metastatic disease by DNA ploidy demonstrates that those with diploid primary tumors have a better prognosis than those with nondiploid primary tumors. The presence or absence of aneuploidy in the metastatic lesion also has prognostic significance.[18,48,51]

Ljungberg, Stenling, and Roos studied 59 patients with renal cell carcinoma followed for 2 years.[51] Of these patients, 23 had metastatic disease at the time of diagnosis. Ten of 23 had diploid primary tumors, and 13 had aneuploid primary tumors. Nine of the 10 patients with diploid tumors were alive at the end of follow-up, whereas only 1 of 13 patients with an aneuploid tumor was alive.

Furthermore, 7 of the 23 patients with metastatic disease had aneuploidy in the metastatic lesion, and all of them died during follow-up. Most of the patients with diploidy in the metastatic lesion were alive at the end of the follow-up. From these data Ljungberg and co-workers concluded that if a patient has a diploid primary tumor, aggressive treatment with surgical excision of all apparent metastases is indicated. However, in the presence of aneuploidy in a primary or metastatic lesion, aggressive therapy does not influence survival.[51]

Ljungberg, Stenling, and Roos examined ploidy in primary and metastatic renal cell carcinoma with respect to its predictive value for the development of metastatic disease.[52] The primary tumors were diploid in 47% of the patients and aneuploid in 53%. Among 32 metastatic lesions, 10 were diploid and 22 were aneuploid. The 15 diploid primary tumors spawned 9 aneuploid metastatic lesions, and 4 of the 17 aneuploid tumors produced diploid metastatic lesions. This is a further example of the tremendous heterogeneity found in renal cell carcinoma. When various predictors of survival were examined, the only parameter of statistical significance was the ploidy of the metastatic deposit. Patients with diploid metastasis survived an average of 31 months, whereas those with aneuploid metastatic lesions survived only 11.5 months ($p = 0.0004$).[52]

In contrast to the preceding data, two studies have claimed lack of correlation between ploidy and outcome. Ljungberg, Stenling, and Roos studied 32 patients with metastatic renal cell carcinoma and found no difference in the ultimate outcome between diploid and aneuploid tumors, although a significantly longer survival time was observed in the diploid group.[53] Chin and co-workers studied 54 renal cell carcinomas in 50 patients.[47] They found an overall incidence of aneuploidy of 74%. The percentage of aneuploid tumors did not vary significantly between the clear and granular cell types, between primary and metastatic tumors, or between stage III and IV tumors. Forty-five percent of patients with diploid tumors and 69.7% of patients with aneuploid tumors died of disease. Even though patients with diploidy had a slight advantage for survival, the authors could not firmly state that flow cytometry of renal cell carcinoma helped predict survival. Ljungberg's and Chin's failure to demonstrate a correlation between DNA ploidy and survival may be due in part to patient selection.[47,53] The patients Ljungberg studied already had metastatic disease. Chin's study looked at patients in higher stages (III and IV), and therefore these patients were known to have poor prognoses even without the use of flow cytometry.

Stage at diagnosis remains the most important determinant of survival in patients with renal cell carcinoma. However, DNA ploidy is an independent, statistically significant variable. The ploidy of the primary tumor correlates with the development of metastatic disease, and the ploidy of the metastatic lesion correlates with survival.

RENAL SARCOMA

Primary sarcomas of the kidney account for only 1% of all primary renal malignancies. Because of the tumor's rarity, only a few reports of DNA ploidy in renal sarcoma exist. Grignon and colleagues at M.D. Anderson, Houston, studied the ploidy of 17 renal sarcomas.[54] They found 7 aneuploid, 5 diploid, and 5 unclassified. The presence of aneuploidy correlated with tumors of higher histologic grade, higher mitotic rate, and increased nuclear pleomorphism. Ploidy, however, did not correlate with prognosis or survival. This finding may be due to the overall poor prognosis of renal sarcomas or to the small number of tumors studied.

ONCOCYTOMA

Renal oncocytomas account for 5% of renal parenchymal tumors and are generally considered benign. However, disease progression has been reported in patients thought to have benign renal oncocytomas. Rainwater, Farrow, and Lieber studied 51 oncocytomas classified as grade I (histologically very well differentiated) with flow cytometry for DNA ploidy.[23] They found that 50% had a normal diploid DNA pattern, 39% had a polyploid-tetraploid pattern, and 11% were aneuploid. In patients with diploidy or aneuploidy, no tumor progression or deaths were observed. Of the patients with polyploid and tetraploid tumors, 3 had the development of metastatic disease and 2 died of their disease. Since renal oncocytomas have a low malignant potential, the finding of such a high percentage of tumors with an abnormal DNA ploidy is surprising. The significance of this is unclear, especially since it was not the tetraploid but the nontetraploid aneuploid tumors that progressed. Perhaps this could be explained by tumor volume. Further work on oncocytomas is necessary before DNA ploidy determinations will be meaningful in the evaluation of their malignant potential and the determination of their natural history.

MULTICYSTIC DYSPLASTIC KIDNEY

The long-term natural history of multicystic dysplastic kidney is not known. Therefore the management of multicystic dysplastic kidney is controversial. Six cases of malignancy have been reported, and the incidence of nephroblastomatosis is 5% to 7%. To determine whether DNA ploidy might be useful in identifying kidneys prone to malignant disease, Jung and colleagues studied 30 archival multicystic dysplastic kidneys with flow cytometry.[55] None had evidence of malignancy, and all were found to be diploid. Whether an abnormality of DNA ploidy might herald malignant transformation in this population remains unknown.

PROSTATE CANCER

Cancer of the prostate varies greatly in biologic behavior.[5,18,56,57] In some cases the cancer is an incidental finding at postmortem examination and had no impact on the patient's life. When clinically manifest, it may run a long and uneventful course with the patient dying with rather than from his prostate cancer. In other patients, however, it is a highly aggressive and rapidly fatal disease. Since prostate cancer is most common in elderly men (average age at diagnosis 70 years), a decision to treat a patient with prostate cancer must be realistically aimed at increasing life expectancy without worsening quality of life.[58] Thus an important problem in the management of prostate cancer is predicting an individual tumor's malignant potential, especially its likelihood of spreading outside the prostate gland and metastasizing.

Many grading systems employing subjective and objective pathologic criteria have been used in attempts to predict the malignant potential of prostate cancer.[59-61] However, malignant potential is only partly reflected by morphologic criteria, particularly in the large group of patients with moderately differentiated tumors.[62] Thus DNA ploidy has been used in the search for meaningful predictors of patient prognosis.[18,56,57,63-69] Many studies support the value of flow cytometry DNA ploidy for predicting prognosis of the prostate cancer, especially when the degree of glandular differentiation is considered together with ploidy.[18,56,57,63-69]

Prostate cancer presents unique challenges to assessment by flow cytometric DNA ploidy. Like renal cell cancer, the tumor can have a long clinical course, which makes prospective clinical studies difficult to interpret. This problem can be overcome by retrospective analysis. Second, and more difficult to overcome, are the problems encountered in obtaining an appropriate sample of pure tumor. Primary prostate cancer, even when purely differentiated, is surrounded by a large stromal component and nonmalignant prostatic epithelium. Although all tumors have supporting stroma, the stromal component in prostate cancer may greatly exceed the epithelial tumor. Even when nontumor areas are carefully excised, the signal to noise ratio (tumor cell to stroma) may be very low. Nonmalignant prostatic epithelium and benign prostatic hyperplasia are usually diploid. The incidence of tetraploidy is approximately 2% to 5%.

DNA Patterns in Prostate Cancer

The use of DNA ploidy to portend prognosis has focused on two categories of patients. The first are patients with localized disease. In this setting, flow cytometric DNA ploidy has had mixed results. Some studies demonstrate a clear ability to stratify patients into high- and low-risk groups, whereas others have shown flow cytometric DNA ploidy to be no better than, and in some instances worse than, pathologic grading.[56,57,64,68,70-73] The second category represents patients with documented metastatic disease. In this group, flow cytometric DNA ploidy can recognize biologic aggressiveness not identifiable by standard histopathology.[56,57,66,67,70,74-77]

Localized Prostate Cancer

Cancer Treated by Radical Surgery. The apparent inability of flow cytometry to uniformly identify patients at increased risk for progressive disease might suggest that adverse DNA ploidy does not have a negative impact on survival. However, the inconsistency of results found in patients with localized disease can be partly explained by the heterogeneous therapeutic modalities employed.[56,57,64,68,70-73] If only series in which each patient's pathologic stage is correlated with ploidy and prognosis are considered, the results are clearer.[63,64,73] Among patients treated with radical prostatectomy and pelvic lymph node dissection, the presence of aneuploidy in pathologic stage B (negative margin, negative node) specimens does not seem to worsen overall survival.[63,64,73] A study by Montgomery and associates from the Mayo Clinic demonstrated a statistically significant difference in disease-specific survival but no difference in overall survival.[63]

Using archival material, Montgomery and coworkers examined the relationship of ploidy to progression rate and survival in localized (stage B) prostate cancer.[63] Among 261 patients with pathologic stage B disease, 177 (68%) had diploidy, 74 (28%) had tetraploidy, and 10 (4%) had aneuploidy. These patients had an average follow-up of 9.4 years. In 53 patients (20%) the disease progressed during follow-up. Progression occurred in 15% (27 of 177) of patients with diploid tumors and in all 10 patients with aneuploid tumors. Multivariate analysis of this population revealed that progression and cause-specific survival were significantly worse for patients with aneuploidy than for those with diploidy or tetraploidy ($p \leq 0.0001$). Although tetraploidy was not an unfavorable prognostic sign in pathologic stage B cancer, it was in stage C and D prostate cancer.

In contrast to the preceding study, Ritchie and associates found that DNA ploidy did not affect prognosis in pathologically localized prostate cancer.[64] They retrospectively studied 109 patients using flow cytometry. Fifty-nine (54%) had diploidy, 44 (40%) had tetraploidy, and 6 (6%) had aneuploidy. Twenty-one patients had recurrence, but none of the 6 with aneuploidy did. In this study, grade was a more significant determinant of prognosis than DNA ploidy. However, the mean follow-up was only 5 years and the number of patients was small, so these data may not be conclusive.

A study from our institution also failed to support the Mayo Clinic series. Fifty-four patients undergoing a radical prostatectomy and pelvic lymphadenectomy for clinical stage A and B disease were examined, DNA ploidy was correlated with pathologic grading, and both were correlated with disease status.[73] Aneuploidy was identified in three tumors (5.6%); none have recurred. Abnormally increased cell replication (>15% of the total population in the G-2+M phase) was noted in 22 patients (41%); recurrent disease developed in 5 of these patients (23%). Diploid tumors were present in 29 patients (59%); recurrence developed in 3 of these patients (10%). Seminal vesicle invasion and positive surgical margins were also related to the development of recurrent disease ($p < 0.01$ and $p < 0.05$, respectively). For pathologically confined prostate cancer, DNA ploidy failed to enhance the ability of standard histopathologic grading to predict disease recurrence. If, however, these patients had either positive margins or positive nodes at the time of surgery (pathologic stage C or D-1), aneuploidy portended a worse prognosis.

Aneuploidy in pathologically localized prostate cancer may signal a worse prognosis. However, this conclusion is based on only 10 patients in one study. In other studies with shorter follow-up, the significance of aneuploidy was less dramatic. Patients with aneuploid tumors not treated by radical surgery or those with positive margins do appear to be at a disadvantage compared with those who have diploid tumors.[56,57,67,70,74-79]

Cancer Treated by External Radiation Therapy. The available data on patients treated with radiation therapy is more limited than the data from patients treated with radical surgery. Retrospective studies are more difficult to perform on biopsy cores, where significantly less material is available for analysis. The effect of ploidy on those failing to respond to radiation therapy has been studied at the Mayo Clinic, and DeVere White and colleagues have an ongoing study prospectively examining the relationship between ploidy and radioresponsiveness.[68,69]

Rainwater and Zincke examined the association of DNA ploidy with progression and survival in patients treated with radiation therapy.[68] Thirty patients underwent either a radical prostatectomy or cystoprostatectomy. In 17 the tumor failed to respond locally to radiation therapy with curative intent, and 13 patients had surgery within 2 months after planned radiation therapy. Among the entire population, 5 had diploidy, 20 had tetraploidy, and 5 had aneuploidy. Recurrence after surgery took place in 1 of 5 (20%) with diploidy, 8 of 20 (40%) with tetraploidy, and 3 of 5 (60%) with aneuploidy. All three who had aneuploidy and recurrence died of prostate cancer. In a multivariate study of this population, Rainwater and Zincke concluded that only ploidy correlated with prognosis and survival. The population was not stratified based on whether prior radiation therapy had failed.

DeVere White and co-workers examined preradiation and postradiation DNA ploidy to determine predictability of response to radiation therapy in prostate cancer.[69] Using flow cytometry, they studied 48 patients before radiation therapy and 2 years after radiation therapy. Before therapy 38 (79%) had diploidy and 10 (21%) had aneuploidy. Two years after therapy, 27 (56%) had diploidy and 21 (44%) had aneuploidy. When the preradiation and postradiation histograms were compared, 17 (35%) were unchanged, 3 (6%) were improved, and 28 (58%) were worse. In this preliminary report, pretreatment histograms did not identify those likely to respond to radiation therapy. Of concern, however, was the dramatic increase in aneuploidy after radiation therapy. Whether this represents evolution or clonal selection is unknown.

Cancer Treated by Endocrine Therapy. In a study of fine-needle aspiration biopsies performed at the Karolinska Institute, 43 patients with similar grade (I to III) and stage (B and C) characteristics were retrospectively selected based on their response to endocrine treatment. Twenty-one patients were known to have survived more than 5 years, and 22 had died within 3 years. Fourteen of the 21 surviving patients demonstrated predominantly diploid tumors, compared with only 4 of the 22 patients living less than 3 years.[79]

Stage C Prostate Cancer

Frankfurt and associates studied ploidy pattern as a function of clinical stage in 45 cancers.[56] The frequency of aneuploidy increased with increasing stage and with increasing Gleason score. There were significant relationships between Gleason score and stage and between ploidy and stage. In this study no tumor in stage B had aneuploidy but 46.7% of stage C tumors were aneuploid.

The DNA patterns in stage C prostate cancer have also been examined by Nativ and co-workers at the Mayo Clinic.[65] Among 146 patients with stage C prostate cancer, 46% had diploidy, 47% had tetraploidy, and 7% had aneuploidy. Recurrence developed in 13 of 67 (19.4%) with diploidy, 34 of 68 (50%) with tetraploidy, and 7 of 11 (63.6%) with aneuploidy. At 10-year follow-up, 10% of patients with diploidy, 28% with tetraploidy, and 36% with aneuploidy had died of cancer of the prostate. Thus, in stage C prostate cancer, both tetraploid and nontetraploid aneuploidy are predictive of disease recurrence and poorer survival.

Metastatic Prostate Cancer

In patients with metastatic disease, survival is almost uniformly worse if aneuploidy is present. Volume of disease is an independent variable that should be considered when analyzing these data and designing studies.[56,57,66,67,70,74-77]

Stage D1. Stephenson and associates from Memorial Hospital found that patients with aneuploid tumor in the lymph nodes at the time of pelvic lymph node dissection before ^{125}I seed implantation had a worse prognosis.[67] Between 1970 and 1978, 133 of 366 patients were found to have lymph node involvement. Of these, 82 had archival material suitable for analysis. Thirty-three of 82 (40%) tumors were diploid and 49 (60%) were aneuploid. At 5 years disease-free survival in these patients was 33.4% and 13.9% for diploid and aneuploid tumors, respectively. The overall 5-year survival was 87.9% for diploid tumors and 49.5% for aneuploid tumors.

The DNA patterns of patients with stage D1 prostate cancer have also been examined by Winkler and colleagues at the Mayo Clinic.[66] Using archival material, they studied 91 patients with stage D1 prostate cancer. Forty-two percent of the tumors were diploid, 45% were tetraploid, and 13% were aneuploid. Cancer recurred in 75% of patients with nondiploid tumors (tetraploid and aneuploid) but in only 15% of those with diploid tumors. In addition, 43% of tetraploid, 44% of aneuploid, and none of diploid patients died of prostate cancer within 10 years. At 15 years 65% of diploid, 12% of tetraploid, and none of aneuploid patients were alive. All of these patients received endocrine therapy.

Thus, in stage D1 prostate cancer, a nondiploid DNA pattern correlates with a significantly worse disease recurrence rate and survival. This result is similar to the findings in clinical stage C disease, in which many patients can be expected to have node involvement.

Stage D2. There is a paucity of data correlating survival and stage D2 cancer for the same reason that limited data are available on ploidy and survival for patients treated with radiation therapy: retrospective analysis of biopsy material is necessary. Nevertheless, sufficient data are available to state that aneuploidy portends a worse prognosis.

In a study of 419 patients with prostate cancer, Tribukait found 80 patients with bone metastases.[80] Among them, 7% had diploidy, 17% had nontetraploid aneuploidy, 28% had aneuploidy, and 52% had aneuploidy with multiple cell lines. Length of survival decreased from diploidy to tetraploidy to nontetraploid aneuploidy and aneuploidy with multiple stem lines.

DNA Patterns and Survival in Prostate Cancer

The previous review demonstrates that ploidy is an important prognostic indicator of survival. Its value is potentiated when glandular differentiation is added. The 4-year survival has been reported to be 95% for diploid tumors and 25% for aneuploid tumors.[18] Fordham and co-workers added Gleason score to their analysis of prognosis.[57] They found that in patients with prostate cancer, a Gleason score of 2 to 6, and diploidy the average survival was 104 months, whereas those with the same Gleason score but aneuploidy had an average survival of 68 months. Similarly, in patients with a Gleason score of 7 to 10, diploidy was associated with an average survival of 55.2 months and aneuploidy with an average survival of 22.4 months. These differences were statistically significant.[57] The effect of stage was not determined because most patients did not undergo a thorough staging evaluation.[57]

Flow Cytometric Determination of Morphology

As cells pass through the laser beams of a flow cytometer, incident light reflects, diffracts, and refracts from the surface and internal structures of the cell. The combination of these phenomena is known as light scatter. Although light scatter could be measured at any angle from the incident light source, the commercially available flow cytometers are designed to measure light scatter in the forward and perpendicular directions. In flow cytometric systems, forward light scatter (FLS) has been shown to correspond directly to the size of the object being studied.[81] Thus the larger the cell, the more intense the FLS signals.

Perpendicular light scatter (PLS) intensity is also related to cell size, but more important, it measures internal cellular structure.[81-83] Because the largest internal structure in prostate cancer cells is the nucleus, PLS predominantly measures nuclear surface area.[82] Although PLS and FLS have not been widely used in the study of human prostate cancer, evidence in animal studies suggests that the combination of these parameters can be used in quantitative grading of tumor on the basis of cell size and nuclear shape.[84] Preliminary studies in humans undergoing radical retropubic prostatectomy demonstrated that the combination of FLS and PLS can help predict pathologic stage.[85]

Quantitative cytologic analysis by flow cytometry has been successfully applied to prostate cancer. Quantitative cytology appears useful in portending patient prognosis. These techniques have predictive value independent of and in some cases beyond that of cytologic analysis or Gleason score and tumor stage. The conclusion that aneuploidy is less of a threat when radical surgery is employed is provocative and requires continued observation of the populations at risk and expanded studies. The emergence of aneuploidy after radiation therapy for localized diploid tumors may be secondary to selection of preexisting clones or genotype alteration caused by the radiation therapy. Regardless, if this finding is confirmed in other prospective studies, it may influence use of radiation therapy in some populations.

Summary

The conclusion that aneuploidy is significant only if the tumor is not removed is provocative. Before such a conclusion can be reached, careful and detailed analysis of larger series of patients is necessary. Also, the effect of external radiation therapy on prostate cancer and the relationship between ploidy and survival need further analysis. The ongoing study by DeVere White should aid us substantially. The relationship between ploidy and survival for stage D2 prostate cancer is being elucidated by the Southwest Oncology Group, which is analyzing the efficacy of flutamide in patients treated by orchiectomy.

ADRENAL TUMORS

The classification of adrenocortical and adrenomedullary tumors as benign or malignant is difficult because histologic appearance is not always a reliable means of distinguishing the two. Certain histologic features such as marked nuclear atypia or a high mitotic index suggest malignancy, but some pathologists label a tumor malignant only if venous or capsular invasion is present or if metastatic disease is identified.[86,87] Flow cytometric DNA ploidy has been used in attempts to diagnose and predict the natural history of these tumors.

Klein and colleagues studied samples of seven adrenal neoplasms and four normal adrenal glands obtained at radical nephrectomy.[86] Among the seven adrenal neoplasms were four adrenocortical carcinomas, two adrenal adenomas, and one pheochromocytoma. All four carcinomas were aneuploid, and the four normal adrenal glands were diploid. The two adenomas and the pheochromocytoma had variable proportions of tetraploid cells, but none had nontetraploid aneuploidy. In three of the four patients with carcinomas, the disease metastasized during the follow-up. Klein and associates concluded that DNA flow cytometry is useful for the diagnosis of adrenocortical carcinoma, since aneuploidy was seen only in malignant tumors.

Slightly different observations and conclusions were made by Rainwater and colleagues.[87] They studied 20 benign aldosterone-producing adrenal adenomas and 6 malignant aldosterone-producing adrenocortical carcinomas. Seventeen of the 20 benign adrenal tumors had normal DNA histograms. However, 3 of what were thought to be benign adrenal tumors had abnormal DNA ploidy. Two were tetraploid and 1 was aneuploid; all 3 had clinically benign courses. All 6 of the histologically malignant tumors had abnormal DNA histograms. Three had tetraploidy or polyploidy, and 3 others had aneuploidy. Only the 3 patients with aneuploid malignant tumors subsequently died of the disease. From this study, Rainwater and associates concluded that DNA ploidy determined by flow cytometry can help predict the prognosis of patients with adrenocortical carcinomas but that it is not helpful in distinguishing benign from malignant tumors.

These two studies demonstrate that as with many other cancers, aneuploidy is associated with a worse prognosis. Unlike Rainwater and associates, however, Klein and colleagues did not consider tetraploidy abnormal. This reinforces the necessity of considering the methods employed before making conclusions about the significance of DNA ploidy. To state that since the disease did not progress or recur, the tumor was benign is incorrect in our opinion. This implies that no malignant tumor is curable. Historically this was true, since adrenal malignancy was not diagnosed in the absence of invasion or metastasis. Probably no malignant tumor that has invaded beyond the adrenal gland is surgically curable. The preceding studies do support the conclusion that aneuploidy is associated with a worse prognosis. Whether some aneuploid tumors are benign and some malignant cannot be determined by the patient's clinical course, since as is the case for other cancers, some malignant adrenal tumors may not have the capacity to metastasize.

GERM CELL TUMORS

Carcinoma in Situ

Carcinoma in situ of the testis is presumed to be the precursor of invasive germ cell cancer. The incidence of carcinoma in situ in a contralateral testicle following orchiectomy for a germ cell malignancy is approximately 5%.[88] Flow cytometric DNA ploidy analysis of ejaculate has been used to improve early detection of carcinoma in situ and to diagnose testicular cancer. Giwercman, Clausen, and Skakkebaek compared the semen from 8 patients with diagnosed carcinoma in situ of the testis with that of 26 normal healthy men.[89] They found aneuploidy in the semen of 4 of 8 men with carcinoma in situ, whereas none of the healthy men had aneuploidy. At 1 year after orchiectomy, none of the four men who previously had aneuploidy demonstrated aneuploidy in the ejaculate. The use of flow cytometric DNA ploidy to screen high-risk populations (i.e., those with prior germ cell tumors) for the occurrence of carcinoma in situ may be justified. However, it should not be considered a good screening modality for testicular cancer. In Giwercam's study only 50% of the patients with carcinoma in situ had aneuploid tumors. In addition, a significant incidence of false negative results can be expected owing to blockage of sperm transit by the mass effect in the testes.

Invasive Germ Cell Tumors

The DNA ploidy and proliferative fraction of testis cancer have been studied with flow cytometry. The incidence of diploid germ cell tumors among all germ cell tumors of the testis varies between 5% and 30%.[90-92] Oosterhuis and associates examined 10 infantile yolk sac tumors and 72 germ cell tumors of adults and found only 3 of 10 yolk sac tumors and 1 of 71 germ cell tumors to be diploid.[93] This high incidence of aneuploidy is supported by Kleinhans and co-workers, who found 95% aneuploidy in 75 malignant testicular germ cell tumors.[94] Noting that 3 of 3 testicular lymphomas and 2 of 3 Leydig cell tumors were diploid, Oosterhuis and associates concluded that when a testicular tumor is diploid, the diagnosis of nonseminomatous germ cell tumor should be reviewed.[93]

Prognosis in Testicular Cancer

The prognosis of patients with advanced germ cell cancer has been examined by Sledge and colleagues.[95] They examined 50 patients with disseminated germ cell tumors of the testis with respect to DNA index, tumor marker levels, treatment modality, proliferative index, and "pathology score." DNA index was not correlated with survival, since 95% of patients had aneuploid tumors. However, a high proliferative fraction (S phase percentage) was associated with a significantly shorter survival than a low proliferative fraction (37.7 versus 85.6 months; $p < 0.001$).

Watson and colleagues used flow cytometry to study the expression of the p62 c-*myc* oncoprotein in patients with testicular cancer.[96] They examined nuclei extracted from paraffin-embedded testicular cancer using a monoclonal antibody to the p62 c-*myc* oncoprotein. They found that the patients with higher expression of this oncoprotein had better prognoses than those with lower expression. In addition, the oncoprotein level increased significantly with increasing teratoma differentiation and decreased for the intermediate and undifferentiated tumors.

Flow cytometric DNA ploidy can be used to detect carcinoma in situ but is of little value in portending prognosis, since virtually all nonseminomatous germ cell tumors are aneuploid. Flow cytometry has been used to predict prognosis in testicular cancer by assessment of the p62 c-*myc* oncoprotein.

FLOW CYTOMETRY OF SPERM AND MALE GERM CELLS

Flow cytometric DNA ploidy analysis has been applied to the complex process of sperm development in both normal and perturbed circumstances.[97,98] Spermatogenesis is divided into three major phases: (1) spermatogonial proliferation and renewal, (2) mitosis and meiosis, and (3) spermiogenesis. On the basis of cellular DNA content, one expects to see spermatogonia and spermatocytes cycling between 2C and 4C equivalents and all spermatids and sperm stages at 1C. In reality, however, a minimum of five distinct peaks can be distinguished and sorted. These populations correspond to diploid and tetraploid cells, round and elongated spermatids, and mature sperm.

Flow cytometry has been used to evaluate fertility. However, these studies are often complicated by the extreme heterogeneity of sperm in human ejaculates. The findings show that fertile donors have sperm with relatively homogeneous chromatin structure, whereas infertile donors have a higher variability in chromatin structure. In a study of 40 infertile men, immature DNA pattern was observed and postulated to be due to a lack of haploid cell formation.[99]

Flow cytometric DNA ploidy has also been used to evaluate the sperm characteristics of patients after orchiectomy for testicular cancer. Many patients with testicular cancer have poor-quality semen even before therapy. In addition, infertility is a significant side effect of therapy for testicular cancer.[100] Fossa and co-workers examined the ejaculate of 85 patients with testicular cancer 3 to 60 days after orchiectomy but before any further therapy.[100] The patients were compared with an age-matched healthy control group. DNA ploidy of ejaculate revealed that the cancer group had a significantly lower percentage of condensed haploid sperm cells and a significantly higher percentage of diploid cells than did the control subjects. Fossa and associates postulate that this may be due to a maturational defect during spermatogenesis in the testis remaining after orchiectomy for testicular cancer.

REFERENCES

1. Papanicolaou GN, Traut HF: The diagnostic value of vaginal smears in carcinoma of the uterus. Am J Obstet Gynecol 42:193, 1941.
2. Fulwyler MJ: Electronic separation of biological cells by volume. Science 150:910, 1965.
3. Kamentsky LA, Melamed MR: Spectrophotometric cell sorter. Science 156:1364, 1967.
4. Shapiro HM: Practical flow cytometry, ed 2. New York: Alan R Liss, 1988.

5. Benson MC: The application of flow cytometry to the study of prostate cancer. In Coffey DS, Bruchovsky N, Gardner WA, et al (eds): Progress in clinical and biological research, vol 239. New York: Alan R Liss, 1987, pp 765-778.
6. Pretlow TG, Pretlow TP: Cell separation: methods and selected applications. New York: Academic Press, 1982.
7. Dietch AP, Law H, DeVere White RW: A stable propidium iodide staining procedure for flow cytometry. J Histochem Cytochem 30:967-970, 1982.
8. Hedley DW, Friedlander ML, Taylor IW, et al: Method for analysis of cellular DNA content in paraffin embedded pathological material using flow cytometry. J Histochem Cytochem 31:1333, 1983.
9. Meyers FJ, Gumerlock PH, Teplitz RL, et al: Sequential flow cytometry and single gene analysis by enzymatic amplification and allele specific oligonucleotide hybridization of urothelial cells. J Urol 142:1599-1601, 1989.
10. Melamed MR, Lindmo T, Mendelsohn ML (eds): Flow cytometry and sorting, ed 2. New York: Wiley-Liss, 1990.
11. Steinkamp JA: Flow cytometry. Rev Sci Inst 55:1375, 1984.
12. Wheeless LL, Coon JS, Cox C, et al: Measurement of variability in DNA flow cytometry of replicate samples. Cytometry 10:731-738, 1989.
13. Julius MH, Musuda T, Herzenberg LA: Demonstration that antigen binding cells are precursors of antibody producing cells after purification with a fluorescence. Proc Natl Acad Sci USA 69:134, 1972.
14. Kraemer PM, Tobey RA, Van Dilla MA: Flow microfluorometric studies of lectin binding to mammalian cells. J Cell Physiol 81:305, 1973.
15. Kerker M, Van Dilla MA, Brunsting A, et al: Is the central dogma of flow cytometry true: that fluorescence intensity is proportional to cell dye content? Cytometry 3:71, 1982.
16. Traganos F: Single and multiparameter analysis of the effects of chemotherapeutic agents on cell proliferation in vitro. In Melamed MR, Lindmo T, Mendelsohn ML (eds): Flow cytometry and sorting, ed 2. New York: Wiley-Liss, 1990.
17. Gray J, Pallavicini M: Quantitative cell-cycle analysis. In Melamed MR, Lindmo T, Mendelsohn ML (eds): Flow cytometry and sorting, ed 2. New York: Wiley-Liss, 1990.
18. Tribukait B: Flow cytometry in assessing the clinical aggressiveness of genito-urinary neoplasms. World J Urol 5:108-122, 1987.
19. Barlogie B, Raber MN, Schumann J, et al: Flow cytometry in clinical cancer research. Cancer Res 43:3982-3997, 1983.
20. Baisch H, Otto U, Konig K, et al: DNA content of human kidney carcinoma cells in relation to histological grading. Br J Cancer 45:878-886, 1982.
21. Feichter GE: DNA flow cytometry in diagnostic cytopathology: methodologic consideration and current state of clinical applications. In Goerttler K, Feichter GE, Wittes S (eds): New frontiers in cytology. Berlin, Springer-Verlag, 1988.
22. Collste L, Darzynkiewicz Z, Traganos F, et al: Flow cytometry in bladder cancer detection and evaluation using acridine orange metachromatic nucleic acid staining of irrigation cytology specimens. J Urol 123:478-485, 1980.
23. Rainwater LM, Farrow GM, Lieber MM: Flow cytometry of renal oncocytoma: common occurrence of deoxyribonucleic acid polyploidy and aneuploidy. J Urol 135:1167-1171, 1986.
24. Laerum OD, Farsund T: Clinical application of flow cytometry: a review. Cytometry 2:1-13, 1984.
25. Tribukait B, Esposti PL: Quantitative flow-microfluorometric analysis of the DNA in cells from neoplasms of the urinary bladder: correlation of aneuploidy with histological grading and the cytological findings. Urol Res 6:201, 1978.
26. Melamed MR: Flow cytometry of the urinary bladder. Urol Clin North Am 11(4):599-608, 1984.
27. Badalament RA, Hermansen DK, Kimmel M, et al: The sensitivity of bladder wash flow cytometry, bladder wash cytology and voided cytology in the detection of bladder carcinoma. Cancer 60:1423-1427, 1987.
28. Devonec M, Darzynkiewicz Z, Kostyrka-Claps ML, et al: Flow cytometry of low stage bladder tumors. Cancer 48:109-118, 1982.
29. Hermansen DK, Badalament RA, Fair WR, et al: Detection of bladder carcinoma in females by flow cytometry and cytology. Cytometry 10:739-742, 1989.
30. Klein FA, Herr HW, Whitmore WF Jr, et al: An evaluation of automated flow cytometry in detection of carcinoma in situ of the urinary bladder. Cancer 50:1003-1008, 1982.
31. Giella JG, Ring KS, Olsson CA, et al: The predictive value of flow cytometry and urinary cytology in the follow-up of patients with transitional cell carcinoma of the bladder. Submitted, J Urol, 1990.
32. Ring KS, Karp F, Benson MC: Enhanced detection of bladder cancer using the epithelial surface marker, EMA: preliminary results. J Occup Med 32:904-909, 1990.
33. Farsund T, Hoestmark JG, Laerum OD: Relation between flow cytometric DNA distribution and pathology in human bladder cancer. Cancer 54:1771, 1984.
34. Melicow MM, Hollowell JW: Intra-urothelial cancer: carcinoma in situ, Bowen's disease of the urinary system; discussion of thirty cases. J Urol 68:763, 1952.
35. Gustafson H, Tribukait B, Esposti PL: The prognostic value of DNA analysis in primary carcinoma in situ of the urinary bladder. Scand J Urol Nephrol 16:141-146, 1982.
36. Heney NM, Ahmed S, Flanagan MJ, et al for National Bladder Cancer Collaborative Group A: Superficial bladder cancer: progression and recurrence. J Urol 130:1083-1086, 1983.
37. Gustafson H, Tribukait B, Esposti PL: DNA profile and tumor progression in patients with superficial bladder tumors. Urol Res 10:12, 1982.
38. DeVere White RW, Deitch AD, West B, Fitzpatrick JM: The predictive value of flow cytometric information in the clinical management of stage 0 (Ta) bladder cancer. J Urol 139:279-282, 1988.
39. Gustafson H, Tribukait B, Esposti PL: DNA pattern, histological grade and multiplicity related to recurrence rate in superficial bladder tumours. Scand J Urol Nephrol 16:135-139, 1982.
40. Fradet Y, Tardif M, Bourget L, Robert J, and the Laval University Urology Group: Clinical cancer progression in urinary bladder tumors evaluated by multiparameter flow cytometry with monoclonal antibodies. Cancer Res 50:432-437, 1990.
41. Wijkstrom H, Gustafson H, Tribukait B: Deoxyribonucleic acid analysis in the evaluation of transitional cell carcinoma before cystectomy. J Urol 132:894-898, 1984.
42. Fossa SD, Kaalhus O, Scott-Knudsen O: The clinical and histopathological significance of Feulgen DNA values in transitional cell carcinoma of the human urinary bladder. Eur J Cancer 13:1155-1162, 1977.
43. Klein FA, Whitmore WF Jr, Wolf RM, et al: Presumptive down-staging from preoperative irradiation for bladder cancer as determined by flow cytometry: preliminary report. Int J Radiat Oncol Biol Phys 9:487-491, 1983.
44. Murphy WM, Chandler RW, Trafford RM: Flow cytometry of deparaffinized nuclei compared to histological grading for the pathological evaluation of transitional cell carcinomas. J Urol 135:694-697, 1986.
45. Oldbring J, Hellsten S, Lindholm K, et al: Flow DNA analysis in the characterization of carcinoma of the renal pelvis and ureter. Cancer 64:2141-2145, 1989.
46. Grignon DJ, Ayala A, El-Naggar A, et al: Renal cell carcinoma. Cancer 64:2133-2140, 1989.
47. Chin J, Pontes J, Frankfurt O: Flow cytometric deoxyribonucleic acid analysis of primary and metastatic human renal cell carcinoma. J Urol 133:582-585, 1985.
48. Otto U, Baisch H, Huland H, Kloppel G: Tumor cell de-

oxyribonucleic acid content and prognosis in human renal cell carcinoma. J Urol 132:237-239, 1984.
49. Schouman M, Warter A, Roos M, Bollack C: Renal cell carcinoma: statistical study of survival based on pathological criteria. World J Urol 2:109-113, 1984.
50. Baisch H, Otto U, Kloppel G: Malignancy index based on flow cytometry and histology for renal cell carcinomas and its correlation to prognosis. Cytometry 7:200-204, 1986.
51. Ljungberg B, Stenling R, Roos G: Prognostic value of deoxyribonucleic acid content in metastatic renal cell carcinoma. J Urol 136:801-804, 1986.
52. Ljungberg B, Stenling R, Roos G: DNA content and prognosis in renal cell carcinoma. Cancer 57:2346-2350, 1986.
53. Ljungberg B, Stenling R, Roos G: DNA content in renal cell carcinoma with reference to tumor heterogeneity. Cancer 56:503-508, 1985.
54. Grignon DJ, Ayala A, Ro J, et al: Primary sarcomas of the kidney. Cancer 65:1611-1618, 1990.
55. Jung WH, Peters CA, Mandell J, et al: Flow cytometric evaluation of multicystic dysplastic kidneys. J Urol 144:413-415, 1990.
56. Frankfurt O, Chin J, Englander L, et al: Relationship between DNA ploidy, glandular differentiation and tumor spread in human prostate cancer. Cancer Res 45:1418-1423, 1985.
57. Fordham M, Burdge A, Matthews J, et al: Prostate carcinoma cell DNA content measured by flow cytometry and its relation to clinical outcome. Br J Surg 73:400-403, 1986.
58. Johansson JE, Adami HO, Andersson SO, et al: Natural history of localised prostatic cancer: a population based study in 223 untreated patients. Lancet 1:799-803, 1989.
59. Gaeta JF, Asirwatham JE, Miller G, Murphy GP: Histologic grading of primary prostate cancer: a new approach to an old problem. J Urol 123:689-693, 1980.
60. Mostofi FK: Problems of grading carcinoma of prostate. Semin Oncol 3:161-169, 1976.
61. Utz DC, Farrow GM: Pathologic differentiation and prognosis of prostate carcinoma. JAMA 209:1701-1703, 1969.
62. Benson MC: Application of flow cytometry and automated image analysis to the study of prostate cancer. NCI Monogr 7:25-29, 1988.
63. Montgomery BT, Nativ O, Blute ML, et al: Stage B prostate adenocarcinoma. Arch Surg 125:327-331, 1990.
64. Ritchie AWS, Layfield LJ, Hannah J, et al: Relationship of DNA content to conventional prognostic factors in clinically localized carcinoma of the prostate. Br J Urol 62:254-260, 1988.
65. Nativ O, Winkler HZ, Raz Y, et al: Stage C prostatic adenocarcinoma: flow cytometric nuclear DNA ploidy analysis. Mayo Clin Proc 64:911-919, 1989.
66. Winkler HZ, Rainwater LM, Myers RP, et al: Stage D1 prostatic adenocarcinoma: significance of nuclear DNA ploidy patterns studied by flow cytometry. Mayo Clin Proc 63:103-112, 1988.
67. Stephenson RA, James BC, Gay H, et al: Flow cytometry of prostate cancer: relationship of DNA content to survival. Cancer Res 47:2504-2509, 1987.
68. Rainwater LM, Zincke H: Radical prostatectomy after radiation therapy for cancer of the prostate: feasibility and prognosis. J Urol 140:1455-1459, 1988.
69. DeVere White RW, Deitch A, Myer-Haass G, et al: DNA ploidy in irradiated prostate. AUA abstract No 52, 1990, p 201A.
70. Dejter SW Jr, Cunningham RE, Noguchi PD, et al: Prognostic significance of DNA ploidy in carcinoma of the prostate. Urology 33:361-366, 1989.
71. Lee SE, Currin SM, Paulson DF, et al: Flow cytometric determination of ploidy in prostatic adenocarcinoma: a comparison with seminal vesicle involvement and histopathological grading as a predictor of clinical recurrence. J Urol 140:769-774, 1988.
72. Pontes JE, Wajsman Z, Huben RP, et al: Prognostic factors in localized prostatic cancer. J Urol 134:1137-1139, 1985.
73. Ring KS, Karp FS, Olsson CA, et al: Flow cytometric analysis of localized adenocarcinoma of the prostate: the use of archival DNA analysis in conjunction with pathological grading to predict clinical outcome following radical retropubic prostatectomy. Submitted, Prostate.
74. DiSilverio F, Sciarra F: Therapeutic approach in prostatic cancer. J Steroid Biochem 25:773-779, 1986.
75. Lundberg S, Carstensen J, Rundquist I: DNA flow cytometry and histopathological grading of paraffin-embedded prostate biopsy specimens in a survival study. Cancer Res 47:1973-1977, 1987.
76. Muntzing J: DNA determinations for prognosis and therapy control in prostatic cancer. Semin Oncol 10(suppl):16-20, 1983.
77. Taveres AS, Costa J, Costa-Maia J: Correlation between ploidy and prognosis in prostatic carcinoma. J Urol 109:676-679, 1973.
78. Ronstrom L, Tribukait B, Esposti PL: DNA pattern and cytological findings in fine-needle aspirates of untreated prostatic tumors: a flow-cytofluorometric study. Prostate 2:79-88, 1981.
79. Zetterberg A, Esposti PL: Prostatic significance of nuclear DNA levels in prostatic carcinoma. Scand J Urol Nephrol 55(suppl):53-56, 1980.
80. Tribukait B: Flow cytometry in surgical pathology and cytology of tumors of the genito-urinary tract. In Koss LG, Coleman DV (eds): Adv Clin Cytol 2:163, 1984.
81. Kerker M: Elastic and inelastic light scattering in flow cytometry. Cytometry 4:1-10, 1983.
82. Benson MC, McDougal D, Coffey DS: The application of perpendicular and forward light scatter to assess nuclear and cellular morphology. Cytometry 5:515-522, 1984.
83. Brunsting A, Mullaney PF: Differential light scattering from spherical mammalian cells. Biophys J 14:439-453, 1974.
84. Benson MC, McDougal D, Coffey DS: The use of multiparameter flow cytometry to assess tumor cell heterogeneity and grade prostate cancer. Prostate 5:27-45, 1984.
85. Benson MC, Walsh PC: The application of flow cytometry to the assessment of tumor cell heterogeneity and the grading of human prostate cancer: preliminary results. J Urol 135:1194-1198, 1986.
86. Klein FA, Kay S, Ratliff J, et al: Flow cytometric determinations of ploidy and proliferation patterns of adrenal neoplasms: an adjunct to histological classification. J Urol 134:862-866, 1985.
87. Rainwater LM, Young W, Farrow G, et al: Flow cytometric analysis of deoxyribonucleic acid ploidy in benign and malignant aldosterone-producing neoplasms of the adrenal gland. Surg Gynecol & Obstet 168:491-496, 1989.
88. Skakkebaek NE: Possible carcinoma-in-situ of the testis. Lancet 2:516-517, 1972.
89. Giwercman A, Clausen OP, Skakkebaek NE: Carcinoma in situ of the testis: aneuploid cells in semen. Br Med J 296:1762-1764, 1988.
90. Fossa SD, Pettersen EO, Thorud E, et al: DNA flow cytometry in human testicular cancer. Cancer Lett 28:55, 1985.
91. Quirke P, Dyson JED, Sutton J, et al: Assessment of germ cell tumours of testis by flow cytometry and histopathology. Adv Biosci 55:45, 1986.
92. Sledge GW Jr, Eble JN, Roth JB, et al: Flow cytometry derived DNA content of the primary lesions of advanced germ cell tumours. Int J Androl 10:115, 1987.
93. Oosterhuis JW, Castedo SMMJ, De Jong B, et al: Ploidy of primary germ cell tumours of the testis. Lab Invest 60:14-21, 1989.
94. Kleinhans G, Hacker KU, Gohde W, et al: Studies of the cell kinetics of human malignant testicular tumors. Urologe A 25:294-297, 1986.
95. Sledge GW Jr, Eble JN, Roth BJ, et al: Relation of proliferative activity to survival in patients with advanced germ cell cancer. Cancer Res 48:3864-3868, 1988.
96. Watson JV, Stewart J, Evan GI, et al: The clinical sig-

nificance of flow cytometric c-*myc* oncoprotein quantitation in testicular cancer. Br J Cancer 53:331-337, 1986.
97. Gledhill BL, Evenson DP, Pinkel D: Flow cytometry and sorting of sperm and male germ cells. In Melamed MR, Lindmo T, Mendelsohn ML (eds): Flow cytometry and sorting, ed 2. New York: Wiley-Liss, 1990.
98. Otto FJ, Hacker U, Zante J, et al: Flow cytometry of human spermatozoa. Histochemistry 61:249, 1979.
99. Thorud E, Clausen OPF, Abyholm T: Fine needle aspiration biopsies from human testes evaluated by DNA flow cytometry. In Laerum OD, Lindmo T, Thorud E (eds): Flow cytometry IV. Bergen-Oslo-Trondheim: Universitetsforlaget, 1980.
100. Fossa SD, Melvik JE, Juul NO, et al: DNA flow cytometry in sperm cells from unilaterally orchiectomized patients with testicular cancer before further treatment. Cytometry 10:345-350, 1989.

CHAPTER 11

ADVANCES IN DIAGNOSING AND TREATING SPERM PROBLEMS AND ADVANCED REPRODUCTIVE TECHNIQUES

RONALD L. URRY

The last decade has witnessed an explosive growth in the techniques for diagnosis and treatment of certain fertility disorders. Before 1980 little progress was made in this area, and little indicated that techniques would be developed to revolutionize reproductive health care. Despite the enormous advances, many laboratories and physicians in reproductive health care have not used or understood methodologies available for work with infertile couples. An example of this is the standard semen analysis, which remains one of the most poorly performed tests for providing information to help treat males with fertility problems.

This chapter outlines many of the advances in reproductive technology and emphasizes the importance of knowing which techniques are useful to diagnose and treat fertility defects in males. Advances in reproductive care include sperm collection techniques with the rebirth of electrical ejaculation for use with spinal cord–injured patients. This advance has given new fertility hope to couples who had few options. Improvement in sperm manipulation techniques has yielded better methods of assisting individuals with retrograde ejaculation and improving their chances of contributing to pregnancy.

Microsurgical advances allow more precise anastomosis of the vas deferens during vasovasostomy and better anastomosis with epididymovasostomy. Direct sperm aspiration from the epididymis has given new hope to individuals with congenital absence of the vas deferens and has raised the possibility that some of these men might become fertile. A combination of sperm aspiration with advanced reproductive techniques, such as in vitro fertilization, has further improved the success rate of these procedures.

One of the biggest advances in the last decade has been in techniques that improve sperm quality before the sperm are used for artificial insemination, in vitro fertilization, and related techniques. This chapter discusses these techniques and correlates the diagnostic findings of sperm quality with the treatment that best improves sperm with a given type of defect. The biggest and most unexpected advance in treating human infertility has been the ability to perform in vitro fertilization and similar techniques. These techniques have led to tremendous advances in the ability to treat the infertile male who previously had little hope. The techniques are discussed to show how they should be integrated into treatment.

The developments in infertility technology have created an ever-widening gap between the specialist in infertility who has kept up with the technology and the urologist in general practice. Because of this, male infertility services are more frequently being taken over by obstetrics and gynecology programs and the urologist is playing a smaller role in this traditional urologic area. This chapter attempts to outline the technologies that are necessary to diagnose and treat male fertility disorders that might help the practicing urologist to regain the responsibility for treating male infertility.

ADVANCES IN DIAGNOSING MALE FERTILITY DISORDERS

Getting to the Egg

Numerous tests are available to diagnose male fertility disorders, and many advances have been made in testing the probability that sperm will reach the fertilization site. The tests include a series of carefully performed semen analyses, mucus-sperm interaction tests, and antibody analyses when indicated.

Semen Analysis

Semen analysis is poorly performed by most laboratories that do not specialize in fertility evaluation. The traditional laboratory report assessing total sperm motility and sperm concentration and giving a best estimate of sperm morphology is virtually worthless in predicting an individual's fertility. A carefully performed semen analysis is critical to the technologic advances outlined in this chapter.[1,2] Without adequate data the practitioner cannot select the techniques most useful for treating a given male. Therefore the assessment of sperm quality via semen analysis is stressed and the minimum information necessary to diagnose infertility is outlined.

A semen analysis has traditionally measured ejaculate volume. It is doubtful that volume plays much of a direct role in infertility except when it is low (less than 1 ml) because lack of volume may cause failure to make adequate contact with the woman's cervical mucus during intercourse. The volume assessment allows calculation of total sperm per ejaculate.

Upon adequate liquefaction (usually at least 20 minutes after sperm collection) a drop of well-mixed seminal fluid should be observed to determine seminal viscosity, the presence of white blood cells, and sperm agglutination if present. Semen viscosity may be the quality most often incorrectly assessed in an analysis. Many laboratories report high viscosity in most sperm samples because of the laboratories' misunderstanding of seminal liquefaction characteristics. A technique has been developed to assess semen viscosity based on both liquid viscosity and undissolved particulate debris. Liquid viscosity is rated as 0 (normal), 1 (slight viscosity; semen forms trailing streamers when expelled from a pipette), 2 (moderate viscosity; semen forms a steady stream when expelled from a pipette), and 3 (severe viscosity; semen is difficult to expel from pipette). High semen viscosity probably does not play a significant role in infertility if the sample has normal sperm motility. However, high viscosity can impair the ability to accurately complete the rest of the analysis, as well as to use some sperm preparation techniques. High viscosity makes separation of the sperm from the seminal fluid more difficult and increases the possibility that a larger number of sperm will be lost. This can be easily overcome by thoroughly mixing the seminal fluid with artificial media, as described in the sperm manipulation section of this chapter, and then aspirating the mixture into and out of a 3 ml syringe with a 20-gauge needle. This mixes the fluids thoroughly, and the sperm separates better during centrifugation of the sample. High viscosity can be treated for diagnostic purposes by adding alpha-amylase powder 2 mg/ml to the seminal fluid. The sample is then mixed and usually liquefies enough to allow a more accurate semen analysis.

A drop of semen is observed with a microscope, and areas of sperm agglutination are recorded. Agglutination should be differentiated from sperm clumping, which almost always occurs with high sperm density. Agglutination typically occurs in an organized fashion and is rated in our laboratory on a three-point scale with 1 equaling slight agglutination (agglutinated areas of sperm every three to five microscopic fields), 2 equaling moderate agglutination (agglutinated areas every one to three fields), and 3 equaling severe agglutination (massive agglutination present in every field). In addition to the severity of the agglutination, the pattern of agglutination (i.e., head to head, head to tail, or tail to tail) is carefully recorded. Moderate or severe agglutination in an organized pattern can indicate the presence of antisperm antibodies and the necessity of testing for antibodies.[3]

During observation of the initial drop of semen the presence of white blood cells in seminal fluid is documented to indicate whether the patient needs additional examination to rule out infection. A typical laboratory performing a semen analysis reports white blood cells any time the technicians see round cells in the ejaculate. Many of these round cells are spermatocytes or spermatids, not white blood cells. Such laboratory reports have led many physicians to attempt to treat round cells with antibiotics when the round cells were probably spermatocytes. Peroxidase-sensitive leukocytes (multinuclear leukocytes) can be detected by peroxidase staining. Whenever round cells are seen in the seminal fluid, peroxidase staining can be a quick way to differentiate polynuclear cells. The semen sample can also be stained with the methods used for morphology assessment, and an experienced observer can view the slide to determine the relative concentration of polynuclear cells in the ejaculate.

Advances in immunology have enabled the formation of antibodies directed against the leukocyte surface, which when coupled with fluorescence assays enables the differentiation of all leukocytes from sperm. Likewise, antibodies to spermatocyte-surface proteins have been developed, and these can be used to differentiate spermatocytes from leukocytes.[4] Completion of these techniques is necessary before it can be assumed that the semen sam-

TABLE 11–1. Sample Estimation of Sperm Motility

Motility Level	Description of Motility	Motility Percent	Motility Score
0	Nonmotile	40	5
1	Shaking motion ("in place motion")	5	5
2	Random, nonlinear, sluggish motion	10	20
3	Moderate velocity, linear direction	20	60
4	Rapid velocity, linear direction	25	100
		TOTAL MOTILITY SCORE	185

The percentage of sperm moving at each motility level is estimated after observing more than 50 fields at 200× magnification. The percentage of sperm at each level is multiplied by the level, and the resulting numbers are added to obtain the sperm motility score.

ple contains white blood cells. An individual with semen containing documented white blood cells should be thoroughly evaluated for prostatitis and *Chlamydia* infection, and semen cultures should be done. This is particularly true if the sample will be used for intrauterine insemination or advanced reproductive techniques. White blood cells should be removed from the sample before the sperm is placed in the uterus. The technologies to accomplish this are described in subsequent sections on sperm processing.

Sperm motility can be one of the most useful factors measured in the semen analysis. Although the factors in a semen analysis that correlate with fertility prediction have not been conclusively established, sperm motility is almost always listed as a factor that has one of the highest correlations with predicting future fertility.[5-7] As mentioned previously, total sperm motility rarely has been shown to have any predictive value for male fertility. Despite this, many laboratories report only total sperm motility. The highest fertility predictive correlate with respect to sperm motility has always been a measurement of progressive sperm motility.[8] This can be done subjectively to determine quantitative motility measurements, as in the technique we use (Table 11–1), or can be performed with the relatively new technology using computer-assisted analysis of sperm motility. Computer-assisted analysis allows measurement of the linearity of sperm movement, sperm head beat frequency, mean and maximum amplitude of lateral sperm head displacement, sperm velocity, and mean tail beat amplitude. We have correlated our technique for sperm motility assessment with time-lapse photography, as well as computer-assisted techniques, and our technique, when used by an experienced observer, correlates with all of the other quantitative methods. The important information is the percentage of sperm moving with reasonable speed in a relatively linear direction. These are the sperm likely to reach the fertilization site with the motility characteristics necessary to enter the egg.

Many laboratories still attempt to assess sperm motility throughout a multihour period while the sperm remain in seminal fluid. This examination does nothing to predict fertility problems, since it is clear that sperm eventually die as they incubate in seminal fluid. A sperm longevity test can be done, however, by removing sperm from the seminal fluid and suspending them in an artificial medium.[9] The sperm sample is incubated in a carbon dioxide incubator for 12 to 24 hours, and sperm motility is observed. The longevity assay can give useful information about the likelihood of the sperm fertilizing the egg.

Assessment of progressive sperm motility is important whether this is manually accomplished or performed with an automated semen analyzer. This measurement aids in the decision of which advanced reproductive technique to use for a given patient.

Sperm morphology is another factor that is usually reported to have a high correlation with male fertility. Unfortunately, most laboratories give only a best estimate of the number of normal or abnormal sperm, which is not helpful in diagnosing male fertility problems. Spermatozoa should be stained and then counted by head shape category to determine their ability to get to and get into the egg. We prefer to use a hematoxylin-eosin stain, but many other stains are adequate for the assessment of sperm morphology.

Once appropriate smears from a semen specimen have been stained, several hundred sperm should be counted. We prefer to divide sperm into seven head shape categories and seven tail shape categories (Table 11–2).[1,2] Both head and tail shape defects correlate with the prediction of infertility. The presence of more than 20% tapered sperm in a patient gives the best prediction of subsequent infertility. Whatever technique is used, quantitative morphology assessment not only gives predictive values for future fertility but also indicates the

TABLE 11–2. Sperm Morphology Categories for Head and Tail Shape Determination

Sperm Head Shape	Sperm Tail Shape
Oval (normal)	Normal
Large	No tail
Small	Short tail
Tapered	Coiled tail
Immature	Bent tail
Duplicate	Duplicate tail
Amorphous	Midpiece defect

Two hundred sperm are analyzed under high-power magnification for both head and tail shape categories.

likelihood of a varicocele. As pointed out nearly three decades ago,[10-12] men with varicoceles often have higher numbers of tapered sperm, although such sperm may also be increased in men without varicoceles.

Large numbers of amorphous sperm, particularly sperm with round heads, may indicate abnormalities in the acrosome. Whenever large numbers of abnormally shaped sperm are present, a hamster egg penetration test, as discussed later in the chapter, may be useful to assess the capability of the sperm to penetrate an egg.

Assessment of sperm membrane function is important in detecting the presence of antisperm antibodies. Two techniques are used: the viability stain and the hypoosmolarity (HOS) sperm test. The viability stain we prefer is the eosin-nigrosin stain, which allows assessment of the sperm membrane's ability to exclude the stain.[1,2,13] Live sperm occasionally allow the stain to pass through, but this stain does indicate a sperm membrane permeability defect.

The HOS sperm test is a new technology that we have found helpful in evaluating sperm membrane function.[14-17] Several studies have shown this test to correlate with the prediction of subsequent fertility and the success of in vitro fertilization, whereas others have found no such correlation.[16-18] The HOS test and viability test methods are outlined in Table 11–3. We have found that three alterations in the sperm membrane have a high correlation with the presence of antisperm antibodies. These factors are low sperm viability, alterations in HOS test findings, and increased numbers of sperm either not moving or moving with immobilizing (shaking) motion. When these three factors exist simultaneously, the patient has more than a 70% chance of having antisperm antibodies.

Sperm density is the last item to be discussed under semen analysis and probably the least important in predicting subsequent fertility. Sperm are usually counted manually in a hemocytometer, a Mackler chamber, or more recently a microscope slide containing a laser-formed channel. Because sperm density assessment can vary within a given individual and between technicians, density values should be considered in their proper perspective. Recent developments in automated technology and computer-assisted analysis permit rapid and automatic sperm density assessment. The accuracy of these instruments is in question, however, particularly with exceptionally low or high sperm count ranges.[20-22] In any case the only useful assessment of sperm density is motile sperm density or progressively motile sperm density.[23-25] The progressive motile sperm density gives the physician an idea of how many sperm could reach and penetrate the egg. Numerous studies have indicated a strong correlation between progressive motile sperm density and fertility outcome.[24-28] It appears that at least 20 to 30 million progressively motile sperm per ejaculate are needed and that the higher numbers used in the past are unrealistic.[24] A man with low sperm numbers should not be advised that he has no chance of contributing to a pregnancy, since pregnancies have been documented with extremely low sperm concentrations.[29]

Mucus-Sperm Interaction

The ability of the sperm to penetrate cervical mucus is important in determining the likelihood that the sperm will reach the egg. Techniques for assessing the ability of sperm to reach the egg include the postcoital test, mucus-slide sperm inhibition test, and bovine mucus-sperm penetration test.

The most widely used mucus test is the postcoital test, in which the gynecologist estimates when the woman is ovulating based on the length of her cycles, basal body temperature charts, or other information. The gynecologist asks the couple to have intercourse on the suspected day of ovulation and examines the woman between 2 and 24 hours after intercourse.[30] Cervical mucus is aspirated, assessed for its quantity, clarity, and stretchability, and observed under the microscope to count the sperm in

TABLE 11–3. Methods to Determine Sperm Membrane Defects

Test	Principle	Result: Normal	Result: Abnormal
Viability stain	Normal viable plasma membrane excludes nigrosin	White	Pink-red
HOS reaction	Functional plasma membrane will respond to hypoosmotic solution with sperm head swelling and coiled sperm tail	Coiled tail	Straight tail
Triple stain (or fluorescein-labeled agglutinins or monoclonal antibodies)	Rose bengal stains the acrosome of sperm if present	White acrosomal regions	Absent acrosome or nonreacted

Structural defects can be analyzed with use of the eosin-nigrosin viability stain, and functional defects can be analyzed with use of the HOS reaction assay. The triple stain or other acrosomal stains can be used to analyze normal acrosome morphology and the ability to undergo the acrosome reaction.

each microscopic field. Sperm motility is also evaluated; ideally more than five sperm exhibiting forward progression are seen in each field. The problem with the postcoital test is that if it is poor, which it often is, the gynecologist has to guess why the result is abnormal. Often, if the mucus quality appears adequate, the gynecologist tells the woman that her husband has a sperm problem and that this must be remedied before any further female testing is done. In fact, the woman is often told that female testing will stop if any sperm defects that may alter the couple's fertility are found. This is why adequate urologic assessment is so important.

A different method for evaluating sperm-mucus compatibility consists of obtaining cervical mucus from the woman on the day of ovulation. The day of ovulation can be determined by having the woman measure urine luteinizing hormone (LH) starting a couple of days before expected ovulation. Using an accurate home LH timing kit, a woman knows approximately 1 to 1½ days before ovulation that she is going to ovulate. Cervical mucus is obtained on the day of ovulation, and a drop of the mucus is placed in the center of a warm microscope slide. Next to this is placed a drop of test sperm from a suitable donor who has been previously evaluated for mucus penetration capability, and on the other side of the mucus is placed a drop of the husband's sperm.[31] The slide is covered with a large coverslip (22 × 60 mm) and incubated in a humidified chamber. The initial sperm motility of both the test sample and the husband's sample is observed, and the sperm motility and relative numbers of sperm that have penetrated the mucus are recorded every 20 to 30 minutes for 2 hours. If the husband's sperm exhibits poor mucus-sperm compatibility but the test sperm interacts well with the woman's mucus, the husband's sperm must develop better motility characteristics or be placed beyond the cervical mucus for the couple to have a better chance of pregnancy. If both samples have good interaction with the mucus, intercourse around the day of ovulation should give the couple a chance of pregnancy, at least as far as the mucus-sperm compatibility is concerned. If neither sperm sample exhibits compatibility with the woman's mucus, the woman should be tested for mucus and serum antisperm antibodies. Although simple, this test gives useful information about the couple's chances of achieving pregnancy with intercourse. An adequate supply of test sperm must be available on the day the test will be done, and like any other test of fertility, the test should be repeated to verify the results.

Over the last decade bovine cervical mucus has been used to evaluate the ability of human sperm to penetrate mucus.[32,33] This test has some correlation with the ability of sperm to penetrate human mucus but is not a substitute for assessing the woman's own mucus with her husband's sperm. The test can be done to indicate how well the sperm interact with mucus in general and how well a given sperm sample can move through viscous fluids. As an adjunct to a series of semen analyses, this can provide useful information about sperm function.

Antisperm Antibodies

The concept of antisperm antibodies is not new, but recently several tests to detect these antibodies in men and women have been developed.[34-37] A great deal of controversy remains in the literature with respect to the importance of antisperm antibodies in men or women and their relationship to infertility.[35-39] Antisperm antibodies should be measured in any male patient whose sperm shows significant and consistent agglutination, low motility, low viability, or hypoosmolarity. Clinical evidence of an adverse effect of antisperm antibodies is almost always accompanied by increased numbers of nonactive sperm, immobilizing sperm motility (in-place shaking motion), low HOS values (<50% reacted), and low viability scores (<40% live), as previously discussed. Clinical manifestations of antibodies should lead to measurement of antibody levels in male patients. This can be done with a variety of tests, including enzyme-linked immunosorbent assay (ELISA) tests, microagglutination and macroagglutination tests, sperm-immobilizing tests, and measurement of the binding of IgG, IgA, and IgM immunobeads. The immunobead test can be completed as a direct or indirect assay. In the direct assay the patient's own sperm are incubated with the immunobeads. If antibodies are present, the respective bead type binds to the antibody on the sperm surface. The percentage of sperm bound and the location of the beads' binding to the sperm are recorded. Typically, tests in which more than 20% of the sperm are bound to beads are considered positive. We prefer to perform a combination of antibody tests, including the Kibrick agglutination test, Isojima immobilization test, and immunobead test. Results from all three tests are correlated with clinical findings to assess whether the patient might have significant levels of antibodies interfering with fertility. Antibodies interfere with the ability of the sperm to get to the egg but may also decrease their ability to get into the egg because of the impaired sperm motility. Antibodies also alter sperm membrane permeability and function, which may adversely affect the quality of the sperm in a patient with significant levels of antisperm antibodies.

Men who are contemplating a vasectomy reversal should be tested for antisperm antibodies to determine whether they could adversely affect the reversal outcome. Other men with clinical evidence of antibodies, as described previously, should also be tested for antisperm antibodies.

Getting Into the Egg

Once sperm are at the fertilization site, they must be able to release hyaluronidase, which assists the sperm in digesting through the egg vestments to reach the egg itself, and then undergo capacitation and bind with and be incorporated through the zona pellucida and subsequently the vitelline membrane. Capacitation potential can be measured in a variety of ways. Although none of the techniques is as accurate as placing human sperm with human eggs and determining whether a given male's sperm can fertilize a given woman's eggs, some tests provide information about the sperm's ability to enter the egg. These tests include the hamster egg penetration test, the hemi-zona assay, and evaluation of the sperm acrosome.

The hamster egg penetration test has been used for the last 10 to 12 years (Figure 11–1).[40-42] This assay involves injecting hamsters with pregnant mare's serum gonadotropin (mostly follicle-stimulating hormone [FSH]) on the appropriate day of their cycle to induce the development of multiple follicles. Approximately 48 hours later the animals are injected with human chorionic gonadotropin (hCG), which completes egg maturation and causes the animals to ovulate. At about 14 to 16 hours after the hCG injection, eggs are recovered from the fallopian tubes and placed in hyaluronidase to separate the eggs from the cumulus mass. The eggs are subsequently placed in a dilute trypsin solution to remove the zona pellucida. The zona-free eggs are then placed with human sperm that have been incubated several hours or overnight, and the sperm-egg mixture is allowed to incubate for 2 to 5 hours. The eggs are then removed, carefully prepared, and observed under a phase-contrast microscope for evidence of sperm penetration. The sperm heads swell after they penetrate the egg, as with penetration of a human egg, and the eggs are observed for this phenomenon.

One problem with the hamster test is that it is difficult to perform, and therefore the correlation and predictive value of this test have been subject to a great deal of controversy.[43-46] We have had the same individual perform the assay for 12 years, and the results are consistent and have a high predictive value for subsequent patient fertility as well

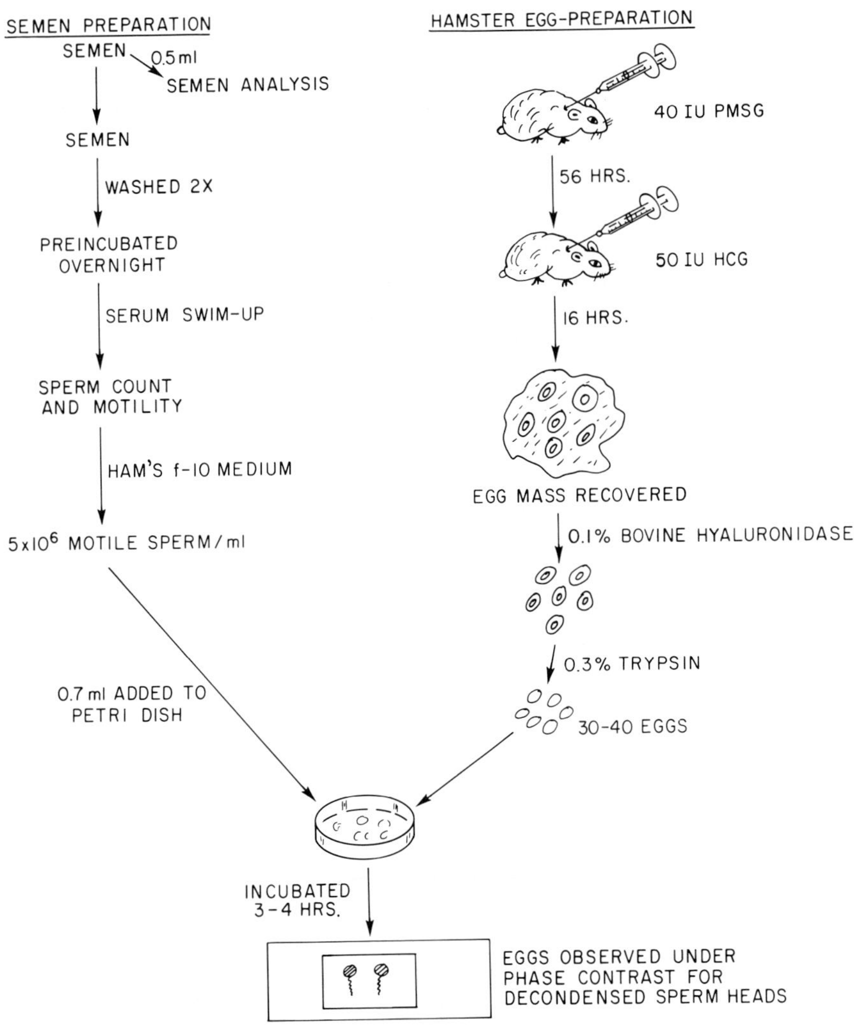

FIGURE 11–1. Procedure for the hamster egg–human sperm penetration assay.

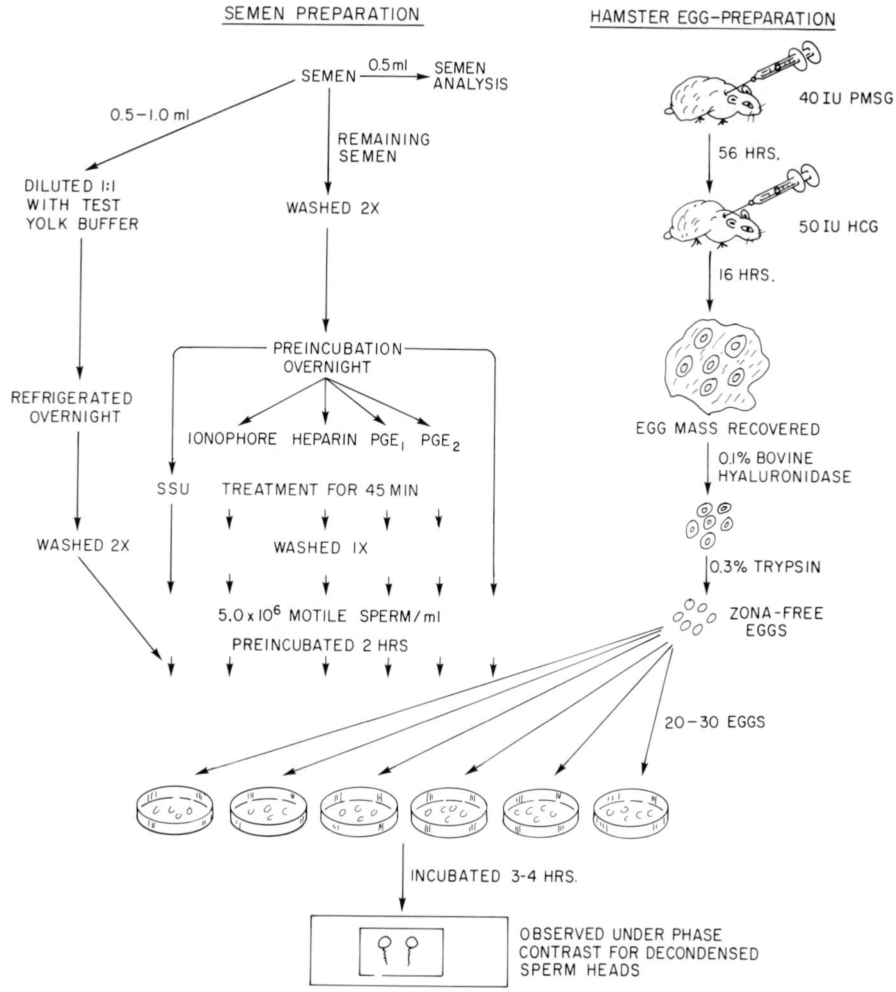

FIGURE 11–2. Procedure for the repeat hamster egg–human sperm penetration assay.

as in vitro fertilization outcome. We therefore consider the hamster test useful for predicting whether the sperm can enter the egg, and we routinely perform a hamster test on couples with unexplained infertility, men with normal sperm quality who have moderate to large varicoceles, and couples contemplating in vitro fertilization or related procedures.

A recent advance in treating male infertility is an assay to repeat the hamster egg penetration test when it is decreased. The normal value for the hamster test remains controversial but appears to be penetration of more than 15% of the eggs. Whenever the penetration value is 10% or less, we repeat the test on another occasion as outlined in Figure 11–2. With this assay, hamster eggs are obtained as described previously. Aliquots of sperm undergo incubation with heparin or calcium ionophore, or a portion of the sperm is incubated overnight with refrigeration after an appropriate cryoprotective is added. Eggs are then placed separately with sperm from each of the preparation techniques and the penetration is assessed. Typically unassisted hamster test results in penetration of zero to 6%, improvement with heparin 15% to 20%, calcium ionophore 10% to 30%, and refrigeration 50% to 70% when the treatment is effective. If we have an individual with low penetration (less than 10%) and none of the preceding treatments improve the penetration capacity, we advise the couple that the penetration defect might be contributing to their fertility problem and that it currently cannot be easily treated (see "Micromanipulation"). If, on the other hand, one or more of the techniques appears effective in improving penetration capacity, they are used to prepare the sperm for whatever procedure the couple will undergo. An example is a man with 6% penetration in the initial and repeat tests, which was improved to 25% penetration with heparin and 65% penetration with refrigeration. If this couple was going to undergo intrauterine insemination, a sample would be obtained for refrigeration the day before the insemination. Another sample would be obtained the next day, on the day of insemination, and this sample would be prepared with heparin incubation as described in the section on chemical incubation. The refrigerated and heparin-incubated samples would be combined and used for the insemination. These techniques are also applicable to couples undergoing in vitro fertilization. We consider improvement in penetration capacity to be one of the most useful advances in useful advances in sperm manipulation procedures. It has helped a number of couples to achieve fertilization when penetration capacity was essentially zero, as explained in the section on in vitro fertilization.

The hemi-zona assay uses immature human eggs obtained from ovaries at the time of oophorectomy or ovarian dissection. The zona pellucida is removed from the eggs and cut into two portions.[47] These portions are incubated with spermatozoa to determine the binding potential of the human sperm to the zona pellucida. Failure to bind to the zona pellucida may correlate with a diminished ability of sperm to capacitate and subsequently fertilize the egg.

The status of the sperm acrosome can be determined by a number of techniques. A triple-stain technique[48] can be used to evaluate the presence of the acrosome and is particularly useful when a large number of amorphous sperm (especially those with completely round heads) are noted during morphology assessment. The technique can also be used to count the sperm that have undergone capacitation reactions after stimulation.

The acrosome can be detected and acrosomal status evaluated by using antibodies that bind to the acrosome[49] or with additional fluorescence techniques.[50] In our experience, all these techniques give similar, but not identical, results in evaluating acrosomal status. Some groups have reported that acrosomal status has a high correlation to subsequent prediction of fertility, but others have found a minimal correlation.[51,52]

Sperm Collection

The last decade has brought advances in techniques for collecting sperm from men who previously had little hope of becoming fertile.

The procedure for normal collection of semen is well known and basically requires the individual to collect the sample in a clean, sterile container free of chemical or soap residues. Masturbation, with collection of the entire sample into the container, is the preferred technique for laboratory analysis, but the method most comfortable for the individual should be used. When the specimen is collected away from our institution, we typically have the individual use our container, making sure that the lid is placed on tightly after the sample is in the container. The entire container is then wrapped in a dry hand towel, and this is put into a sack. This wrapping usually keeps the sample adequately warm for transportation to the laboratory. The sample should be processed within 1 hour of collection. Samples can also be collected in a nonspermatocidal condom during intercourse. The physician should keep a small stock of these condoms on hand in the office so they can be distributed to patients. After sample collection the condom is put into a sterile container and brought into the laboratory within 1 hour.

Patients with retrograde ejaculation have been treated in a variety of ways. Any patient who has no ejaculate should be asked to provide a urine sample after sexual activity to check for sperm. In the past, the patient was catheterized to remove the urine, the bladder was irrigated, and after the patient had sexual activity, the bladder was recatheterized to collect the seminal fluid in the residual irrigation fluid.[53,54] Unfortunately, the trauma of the catheterization often resulted in a poor specimen collection, and patients were not enthusiastic about attempts to repeat the procedure. We have developed a technique that allows some patients with retrograde ejaculation to achieve pregnancy with their partner.[55] In the initial assessment of the retrograde ejaculation the patient is asked to urinate, have sexual activity, and urinate again into one of our containers. This eliminates the large amount of urine that would be obtained without the initial voiding. The sample is then mixed with artificial fluid, as described in the sperm processing section, and washed, and the sperm are resuspended in artificial fluid. A full semen analysis is then completed. The patient is asked to complete this procedure at least twice, since samples from an individual with retrograde ejaculation usually vary. After this assessment, if enough sperm can be obtained on at least one occasion, the wife is evaluated and her ovulation timed with urine LH assessment as described previously. On the day of ovulation the patient is told to make the urine alkaline by taking sodium bicarbonate tablets the night before specimen collection and again 2 to 4 hours before specimen collection. The patient voids, has sexual activity, and voids again, and the sperm are quickly removed by means of the washing technique. The sperm are suspended in 0.5 ml of fluid, which is then placed directly into the uterus. The couple should be advised that because sperm quality varies with retrograde ejaculation, the procedure may have to be repeated in numerous cycles before five to six reasonable cycles are obtained. We have had a dramatic pregnancy rate when patients have at least five to six good attempts based on final sperm quality. When an individual rarely has reasonable sperm quality, this technique is ineffective and may have to be combined with advanced reproductive techniques to increase the chance of fertilization.

Another advance in sperm collection has been the ability to aspirate sperm directly from the epididymis in men who have a congenital absence of the vas deferens.[56,57] This technique is usually combined with in vitro fertilization or related procedures because the aspirated sperm often shows poor concentration, morphology, and motility. The technique occasionally results in fertilization when combined with in vitro fertilization. It is not a substitute for vasectomy reversal, despite recent reports to the contrary in the popular press, and should be reserved for men with congenital absence of the vas deferens.

Electrical ejaculation is a technique that has been revived from the early 1970s because of advances in electronics and a better understanding of the coupling of this equipment to stimulation of ejaculation in primates. Electrical ejaculation is used to obtain semen samples from men with spinal cord injuries.[58-60] Although success rates vary, all reports indicate that this technique has great promise for selected cord-injured patients.[58-61] The time from injury and the patient's age, within a fairly large range, have relatively little relationship to the ability to obtain an ejaculate. Thoracic cord–injured patients are more likely to have viable sperm than those with injuries in other parts of the spinal cord.[60] Additional research to select the best candidates will mean that a greater percentage of spinal cord injury patients can have fertility restored through electrical ejaculation.

TREATMENT OF MALE INFERTILITY

Medications

It would be encouraging to report that medical advances in the last decade have led to the improvement of sperm defects and increased the urologist's ability to treat infertility. Unfortunately, no such advances have been made and none are on the horizon. The occasional patient who has hypogonadotropic hypogonadism (low FSH, LH, and testosterone levels) can be effectively treated with gonadotropin-releasing hormone and gonadotropins.[62] Most men with sperm defects have normal levels of FSH, LH and testosterone, although some have elevations in FSH and occasionally in LH levels, with perhaps lower testosterone levels. Only the combination of low FSH, low LH, and low testosterone levels is amenable to drug treatment, as described previously. Clomiphene citrate has been used in attempts to restore fertility to men with sperm defects but has not been effective.[63] hCG injections and testosterone rebound therapy have rarely improved sperm quality enough to restore fertility.[64]

Immunosuppressive therapy with prednisone or similar drugs has been used to reduce levels of antisperm antibodies.[65,66] Results have been variable, and patients have needed careful follow-up because of the many possible side effects of immunosuppression.

Surgery

The biggest improvement in the surgical correction of male infertility has resulted from incorporation of microsurgical techniques into reproductive surgery.[67,68] These techniques have particularly improved the ability to connect the vas deferens at vasectomy reversal and the technique of epididymovasostomy. More precise anastomosis of the vas, as well as the epididymis, has increased the percentage of men with sperm and probably increased the time of patency after surgery.

The sperm aspiration technique, mentioned previously, has enabled the urologist to aspirate sperm directly from the epididymis by puncturing the tubule with a long sterile Pasteur pipette. Epididymal fluid is then allowed to rise in the tubule by capillary action or with gentle suction, and the fluid is examined for spermatozoa. If sperm are found in the fluid, they can be recovered with washing techniques, incubated to improve their motility, and used for insemination or advanced reproductive procedures.

Other improved surgical techniques in reproductive surgery include tightening of the bladder neck muscle to restore normal ejaculation in the individual with retrograde ejaculation[69] and using needle biopsy to collect specimens from the testes by a minimally traumatic procedure.[70]

Advanced Reproductive Techniques

Most of the explosive growth in the area of reproduction has occurred with the development of advanced reproductive techniques. Such techniques allow direct placement of improved sperm in the vicinity of the egg or even into the egg, which increases the probability that the egg(s) will be fertilized.

Sperm Manipulation Procedures

Rapid advances in the development of new fluids in which to suspend the sperm removed from seminal plasma, and in the ability to manipulate sperm to improve their function before use, have greatly enhanced the ability to treat infertile men. These techniques are discussed here in detail. By gaining an in-depth knowledge of the various techniques and their use for particular defects, the urologist can advise the laboratory about the best technique for preparing the sperm. Sperm manipulation procedures can be used to concentrate sperm, improve sperm motility, isolate sperm with the best head shapes, and increase the ability of sperm to penetrate the egg.

Sperm Processing

Many techniques can be used to process sperm, and a variety of media can be used for suspension of the sperm. We prefer using a modified Ham's F-10 medium that we prepare in our laboratory.[71] A comparison of different solutions is shown in Table

TABLE 11–4. Progressive Sperm Motility Before and After Washing in Various Solutions (50 Samples Per Medium)

Media	*Percent Prewash Progressive Sperm Motility*	*Percent Postwash Progressive Sperm Motility*
Tyrode's buffer	20.42 ± 4.1	21.67 ± 7.7
Earle's MEM	16.92 ± 3.23	19.81 ± 2.51
BWW	28.29 ± 2.47	32.71 ± 2.11
Modified Ham's F-10	32.41 ± 2.7	39.68 ± 2.88*

*$p < 0.05$ when compared with prewash motility.

11–4 and indicates that the modified Ham's F-10 provides better sperm function than the other solutions. We have also evaluated sperm quality in other solutions, including human tubal fluid, and still prefer the modified Ham's F-10 medium.

The following processing procedures can improve sperm function for use of the sperm with insemination or advanced reproductive techniques.

Sperm Washing. Sperm washing is the simplest sperm processing technique and is accomplished as follows:

1. Liquefy the semen at 37° C for 15 to 30 minutes.
2. After liquefaction, pour the semen into a sterile 15 ml centrifuge tube. Measure and record the volume.
3. With a sterile syringe, withdraw some mixed semen from the 15 ml centrifuge tube and place 1 drop on a glass slide. Place a coverslip over the specimen.
4. Record the motility using the motility procedure.
5. Add pH-adjusted Ham's F-10 medium to the specimen in a ratio of 3 parts medium to 1 part semen. Gently invert the tube several times to ensure gentle mixing. NOTE: If the initial volume is large (>6 ml), it is better to split the specimen in half and use two centrifuge tubes for washing.
6. Centrifuge for 10 minutes at 250 to 300 × g.
7. Carefully decant the supernatant.
8. Using a syringe, resuspend the semen pellet in Ham's F-10 medium. If intrauterine insemination is to be performed, a total volume of 0.5 ml is used. If a cervical insemination is to be performed, the total volume is 1 ml.
9. Draw all suspended material into a sterile syringe. Make sure the syringe has the patient's name on it.
10. Place 1 drop of the semen mixture on a slide and cover with a coverslip.
11. Record the final motility. The specimen should be more motile and more concentrated.
12. Wrap the syringe in a paper towel. Make sure everything is labeled with the patient's name, and hand it to the patient to take for insemination.

This technique is used primarily to concentrate sperm from a man with fewer than 20 to 30 million progressively motile sperm per ejaculate before intrauterine placement. The wash is also the best choice for frozen samples, which usually are more fragile than fresh samples, for samples with antisperm antibodies, or for samples from men with retrograde ejaculation. These samples are more gently mixed with the Ham's medium and centrifuged for a shorter time and at a slightly slower speed, all of which improves the recovery of motile sperm after the washing procedure when the sperm are more susceptible to damage. Washing is a reasonable technique for individuals with antisperm antibodies, which may require more than one wash. Samples with clinical evidence of antisperm antibodies, however, have more initial membrane damage and are more easily damaged during washing procedures. Often the antibodies cannot be displaced from the sperm, and a test wash procedure or a one-cycle insemination trial may be necessary to determine how much the sperm can be improved. We also use washing techniques for economic reasons, although, as shown in Table 11–5, washing yields lower pregnancy rates than such techniques as serum swim-up.[72] In summary, washing is useful for the simple concentration of sperm for intrauterine placement; for the preparation of sperm from frozen samples, from retrograde ejaculators, or from men with antisperm antibodies; and for economic reasons.

Incubation and Swim-up. Another popular sperm preparation technique is the serum incubation, serum swim-up, or incubation or swim-up without serum. This technique is outlined as:

1. One to 3 days before ovulation, draw 15 ml of blood from the woman into a 15 ml red top tube. Label the tube with the patient's name, the date, and the procedure.
2. Allow the blood to clot at room temperature for 15 to 60 minutes.
3. After the blood is clotted, centrifuge for 10 minutes at 3000 rpm (500 × g).
4. Draw the serum off using a sterile syringe. Carefully remove the needle, and place a filter assembly (0.22 μm) on the syringe. Gently push the serum through the filter assembly and into a sterile 15 ml centrifuge tube (less than 5 ml per filter).

TABLE 11–5. Pregnancy Rate Comparison in 24 Patients Undergoing a Four-Cycle Insemination Protocol with Sperm Washing and Serum Swim-up

Sperm Preparation Method	*Pregnancies* No.	*Pregnancies* Percent
Sperm washing	15	62
Serum swim-up	9	38

The tube must be labeled with the patient's name, the date, and the procedure.

5. Heat inactivate the serum in a 56° C water bath for 30 minutes.
6. Freeze the serum until the day of insemination.
7. On the day of insemination, thaw the serum at 37° C.
8. Label another sterile 15 ml centrifuge tube with the patient's name, the date, and the words "Serum Mix" or "Serum Swim-up."
9. Using a 1 ml sterile pipette, transfer 0.8 ml of the heat-inactivated serum into the labeled sterile centrifuge tube. Add Ham's F-10 medium, which has been bubbled with 5% CO_2 (in air), up to the 10 ml mark on the tube (8% serum mixture). This serum mixture will be used to prepare the sperm.
10. Before using the semen specimen, make sure it has been liquefied. To liquefy the specimen, place it in a 37° C incubator for 15 to 30 minutes.
11. After an adequate time for liquefaction, label another sterile 15 ml centrifuge tube with the patient's name, the date, and the words "Sperm Sample." Place the semen in the labeled centrifuge tube and record the volume. Handle the sample with sterile equipment in all steps.
12. Take a drop of semen, place on a clear slide, cover with a coverslip, record the initial motility, and prepare another slide for morphology. The slides must be labeled with the date, the patient's name, and whether the smear is an initial or the final slide of the test. Use a frosted end slide for the morphology smears.
13. Wash the semen twice using the semen wash procedure. Use the previously prepared Ham's F-10 serum mixture (the tube labeled "Serum Mix") to wash the sperm.
14. After the second wash, resuspend the sperm pellet in 0.5 to 0.8 ml of Ham's F-10 medium. Record the postwash motility.
15. Gently layer 1.5 ml of medium on top of the 0.5 ml of sample. A clean interface must be created between the sample and the 1.5 ml of Ham's F-10 serum mixture.
16. Let stand at an angle (in a beaker) in the 37° C incubator for 1 to 1½ hours.
17. Remove the top 1 ml of the fluid in the centrifuge tube. Record the final motility and concentration. If necessary mix the sample with the bottom layer to increase the sperm count. Make a final morphology smear.
18. Wrap the syringe in a paper towel and place in the incubator until given to the patient.

The serum enhances sperm function and yields a sample with better sperm motility and usually better sperm morphology as the sperm move into the clear layer above the sperm suspension. If the sperm concentration is diminished in the initial sample (fewer than 50 million progressively motile sperm per ejaculate), the technique is converted into a serum incubation. In the serum incubation technique, sperm are suspended in approximately 1 ml of fluid after two washes and allowed to incubate in a CO_2 incubator for at least 1 hour. The entire sample is then used for intrauterine insemination, or a portion of the sperm is used for advanced reproductive procedures. We prefer using the serum swim-up technique because results from a pilot project demonstrated that more than 60% of the pregnancies obtained with insemination were produced by a serum swim-up.[72] The serum swim-up results in better motility, capacitation, and morphology than the wash. Recent studies have indicated that the timing and the source of the serum are less important than having serum in the fluid and that human serum appears to work better than serum substitutes for improving sperm quality.[73]

Swim-down. Another method of sperm preparation is the swim-down technique, in which sperm are washed, resuspended in fluids, and carefully layered on thick solutions into which they are allowed to swim down. Albumin solutions are commonly used; we often use bovine serum albumin with the following technique:

1. Use sterile techniques for all steps.
2. Record the initial sperm motility and make a morphology slide.
3. Prepare the following solutions:
   a. 10% bovine serum albumin (BSA)
   b. 1 g BSA to 10 ml Ham's F-10 solution (pass through with 0.22 μm filter)
4. Place the sperm in a sterile centrifuge tube and wash once with Ham's F-10 medium. Centrifuge at 250 to 300 × g for 10 minutes. Decant the supernatant and resuspend the sperm pellet in 1 ml of Ham's F-10 medium.
5. With a sterile syringe, fill five sterile 6 × 50 mm tubes half full of 10% BSA. Mark the top of this layer with a marking pen. Layer 0.2 ml of the resuspended sperm solution on top of the BSA layer in each tube. Add slowly to create an interface and two distinct layers.
6. Incubate all tubes at 37° C for 1 hour.
7. After 1 hour remove the top sperm layer and discard.
8. Pool the remaining 10% BSA layers from each tube and place in a sterile centrifuge tube. Add Ham's F-10 medium to obtain 10 ml total volume and invert gently to mix. Centrifuge at 250 to 300 × g for 10 minutes. Decant the supernatant and resuspend the pellet in 0.5 to 1 ml of Ham's F-10 medium.
9. Record the final motility and make a morphology slide.
10. Wrap the syringe containing sperm in a paper towel for transportation.

This technique is useful to improve sperm motility, sperm morphology, and capacitation. It is also used in the first stages of separating X- and Y-bearing sperm.[75] The latter technique has been reported to increase male birth rates by 60% to 70% in some studies, although other studies have found no difference in birth rates with the technique.[75] With either the swim-down or swim-up technique, 30% to 60% of the initial sperm concentration is lost. At the end of any preparation process we attempt to recover at least 30 million progressively motile sperm for intrauterine placement. The technique used to prepare sperm remains a matter of individual preference, since no technique is clearly superior in contributing to pregnancies.

Percoll Suspension. Percoll, a silica-based solution, can be used to separate sperm with better motility and quality. Either the sperm are washed, or the semen is placed directly in tubes on top of varying concentrations of Percoll.[76] This suspension is then centrifuged for 10 to 30 minutes, after which the sperm are isolated from the lower one to two layers of Percoll, washed, and resuspended for use. Many groups prefer the Percoll suspension method for preparing sperm before intrauterine insemination or for advanced reproductive techniques. Similar to the swim-up and swim-down procedures, 20% to 60% of the initial sperm concentration is lost during the sperm separation process. We prefer to use a two- to three-layer gradient Percoll technique as follows:

1. Prepare 10 × concentrated Ham's F-10 medium by adding 1 packet of Ham's F-10 powder in 30 ml 5 × distilled water. Add to the above:
   a. 18.75 mg of penicillin G in 10 ml 5 × distilled water
   b. 12.5 mg of streptomycin in 10 ml 5 × distilled water
   c. 245.2 mg of calcium lactate in 10 ml 5 × distilled water
   d. 1260 mg of sodium bicarbonate in 10 ml 5 × distilled water
   e. 507.6 mg of potassium bicarbonate in 10 ml 5 × distilled water

   Bring volume to 100 ml and filter.
2. Prepare an isotonic Percoll solution (to be known as 100% Percoll) by adding 6 ml of 10 × concentrated Ham's F-10 medium to 75 ml of Percoll. Sterile techniques should be used in all steps.
3. Measure the osmolarity and adjust to 278 mOsm/kg by adding either 10 × concentrated Ham's F-10 medium or more Percoll.
4. Prepare the following concentrations of Percoll solution to be used in the Percoll gradient:
   a. 90% Percoll: add 1 ml of regular Ham's F-10 medium to 9 ml of 100% Percoll.
   b. 65% Percoll: add 3.5 ml of regular Ham's F-10 medium to 6.5 ml of 100% Percoll.
   c. 35% Percoll: add 6.5 ml of regular Ham's F-10 medium to 3.5 ml of 100% Percoll.
5. Prepare the Percoll gradient by carefully and slowly adding the following to a sterile 15 ml conical centrifuge tube:
   a. 1.5 ml of 90% Percoll
   b. 1.5 ml of 65% Percoll
   c. 1.5 ml of 35% Percoll

   If a two-layer gradient is desired, the 65% Percoll layer is omitted.
6. Prepare initial slides for sperm motility and morphology. Save approximately 0.2 ml of semen for a sperm count.
7. Wash the remaining portion of the semen sample at 250 × g, then resuspend the pellet in 1 ml of Ham's F-10 medium. Record the postwash motility.
8. Carefully layer the sperm suspension onto the previously prepared gradient.
9. Centrifuge the gradient at 250 × g for 15 minutes.
10. Using a 3 ml sterile syringe, carefully remove the sperm suspension layer and save. With another syringe carefully remove the 35% and 65% Percoll layers. (If a two-layer gradient is used, remove the 35% Percoll layer and proceed as described in the following steps.)
11. Add 6 to 8 ml of Ham's F-10 medium to the remaining 1.5 ml of 90% Percoll. Gently mix and centrifuge at 250 × g for 10 minutes.
12. Resuspend the pellet in approximately 0.7 ml of Ham's F-10 medium. Prepare a final motility and morphology slide and count the sperm.
13. If the initial sperm concentration is decreased or the progressive motility is less than 25%, a two-layer gradient (90% and 35%) should be used.
14. If the final sperm concentration is less than 30×10^6 progressively motile sperm, the sperm suspension layer (step 10) may be added to the final preparation to increase the motile density.

This technique is simple and works in essentially the same way as the multilayered Percoll techniques used by some groups.[77]

Other Techniques. Sperm have been processed by having them swim through glass wool.[78] We have not found this technique to be as useful as the preceding techniques and therefore do not recommend it. Sperm can also be placed on columns of Sephadex or similar solutions to separate the most motile sperm, but these techniques are less reliable and less widely used than the preceding processing techniques.

Purpose of Sperm Processing. The purpose of sperm processing is to improve the sperm sample before its use for insemination. Insemination

TABLE 11–6. Comparison of Methods for Sperm Freezing With Complex or Simple Cryoprotectants

Freezing	*Cryoprotectant*	*Method*
Simple	7.5% Glycerol	18 Drops cryoprotectant added in three steps to 0.9 ml semen frozen in liquid nitrogen vapor
Complex	20% Fresh egg yolk in TEST buffer	Semen mixed 1:1 with cryoprotectant and frozen in vapor

should be done near the time of ovulation, which, as mentioned above, the woman can determine at home with an accurate LH timing predictor kit. The woman starts testing her urine a couple of days before expected ovulation. We prefer to have the woman test twice daily, in the morning and early evening. If the morning sample indicates an LH surge, the insemination is typically done in the afternoon of the next day. If the early evening sample indicates an LH surge, the insemination is done not the next morning but the morning after that. The insemination therefore is done approximately 36 hours after the LH surge. We perform just one insemination per cycle, although some groups do two. No one has proved that two inseminations give a better pregnancy rate than one insemination, and furthermore doing two increases the cost to the couple. Insemination appears to make sense for couples who have poor mucus-sperm compatibility and is probably useful for men with sperm defects.[79] Inseminations do not give a high pregnancy rate in couples with unexplained infertility, as might be expected, or when the female partner has other significant defects.[80] Our data indicate that five or six cycles of insemination should be tried and that if no pregnancy results by then, other techniques should be considered.

Concentration and Combination

Many patients, when told they have diminished sperm concentration, ask about the possibility of preserving a number of samples, thawing them, and adding them together to increase the effective concentration. The problem with this proposal is that men with low sperm density often also have low sperm motility and altered morphology. Freezing and thawing samples from such patients would not provide enough viable sperm at the end of the process to significantly improve the chances of conception. Freezing sufficient samples to make a difference in the effective sperm concentration would be extremely expensive. Occasionally an individual with low sperm density has excellent sperm motility, and in this case a few samples can be frozen, combined, and used for intrauterine insemination or advanced reproductive techniques. We occasionally obtain a sperm sample from a man with low sperm density on the day before his partner ovulates, refrigerate the sample overnight using techniques described in the section on refrigeration, and combine the sample with a fresh sample the day of the insemination. The combined sample is washed, concentrated, and used for intrauterine insemination. Refrigeration is less harsh than freezing and can occasionally be used to combine at least two samples from a given individual for insemination. The technique is also used to enhance capacitation as mentioned previously and described later.

Several techniques can be used to freeze sperm for short- or long-term preservation. Table 11–6 compares two commonly used techniques for cryopreserving sperm. We have used both techniques and believe that they work equally well. Generally the complex cryoprotectant yields better sperm motility and viability, but in a preliminary study the glycerol technique yielded better sperm membrane function (Table 11–7).

Chemical Incubation

For many years investigators have suggested that sperm could be incubated with various chemicals to improve their function during insemination or advanced reproductive techniques.[81] Chemicals have been used in attempts to improve sperm motility and penetration capacitation. A number of articles have reported that caffeine incubation improves sperm motility, although caffeine has never

TABLE 11–7. Recovery in Progressive Sperm Motility, Viable Sperm, and Hypoosmolarity Score After Cryopreservation with Three Different Cryopreservation Techniques

Type of Cryopreservation	*Decrease in Progressive Sperm Motility (%)*	*Decrease in Live Spermatozoa (%)*	*HOS Score Decrease (%)*
Refrigeration	−8.3*†	−27.4	+3.2‡§
Complex protectant	−13.6‡	−30.4	−21.4‡
Glycerol protectant	−24.5	−37.4	−11.1

*Value represents mean percent change from precryopreservation values.
†p at least <0.05 compared with simple protectant.
‡p at least <0.05 compared with simple protectant.
§p at least <0.05 compared with complex protectant.

been shown to improve pregnancy rates when used with sperm incubation.[82] Similar-acting chemicals have also been suggested to improve sperm motility, although so far none has been shown to change pregnancy rates.[83]

We routinely use heparin incubation, as mentioned previously, to improve sperm capacitation if the patient has a demonstrated diminished capacitation, based on a hamster test, and if results of a repeat hamster test can be improved with heparin incubation. In these individuals the following heparin incubation procedure may prove useful:

1. Determine the sperm motility and morphology. Wash the sperm in Ham's F-10 medium. Make sure the medium has been bubbled with 5% CO_2.
2. Resuspend the pellet in Ham's medium.
3. Wash the sperm a second time using Ham's medium with 8% female preovulatory heat-inactivated serum.
4. Determine the sperm motility, and resuspend the sperm in 1 to 2 ml Ham's medium with female preovulatory serum containing 53 U.S.P. units per milliliter of heparin.
5. Allow this mixture to incubate in a CO_2 incubator for 1 hour. Determine sperm motility.
6. Wash the sample in the medium containing the serum.
7. Resuspend the sample for the insemination with the Ham's medium and serum mixture and determine sperm motility.

This technique has improved sperm capacitation, as judged by improved hamster test results, in approximately 30% of the individuals we have tested. Among the other chemicals used in attempts to improve sperm capacitation and sperm motility are calcium ionophore, prostaglandin E_1, and prostaglandin E_2.[84]

Refrigeration

Refrigeration of sperm after addition of an appropriate cryoprotectant can be used to improve sperm capacitation and to preserve sperm for short periods (up to 3 days) before use. The complex cryoprotectant outlined in Table 11–6 is used with refrigeration according to the technique described below. Refrigeration has improved sperm penetration capacity in approximately 60% to 65% of our patients with abnormal penetration values. Because the cryoprotectant medium is an ideal fluid for bacterial growth, meticulous care and sterile techniques are necessary when working with these solutions. The refrigeration technique is accomplished as follows:

1. Media preparation
    a. Add 150 ml H_2O to:
       TES—4.32 g
       TRIS—1.02 g
       Sodium citrate—2.86 g
       Fructose—0.116 g
       Streptomycin—0.025 g
       Penicillin—0.015 g
    b. Adjust the osmolarity to between 320 and 325 mOsm by adding TRIS, and adjust pH to 7.4.
    c. Add 7.4 ml of the above TEST solution to 0.6 ml of glycerol and filter with a micropore filter.
    d. To the 7.4 ml of sterile TEST-glycerol solution add 2 ml of fresh egg yolk. Mix well.
    e. Centrifuge at high speed (800 × g) for 5 minutes.
    f. Pour supernatant into a sterile 15 ml conical centrifuge tube. Discard the pellet. Store in refrigerator.
2. Refrigeration
    a. When using the refrigeration solution, first warm to room temperature. Fill a semen specimen container three-fourths full with H_2O at room temperature.
    b. Measure and record semen volume and sperm motility.
    c. Place the semen in a sterile 15 ml conical centrifuge tube and add an equal aliquot of the refrigeration solution. Gently mix.
    d. Place the tube containing the semen–refrigeration solution mixture in the container filled with H_2O at room temperature.
    e. Place the container in the refrigerator.
    f. Store at 4° to 5° C for a maximum of 96 hours.
3. Preparation before insemination
    a. Remove the container from the refrigerator and place in 37° C incubator. (Leave tube in H_2O bath.)
    b. Let sample slowly warm to 37° C, then wash two times with Ham's F-10 medium.

The refrigeration and heparin techniques have improved fertilization rates in patients with zero values on hamster egg penetration tests repeated at least twice. Refrigeration and heparin incubation were used to prepare the sperm before addition to eggs during in vitro fertilization. Patients were included in this protocol if enough eggs were obtained so that some would have sperm added that were prepared from a serum swim-up technique and some would have sperm added that were prepared with refrigeration or heparin or both. As can be seen from Table 11–8, all the patients had at least some fertilization when refrigerated or heparin-incubated sperm were used, whereas sperm prepared with the serum swim-up process gave a lower fertilization rate. Additional studies are necessary to determine the full role of refrigeration in improving male fertility, but at this point these techniques have exciting potential to benefit at least some men with concentration or penetration defects.

TABLE 11–8. In Vitro Fertilization of Human Oocytes by Either Fresh Sperm Prepared by Serum Swim-up or the Refrigeration and Heparin Techniques in Patients With Initial Sperm Penetration Assay Value of Zero Penetration

	Percent of Human Oocytes Fertilized	
Patient No.	*Refrigeration Plus Heparin*	*Serum Swim-up (Fresh)*
1	62 (5/8)	0 (0/5)
2	50 (1/2)	0 (0/2)
3	20 (1/5)	0 (0/4)
4	25 (2/8)	0 (0/7)
5	50 (2/4)	75 (3/4)
6	100 (5/5)	75 (3/4)
Mean + standard error	51.2 ± 12.5*	25.0 ± 16.8

*$p < 0.001$ compared with serum swim-up.

ADVANCED REPRODUCTIVE TECHNOLOGIES

The explosive growth in advanced reproductive procedures has kindled excitement about the ability to treat previously insoluble male fertility problems. These techniques allow the placement of sperm near the egg and increase the likelihood of fertilization. Techniques discussed in this section include in vitro fertilization (IVF), gamete intrafallopian tubal transfer (GIFT), zygote intrafallopian tubal transfer (ZIFT), pronuclear intrafallopian tubal transfer (PROST), intratubal placement of sperm, micromanipulation of eggs to enhance the ability of poor-quality sperm to fertilize the egg, embryo freezing, and embryo biopsy procedures.

In Vitro Fertilization

IVF has revolutionized the treatment of infertility. For many years the success rate with IVF was low enough (<10% pregnancy per attempt) to make the technique interesting but not particularly useful to the treatment of infertility. The pregnancy rate in some programs is now closer to 20% to 30% per attempt, which makes the process more useful as a routine treatment. Advances in the ability to induce multiple follicles to develop so that several eggs are available, as well as advances in egg recovery, fertilization, and embryo transfer, have improved the success rate.

Couples who have exhausted all other treatment options to achieve conception are considered candidates for IVF. The ideal candidates are couples in which the woman has irreversibly blocked fallopian tubes and a history of previous pregnancies and the man has normal sperm. This group of patients can achieve a high rate of pregnancy with IVF, particularly after multiple attempts. Patients with other types of fertility defects can also benefit from IVF but generally have a lower success rate. Before IVF the couple's fertility history must be thoroughly reviewed and all applicable tests must be completed. These tests might include the assessment of female antisperm antibodies and a series of carefully conducted semen analyses to obtain the information discussed previously in this chapter. We also require a hamster egg penetration test, which must be repeated if the initial value is less than 10%.

Several medications are used to induce multiple follicular development, including clomiphene citrate, clomiphene citrate coupled with injections of drugs containing FSH and LH, and pure FSH.[85] Many programs begin with a suppression period of Lupron and then add the FSH and LH or pure FSH preparations to stimulate multiple follicular development.[86] Follicular maturation is carefully observed with a combination of ultrasound and estradiol measurements to assess egg maturity. When the follicles are 1.7 to 2 cm and the estradiol level is appropriate for the number of mature follicles, the woman is given an injection of hCG to complete egg maturation. Approximately 34 hours after the hCG injection the follicles are aspirated and the oocytes obtained. For several years eggs were recovered via laparoscopy, but this was eventually replaced by ultrasound-directed aspiration.[87] Transvaginal ultrasound with the patient lightly sedated permits rapid aspiration of the follicles in a relatively noninvasive fashion. Once the follicles have been aspirated, oocytes are identified, graded with respect to maturity, and incubated in a petri dish or test tube. We incubate recovered oocytes in modified Ham's F-10 medium that has been supplemented with 8% female preovulatory serum. For women who have been shown to have antisperm antibodies, the medium is supplemented with 8% fetal cord serum that has been tested for sexually transmitted diseases. The eggs are allowed to incubate for approximately 5½ hours, during which time the sperm sample is obtained and prepared. If the sperm sample and hamster egg penetration test findings are relatively normal, the sperm sample is prepared with the serum swim-up technique described previously. If the penetration capacity is significantly low or the sperm have significantly reduced sperm quality (motility, density, or morphology), a sample is obtained the day before egg recovery and refrigerated overnight using the previously described techniques. An additional sample is obtained the day of egg recovery and incubated with heparin. These samples are combined to make a final sample for fertilization. We typically add 200,000 to 900,000 progressively motile sperm per egg depending on the data from the initial semen analyses, the hamster test information, and the quality of the IVF sample, which unfortunately is often poorer than the samples obtained previously for diagnostic purposes. All of this information determines how many sperm are finally added to each egg. Once the sperm have been added at about 5½ hours after egg recovery, the eggs are allowed to incubate for approximately 16 to 20 hours. The eggs are then gently removed and placed into a petri dish on a warmer under the microscope, and the cumulus cells are carefully teased from the egg with fine needles. This takes approximately 60 to 120 seconds, after which time the egg is observed for the presence or absence of two pronuclei. If the egg contains two pronuclei, it is placed in a separate petri dish with 3 to 4 ml of solution containing modified Ham's medium plus 16% heat-inactivated preovulatory serum from the woman. These dishes are allowed to incubate for 24 to 28 additional hours. The eggs that do not have evidence of fertilization are refertilized with the patient's backup frozen sample, the sample prepared from the patient the previous day, or a new sample that is obtained for the attempt at refertilization. Although some of the eggs are fertilized after a refertilization attempt, the pregnancy outcome when these eggs are used is relatively poor.[88] Couples in which the man has severe sperm defects are counseled before undergoing IVF to determine whether they want a percentage of the eggs mixed with donor sperm. Some programs add the husband's sperm to all of the eggs and then follow up with donor sperm 4 to 6 hours later. The problem with this technique is that the couple never knows whether the husband's sperm were able to fertilize the egg. Part of the IVF process should be enabling the couple to learn whether they can make fertilized eggs together and evaluating the quality of the embryo they have together. When donor sperm are added to all the eggs, this information is lost. If the couple so desires, donor sperm can be added to some of the eggs to increase the chance that at least some eggs will be fertilized. Approximately 24 hours after the pronuclear eggs have been put into the incubator, the embryos are pooled and the quality of each embryo is determined. We typically rate embryo quality on a quantitative scale, which allows us to calculate an embryo score according to the following criteria:

1. Embryos are given a number of points based on the extent of cell division. For example, a two-cell embryo is given 2 points; a one-cell fertilized embryo but not yet divided, 1 point; a three-cell, 3 points; and a four-cell, 4 points.
2. Points are subtracted from the above embryo level score based on the quality of the embryo. Embryos having equal size blastomeres with no cytoplasm fragmentation are called level one embryos and do not have any points subtracted. Embryos with moderate fragmentation or some difference in size of the blastomeres are called level two embryos and have 2 points subtracted. Embryos with significant fragmentation are called level three embryos and have 3 points subtracted.
3. The resulting modified embryo scores for each embryo are added together to give a total embryo score for the embryos that will be transferred into the uterus. The embryo score is subsequently modified to give a final score based on the difficulty of the embryo transfer. If the transfer is easy, the embryo score equals the final score. If the transfer is moderately difficult, the embryo score is divided by two and the resulting number equals the final score. If the transfer is extremely difficult, the embryo score is divided by three and the resulting number equals the final score.

We try to obtain an embryo score between 12 and 16, and therefore we transfer the number of embryos that equals a score in this range. The resulting embryo score and final score have a high correlation to prediction of whether pregnancy will occur.

The embryo transfer is done by aspirating 5 μl of fluid in a small plastic catheter (tomcat) after the catheter has been flushed numerous times with media. The embryos are then aspirated into the catheter, which contains an additional 5 μl, making a total volume of 10 μl. Between 2 and 3 μl of air is aspirated into the end of the catheter, which is then gently inserted into the uterus to a premeasured depth of 0.5 cm from the fundus of the uterus. The embryos are gently expelled into the uterus, and the catheter is removed. The catheter is flushed to ensure that embryos have not adhered to the catheter, and the transfer process is complete. The transfer is done under quiet conditions with the patient in the supine position to minimize uterine contractility. Generally the patient has luteal phase supplementation with injectable progresterone. Two weeks after embryo transfer a quantitative hCG measurement is performed to determine pregnancy.

With the preceding technique our pregnancy per retrieval rate is approximately 30% to 35% and the take home baby rate generally is between 20% and 28%. Most patients have at least one fertilized egg for an overall fertilization rate of approximately 60%. Concentration of sperm from individuals with sperm defects, manipulation of the sperm before addition, and micromanipulation procedures (which are discussed subsequently) have all improved the likelihood of fertilization. Accurate data before a couple undergoes IVF is essential for an optimal patient outcome. We have had pregnancies when the father had a total ejaculate sperm density of approximately 200,000 progressively motile sperm, but success with individuals who have sperm in this range is far more elusive than with normal sperm or more subtle defects in sperm quality.

Gamete Intrafallopian Tubal Transfer

The GIFT technique is designed for couples with essentially unexplained fertility problems.[89] The basic premise of the technique is that unfertilized eggs and sperm can be placed together in the high part of the fallopian tube, where conditions may be more conducive to fertilization and gradual movement of the fertilized egg and subsequent embryo into the uterus, ensuring more appropriate timing. The rationale for GIFT is that it eliminates the necessity of culturing oocytes and embryos in the laboratory where adverse influences on the embryo may occur. The GIFT process is similar to IVF but must be performed in a woman with normal tubal anatomy and function. The woman is given drugs to induce multiple follicular development; the follicle maturity is monitored with ultrasound and estrogen, as described previously; and when the follicles are mature, the woman is given an injection of hCG. Approximately 34 hours later, laparoscopy is performed and the eggs are recovered from the ovaries. Approximately two eggs and between 200,000 and 800,000 progressively motile sperm in about 50 to 100 μl of fluid are placed into each fallopian tube. This completes the procedure; the hope is that one or more eggs will be fertilized normally and implanted in the uterus. The GIFT technique is more acceptable to some religious groups because they believe that the process is more natural, with eggs fertilized in the body instead of the laboratory. The average GIFT pregnancy rate is approximately 20% to 30%.

A problem with GIFT has been that couples did not learn much from this process if they failed to achieve pregnancy. With IVF couples find out whether they can make fertilized eggs and embryos together and whether the quality of the embryo is good. With GIFT, this has not been possible. Now, however, extra eggs from the GIFT procedure can be fertilized with IVF and cultured to embryos as described previously. These embryos can be frozen in a programmable liquid nitrogen freezer (discussed later), and this enables the couple to learn whether they achieved fertilization and embryo development. The outcome of these extra eggs fertilized in the laboratory has a high correlation to the couple's chance of subsequently achieving pregnancy.[90]

Another disadvantage of GIFT is that the woman must have general anesthesia and be exposed to the surgical process of laparoscopy. Recovery from this process is more difficult than recovery from transvaginal ultrasound aspiration. Since the GIFT pregnancy rate is higher overall than the average for IVF (approximately 25% versus 11% to 15%), GIFT may be a better choice for the couple with unexplained fertility if the aforementioned limitations are taken into account.

Zygote Intrafallopian Tubal Transfer and Pronuclear Intrafallopian Tubal Transfer

The processes of ZIFT and PROST were developed to put fertilized eggs (PROST) or embryos (ZIFT) back into the fallopian tube in a more natural environment. These procedures are accomplished by obtaining eggs under ultrasound guidance, fertilizing the eggs in vitro, and placing the eggs or embryos into the fallopian tube at the single-cell fertilized stage (PROST) or the embryo stage (ZIFT). The fertilized eggs or embryos are put back in a laparoscopy procedure, so the biggest disadvantage of the process is that it requires two procedures, one to obtain the eggs and another to put the eggs or embryos back. Early reports of high success rates will have to be documented with larger numbers of patients and numerous series before meaningful pregnancy statistics can be given. A further disadvantage is that the techniques are significantly more expensive because of the extra procedure to place the eggs or embryos into the tube.

Micromanipulation

Micromanipulation comprises a variety of techniques to increase the probability that a given egg will be fertilized.[91] One of these techniques is zona disruption. With this technique eggs are gently held with a suction pipette and, under visualization with an inverted microscope, a glass needle is used to tear the zona pellucida. This increases the likelihood that sperm with diminished capability of zona penetration will enter the perivitelline space and be incorporated in the ooplasm through the vitelline membrane. This technique is generally used with sperm samples that have poor penetration ability, very low sperm numbers, or poor sperm quality.

Another technique is to aspirate sperm into a fine glass needle and then, using micromanipulators, to inject one or more sperm directly under the zona pellucida into the perivitelline space. With these techniques it is still possible that the sperm will be unable to fertilize the egg, but the likelihood of fertilization is greater than when the zona membrane is left intact.

The third technique involves making small holes in the zona pellucida by microinjecting an acidic trypsin solution that is then flushed from the environment. Injections done at a number of sites leave small holes in the membrane, increasing the likelihood of sperm penetration through the zona.

None of the micromanipulation techniques has been clearly shown to be superior. Additional work is necessary to determine their usefulness in improving IVF rates.

Embryo Freezing

Embryo freezing can be used to freeze extra embryos beyond what can be reasonably placed in the uterus at the time of embryo transfer.[92] Unexpected circumstances may prevent a woman from receiving a transfer of fresh embryos, and in this case they would all have to be frozen for implantation later. Eventually the freezing technique may improve to the point at which it is more advantageous to freeze and subsequently thaw embryos in a natural cycle than to transfer them in a hormonally stimulated cycle. Embryos are generally frozen at the pronuclear stage, two-cell stage, four-cell stage, or a subsequent stage up to the blastocyst stage. We typically freeze embryos at the pronuclear, two-cell, or four-cell stage, using 1.5 M propanediol. This is accomplished in 0.25 ml straws that are placed into a programmable freezer. The embryos are frozen at a decreasing temperature of −0.3° C per minute from −7° C to −30° C, at which point they are immersed directly in liquid nitrogen. Embryos can be placed in the uterus in natural or controlled cycles. Additional work is necessary to improve embryo freezing for better success rates in the future.

Embryo Biopsy

Embryo biopsy is a technique that can be used for couples with known gene defects.[93] In a biopsy procedure the embryo's polar body or one of the blastomeres at the three-cell stage or higher can be removed. Alternatively, the embryo can be allowed to develop to the blastocyst stage and then multiple cells can be sampled. However, only 20% to 30% of embryos in the laboratory develop to the blastocyst stage, and therefore fewer embryos are available to sample. DNA polymerase chain reaction can be used to determine whether a given embryo carries the gene defect. Embryos that do carry the defect are not placed back into the woman. These new procedures offer hope to couples who have avoided pregnancy because of gene defects.

Intrauterine Sperm Placement

Sperm can be inserted into the uterus with a long catheter under ultrasound visualization. With this technique sperm can also be placed beyond the uterus, into the fallopian tube, which theoretically ensures that they will reach the fertilization site. This insemination procedure is new, and additional studies are needed to determine its success rate.

THE FUTURE

The future of reproductive medicine is bright. The last decade has seen advances that could only be dreamed about 15 years ago. Explosive growth is also taking place in genetics. In vitro fertilization procedures will be improved and will be more successful in the future. A variety of techniques will be developed to improve fertilization, embryo development, and pregnancy in couples undergoing these procedures. Although medications that can predictably improve sperm quality are unlikely to appear in the near future, manipulation of sperm to enhance their fertilization success shows great promise. Gene therapy, embryo biopsy procedures, and advances in freezing and thawing embryos will all improve success rates in couples with fertility difficulties. New technologies such as electrical ejaculation will continue to develop. The advances are breathtaking and will ensure that reproductive health care remains exciting for patient and practitioner alike.

REFERENCES

1. Urry RL: Laboratory diagnosis of male infertility. Clin Lab Med 5(2):355, 1985.
2. Urry RL: Seminal fluid. In Kjeldsberg CR, Knight JA (eds): Body fluids. A.S.C.P., 1986, pp 117-127.
3. LaNasa JA Jr, Urry RL: Evaluation and treatment of the infertile male. Semin Reprod Endocrinol 3(2):113, 1985.
4. Wolff H, Anderson DJ: Immunohistologic characterization and quantitation of leukocyte subpopulations in human semen. Fertil Steril 49:497, 1988.
5. Hinting A, Comhaire F, Schoonjans F: Capacity of objectively assessed sperm motility characteristics in differentiating between semen of fertile and subfertile men. Fertil Steril 50:635, 1988.
6. Bongso TA, Ng SC, Mok H, et al: Effect of sperm motility on human in vitro fertilization. Arch Androl 22:185, 1989.
7. Tesarik J, Testart J: Human sperm-egg interactions and their disorders: implications in the management of infertility. Hum Reprod 4:729, 1989.
8. Holt WV, Moore HD, Hillier SG: Computer-assisted measurement of sperm swimming speed in human semen. Fertil Steril 44:112, 1985.
9. Critchlow JD, Matson PL, Newman MC, et al: Quality control in an in vitro fertilization laboratory: use of human sperm survival studies. Hum Reprod 4:545, 1989.
10. MacLeod J: Seminal cytology in the presence of varicocele. Fertil Steril 16:735, 1965.
11. Dubin L, Amelar RD: Etiologic factors in 1294 consecutive cases of male infertility. Fertil Steril 22:469, 1971.
12. Cockett ATK, Urry RL, Dougherty KA: The varicocele and semen characteristics. J Urol 121:435, 1979.
13. Dougherty KA, Urry RL, Cockett ATK: Supravital staining of spermatozoa: relationship of eosin concentration to the percentage of cells staining live. J Urol 118:1008, 1977.
14. Jeyendran RS, VanderVen HH, Perez-Pelaez M, et al: Development of an assay to assess the functional integrity of the human sperm membrane and its relationship to other semen characteristics. J Reprod Fertil 70:219, 1984.
15. Mordel N, Mor-Yosef S, Margalioth E, et al: The human sperm hypoosmotic swelling test: its practical application and suggestions for improvement. Int J Fertil 34:355, 1989.
16. VanderVen HH, Jeyendran RS, Al-Hasani S, et al: Correlation between human sperm swelling in hypoosmotic medium (hypoosmotic swelling test) and in vitro fertilization. J Androl 7:190, 1986.
17. Sjoblom P, Coccia E: On the diagnostic value of the hypoosmotic sperm swelling test in an in vitro fertilization (IVF) program. J In Vitro Fertil Embryo Transf 6:41, 1989.
18. Chan SY, Wang C, Ng M, Ho PC: Multivariate discriminant analysis of the relationship between the hypoosmotic swelling test and the in vitro fertilizing capacity of human sperm. Int J Androl 11:369, 1988.
19. Chan SY, Wang C, Song BL, et al: Computer assisted image analysis of sperm concentration in human semen before

and after swim-up separation: comparison with assessment by haemocytometer. Int J Androl 12:339, 1989.
20. Neuwinger J, Knuth UA, Nieschlag E: Evaluation of the Hamilton-Thorn 2030 motility analyser for routine semen analysis in an infertility clinic. Int J Androl 13:100, 1990.
21. Pedigo NG, Vernon MW, Curry TE Jr: Characterization of a computerized semen analysis system. Fertil Steril 52:659, 1989.
22. Badenoch DF, Moore HD, Holt WV, et al: Sperm motility, velocity and migration. Br J Urol 65:204, 1990.
23. Badenoch DF, Evans SJ, McCloskey DJ: Sperm density measurement: should this be abandoned? Br J Urol 64:521, 1989.
24. Small DR, Collins JA, Wilson EH, Wrixon W: Interpretation of semen analysis among infertile couples. Can Med Assoc J 136:829, 1987.
25. Grunert JH, de-Geyter C, Bordt J, et al: Does computerized image analysis of sperm movement enhance the predictive value of semen analysis for in vitro fertilization results? Int J Androl 12:329, 1989.
26. Gerris J, Khan I: Correlation between in vitro fertilization and human sperm density and motility. J Androl 8:48, 1987.
27. Alper MM, Lee GS, Seibel MM, et al: The relationship of semen parameters to fertilization in patients participating in a program of in vitro fertilization. J In Vitro Fertil Embryo Transf 2:217, 1985.
28. Dunphy BC, Neal LM, Cooke ID: The clinical value of conventional semen analysis. Fertil Steril 51:324, 1989.
29. Horvath PM, Bohrer M, Shelden RM, Kemmann E: The relationship of sperm parameters to cycle fecundity in superovulated women undergoing intrauterine insemination. Fertil Steril 52:288, 1989.
30. Moghissi KS: Postcoital test: physiologic basis, technique, and interpretation. Fertil Steril 27:117, 1976.
31. Urry RL, Middleton RG: Modern concepts in the diagnosis and treatment of male infertility. Urol Clin North Am 13:455, 1986.
32. Urry RL, Middleton RG, Mayo D: A comparison of the penetration of human sperm into bovine and artificial cervical mucus. Fertil Steril 45:135, 1986.
33. Schutte B: Penetration ability of human spermatozoa into standardized bovine cervical mucus (Penetrak) in patients with normal and pathological semen samples. Andrologia 19:317, 1987.
34. Franco JG, Schimberni M, Stone SC: An immunobead assay for antibiodies to spermatozoa in serum: comparison with traditional agglutination and immobilization tests. J Reprod Med 32:188, 1987.
35. Gregoriou O, Vitoratos N, Legakis N, et al: Detection of sperm-bound antibodies in the male partners of infertile couples using the immunobead test. Eur J Obstet Gynecol Reprod Biol 33:235, 1989.
36. Mandelbaum SL, Diamond MP, DeCherney AH: The impact of antisperm antibodies on human infertility. J Urol 138:1, 1987.
37. Naz RK, Deutsch J, Phillips TM. Sperm antibodies in vasectomized men and their effects on fertilization. Biol Reprod 41:163, 1989.
38. Haas GG: How should sperm antibody tests be used clinically? Am J Reprod Immunol Microbiol 15:106, 1987.
39. Urry RL, Coudle MR, Rote NS: Autoimmune infertility and recurrent abortion. In Scott JR, Rote NS (eds): Immunology and obstetrics and gynecology. East Norwalk, Conn: Appleton-Century-Crofts, 1985, pp 77-106.
40. Rogers BJ: The sperm penetration assay: its usefulness reevaluated. Fertil Steril 43:821, 1985.
41. Urry RL, Carrell DT, Hull DB, et al: Penetration of zona-free hamster ova and bovine cervical mucosa by fresh and frozen human spermatozoa, Fertil Steril 39:690, 1983.
42. Rogers BJ, Van Campen H, Ueno M, et al: Analysis of human spermatozoal fertilizing ability using zona-free ova. Fertil Steril 32:664, 1979.
43. Margalioth EJ, Feinmesser M, Navot D, et al: The long-term predictive value of the zona-free hamster ova sperm penetration assay. Fertil Steril 52:490, 1989.
44. Mao C, Grimes DA: The sperm penetration assay: can it discriminate between fertile and infertile men? Am J Obstet Gynecol 159:279, 1988.
45. Bronson RA, Rogers BJ: Pitfalls of the zona-free hamster egg penetration test: protein source as major variable. Fertil Steril 50:851, 1988.
46. Corson SL, Batzer FR, Marmar J, Maislin G: The human sperm-hamster egg penetration assay: prognostic value. Fertil Steril 49:328, 1988.
47. Hodgen GD, Codding CC, Franken DR, et al: The hemizona assay (HZA): finding sperm that have the "right stuff." J In Vitro Fertil Embryo Transf 5:311, 1988.
48. Schill WB, Topfer-Peterson E, Heissler E: The sperm acrosome: functional and clinical aspects. Human Reprod 3:139, 1988.
49. Wolf DP: Acrosomal status quantitation in human sperm. Am J Reprod Immunol 20:106, 1989.
50. Tejada RI, Mitchell JC, Norman A, et al: A test for the practical evaluation of male fertility by acridine orange (AO) fluorescence. Fertil Steril 42:87, 1984.
51. Ibrahim ME, Pedersen H: Acridine orange fluorescence as male fertility test. Arch Androl 20:125, 1988.
52. Byrd W, Tsu J, Wolf DP: Kinetics of spontaneous and induced acrosomal loss in human sperm incubated under capacitating and non-capacitating conditions. Gamete Res 22:109, 1989.
53. Hotchkiss RS, Pinto AB, Kleegman S: Artificial insemination with semen recovered from the bladder. Fertil Steril 6:37, 1955.
54. Scammell GE: Successful treatment of infertility due to retrograde ejaculation. J R Soc Med 74:926, 1981.
55. Urry RL, Middleton RG, McGavin S: A simple and effective technique for increasing pregnancy rates in couples with retrograde ejaculation. Fertil Steril 46:1124, 1986.
56. Silber SJ, Balmaceda J, Borrero C, et al: Pregnancy with sperm aspiration from the proximal head of the epididymis: a new treatment for congenital absence of the vas deferens. Fertil Steril 50:525, 1988.
57. Silber SJ, Patrizio P, Asch RH: Quantitative evaluation of spermatogenesis by testicular histology in men with congenital absence of the vas deferens undergoing epididymal sperm aspiration. Hum Reprod 5:89, 1990.
58. Randolph JR, Ohl DA, Bennett CJ, et al: Combined electroejaculation and in vitro fertilization in the evaluation of anejaculatory infertility. J In Vitro Fertil Embryo Transf 7:58-62, 1990.
59. Ohl DA, Bennett CJ, McCabe M, et al: Predictors of success in electroejaculation of spinal cord injured men. J Urol 142:1483, 1989.
60. Bennett CJ, Seager SW, Vasher EA, McGuire EJ: Sexual dysfunction and electroejaculation in men with spinal cord injury: review. J Urol 139:453, 1988.
61. Perkash I, Martin DE, Warner H, Speck V: Electroejaculation in spinal cord injury patients: simplified new equipment and technique. J Urol 143:305, 1990.
62. MacLeod J: The effects of urinary gonadotropins following hypophysectomy and in hypogonadotropic eunuchoids. In Rosenberg E, Paulsen CA (eds): The human testis. New York: Plenum Press, 1970, pp 135-156.
63. Newton R, Schinveld JS, Schiff I: Clomiphene treatment of infertile men: failure of response with idiopathic oligospermia. Fertil Steril 34:399, 1980.
64. LaNasa J, Lang E: Disorders of the scrotum and its contents. In Resnick MI, Older RA (eds): Diagnosis of genitourinary disease. New York: Thieme-Stratton, 1982, pp 433-486.
65. Hendry WR, Stedronaska J, Parslow J: The results of intermittent high-dose steroid therapy for male infertility due to anti-sperm antibodies. Fertil Steril 36:351, 1981.
66. Mathur S, Baker ER, Williamson HD, et al: Clinical significance of sperm antibodies in infertility. Fertil Steril 36:486, 1981.

67. Silber SJ: Microsurgery for male infertility. Microsurgery 9:251, 1988.
68. Southwick GJ, Temple-Smith PD: Epididymal microsurgery: current techniques and new horizons. Microsurgery 9:226, 1988.
69. Middleton RG, Urry RL: Young-Dees operation for the correction of retrograde ejaculation. J Urol 136:1208, 1986.
70. Cohen MS, Warner RS: Needle biopsy of testes: a safe outpatient procedure. Urology 29:279, 1987.
71. Jones KP, Keye WP, Poulson AM, et al: Summary of the University of Utah in vitro fertilization program. J In Vitro Fertil Transf 1:80, 1984.
72. Urry RL, Cropper D, McReynolds L, et al: Artificial insemination: a comparison of pregnancy rates with intrauterine versus cervical insemination and washed sperm versus serum swim-up sperm preparations. Fertil Steril 49:1036, 1988.
73. Hammitt DG, Walker DL, Williamson RA: Survival and in vitro fertilization potential of sperm following washing and incubation with different protein supplements. Int J Fertil 35:46, 1990.
74. Urry RL, Middleton RG, McNamara L, Vitari CA: The effect of single-density bovine serum albumin columns on sperm concentration, motility and morphology. Fertil Steril 40:666, 1983.
75. Zarutskie PW, Muller CH, Magone M, Soules MR: The clinical relevance of sex selection technique. Fertil Steril 52:891, 1989.
76. Tanphaichitr N, Millette CF, Agulnick A, Fitzgerald LM: Egg penetration ability and structural properties of human sperm prepared by Percoll-gradient centrifugation. Gamete Res 20:67, 1988.
77. Iizuka R, Kaneko S, Kobanawa K, Kobayashi T: Washing and concentration of human semen by Percoll density gradients and its application to AIH. Arch Androl 20:117, 1988.
78. Rhemrev J, Jeyendran RS, Vermeiden JP, Zaneveld LJ: Human sperm selection by glass wool filtration and two-layer, discontinuous Percoll gradient centrifugation. Fertil Steril 51:685, 1989.
79. Confino E, Friberg J, Dudkiewicz AB, Glecher N: Intrauterine inseminations with washed human spermatozoa. Fertil Steril 46:55, 1986.
80. Yovich JL, Matson PL: The treatment of infertility by the high intrauterine insemination of husband's washed spermatozoa. Hum Reprod 3:939, 1988.
81. Schill WB, Littich M: Split ejaculate insemination with and without the addition of kallikrein. Andrologia 13:121, 1981.
82. Barkey J, Bartoov B, Ben-Ezra S, et al: The influence of in vitro caffeine treatment on human sperm morphology and fertilizing capacity. Fertil Steril 41:913, 1984.
83. Gerhard I, Roth B, Eggert-Kruse W, Runnebaum B: Effects of kallikrein on sperm motility, capillary tube test, and pregnancy rate in an AIH program. Arch Androl 24:129, 1990.
84. Carrell DT, Bradshaw WS, Jones KP, Urry RL: An evaluation of various treatments to increase sperm penetration capacity for potential use in an IVF program. Fertil Steril, 1990, in press.
85. Quigley MM: The use of ovulation-inducing agents in in vitro fertilization. Clin Obstet Gynecol 27:983, 1984.
86. Frydman R, Forman R, Rainhorn J-D, et al: A new approach to follicular stimulation for in vitro fertilization: programmed oocyte retrieval. Fertil Steril 46:657, 1986.
87. Lenz S, Lauritsen JG: Ultrasonically guided percutaneous aspiration of human follicles under local anesthesia: a new method of collecting oocytes for in vitro fertilization. Fertil Steril 38:673, 1982.
88. Pampiglione JS, Mills C, Campbell S, et al: The clinical outcome of reinsemination of human oocytes fertilized in vitro. Fertil Steril 53:306, 1990.
89. Barlow DH: IVF, GIFT et al. J R Soc Med 81:622, 1988.
90. Hinting A, Comhaire F, Vermeulen L, et al: Value of sperm characteristics and the result of in-vitro fertilization for predicting the outcome of assisted reproduction. Int J Androl 13:59, 1990.
91. Ng SC, Bongso A, Sathananthan H, Ratnam SS: Micromanipulation: its relevance to human in vitro fertilization. Fertil Steril 53:203, 1990.
92. Friedler S, Giudice LC, Lamb EJ: Cryopreservation of embryos and ova. Fertil Steril 49:743, 1988.
93. Monk M, Handyside AH: Sexing of preimplantation mouse embryos by measurement of X-linked gene dosage in a single blastomere. J Reprod Fertil 82:365, 1988.

CHAPTER 12

RECENT ADVANCES IN IMMUNOLOGY AND MOLECULAR BIOLOGY

MONICA LIEBERT and H. BARTON GROSSMAN

In the past two decades, advances in the basic sciences have elucidated the pathogenesis of urologic disease and formed the framework for the development of new methods of diagnosis and therapy. Immunology comprises a major part of this effort. Two seminal events in immunology that have been important for routine urologic care were the development of monoclonal antibodies (for which the Nobel Prize in Physiology or Medicine was awarded in 1984) and the cloning and characterization of cytokines, such as interleukin-2 (IL-2) have contributed significantly to cellular immunotherapies for cancer. A relatively recent but rapidly growing science, molecular biology has made extraordinary contributions in many areas. In this chapter we focus on advances in immunology and molecular biology that have particular relevance for the urologist.

IMMUNOLOGY

Immune System

The immune system defends the body against disease, and the body's major warriors in this continuous battle are the fluid mediators and the cells of the immune system.[1-3] The fluid phase components include antibodies, cytokines, complement, and other chemical mediators of inflammation. This arm of the immune system is called humoral immunity.

Antibodies are relatively high molecular weight proteins that are produced in response to immune stimulation by antigens. Antibodies are composed of heavy and light chains and can be divided into classes called isotypes based on the composition of the heavy chain. Antibody isotypes differ in molecular weight, time of production after stimulation, site of production, and function, as shown in Table 12–1. Some of the antibody isotypes have subtypes, which are the result of biochemical differences that may also contribute to functional and pharmacokinetic differences. The structure of an idealized IgG molecule is shown in Figure 12–1. The Fc portion of the molecule contains the protein structure that defines isotype and subtype and affects function. The Fc portion also has a consistent amino acid sequence within isotypes and subtypes and is therefore called the constant region of the molecule. The Fab portion of the molecule contains the amino acid structure responsible for antigen binding. The amino acid sequence of this portion of the molecule varies depending on the antigenic specificity of the antibody. Thus the Fab portion is called the variable portion of the molecule. Antibodies can also act as immunogens or immunostimulatory antigens. Under certain circumstances, antibodies to the antigen-combining amino acid sequences in the Fab portion of the molecule are produced. The antigen present in this portion of antibody molecule is called an idiotype, and the antibodies produced are called antiidiotypic antibodies.[1-3]

How a limited number of genes could be responsible for the vast diversity of antibody molecules was a question that plagued immunologists for many years. Recently it has been shown that even though a limited number of genes are present, a great diversity of antibodies can be generated by rearrangement of the DNA. The DNA coding for antibody molecules consists of multiple sequences for the variable portion (V genes), segments responsible for joining sequences (J sequences in light chains, and J and D [for diversity] sequences in heavy chains), segments responsible for class

TABLE 12–1. Human Antibody Classes

Class	Subtypes	Molecular Weight	Function
IgM	None	800,000	Virus neutralization; primary antibody responses
IgG	1, 2, 3, 4	150,000	Secondary antibody responses
IgA	1, 2	160,000 385,000*	Mucosal immunity
IgD	None	170,000	Membrane receptor
IgE	None	170,000	Allergic responses

*Dimer with secretory piece.

switching (S segments), and segments coding for constant portions of the molecule (C segments). An S segment immediately precedes each heavy chain C segment. Multiple segments for each type of sequence are present. The diversity of antibody specificity is produced by different combinations of V genes expressed with the same C genes. Further complexity is developed by mutational events in the V genes. In the generation of an antibody with a particular specificity, the genes for an intact antibody are rearranged to be in proximity with each other in the sequence V-J-(D in heavy chain)-S-C, with deletion of the sequences that had been in between the coding sequences. As an antibody-producing cell (B cell) differentiates, the antibody produced switches from IgM to IgG and the genes again are rearranged, going from V-J-D-$S_{(M\ heavy\ chain)}$-$C_{(M\ heavy\ chain)}$ to V-J-D-$S_{(G\ heavy\ chain)}$-$C_{(G\ heavy\ chain)}$, again with deletion of many of the intervening sequences.[4,5]

Cytokines have a much smaller molecular weight than antibodies and are soluble mediators of inflammation and cell activation that are produced by cells participating in immune reactions. Many of the cytokines were originally described as lymphokines or monokines, or as materials associated with specific functions, such as T cell growth factor. With the application of molecular biology techniques, many cytokines are now well characterized, have been renamed to reflect their diverse functions, and have been produced in bulk from bacteria transfected with the cytokine genes. Some of the defined cytokines are described in Table 12–2. This field is rapidly expanding, and many new developments will be forthcoming over the next several years. Included in the list are some other bioactive peptides (colony-stimulating factors) that stimulate the growth of hematopoietic progenitors.[1-3]

Complement is a series of proteins that were originally described as "complementary" to antibody function, especially in lytic activity. These 20 plasma proteins are activated in a sequence shown in Figure 12–2 and serve important functions in the immune response and inflammation.[6] Besides these proteins, another group of proteins and cell receptors that regulate complement activation also exists.[7]

Activation of complement via the "classical pathway" begins as an antibody binds to its antigen, exposing sites on the Fc portion of the antibody molecule that activate C1 (composed of three chains, C1q, C1r, and C1s). Activated C1s acts as an enzyme and cleaves the next two components, C4 and C2, releasing C4a and C2b fragments and generating the stable C4b-C2a complex at the activation surface. This complex is also enzymatic and splits the next component, C3, resulting in the release of C3a fragment and the addition of C3b fragment to the complex. C5 serves as the substrate for the C4b-C2a-C3b complex. C5 is fragmented to C5b, which becomes part of the active complex, and the C5a fragment is released. The activation of C5 to C5b results in the formation of a "membrane attack complex" of C5b-C6-C7-C8-C9, which forms

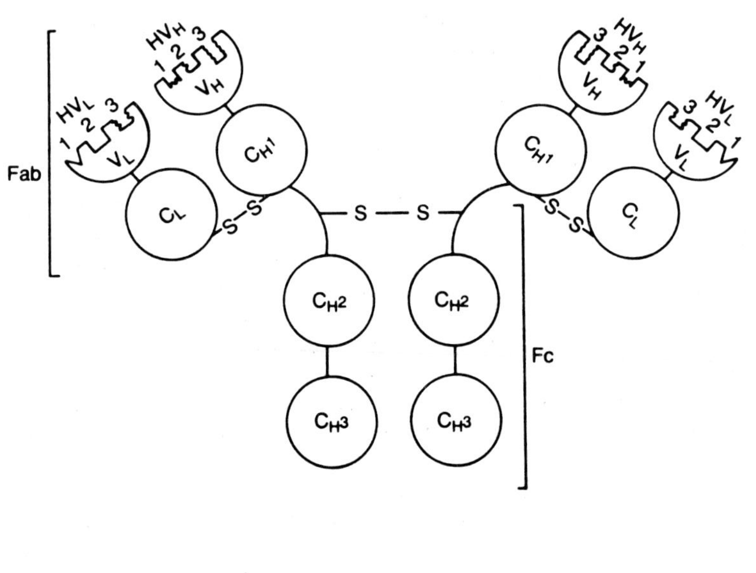

FIGURE 12–1. An idealized illustration of the antibody molecule. This figure is of an IgG-type antibody, composed of two identical heavy chains *($C_H1, 2, 3; V_H$)* and two identical light chains *($C_L; V_L$)*, held together by disulfide *(S—S)* bonds. The antigen-binding portion *(Fab)* is present at one end of the molecule, at the site of the variable portions of the chains (V parts of the chains). The Fc portion is at the other end of the molecule. (From Mayforth RD, Quintans J: Designer and catalytic antibodies. N Engl J Med 323:174, 1990. Reprinted by permission of the New England Journal of Medicine.)

TABLE 12–2. Cytokines

Type	Members	Action
Interferon	IFN-alpha IFN-beta IFN-gamma	Diverse effects on a variety of cells
Tumor necrosis factor	TNF-alpha TNF-beta	Cytotoxic, with other diverse effects on various cells
Transforming growth factor	TGF-beta	Diverse effects on a variety of cells
Interleukins	IL-1 alpha IL-1 beta	Diverse effects on a variety of cells
	IL-2	T and NK cell growth, B cell development
	IL-3	Mast cell growth, differentiation of cells from the bone marrow
	IL-4	T and B cell growth and differentiation
	IL-5	B cell growth and development, increased antibody production
	IL-6	Diverse effects on various cells
	IL-7	Growth of B cell precursors in marrow
	IL-8	Neutrophil and lymphocyte chemotaxis and activation (NAP-1; NCF)
	IL-9	T cell and mast cell growth (P40)
Colony-stimulating factors	GM-CSF	Growth in all cell lineages from bone marrow
	G-CSF	Growth and maturation of granulocyte lineage from bone marrow
	M-CSF	Growth and maturation of macrophage lineage from bone marrow
	Erythropoietin	Growth and maturation of red cells and platelets from bone marrow

a hole or pore in a cell membrane and can cause lysis of the cell on which the complex is deposited.[6]

In the "alternative" pathway (sometimes called the properdin pathway) of complement activation, C3 is directly activated by spontaneous hydrolysis of an internal thioester bond. This activation can occur by interaction with microbes or other activating surfaces. This activated C3 binds a plasma protein called protein B, resulting in a C3bB complex that is fragmented by protease D, generating a C3bBb complex. C5 is the substrate for the enzymatic action of the C3bBb complex, which is stabilized by the presence of another protein, properdin. This complex activates C5 through C9 to generate the membrane attack complex just as the C4b-C2a-C3b does in the "classical" pathway described previously.[6,7]

Several of the fragments generated during this cascade have biologic activity. Soluble fragments of C4, C3, and C5, that is, C4a, C3a, and C5a, are chemotactic for neutrophils and activate neutrophils as well as a variety of other white blood cells. These three fragments are also called anaphylotoxins because of their association with anaphylaxis. They cause smooth muscle contraction, increased vascular permeability, and release of vasoactive amines.[6,8]

The complement cascade is closely regulated by a variety of inhibitory proteins and cell receptors. These inhibitors include membrane receptors CR1 (for C3b), CR2, CR3, and two other cellular membrane cofactors.[9,10] The complement receptors CR1, CR2, and CR3, present on a variety of cells, improve phagocytosis of complement-coated materials, which is essential for the development of immune processing. The CR1 receptor binds to C3b. CR2 and two integrin family receptors, CR3 (Mac-1) and p150,95, bind to a fragment of C3b called iC3b. All

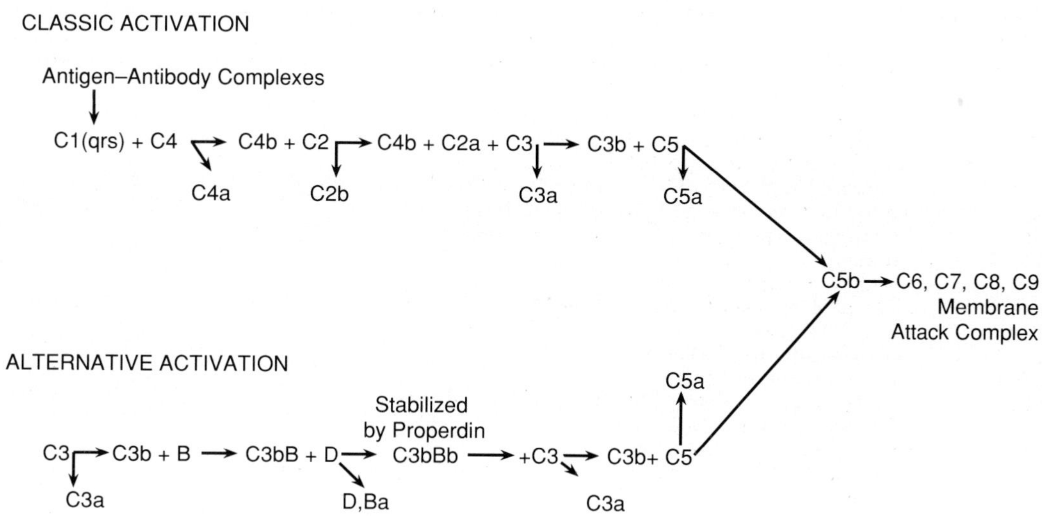

FIGURE 12–2. Complement components and their activation sequence.

of the complement receptors are involved in phagocytosis of coated materials.[10] CR2 is also the B cell receptor for Epstein-Barr virus.[10] Soluble (fluid phase) inhibitors of complement activation also exist, including a C1 inhibitor that is lacking in hereditary angioedema.[7,9-11]

Patients with complement component deficiencies show a lack of immune response, have problems with persistent infections, and in some cases develop autoimmune diseases.[10,12] Thus complement activation also plays a role in the immune network for the development of specific immunity. Complement activation can be demonstrated in a variety of conditions, including the active phases of autoimmune diseases and following an incompatible blood transfusion. This activation can be measured by a drop in the total complement activity (called CH_{50}), decreases in specific components such as C3, increased production of fragments such as C4a, and in some cases changes in the expression of cellular complement receptors CR1 or CR2.[10,13]

Activation of complement also interacts with other biologic cascades. The C1 inhibitor, besides downregulating C1 activity, also downregulates Hageman factor in the coagulation pathway, inhibits plasmin in the plasmin pathway, and downregulates kallikrein in the kinin system.[11,12] Kallikrein activates bradykinin, which is a peptide responsible for increased vascular permeability, pain, and leukocyte chemotaxis.[12] Other kinins, through phospholipase A activation, cause the formation of prostaglandins and leukotrienes.[12,14] Besides having direct effects on nearby tissues, prostaglandins and leukotrienes activate neutrophils which can result in the local generation of oxygen free radicals and proteases.[12] These biologic cascades are responsible for generating and regulating important local reactions in inflammation.[11,12,14]

Cells are the heart of the immune system. These cellular effectors constitute cellular immunity. A variety of cells produce and respond to the fluid mediators of the immune system.[1-3] Neutrophils are phagocytic cells produced in the bone marrow and are especially active in combatting bacterial infections. Neutrophils are responsive to a number of chemotactic and biologic signals, including cytokines (especially IL-8) and complement fragments (especially C3a and C5a). Neutrophils also release chemical mediators, such as oxygen free radicals, at the site of inflammation. Monocytes and macrophages are other phagocytic cells and are not as abundant as neutrophils. Besides responding to and generating cytokines, macrophages are extremely important as antigen processing cells that are required for the production of antibodies by a class of lymphocytes known as B cells. B cells are named for the bursa, the organ that is their site of origin in birds. Humoral (antibody) immunity depends on normal B cell function.

Another subclass of lymphocytes is known as T cells because they are processed in the thymus. T cells can be further divided by their function and the expression of CD (cluster of differentiation) surface markers, as described in Table 12–3. All T cells express the CD3 marker, which is associated with the T cell receptor (TcR) for antigen. Part of the TcR is structurally similar to immunoglobulin, and the same sorts of gene rearrangements that occur in immunoglobulin genes occur with genes in the TcR and are responsible for antigen specificity of the TcR. The TcR consists of two chains, most often alpha and beta (gamma and delta chains are seen less often), that are associated in a complex with the CD3 antigen. The association of the TcR with CD3 is necessary for the transfer of activation signals inside the cell.[4] The alpha and beta units of the TcR also have a V-J-C (and for the beta unit, V-J-D-C) structure, which is rearranged as the T cell matures. Again, diversity is produced by the presence of multiple possible V and J gene seg-

TABLE 12–3. CD Antigens

Designation	*Functions*	*Previous Names*
CD2	LFA-3 ligand	E-receptor
CD3	Associated with T cell receptor for antigen	OKT3
CD4	Antigen recognition with MHC class II antigen; HIV receptor	
CD8	Antigen recognition with MHC class I antigen	
CD11a	Integrin receptor for intercellular adhesion molecule-1 (ICAM-1; CD54)	LFA-1
CD11b	Integrin receptor for iC3b complement fragment	CR3
CD11c	Integrin receptor for iC3b complement fragment	gp 150/95
CD16	Receptor for IgG Fc	FcR III
CD18	Beta chain for CD11 family	
CD21	Receptor for C3d complement fragment; EBV receptor	CR2
CD23	IgE Fc receptor	
CD25	IL-2 receptor (55 kd beta chain)	Tac
CDw32	Immunoglobulin Fc receptor	FcRII
CD35	Receptor for complement fragments (C3b, C4b)	CR1
CD46	Complement membrane cofactor	MCP
CD54	Intercellular adhesion molecule-1	ICAM-1
CD56	Neural cell adhesion molecule, natural killer (NK) cell marker	HNK-1
CD58	Receptor for CD2	LFA-3
CD64	Fc receptor	FcR I

ments, of which only one type is expressed in conjunction with common C gene products.[4,15] Several other accessory molecules, CD2, CD4, and CD8, may also play roles in T cell–antigen recognition.[4,16] Antibodies to CD2 can sometimes prevent T cell activation through the TcR/CD3 molecule, and CD2 can synergize T cell activation.[15,17] CD2 is the ligand for another T cell receptor, LFA-3 (CD58), and may act by mediating cell-cell adherence.[18] CD4 and CD8 function in T cell activation by coordinating interactions with antigens of the major histocompatibility complex (MHC).

The MHC is a gene complex that includes genes coding for histocompatibility (tissue type) antigens.[19-22] MHC histocompatibility antigens have two major classes. The class I MHC antigens (HLA-A, B, C) are composed of two chains, a larger one of 44 kDa and a smaller 12 kDa beta$_2$ microglobulin molecule, and are found on a wide variety of tissues in the body. Class II MHC antigens (also called HLA-DR antigens) are composed of two chains of 35 and 28 kDa and have a restricted tissue distribution. These molecules play an essential role in the presentation of antigen to reactive cells, such as T cells.[21,22] The MHC antigens have a "groove" in the center of the molecule that serves as a resting place for peptide antigens and interacts with T and B cells to generate immune responses.[20-22] In some cases foreign antigen is associated with the MHC antigen at sites outside this groove.[21]

Both antibody production and generation of specific cytotoxic T lymphocytes depend on helper T cells, which usually recognize foreign antigens in association with autologous HLA class II antigens and express a surface marker called CD4. Cytotoxic T cells most frequently recognize foreign antigens in association with autologous HLA class I antigens and express the CD8 marker.[23] Antigen presentation for T cell activation probably uses this pathway. Therefore this function is an important part of T cell recognition of antigen.[16,23] Another cell-cell adhesion associative complex consisting of intercellular adhesion molecule-1 (ICAM-1 or CD54) and LFA-1 (the complex of CD11a and CD18) also brings cells into contact and plays a role in T cell activation.[23]

Cellular activation is associated with the expression of genes that were previously silent. Two genes that are expressed as part of T cell activation are the genes for IL-2 and for the IL-2 receptor.[15,24] The IL-2 receptor is a dimer of two chains, one of 55 kDa and the other of 75 kDa. The 55 kDa receptor (CD25; identified by anti-Tac antibodies) has a relatively low affinity for IL-2. However, once IL-2 is bound by the 55 kDa receptor, the 75 kDa chain binds to IL-2 with high affinity and transmits the activation signal to the interior of the cell.[24]

Another population of lymphocytes is the natural killer (NK) cells. These cells lack the CD3 T cell marker but are capable of target cell lysis.[18,25] NK cells respond to IL-2 through continuous expression of the low-affinity IL-2 receptor (CD25; 55 kDa Tac antigen[24]). Like T cells, NK cells express CD2 and some also express the CD8 marker.[18]

The expression of cell surface for Fc portion of immunoglobulin receptors permits various types of leukocytes to interact with antibodies. Such leukocytes can bind antibody through the Fc receptor and use the antibody specificity for cellular targeting and activation. This process can be measured in assays evaluating antibody-dependent cellular cytotoxicity (ADCC). Three Fc receptors for IgG and one for IgE have been identified and given "CD" designations (CD16, CDw32, and CD64 for IgG; CD23 for IgE).

Acquired Immunodeficiency Syndrome

Although a number of immunodeficiency disorders exist, no more dramatic example of the importance of immunity to health is the current epidemic of the acquired immunodeficiency syndrome (AIDS). The AIDS agent, the human immunodeficiency virus (HIV), infects cells by attaching to its receptor, the CD4 molecule.[26,27] immediately after infection, the levels of CD4-positive T cells drop, but then recover. In most cases, after a time the numbers of CD4 positive cells fall again and the patient loses the ability to fight off infection.[28]

Several aspects of the HIV epidemic are important for the urologist. During the time that numbers of CD4-positive T cells are falling, but before the development of AIDS or AIDS-related complex (ARC, another group of infections seen in less severe immunosuppression caused by HIV infection), the patient may experience subclinical immune dysfunctions with an increased number of infections.[28] These infections may include diseases commonly treated by urologists, such as urinary tract infections, epididymitis, and prostatitis.[29-31] In addition, susceptibility to tuberculosis infections is increased. Patients with AIDS often have activation of previously subclinical infections with *Mycobacterium tuberculosis* and may develop infections with other species of *Mycobacterium* as well.[32,33] Extrapulmonary disease requiring surgical intervention can occur in these patients.[33] These infected patients may also be a source of tuberculosis infection for others in the population. In fact, the incidence of tuberculosis increased in the period 1984-1988 after years of decline.[32]

The urologist may also be consulted because of neoplastic problems in patients with recognized or undiagnosed AIDS. Kaposi's sarcoma of the penis may rarely be the initial manifestation of AIDS.[34] Furthermore, patients with HIV infection may be at increased risk for testis cancer.[35] The treatment of infertility by artificial insemination is also cause for concern. Donor semen may transmit infection, and increased screening of potential donors is warranted.[36]

Appropriate precautions are mandatory when treating HIV-infected patients.[37,38] The highest concentrations of virus are found in CD4-positive tissues, including blood. Other tissues that express the CD4 antigen and may contain significant quantities of HIV are the brain, colon, testes, prostate gland, and seminal fluid.[26,37-39] Other body fluids, such as urine and tears, may contain low levels of HIV.[37,38] The use of autologous blood for surgery is increasing because of the fear of AIDS in the community. Recombinant erythropoietin can safely increase the red blood cell volume obtained from patients donating autologous blood.[40]

Monoclonal Antibodies

A number of different antibody-producing cells, or B cells, respond to an antigenic stimulus, resulting in the production of a variety of antibodies of different specificities. The progeny of a single cell is called a clone, and this response is called a polyclonal response because more than one clone of B cells is responding. Normal B cells die after a short time in tissue culture. However, the genetic information causing these B cells to respond can be "captured" by fusion with an immortalized myeloma cell. The resulting hybrids can be isolated by appropriate selection techniques, so that the cells from a single clone can be propagated indefinitely in culture. Because these cells are the progeny of a single clone, the antibodies produced are monoclonal antibodies. A monoclonal antibody has a single isotype with a single antigen-binding specificity. Because only one kind of amino acid sequence is present at the Fab region, only a single idiotype, or antigenic specificity at the Fab region, is present in these antibodies. Since the cells are now immortalized, a theoretically unlimited supply of chemically pure antibody with a defined specificity is available from these cultures.

The production of monoclonal antibodies has contributed significantly to the current biotechnology revolution. These antibodies have been used in vitro for the detection of tumor-associated antigens and improved radioimmunoassays and in vivo for the diagnosis and treatment of graft rejection and cancer.

Monoclonal Antibodies to Urologic Tumor–Associated Antigens

Renal Cancer. The reports of spontaneous regression in renal cancer have long supported the hypothesis that some renal cancer cells express antigens that could be immunologically detected and result in tumor rejection. Because of this, renal carcinoma has been the target of a significant research effort to produce monoclonal antibodies with tumor specificity. Many antibodies that define antigens expressed by both renal carcinoma and normal kidney cells have been produced.[41-43] Two of these antibodies, URO-4 (S27) and URO-4a, bind to adenosine deaminase–binding protein. The presence of this proximal tubular protein in urine has been useful in the evaluation of acute tubular necrosis, allograft rejection, and cyclosporine toxicity in renal transplantation.[44] Other monoclonal antibody–defined markers have been valuable in the pathologic evaluation of renal cancer.[45-47] A recent report has shown a relationship between the expression of a monoclonal antibody–defined renal differentiation antigen, gp160, and the response to interferon treatment both in vitro and in vivo with human renal carcinoma cell lines.[48] Absence of gp160 appears to predict tumor responsiveness to alpha interferon. A clinical trial using this marker as a predictor for therapeutic response to interferon treatment of renal cell carcinoma is under way (N. Bander, personal communication).

The use of radiolabeled anti–renal cell carcinoma monoclonal antibodies for in vivo localization has been evaluated both in animal models and in human clinical trials. Ballou and his co-workers demonstrated that cross-reactivity with normal components of the kidney did not preclude the in vivo use of monoclonal antibodies.[49] This point is important because many of the antibodies that have been described are not restricted to kidney tumors and are often found on normal kidney cells as well. The AH6 antibody, first described by Vesella and his co-workers, showed promise as a tumor-targeting monoclonal antibody with excellent in vivo localization in animals that had received xenografts.[50] The same xenograft model was subsequently used to document the success of AH6 as a radioimmunotherapeutic agent.[51] However, the preliminary human trials with AH6 were not impressive. Further study showed that AH6 localization in xenografts was influenced by high vascular permeability in the renal tumors.[52] Other trials of monoclonal antibodies[53] in renal cell carcinoma have been reported but so far have met with little success (N. Bander, personal communication).

Technical methods to enhance the therapeutic effectiveness of monoclonal antibodies to renal cancer have been reported. For example, methotrexate has been conjugated both directly and in liposomes to a monoclonal antibody that binds to renal cancer.[54,55]

Bladder Cancer. Bladder cancers vary significantly in their biologic characteristics and response to therapy. Correlation of the loss of blood group (A, B, H) antigen expression and progression was originally noted in mixed hemadsorption tests and subsequently was confirmed with monoclonal antibodies.[56-58] Other bladder tumor markers that have been evaluated with monoclonal antibodies include the Thomsen-Friedenreich (T) antigen, expression of which is also correlated with poorer outcome,[58] and cytokeratin 18, which is highly expressed in bladder cancer.[59] High levels of expression of the epidermal growth factor receptor have also been correlated with more aggressive disease and a poorer prognosis.[60,61] Recently another bladder cancer–associated cell marker, the transferrin receptor, has been reported to correlate with an increased risk of recurrence in low-grade bladder cancer.[62] Other monoclonal antibody–defined antigens have also been associated with the biologic aggressiveness of bladder cancer. Om5 is expressed on some normal urothelial cells and on superficial bladder cancers, whereas T138 and T43 are more commonly found on muscle-invasive and metastatic tumors.[63] The expression of monoclonal antibody–defined antigens T43 and T16 is related to the growth characteristics of bladder cancer cells. T16 is expressed at a high concentration by resting cells, and T43 is expressed at high levels by actively dividing cells.[64] The Ki-67 antibody, which binds to a nuclear protein associated with active cell division, has been used to evaluate proliferation in bladder cancers of differing stage and grade. As might be expected, significantly more staining was observed in higher grade and higher stage bladder cancers than in normal bladder mucosa or low-grade and low-stage tumors, and in nonpapillary tumors compared with papillary tumors.[65] These types of monoclonal antibody–defined antigens may be useful in evaluating the growth fraction of bladder cancer cells, which in turn may be correlated with metastatic potential and facilitate selection of appropriate therapy.

A major application of monoclonal antibodies in bladder cancer has been in improving the detection of tumor cells in urine by immunocytology.[63,66-68] Flow cytometric analysis of bladder washings with antibodies, sometimes in conjunction with ploidy analysis, has also been performed. Although flow cytometry is a powerful technique for detecting neoplastic cells in urine and bladder washings, the presence of nonneoplastic cells, either normal urothelium or inflammatory cells, decreases the sensitivity of this approach. The selection of only bladder tumor cells through the use of the monoclonal antibody DU83.21 improves the sensitivity of flow cytometry.[69] DU83.21 binds to bladder and prostate cancer cells but not to normal tissue. Immunoselection with DU83.21 and flow cytometry was more sensitive than flow cytometry alone or flow cytometry and immunoselection with an anticytokeratin antibody. The fact that DU83.21 does not bind to all bladder cancer cells is a limitation of this technique.

Other studies have evaluated bladder washings by flow cytometry with cytokeratin 18 antibodies,[59,70] anti-T antigen,[71] and T16, T43, and T138 antibodies.[72] In the last study 68 patients with bladder cancer were monitored with flow cytometry using antibody binding and DNA analysis. The T16 antigen was used to identify urothelial cells and exclude white blood cells from the analysis. The monoclonal antibody–identified tumor-associated antigens T43 and T138 were used to identify tumor cells, even when diploid. Patients with T138-negative cells survived longer than those with positive cells, even when the tumors were diploid.[72]

The expression of monoclonal antibody–defined antigens in bladder washings has been used to follow the responses to intravesical bacille Calmette-Guérin (BCG) therapy for bladder cancer.[68,73] In the study by Huffman and his co-workers, the monoclonal antibody to the Om5 antigen (expressed on cells of superficial bladder cancers, cells of carcinoma in situ, and some normal urothelial cells) was used to monitor BCG therapy in 15 patients. In 4 patients, Om5 positive cells were observed before BCG treatment but were no longer found after treatment. These results suggest that only the tumor cells in these cases expressed the Om5 antigen, and that the patients, after responding to the BCG, no longer had tumor cells expressing Om5.[68] In a study of 20 patients with superficial bladder cancer or carcinoma in situ treated with BCG, tumor tissues were evaluated with monoclonal antibody staining. The antibodies used were G4, E7, anti–blood group, anti–epidermal growth factor receptor, and anti–cytokeratin 18. In this small study no correlation was found between the response to BCG therapy and the binding of anti–blood group, anti–epidermal growth factor receptor, E7, or G4 antibodies, although other studies have shown that the loss of blood group antigens and expression of epidermal growth factor receptor are correlated with higher grade tumors that are more likely to be invasive. Significant differences were seen with anti–cytokeratin 18 antibodies. Patients whose tumors responded to BCG had higher levels of cytokeratin 18 staining (7/10), whereas those whose tumors failed to respond to BCG treatment had lower levels (only 2/10 positive of cytokeratin 18). Furthermore, tumors that became invasive were more often cytokeratin 18 negative (5/11 in the cytokeratin-negative group had invasive tumors compared with 1/9 in the cytokeratin-positive group).[73]

Various monoclonal antibodies have been evaluated in xenograft animal tumor models for immunolocalization,[74-77] and one has been used in mice for radioimmunotherapy and for targeted drug therapy as an immunoconjugate with doxorubicin.[78,79] The localized nature of superficial bladder cancer invites intravesical therapy, and this method of delivery has been reported.[80] Other monoclonal antibodies have been linked with a photosensitizer for local phototherapy[81] or used with ricin to produce an immunotoxin.[82] A recent clinical trial of ^{111}In-labeled anti–carcinoembryonic antigen (CEA) for localization of bladder cancer in patients has had some success.[83]

Monoclonal antibodies have also been evaluated as diagnostic agents in the assay of bladder tumor–

associated antigens in urine. A number of substances identified by monoclonal antibodies have been measured as potential urinary bladder tumor markers. It has long been known that some bladder cancer cells express CEA. Urinary levels of CEA may be helpful in monitoring some patients with bladder cancer; 66% of patients were positive for CEA in one study.[84,85] Cytokeratin 18 has also been shown to be shed by bladder tumor cells into the urine.[86,87] A diagnostic assay (IRMAK-18) based on this detection has been evaluated in patients with bladder cancer and demonstrated that 12/26 patients with active disease had significant urinary levels of cytokeratin 18.[86] Fibrin or fibrinogen-like degradation products[88] and oncogene-related products, including *ras* products, have also been found in the urine of patients with bladder cancer.[89,90] Other materials shed by bladder cancer cells are also potentially useful as urinary markers.[91-93]

Biologically active materials have been evaluated as potential urinary bladder tumor markers. Examples include fibroblast growth factor–like material[94] and autocrine motility factor.[95] These last two markers may also have prognostic and biologic significance because their presence may promote the growth or motility of bladder cancer cells. Motility of cancer cells has been associated with greater metastatic capability. Further work with these biologic materials is needed. Unfortunately, no urinary tumor marker for bladder cancer has yet proved reliable in the clinical setting, and the quest for the best tumor marker continues.

Prostate Cancer. Monoclonal antibodies have become an established part of the clinical repertoire through their use in a variety of pathologic analyses, such as serum assays and immunohistologic tests. One prominent example is the measurement of prostate-specific antigen (PSA) as a marker for prostate cancer. This antigen was initially defined through the use of polyclonal antibodies to an extract of human prostatic tissue.[96] Subsequent studies demonstrated the antigen to be present on both primary and metastatic prostatic carcinomas. The two immunoassays currently available for measuring serum levels of PSA yield similar, but not identical, data.[97] The monoclonal antibody–based assay is more commonly used in the United States.

Serum measurements of PSA correlate with the clinical course of prostate cancer, and PSA is a sensitive marker for the follow-up of prostate cancer after surgery, radiation therapy, and hormonal manipulation.[98-101] Although PSA is generally not used to screen asymptomatic men for prostate cancer, evidence suggests that an elevated PSA level (>10 ng/ml measured by monoclonal antibody assay) defines a population with a higher incidence of this disease.[102]

Monoclonal antibodies have also been used to define the biologic characteristics of prostate cancer. Studies have recently identified antibodies to hormone receptors, including those to the androgen receptor[103] and the progesterone receptor.[104] These antibodies will be important reagents in the study of hormonal influences on normal and malignant prostate cell growth. The expression of cytokeratins identified by monoclonal antibodies has been used in the pathologic identification of carcinoma after radiation therapy.[105]

Radioimaging with monoclonal antibodies to prostate cancer–associated antigens has been evaluated with modest success. One early report (1983) indicated that polyclonal antibodies to prostatic acid phosphatase (PAP) could be used to localize metastases.[106] More recently a study of 15 patients injected periprostatically for immunolymphoscintigraphy was reported.[107] This study used ^{123}I-labeled F(ab')$_2$ fragments of anti-PAP antibody PAP 227 and reported success in some patients. The clinical use of another monoclonal antibody to PAP, PAY 276, has been reported with ^{111}In used as the label. As is true for most ^{111}In-labeled antibodies, a high background uptake in the liver and spleen is observed.[108] Intravenous delivery of this antibody into 25 patients resulted in good imaging of the primary tumor.[109] Although imaging of lymphatic metastases was not observed in this study, some metastases to bone were imaged.[109] In contrast, intralymphatic delivery of the same antibody (PAY 276) labeled with ^{111}In in 5 patients showed higher localization of antibody in lymph nodes that lacked tumor than in the lymph nodes that contained tumor.[110] In this study the investigators noted significant retention of the label in unaffected lymph nodes, possibly caused by trapping of ^{111}In, ^{111}In-DTPA complex, or ^{111}In-DTPA-antibody. These results suggest that this antibody labeling technique may not be appropriate for most intralymphatic applications. Another monoclonal antibody, TURP-27, which reacts with a prostate-associated antigen that is not PAP, has shown localization to human prostate cancer xenografts in nude mice.[111] A preliminary clinical trial using ^{131}I-labeled TURP-27 intravenously in 10 patients showed promising results (G. Wright, personal communication). This antibody has been found to react with material resembling neural cell adhesion molecule (NCAM).[112] Further trials of the antibody for localization in patients with prostate cancer are under way (G. Wright, personal communication). Since some prostate cancers express antigens, such as CEA and TAG 72,[113,114] that could be targeted by currently available monoclonal antibodies, additional investigation in this area is likely. Other strategies may employ monoclonal antibodies for therapy. Monoclonal antibodies to PAP have been conjugated to methotrexate and doxorubicin.[115,116] Such conjugates may direct the toxic action of the drug to the cancer cells and provide a new treatment modality.

Testicular Cancer. The monitoring of tumor

markers such as alpha-fetoprotein and beta–human chorionic gonadotropin, which is essential for follow-up of patients with testicular cancer, has been improved significantly by the use of monoclonal antibodies in assays.[117-120] Monoclonal antibodies have also been used to evaluate testicular cancers through the determination of cytokeratins.[121,122]

Although testicular cancer has been the object of intensive evaluation with tumor markers, other uses of monoclonal antibodies for testicular cancer have not been as vigorously investigated, possibly because of the current high level of success in diagnosing and treating this disease. Nevertheless, several reports indicate that radiolabeled monoclonal antibodies localize to testicular cancer. Examples include the use of anti-alpha-fetoprotein[123] and anti–placental alkaline phosphatase antibodies.[124-126] These techniques may be especially useful in the evaluation of a patient with rising tumor markers but no demonstrable disease.

Immunotherapy for Graft Rejection

The field of clinical transplantation is based on an understanding of immunologic principles and has thrived as knowledge of mechanisms that modify immune rejection has increased. Cyclosporine, the major immunosuppressive agent in use today, provides effective immunosuppression with modest side effects at appropriate doses. Cyclosporine binds to a cytoplasmic protein called cyclophilin. This protein has been shown to be a protein isomerase.[127,128] Recently a new immunosuppressive agent, FK 506, has been found to bind to another cytoplasmic protein with similar function.[129] Both FK 506 and cyclosporine function by preventing the synthesis of cytokines, including IL-1, IL-2, IL-3, IL-4, interferon-gamma, and granulocyte-macrophage colony–stimulating factor (GM-CSF).[130,131]

Monoclonal antibody OKT3, which binds to CD3, has been effective in treating acute renal allograft rejection in a multicenter randomized clinical trial and is now routinely used for this purpose.[132] The humoral response to OKT3 administration, that is, anti-OKT3 production, may be suppressed by concomitant low-dose cyclosporine.[133] Recently the use of other monoclonal antibodies for prophylaxis against renal allograft rejection has been reported. Antibodies directed against the IL-2 receptor have been used in clinical trials.[134] The use of these antibodies does not appear to affect circulating lymphocytes but does inhibit the initial cellular activation stages necessary for graft rejection. A similar approach is to target activated IL-2 binding lymphocytes in the recipient by using immunotoxins, such as an anti–IL-2 receptor monoclonal antibody (anti-Tac)–toxin conjugate or an IL-2–toxin conjugate.[24,135] Another antibody that has been used clinically is BMA 031, an IgG_{2b} antibody that binds to human TcR. Preliminary data suggest that BMA 031 can reduce episodes of rejection in high-risk recipients.[136,137] However, BMA 031 appears to result in greater sensitization (i.e., induces higher levels of neutralizing antibodies) than OKT3.[138] Antibodies to the CD4 determinant on T cells have been used in experimental models to induce tolerance to histocompatibility antigens.[139] Anti-CD8 antibodies did not induce tolerance in these models, even though the suspected effector cell in rejection is the cytotoxic T cell, which is usually CD8 positive.[135] In another study kidneys for transplantation were perfused with antibody to CD45 to reduce the immunogenicity of passenger leukocytes. Patients who received treated kidneys had fewer rejection episodes, although graft survival was unchanged.[135]

Problems With In Vivo *Use of Monoclonal Antibodies*

The high specificity of antibodies led to hope that this new technology would finally provide the "magic bullet" against cancer. The goal was to use monoclonal antibodies for tumor targeting, which would make possible new methods of diagnosis or therapy employing radioactively labeled antibodies or antibody-drug conjugates. It was hypothesized that the newly found method for generating unlimited supplies of specific antibody would open up the in vivo localization field, pioneered with polyclonal antibodies by Pressman,[140] Ghose,[141] Order,[142] and Goldenberg.[143] To date, however, in vivo localization with monoclonal antibodies in humans has been poor, with a low amount of antibody localizing to tumors after intravenous injection.[144] Attempts at therapy with monoclonal antibodies have also been disappointing with a few exceptions: R24 in melanoma, anti-GD2 in neuroblastoma, and various antibodies in lymphoma and leukemia.[145] This failure has many causes, including poor antibody specificity (unrealized cross-reactivity), poor expression of the targeting antigen, heterogeneity of antigen expression within tumors, presence of circulating soluble tumor antigen, binding by Fc receptors, and physiologic barriers such as intratumor pressure and vascular permeability.[144,146,147] Furthermore, presenting a foreign protein, such as a mouse or rat monoclonal antibody, to human patients has resulted in the production of human antibodies to the monoclonal antibodies.[147,148] These human anti-mouse antibodies (HAMA) may react with "mouse" foreign determinants on the constant region. However, the human antibody response can also be directed against the idiotype, the variable portion in the Fab region. These antibodies are "antiidiotypic" antibodies that specifically interfere with binding at the antigenic site.[149] These problems have remained a major stumbling block to in vivo applications of monoclonal antibodies.

Biologic Response Modifiers in Cancer Treatment

One of the most effective examples of immunotherapy in urologic oncology is the employment of intravesical BCG in the therapy for superficial bladder cancer. Although BCG is more effective than conventional intravesical chemotherapy,[150] the mechanisms by which BCG achieves tumor prophylaxis remain unclear. A murine model has demonstrated that intravesically administered BCG requires T lymphocytes to be effective.[151] In humans, intravesical BCG increases the number of CD4-positive T cells in the bladder.[152] Futhermore, intravesical BCG increases urinary levels of IL-1, IL-2, and tumor necrosis factor alpha (TNF-α).[153] Patients who respond to therapy tend to have higher urinary levels of IL-2 than those who have tumor recurrence.[154]

Clinical data suggest that direct contact is required for BCG to be effective. Several pieces of evidence support this hypothesis. First, the effectiveness of orally administered BCG remains uncertain.[155,156] Second, BCG has effectively eliminated tumor recurrence in the bladder while progression has been noted in immediately adjacent tissue such as the prostate gland.[157] Third, a prolonged protective systemic immunity does not exist in the conventional sense because ureteral tumors may occur in patients who have had successful intravesical therapy for carcinoma in situ.[158]

Limited animal and human experiments have suggested that other agents may be immunologically active against bladder cancer. These include such diverse substances as interferon, IL-2, and keyhole limpet hemocyanin (KLH). The uses of interferons and IL-2 are discussed in the next section, "Clinical Uses of Cytokines." KLH's activity against bladder cancer was first noted in 1974, when Olsson and associates reported on two groups of patients with bladder cancer who were immunized to KLH and tested for delayed sensitivity to KLH and other agents.[159] The first group had a significant decrease in the bladder tumor recurrence rate after immunization with KLH. In the second group, KLH-immunized patients who had bladder cancer were compared with a nonrandomized age-matched cohort that did not receive KLH. Again the KLH-immunized group had significantly fewer bladder tumors. Subsequent evaluation of KLH in animal models suggested only a minor degree of efficacy. In recent randomized clinical trials, however, intravesical KLH has been effective against superficial bladder cancer. In a trial of intravesical KLH versus mitomycin C in patients with resected superficial tumors, KLH offered significantly better prophylaxis.[160] Another randomized trial, which included only patients who had failed to respond to intravesical treatment with doxorubicin or mitomycin C, compared intravesical KLH with ethoglucid for tumor prophylaxis.[161] The percentage of recurrences, recurrence rate, and tumor progression rate in the two treatment groups were not statistically different. These two clinical trials differ from the study by Olsson and associates because they used both cutaneous immunization and intravesical instillation. The role of KLH in the treatment of superficial bladder cancer remains to be defined. Furthermore, it is still unclear whether both routes of administration (systemic immunization by cutaneous administration and intravesical instillation) are required for a therapeutic effect.

Clinical Uses of Cytokines

Cytokines are low molecular weight proteins, produced by cells, that provide a means of communication between cell populations. At first, most of these materials were identified by their action, such as T cell growth factor or viral interferon. Many of these cytokines were originally identified by their effects on and production by lymphocytes and thus were called lymphokines. Similarly, substances produced by or acting on monocytes were termed monokines. Later, as it became evident that these substances were both produced by and acting on a wide range of blood cell types, the term "interleukin," meaning between white cells, was introduced. Now, however, it is clear that many of these substances are produced by and act on cells that are not blood cells at all, including keratinocytes and endothelial cells. The more general term "cytokine," substances acting between cells, is probably the most descriptive. Unfortunately, the bewildering variety of terms has largely been retained as the field continues to explode with information.

Besides serving as signaling agents between leukocytes, cytokines send communications between leukocytes and endothelial cells, blood vessels, and other tissues.[162] For example, IL-1 and TNF can inhibit smooth muscle contraction, upregulate adhesive molecules on endothelial cells that facilitate leukocyte migration from blood into tissues, and stimulate endothelial cell production of other cytokines such as IL-8.[162] Such interactions resulting from high local concentrations of cytokines can have profound effects on wound healing and tumor metastasis. Some investigators have proposed the existence of a "cytokine network" of communication, in which cytokines interact with the target cells in three steps: (1) induction of the production of other cytokines by the target cell; (2) regulation (either upward or downward) of cell surface receptors for cytokines; and (3) interaction with cell function in a synergistic, antagonistic, or additive fashion.[163] The final message the cell receives may be the total signal from all the cytokines the cell detects.[164]

Investigators hoped that the wide-reaching biologic effects of cytokines would make them useful for increasing the immune response and improving rejection of cancers. Through this approach such agents as alpha and gamma interferon, TNF, and IL-2 are becoming part of the anticancer armamentarium.

Interferons have been used for cancer treatment since the late 1970s.[145] Early trials, sponsored by the American Cancer Society, used "natural" interferon produced by bulk culture of stimulated white blood cells. Although these materials were not pure or completely characterized, preliminary studies were promising.[145,165,166] The availability of materials produced by recombinant DNA techology has allowed large-scale clinical trials of pure, characterized material in cancer treatment.

Three types of interferon have been identified. Alpha interferon (IFN-α) is produced by stimulated leukocytes, beta interferon (IFN-β) is produced by stimulated fibroblasts, and gamma or "immune" interferon (IFN-γ) is produced by activated lymphocytes. Alpha and beta interferons are structurally related and act through a common receptor, while gamma interferon is structurally unrelated.

The mechanisms by which interferons mediate their anticancer action are not clear. Interferons are growth inhibitory in vitro, although this effect is reversible. Direct cytotoxicity has not been demonstrated. Interferons are also known to increase the expression of certain antigens on tumor cells, including histocompatibility antigens and tumor-associated antigens such as TAG 72 and CEA, and to induce the expression of intercellular adhesion molecule-1 (ICAM-1).[167-169] The increased expression of these antigens may help direct a lymphocytic antitumor response. Interferons also activate cellular immunity, particularly through effects on natural killer (NK) and lymphokine-activated killer (LAK) cells.[145,165]

Renal cell carcinoma was a natural target for interferon therapy because spontaneous regressions of this disease hinted at immunologically mediated rejection and no effective therapy for metastatic disease existed. Interferon treatment of metastatic renal cell carcinoma has resulted in partial and complete response rates of approximately 20%.[165,166] In general, alpha interferon has been most effective in the treatment of renal cell carcinoma, with beta and gamma interferons showing less effect.[165,166,170] A recent study using continuous infusion of gamma interferon in renal cell carcinoma showed no response,[171] and a phase I and II clinical trial of a combination of alpha and gamma interferon was unable to detect an increased effect with this combination treatment.[172] Even for alpha interferon, the greatest effect appears to be on distant metastases and the renal primary tumor is less responsive.[165] Preliminary evidence suggests that tumor sensitivity to interferon can be predicted by a monoclonal antibody (see "Monoclonal Antibodies to Urologic Tumor–associated Antigens").

Although a number of effective treatments for superficial bladder cancer exist, efforts to increase the therapeutic efficacy and decrease toxicity continue. A role for interferon treatment has been proposed,[173] and intravesical treatment of superficial bladder cancers with alpha interferon has demonstrated some effect.[166] A randomized study of 85 patients with carcinoma in situ has shown that a high dose of intravesical alpha interferon (100 million units) resulted in 43% complete responses and 23% partial responses, including responses observed in 6 patients who had failed to respond to BCG treatment.[174] Intravesical alpha interferon at these high doses had minimal toxicity.

TNF-α is another cytokine with antitumor activity. Originally described as a serum factor generated during gram-negative sepsis, TNF-α is directly toxic to some tumor cells.[175] TNF-α also has a number of other biologic effects that may affect tumor growth, including activation of endothelial cells, damage to blood vessels in tumors, activation of white blood cells, and generation of a cascade of other cytokines.[175-177] TNF-α has been evaluated in phase I trials.[178,179] Although TNF-α treatment in experimental animal tumors resulted in hemorrhagic necrosis of the tumors, only a few minor tumor responses were seen in patients treated intravenously with TNF-α alone. Furthermore, intravenous TNF-α administration is associated with significant toxic effects, including fever, chills, and rigors. Intravesical delivery of TNF-α has been evaluated in monkeys[180] and a clinical trial of intravesical TNF-α is under way for superficial bladder cancer (M. Ernstoff, R. Bahnson, and T.R. Hakala, personal communication). Because of the toxicity associated with intravenous delivery of TNF-α, most new clinical trials of TNF-α are employing lower doses in combination with other treatments. The use of multimodality therapy has been suggested by the synergistic effects observed with TNF-α in the laboratory setting. TNF-α has been shown in vitro to enhance NK cell activity, which suggests a role for this agent in combination with adoptive immunotherapy.[181] A synergistic effect of TNF-α and etoposide in renal cell carcinoma has been suggsted by in vitro and animal studies.[182,183]

IL-2 is another cytokine that has been used clinically to treat cancers. The mechanism of antitumor action of IL-2 is probably quite different from that of TNF-α or interferons. As described previously, both interferons and TNF-α have direct antitumor effects, as well as other systemic effects that may modify tumor growth. The major effects of IL-2 appear to be on the immune system. IL-2 is produced by activated T cells, and its action is directed to T cells as well.[24] Treatment in vivo with high doses of IL-2 has been shown to increase the number of lymphocytes in the peripheral blood, increase the activity of LAK cells, activate cytotoxic T cells, and cause the generation of other cytokines.[145] These doses of IL-2 are toxic and can be life threatening.[145,184] Trials of IL-2 treatment alone in renal cell carcinoma at the National Institutes of Health (NIH) have shown clinical responses in up to 20% of the patients. Tissues from patients showing responses with IL-2 as a single agent show increases in class II antigen expression on tumors from responding patients, as well as infiltration of the responding tumors with macrophages and both CD4- and CD8-positive T cells.[185] Activation of T cells may be essential for this response. Intralesional injection of IL-2 was associated with tumor regression in a small number of patients with bladder cancer.[186] Huland and Huland have reported the use of continuous intravesical IL-2 for the treatment of five patients with $T_4N_0M_0$ bladder cancer.[187] No toxic effects were observed with this therapy. One patient had a complete response, and all patients showed both local and systemic effects of treatment, including an increased number of activated IL-2 receptor–bearing lymphocytes in their peripheral blood and urine. Even though the response rate was low, this study is significant given the extent of the disease and the lack of toxicity. Because the antitumor effect of IL-2 therapy appears to be due to activation of cell-mediated antitumor cytotoxicity, IL-2 has been combined with a variety of other immunotherapeutic strategies involving the administration of lymphocytes (see "Adoptive Immunotherapy").

Although some clinical responses have been observed with the use of single cytokines for therapy, greater efficacy has been sought through the combination of different cytokines. IL-2 and interferon treatments demonstrated a synergistic effect in murine models[188] and produced a greater than 90% reduction in liver metastases.[188] IL-2 and interferon gamma have been used in combination in a phase I trial in 26 patients, including some patients with renal cell carcinoma.[189] Because IL-2 was used at a reduced dose in this study, the toxicity was less than that of IL-2 alone. IL-2 and interferon gamma showed some synergism in these patients in the activation of cellular immunity tested in vitro.[189] However, only partial and minor responses were noted in the clinical trial, and how much of the effect was caused by interferon gamma remains unclear because the tumors that responded were types known to respond to IL-2 alone. The combination of IL-2 and interferon beta was tested in a clinical trial in 24 patients with renal cell carcinoma.[190] Again, synergy in cellular activation, especially of NK cells, was noted in vitro and in vivo following this therapy. As noted previously, responses to this therapy were most often seen at distant sites, with local disease infrequently affected. Patients who had a previous nephrectomy had more favorable responses, as has been observed in treatments with IL-2 and interferon alpha alone. Toxic effects of the IL-2 and interferon beta included weight loss and fatigue. The study reported a 27% complete plus partial response rate, with a significant increase in LAK cell activity in the responders.[190] TNF-α in combination with IL-2 or interferon gamma has synergistic effects in murine tumor models,[191] and combinations of IL-4 and IL-2 and of IL-2 and GM-CSF have synergistic effects, which suggests that these combinations might also be useful in humans.[191,192] A study of IL-2 and IL-4, which also activates T cells in vitro, has begun.[193]

The use of cytokines with chemotherapeutic agents has been investigated. Most studies have been performed in vitro or in animal models. TNF-α enhances the effectiveness of drugs targeted to DNA topoisomerase I or II[194,195] and can increase the effectiveness of cyclophosphamide, doxorubicin, and 5-fluorouracil.[196] TNF-α also increases the effectiveness of radiation therapy in in vitro models.[195] In a stem cell assay, interferon has been demonstrated to be synergistic with etoposide, doxorubicin, and 5-fluorouracil.[195] Interferon has also shown synergism with 5-fluorouracil in in vitro assays with colon cancer cell lines.[197] The combination of IL-2 with cyclophosphamide or doxorubicin has been observed to be synergistic in animal models.[188] Cyclophosphamide's effect is thought to be due to a reduction in a suppressor cell population, improved T cell access to tumor, or a direct cytotoxic effect.[188]

Cytokines can also be synergistic with monoclonal antibody–based immunotherapy. IL-2 increases the expression of Fc receptors on lymphocytes, which may explain the increased ADCC detected in patients treated with IL-2[198] and in a mouse xenograft model.[199] Thus the administration of a monoclonal antibody and IL-2 may be synergistic if the monoclonal antibody is capable of ADCC.[192,198,199] TNF-α increases the tumor toxicity of drug–monoclonal antibody immunoconjugates both in vitro and in vivo. The in vivo effects may be due to effects of TNF-α on the tumor vasculature.[200,201] Besides the effects on the tumor target cells, cytokine treatment may affect the immune cells of the host. Both interferon and IL-2 cause proliferation of lymphocytes and increase the cytolytic effectiveness of the cells present.[188] Interferon alpha has been shown to improve specific localization of radiolabeled monoclonal antibody in patients with melanoma.[202]

Colony-stimulating factors are glycoproteins that control the production of hematopoietic cells and are named by the cells whose production they increase; for example, GM-CSF is granulocyte-macrophage colony–stimulating factor. Because profound neutropenia and its attendant complications are a common problem with systemic chemotherapy, the use of recombinant colony-stimulating factors is being investigated as a means to limit the toxic effects of treatment and permit the administration of greater amounts of cytotoxic drugs. Granulocyte colony–stimulating factor (G-CSF) decreases the duration of neutropenia in patients receiving M-VAC for advanced transitional cell carcinoma and increases the probability that patients can receive subsequent treatment as scheduled.[203] GM-CSF has permitted the use of escalated doses of M-VAC chemotherapy in a heavily pretreated population.[204] IL-1 can synergize with other colony-stimulating factors to stimulate purified stem cells to form colonies, as can G-CSF with GM-CSF and IL-3 and GM-CSF.[205] GM-CSF may also act therapeutically through the activation of antitumor effects of neutrophils and macrophages.[191] Clinical evaluation of GM-CSF in combination with other cytokines is continuing.

The in vivo administration of cytokines may result in the production of autoantibodies to the cytokine.[206] This response may be considered analogous to the human antimouse antibodies or the antiidiotype antibodies that develop after treatment with monoclonal antibodies. Although anticytokine antibodies have been associated with disease states such as lupus and AIDS, the negative effects of these antibodies are not clearly defined. In fact, Bendtzen and his colleagues have suggested that anticytokine autoantibodies may be beneficial under certain circumstances.[206] The development of anticytokine antibodies during in vivo treatment does not always inhibit the effect of the treatment, in contrast to HAMA and antiidiotype antibodies in monoclonal antibody therapy.

ADOPTIVE IMMUNOTHERAPY

Adoptive immunotherapy is a cancer treatment employing the transfer of immune cells to combat the cancer. The types of cells, which vary among protocols, are obtained from the cancer patient to avoid transplantation barriers. In LAK cell protocols the cells are harvested from the peripheral blood and can be obtained in large quantities from the donor by plasmapheresis. Lymphocyte effectors from the peripheral blood are expanded in tissue culture in the presence of high levels of IL-2. The resulting cultured cells are thereby enriched for a cytotoxic cell called a lymphokine-activated killer cell, or LAK cell. LAK cells are derived from peripheral blood NK cells, are usually negative for CD3, CD4, and CD8, lack the T cell receptor for antigen, and show no specificity in their cytotoxicity (i.e., are not restricted by histocompatibility [MHC] type).[18] LAK cells are CD16 (IgG-Fc receptor) positive and therefore may have the capability of mediating ADCC functions. LAK cells may also express CD2 and CD56. CD56 is related to the neural cellular adhesion molecule and may be important in cell-cell adhesion functions.[18] LAK cells also express LFA-1 (CD11a/CD18), which is an important adhesion molecule binding to ICAM (intercellular adhesion molecule-1 or CD54). Unlike NK cells, LAK cells require stimulation by IL-2 for activation. This activation can be enhanced by IL-1, interferon gamma, and TNF-α. LAK cells are resistant to cyclosporine but can be inhibited by IL-4 or cortisone.[18] Even though LAK cells themselves are not T cells, T cells have been shown to be essential for LAK cell generation in animal models.[18] LAK cells are much more effective in vivo if IL-2 is coadministered.[207]

LAK cell protocols have been investigated extensively by a number of groups, and significant responses have been noted in several types of cancer, including renal cell carcinoma.[208-211] The report from Rosenberg's group at the NIH indicated a 33% complete plus partial response rate in renal cell carcinoma (36 patients) with an overall complete plus partial response rate of 22% (106 total patients with renal cell carcinoma and other tumors). In contrast, treatment with IL-2 alone resulted in only a 5% complete plus partial response in renal cell carcinoma (21 patients).[208] In this protocol the IL-2 was delivered as a bolus. Toxic effects, mostly associated with the IL-2 infusion, were quite significant and included 4 deaths.[145,208] In the report from Oldham's group a continuous infusion of IL-2 was used instead of the bolus administration, which reduced toxicity. This study reported partial responses in 3/6 patients with renal cell carcinoma, with an overall complete plus partial response rate of 32% (13/40 patients).[209] A multicenter phase II clinical trial of LAK cell and IL-2 therapy in patients with renal cell carcinoma was conducted using the protocol developed by Rosenberg's laboratory (i.e., IL-2 bolus). Of the 32 evaluable patients in this study, 5 had complete or partial responses.[210] The toxic effects were somewhat reduced, perhaps because the IL-2 was delivered in an intensive care setting. These investigators summarized the experience with LAK cell and IL-2 therapy in renal cell carcinoma and suggested that responses were seldom observed in intact primary or very large lesions and that patients who had previously undergone nephrectomy were more likely to respond to treatment.[210] Responses were more often seen in distant metastatic sites than in regional recurrence, similar to the responses observed in patients with renal cell carcinoma treated with IFNα alone.[165] Another study has evaluated this issue. In this protocol patients with renal cell carcinoma received nephrectomy and removal of major abdominal tumors before LAK–IL-2 treatment. Although 25% complete plus partial responses were observed in the patients who completed the treatment, a significant proportion (20/53) of the patients entering the trial and undergoing surgery for the primary tumor could not complete the protocol because of various reasons related to tumor growth, the surgical intervention, or other medical factors.[211]

LAK cells have been shown to be cytolytic against both freshly isolated and cultured renal cell carcinoma cell lines in vitro.[212] Effective tumor cell cytolysis has been demonstrated with LAK cells either developed in culture or recovered from the peripheral blood of patients after IL-2 treatment.[213]

In a study of patients with melanona, in vitro lysis of tumor cells by LAK cells generated in vivo was enhanced by the presence of antiganglioside monoclonal antibodies.[214] Use of other cytokines, such as IL-4 in combination with IL-2, may improve the activity of LAK cells and reduce the toxicity of the therapy.[191] Other possible refinements include cotreatment with TNF-α or interferon to increase the expression of target antigens on the tumor cells.[191]

Several other cytokines known to stimulate T cells may improve the development and generation of LAK cells. Examples include IL-1, which is synergistic with IL-2 in stimulating T cells; IL-3, which affects maturation of T cells; IL-4, which is costimulatory for T cells in a variety of settings; IL-5, which improves T cell responses to IL-2 by increasing the expression of the IL-2 receptor; and IL-6, which is stimulatory for T cells and increases IL-2 production. Preliminary results with combinations of IL-2 and IL-4 for LAK cell generation have shown increased cytolytic activity and improved cell recovery.[188,191]

An alternative technique to generate LAK-like effector cells is the use of periodate stimulation along with IL-2 for the in vitro generation of LAK cells.[215] In a clinical trial, infusion of these activated cells accompanied by IL-2 produced significant toxic effects. However, the patients also received maintenance therapy of interferon alpha and in some cases additional LAK–IL-2 treatments. This study reported 22% complete plus partial responses, with 27% complete plus partial responses in the patients who had previous nephrectomy for primary disease. Both the contribution of maintenance therapy to patient survival and the importance of periodate treatment for LAK cell activation remain to be defined.

Exactly how LAK cells are effective in vivo is uncertain because LAK cells have not been found to localize specifically to tumor sites in either experimental animals or human patients.[145,216] LAK cells may affect the tumor vasculature, and a correlation between TNF-α production in the blood and response to LAK cell–IL-2 therapy has been reported.[217] Alternatively, the generation of interferon gamma and TNF-α, along with evidence for monocyte activation, may be central to responses induced during LAK cell–IL-2 therapy.[218] A third possibility is that LAK–IL-2 therapy stimulates tumor-infiltrating T lymphocytes that actually serve as the effector cells.[219] The last hypothesis is suggested by the T cell infiltrates seen in biopsies of responding tumors and the absence of LAK cell localization to tumors in vivo.[216,219] T cell infiltrates are also observed in and may be essential for tumors responding to IL-2 therapy alone.[185]

Although LAK cells used in the preceding protocols are CD3 negative, the role of another cell that is CD3 and CD16 positive has been investigated in vitro.[220,221] The technique to stimulate these cells includes anti-CD3 antibody, which is mitogenic at low concentrations in culture, IL-2, and TNF-α.[221] Greater numbers of cells were generated by this technique with equivalent antitumor lytic effectiveness. The expansion of cytotoxic populations with anti-CD3 may result in a more highly stimulated cell population with a reduced requirement for IL-2 in vivo to maintain effectiveness.

Another immunotherapy approach for renal cell carcinoma with a reportedly lower toxicity is autolymphocyte therapy.[222] In this protocol, peripheral blood cells are removed from patients with renal cell carcinoma and stimulated with anti-CD3 antibody to generate an autologous lymphokine mixture. More peripheral blood cells are removed and are bulk cultured in the presence of the autologous lymphokine mixture along with cimetidine and indomethacin to remove suppressor cell activity. In some cases an extract of the autologous tumor membranes is used during this in vitro stimulation. These cultured cells are then reinfused into the patient. Patients receiving the autolymphocyte therapy showed a significantly longer survival time and a 21% response rate (8/39 partial responses) compared with a survival and response rate of 5% (2/41 partial responses) in a control group receiving cimetidine therapy alone.[222] This report also indicated that more effective generation of IL-1 in the autologous lymphokine mixture correlated with a greater chance of success and that men showed better responses than women. Little toxicity was reported. This type of therapy has become commercially available, so further analysis is likely.

Tumor-infiltrating lymphocyte (TIL) protocols were developed to take advantage of a highly specific antitumor cytotoxic T lymphocyte population that can be identified within malignant tumors.[223] In these protocols a tumor is excised from the patient and the TILs are isolated and expanded in tissue culture in the presence of moderate amounts of IL-2.[207] TILs show specificity in their cytotoxicity and appear to be histocompatibility restricted.[18] TILs are CD3 positive and may express either CD4 or CD8.[18] In these characteristics TILs are similar to cytotoxic T lymphocytes.

Early results with TILs demonstrated that they were 50 to 100 times more effective in tumor cell lysis than LAK cells.[207] Furthermore, unlike LAK cells, TILs have been shown to localize to tumor sites in patients with melanoma.[216] Experimental studies employing TILs against large tumor burdens demonstrated that TIL effectiveness in vivo depended on pretreatment with radiation or cyclophosphamide, possibly by reducing suppressor cell function or permitting homing of the lymphocytes.[224] Evidence from an experimental model indicates that irradiation effect occurs at the tumor site and not systemically, because tumor irradiation is effective whereas whole-body irradiation is not if the tumor field is shielded.[225] The authors hypothesized that the action of cyclophosphamide was due to (1) a reduction in tumor bulk for TILs to attack; (2) slowing of the tumor growth, to give TILs an advantage in tumor destruction; or (3) elimination or reduction of bioactive agents (cytokines) produced by the tumor itself that could be suppressive for TILs.[225] TILs have been harvested and evaluated from renal cell carcinoma,[226] bladder cancer, prostate cancer, and other urologic tumors,[227] raising the possibility that they may be employed in the treatment of a variety of urologic cancers.

Preliminary results of TIL therapy in melanoma have been reported.[228,229] This protocol involved the harvesting of lymphocytes from the tumor and expansion of the lymphocytes in vitro with IL-2. The patients were treated with cyclophosphamide followed 36 hours later by infusion of TILs and therapy with IL-2.[228] These patients were treated with IL-2 for shorter periods (5 days) than those who received LAK plus IL-2 therapy (15 days), so the IL-2 toxicity was reduced. Of the 20 patients in the first report, 11 showed complete or partial responses, although these responses were of short duration.[228] The second report presented an exciting breakthrough in gene therapy. These 5 patients received TILs into which a gene for resistance to a neomycin analog had been introduced by a retroviral vector to allow tracking of the cells in the patient. In this study 3/5 of the patients had complete or partial responses, and the presence of the inserted gene could be found in cells from the peripheral blood and from tumor biopsy specimens (see "Molecular Biology").[229]

A potential problem with TIL therapy is the specificity of the cytolytic reaction. TILs may be reacting with tumor determinants, and specificity (i.e., TIL-mediated lysis of only the stimulating tumor cells) in vitro has been shown in both animal models[230] and human studies.[227] TIL therapy potentially could fail because of tumor heterogeneity or the outgrowth of tumor cell variants lacking the determinants to which the TILs are targeted. Such selection has been demonstrated in vitro.[231] TILs were more effective against the selected resistant variant tumor cells if the tumor cells were pretreated with interferon alpha or gamma or TNF-α, resulting in an increased expression of class II MHC antigens and ICAM-1 (and potentially other tumor target antigens as well). The authors suggested that reculture of newly isolated TILs (from the resistant tumors) might circumvent this problem. Another possible approach to improve the activity of TILs is to provide stimulation with tumor cells.[219]

Synergism of TIL–IL-2 therapy with interferon alpha or with a combination of interferon gamma and TNF-α has been reported in animal models.[188,232,233] Interferon gamma causes increases in both normal (histocompatibility antigens) and tumor antigen expression, which may improve the targeting and cytolytic effectiveness of TILs.[188,232,233] Combinations of TNF-α and IL-2 therapies have been synergistic in mouse models.[188,233] The expression of class I histocompatibility antigens may be important in the ability to generate effective TILs. In a B16 melanoma model, Weber and Rosenberg showed that a class I–deficient cell failed to stimulate TIL production, while a class I–expressing clone generated effective TILs not only against itself, but also against the class I–deficient clone.[232] Cytolysis of either the class I–expressing or the class I–deficient targets by these TILs was seen in vitro, and regression of both tumors was observed in vivo with TIL treatment.[232] These results raise the exciting possibility of improving the quality of harvested TILs by pretreating the patient with interferon, TNF-α, or a combination of agents. Furthermore, in a murine renal cell carcinoma model, the combination of cellular therapy with TIL-like cytotoxic cells and treatment with doxorubicin was effective, supporting the use of other combination therapies.[234]

Another protocol that has been developed to obtain a population of cells for adoptive immunotherapy is in vitro sensitization (IVS). In animal models, IVS cells are obtained from lymphocytes harvested from lymph nodes draining the tumor. These lymphocytes are expanded in tissue culture in the presence of IL-2 and irradiated tumor cells. These cells are highly effective cytotoxic cells that resemble cytotoxic T lymphocytes and can be effective in vivo in the presence of very low levels of IL-2.[235-238] A clinical trial using similar cells in patients with melanoma or renal cell carcinoma is under investigation (S. Shu and A. Chang, University of Michigan Cancer Center, personal communication).

MOLECULAR BIOLOGY

The field of molecular genetics has flourished over the past 15 years and has resulted in dramatic discoveries related to neoplasia and other diseases. The elegant research tools routinely employed in molecular biology laboratories have been made possible by the discovery of specialized nucleases (restriction enzymes) in procaryotic cells that cleave DNA at specific points. The restriction enzymes typically recognize groups of four to six nucleotides and cleave the DNA only if these sequences are present. In 1975 E.M. Southern described a technique whereby DNA fragments separated by gel electrophoresis were transferred to nitrocellulose paper and detected by hybridization with a radiolabeled DNA probe.[239] This method, now known as Southern blotting, is widely used for the detection of known DNA sequences. Because of the power of this blotting technique, similar methods have been developed for the detection of RNA and proteins, and these have been termed Northern and Western blots, respectively.

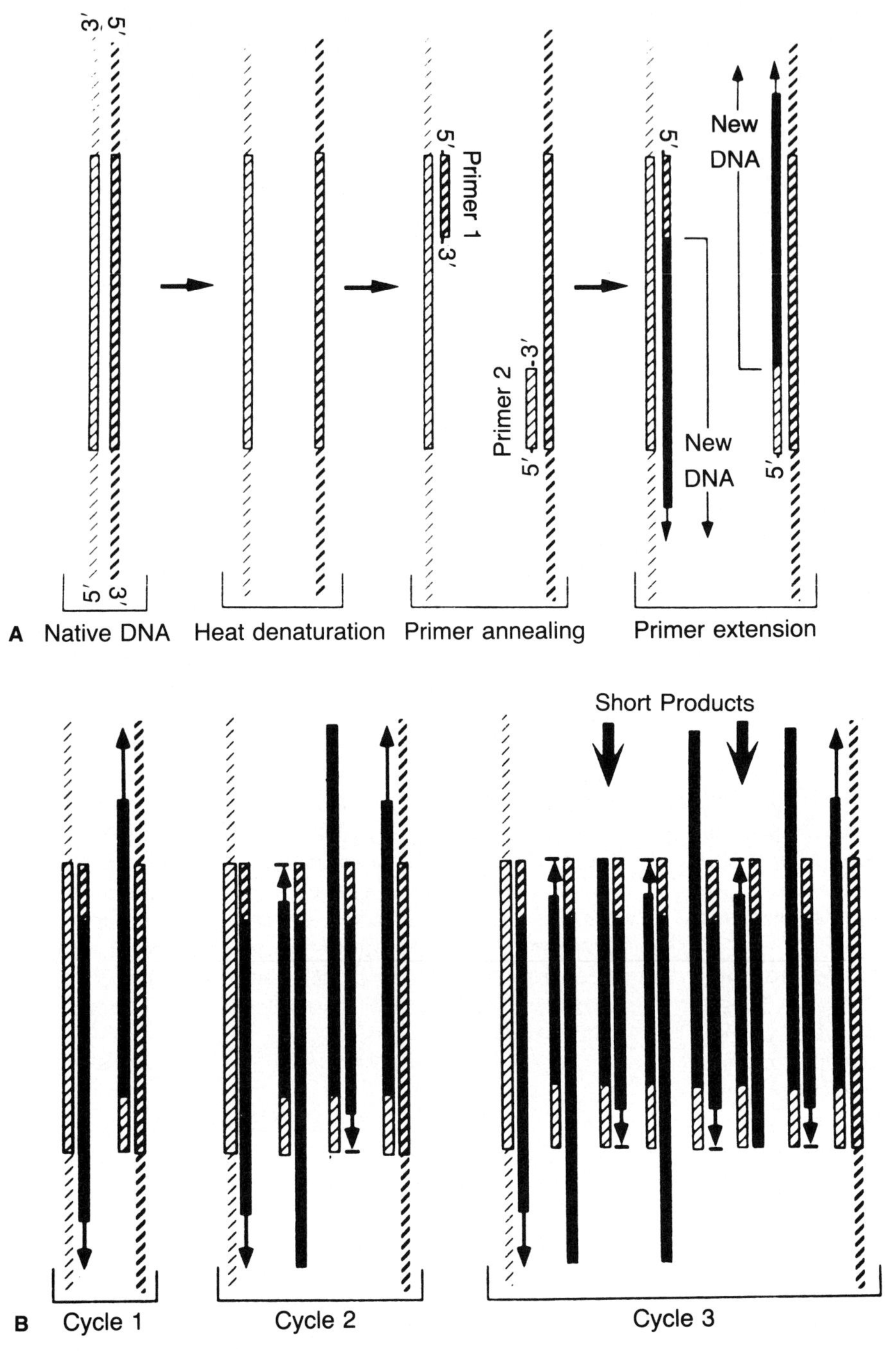

FIGURE 12–3. Polymerase chain reaction. **A,** The reaction is initiated after the two DNA strands are separated by heating from the original material. A "primer" chain with specificity for the sequence of interest is added and anneals to the corresponding sequence in the original material. Then the polymerase enzyme is added and the first round of amplification occurs, producing new complete DNA copies at the site of the primer. The material is heated to separate the chains, and the process is repeated as shown in **B.** (From Eisenstein BI: The polymerase chain reaction. N Engl J Med 322:179, 1990. Reprinted by permission of the New England Journal of Medicine.)

DNA hybridization can be performed in situ, enabling the analysis of DNA structure at the cellular level. The power of this technique is readily appreciated when conventional cytology, flow cytometry, and in situ hybridization are compared. Flow cytometry easily defines tumor subpopulations on the basis of ploidy that are usually undetectable by conventional cytologic analysis. Similarly, in situ hybridization has demonstrated chromosomal heterogeneity indiscernible by flow cytometry.[240]

The discovery of temperature-resistant enzymes has resulted in the automation of an important technique that amplifies specific DNA sequences.[241] The polymerase chain reaction (PCR) employs heat denaturation of double-stranded DNA to produce single strands (Figure 12–3). The temperature is then decreased, and two DNA primers, chosen to encompass the desired sequence, are annealed to complementary sequences on the single-stranded DNA. A heat-stable enzyme, *Taq* DNA polymerase, produces a complementary second strand of new DNA starting at the DNA primer. As the cycle is repeated, the number of DNA templates increases geometrically so that specific DNA sequences can be recovered from small samples such as bladder washings. These can then be analyzed by a variety of techniques, including Southern blotting.

Oncogenes, genes that confer a malignant phenotype, were initially characterized in retroviruses. Normal cellular homologs of these viral oncogenes are called protooncogenes. Protooncogenes appear to play important roles in cell growth and differentiation. Some protooncogenes are related to growth factors or their receptors. In addition to structural changes activating protooncogenes, overexpression of the protooncogene may induce malignant transformation.[242] Genes that inhibit the expression of oncogenes have been characterized. These antioncogenes or tumor suppressor genes appear to be part of the normal genome. The loss of this DNA results in an increased risk of neoplasia.

In 1982 the first human oncogene was cloned from a human bladder cancer cell line.[243-245] This oncogene, H-*ras,* differed from its normal homolog by a single base pair change. The normal allele or protooncogene has been localized to chromosome 11.[246] Although H-*ras* appears to be the dominant oncogene of the *ras* gene family associated with bladder cancer, H-*ras* abnormalities are found in less than 10% of urothelial malignancies.[247-249] Despite this association of the H-*ras* oncogene with urothelial cancer, additional experimental evidence documented that the malignant phenotype could be suppressed in the continued presence of the oncogene.[250] The *ras* oncogene products appear to cause malignant transformation through alterations in signal transduction. This cascade of mitogenic signals has been successfully disturbed with partial reversion of the malignant phenotype through the interruption of downstream signal pathways with antisense-*fos*.[251]

Deletion of 3p, the short arm of chromosome 3, has been associated with the nonpapillary form of renal cell carcinoma.[252] The gene for von Hippel–Landau disease, a genetic disease associated with renal cancer, also maps to this area.[253] It is hypothesized that the 3p deletion may result in neoplasia as a result of loss of suppressor genes that normally inhibit malignant transformation.[254] Similarly, loss of heterozygosity of 11p has been associated with the development of Wilms' tumor, and deletion of 13q is associated with retinoblastoma.[254] Although unconfirmed by genetic linkage data, an association between deletions of 11p and bladder cancer has also been reported.[255] Deletions of 9q and 17p have been found in bladder cancer.[256] Deletions of 17p are more common in high-grade neoplasms. The p53 gene, which is located on 17p, is also mutated in other advanced solid tumors.

Molecular biology has revealed some mechanisms of tumor cell resistance to therapy. The phenomenon of multiple drug resistance (MDR) to chemotherapeutic agents by cancer cells is multifactorial.[257,258] However, one important mechanism of MDR is mediated through the presence of a drug transport membrane protein called P-glycoprotein. P-glycoprotein is coded by a gene called *mdr*-1.[259,260] Additional genes in this family, *mdr*-2 and *mdr*-3, have also been described.[261,262] Increased levels of *mdr*-1 RNA have been associated with a variety of tumors. Renal cell carcinoma has been demonstrated to express high levels of *mdr*-1 RNA without prior exposure to chemotherapeutic drugs.[263] This is not surprising because the kidney is one of several tissues that normally expresses high amounts of *mdr*-1 RNA. Although the function of *mdr*-2 has not yet been defined, *mdr*-3 has been associated with drug resistance in prolymphocytic leukemia.[264] Verapamil and other drugs interfere with MDR mediated by P-glycoprotein. Limited clinical data suggest that the employment of drugs that reverse MDR can improve therapeutic effect.[265] Drugs that reverse MDR are lipophilic, suggesting that improved clinical results with decreased toxicity may be achieved by using several MDR-abrogating agents simultaneously.[266]

The technologic advances that have produced the field of molecular biology have also given research scientists the tools for treating diseases through gene manipulation. Initial attempts at genetic manipulation in people have already been successful. In the first reported experiment, TILs from patients with melanoma were "marked" by the introduction of a gene coding for resistance to the neomycin analog G418 through the use of retroviral gene transduction. These marked TILs were then infused back into the donor patient as part of a course of immunotherapy.[229] Lymphocytes were harvested at various time points and tested for the presence of the introduced gene marker. In some patients the marked TILs survived for up to 2 months after infusion and had no toxic effects. This first experiment demonstrated that human cells could be genetically altered in vitro, retain the functional change from the genetic manipulation in vivo, and not cause any detectable adverse effects in a relatively short observation period. This successful clinical test demonstrated that gene manipulation in humans is technically possible. The first therapeutic trial of human gene manipulation has already begun. It involves virus-mediated transduction of the gene for adenosine deaminase in children congenitally deficient for this enzyme. If this attempt at therapeutic manipulation of the human genome is successful, gene therapy could potentially be used for the treatment of a broad spectrum of diseases.

FUTURE PROSPECTS

Despite the problems in delivering monoclonal antibodies in vivo, the technology has inviting characteristics, including high specificity and biologic activity. Increasing use of multiagent immunotherapy, sophisticated imaging schemes, production of human monoclonal antibodies, and genetic engineering techniques may facilitate the clinical application of monoclonal antibodies. Monoclonal antibodies may be used in immunotherapeutic strategies combining other humoral and cellular therapies, including cytokines and adoptive immunotherapy. Because treatments using monoclonal antibodies have already been shown to be synergistic with some of these approaches, the combination of therapies is an obvious next step.

Novel techniques to improve the delivery of antibodies may significantly improve antibody localization and tumor/background ratios. One approach to this problem is the use of radiolabeled avidin targeted to biotinylated monoclonal antibodies. In this technique the antibody is delivered first and allowed to clear the circulation. Then radiolabeled avidin, a relatively small molecule with high affinity for biotin, is injected. A modification of this technique uses a three-step delivery: biotinylated antibody, avidin, then radiolabeled biotin, which is a much smaller molecule. The two-step technique has been shown to increase the activity accumulating in an animal tumor, and the three-step method improved the ratio of radiolabel clearance.[267] The use of genetic engineering of antibodies to produce smaller or more compatible molecules could also improve in vivo delivery, (Figure 12–4). One example of this approach is the generation of chimeric antibodies, in which the Fab is the well-characterized mouse antibody and the Fc portion is human ("humanized" antibody). This technique takes advantage of the known binding characteristics of the mouse monoclonal antibody and the technology already available to generate these antibodies, while providing a mostly human protein for injection. The lower level of human antimouse antibody produced by injection of this material may make this material superior to entirely murine monoclonal antibodies. These chimeric antibodies have been produced, and preliminary evaluations have been performed.[268-270] The data suggest that greater compatibility (i.e., "humanizing") in the constant region results in lower levels of antiantibody generated, even against the foreign idiotype that is still present.[268-270]

Other genetically engineered molecules that may be of value are also described in Figure 12–4. Single-chain antigen-binding proteins, made of the Fv (only the variable portion) of the antibody molecule, should have a low molecular weight and may overcome some of the access problems that develop when intact monoclonal antibodies are administered. In vivo uptake of such a molecule in an animal model has been evaluated. The localization was quite promising and demonstrated good uptake, comparable to $(Fab')_2$ uptake, even though the clearance from the circulation was quite rapid.[271]

Targeting of drugs and toxins with antibodies has been limited by the complex chemistry needed to link toxins or therapeutic agents to the antibodies. The linking of active agents to antibodies sometimes results in inactivation or aggregation of the

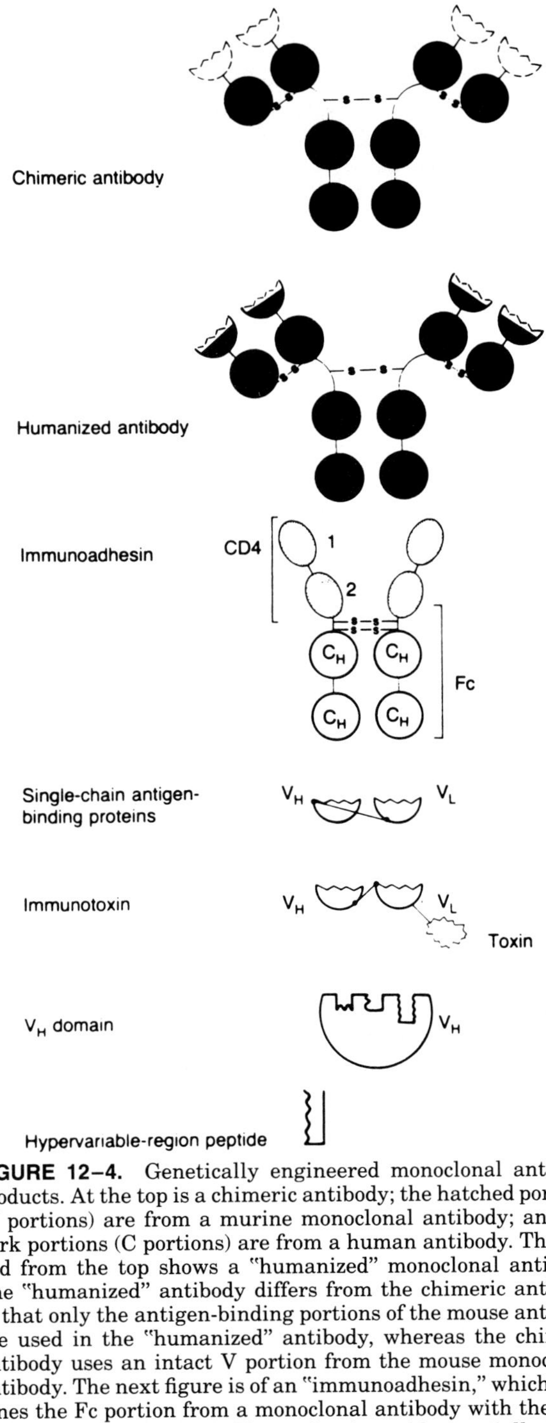

FIGURE 12–4. Genetically engineered monoclonal antibody products. At the top is a chimeric antibody; the hatched portions (V portions) are from a murine monoclonal antibody; and the dark portions (C portions) are from a human antibody. The second from the top shows a "humanized" monoclonal antibody. The "humanized" antibody differs from the chimeric antibody in that only the antigen-binding portions of the mouse antibody are used in the "humanized" antibody, whereas the chimeric antibody uses an intact V portion from the mouse monoclonal antibody. The next figure is of an "immunoadhesin," which combines the Fc portion from a monoclonal antibody with the CD4 determinant of the T cell. This molecule could potentially direct phagocytosis (via the Fc portion) of HIV, which binds specifically to the CD4 molecule. Other constructs with similar function can be imagined. The single-chain antigen-binding protein consists of only the V portions of a monoclonal antibody that are cross-linked to form a single chain. The illustration shows an immunotoxin that comprises a single-chain antibody-binding molecule to which a toxin chain has been added. Finally, at the bottom, are two other components: the V_H domain, which has some antigen-binding activity even in the absence of the V_L domain, and the hypervariable region peptide, which is the shortest peptide retaining antigen-binding activity. (From Mayforth RD, Quintans J: Designer and catalytic antibodies. N Engl J Med 323:175, 1990. Reprinted by permission of the New England Journal of Medicine.)

antibodies, which may negatively affect the localization properties in vivo. Another problem with drug- or toxin-antibody conjugates is the ability to deliver the toxin or drug effectively to the target cell. Special acid-labile linkages have been developed to improve the drug delivery once the antibody is internalized.

A potential problem with toxins is nonspecific killing of cells as the conjugate is cleared. One approach to this problem has been the two-step activation of a toxic compound; that is, the toxin would not be active until the addition of a second signal. Several examples of this approach have been devised or proposed. One is the use of prodrugs, compounds that are not active until a second compound is delivered. Ideally neither the prodrug nor the second compound is toxic. In one system a prodrug is delivered, followed by an antibody-coupled enzyme that activates the prodrug. An example of this system has been tested in an animal model.[272] A novel approach has been suggested by the work of Webb and her co-workers: the development of a two-stage immunotoxin to enhance toxic activity.[273] In this model a bifunctional antibody has been prepared by the fusion of two hybridomas. One "arm" (Fab portion) of the antibody is directed against a toxin, while the other "arm" is directed against a prostate tumor–associated antigen. Additional targeting of the tumor cells is then accomplished with other toxin-antibodies that bind to the toxins employed in the first stage. This technique has resulted in improved targeting of immunotoxins to prostate cancers cells in vitro. Potentially this approach could improve targeting to tumors in vivo, while using toxin molecules (e.g., ricin A chain) that in themselves are not toxic because they lack the ability to bind to cells. Another two-step approach is the use of boronated monoclonal antibodies for localization. The boron is then activated by neutron radiation, releasing locally toxic alpha particles.[274]

Surgical therapy may also be facilitated by the use of radiolabeled monoclonal antibodies. Martin and his co-workers have developed an intraoperative gamma detector that can be used in combination with radiolabeled monoclonal antibodies to detect tumors binding the antibody.[275] This localization technique has been used for more precise excision of metastatic tumors in the liver and lymph nodes. Since the gamma detector probe detects radioactivity and not antibody, this technique could be extended to other radioactive tracers preferentially taken up by tumors. Combining this intraoperative technique with the use of monoclonal antibody fragments or single chain antigen binding proteins would improve the time frame for this analysis and could improve the percentage of the dose taken up by the tumor, which would make the technique more sensitive. Use of the biotin-avidin targeting system may also enhance tumor detection with this technique.

As discussed previously, injection of murine monoclonal antibodies into a patient often results in the patient recognizing the mouse antibodies as foreign and producing HAMA,[144,147,149] including antibodies to the antigen-binding (idiotype) portion, antiidiotype antibodies. It has been suggested that the antigen-binding portion of an antibody (idiotype) should be the "mirror" of the antigen to which it binds, and that antiidiotype antibodies would thus resemble the antigen to which the original idiotype bound.[276] Antiidiotype antibodies might serve as antigenic stimulants for the generation of antibodies against the original antigen. This hypothesis has been proved true in several cases. For example, injection with an antibody to a anti-hepatitis idiotype resulted in the production of anti-hepatitis antibodies.[277] This technique could be used for immunization against infectious agents without exposing the responder to the agent itself and has been proposed as a method for the development of an AIDS vaccine.[278] This idiotypic network could also be used to develop an antitumor response. In a clinical trial 20 patients with colorectal cancer received an antiidiotypic antibody to the CO17-1A anti–colorectal tumor antigen.[279] Many of these patients had specific responses to the antiidiotype. Furthermore, 6 patients had a partial response and 7 had stable disease. Some of these patients also had received chemotherapy. These patients not only had antibody responses, but also developed responsive T cells. Other investigators have also reported this type of response.[149] This method has the potential for improving therapeutic responses through the stimulation of both antibody and cellular immunity.

The area of adoptive immunotherapy is expanding rapidly. As the techniques become less toxic, adoptive immunotherapy with LAK cells or TILs will increasingly become part of the therapeutic armamentarium against some malignancies. This therapeutic approach may also be synergistic with other treatment modalities, including conventional chemotherapy, monoclonal antibody therapy, and radiation therapy. One potential method is the generation of bispecific or heteroconjugate monoclonal antibodies to target killer cells to tumor cells.[280]

Technology is racing ahead as evidenced by the exciting prospect of targeted gene therapy, which has already achieved clinical reality.[229] This new method of treatment offers significant potential not just for cancer therapy, but also for the treatment of many genetic diseases.

REFERENCES

1. Klein J: Immunology: the science of self-nonself discrimination. New York: Wiley Interscience, 1982.
2. Sell S: Immunology, immunopathology and immunity, ed 4. New York: Elsevier, 1987.
3. Paul WE: Fundamental immunology, ed 2. New York: Raven Press, 1989.

4. Reis MD, Griesser H, Mak TW: T cell receptor and immunoglobulin gene rearrangements in lymphoproliferative disorders. Adv Cancer Res 52:45-80, 1989.
5. Honjo T, Nakai S, Nishida Y, et al: Rearrangements of immunoglobulin genes during differentiation and evolution. Immunol Rev 59:33-68, 1981.
6. Muller-Eberhard HJ: Molecular organization and function of the complement system. Annu Rev Biochem 57:321-347, 1988.
7. Hourcade D, Holers VM, Atkinson JP: The regulators of complement activation (RCA) gene cluster. Adv Immunol 45:381-416, 1989.
8. Sharma JN, Mohsin SSJ: The role of chemical mediators in the pathogenesis of inflammation with emphasis on the kinin system. Exp Pathol 38:73-96, 1990.
9. Campbell RD, Law SKA, Reid KBM, Sim RB: Structure, organization, and regulation of the complement genes. Annu Rev Immunol 6:161-195, 1988.
10. Fearon DT: Complement, C receptors, and immune complex disease. Hosp Pract 23:63-72, 1988.
11. Williams LW, Burks W, Steele RW: Complement: function and clinical relevance. Ann Allergy 60:293-301, 1988.
12. Ochs HD, Wedgwood RJ, Heller SR, Beatty PG: Complement, membrane glycoproteins, and complement receptors: their role in regulation of the immune response. Clin Immunol Immunopathol 40:94-104, 1986.
13. Abramson SB, Weissman G: Complement split products and the pathogenesis of SLE. Hosp Pract 23:45-56, 1988.
14. Lewis RA, Austen KF, Soberman RJ: Leukotrienes and other products of the 5-lipoxygenase pathway. N Engl J Med 323:645-655, 1990.
15. Altman A, Coggeshall KM, Mustelin T: Molecular events mediating T cell activation. Adv Immunol 48:227-360, 1990.
16. Davis MM: T cell receptor gene diversity and selection. Annu Rev Biochem 59:475-496, 1990.
17. Moingeon P, Chang H-C, Sayre PH, et al: The structural biology of CD2. Immunol Rev 111:111-144, 1989.
18. Stotter H, Lotze MT: Cytolytic effector cells against human tumors: distinguishing phenotype and function. Cancer Cells 2:44-55, 1990.
19. Charron D: Molecular basis of human leukocyte antigen class II disease associations. Adv Immunol 48:107-159, 1990.
20. Bjorkman PJ, Parham P: Structure, function and diversity of class I major histocompatibility complex molecules. Annu Rev Biochem 59:253-288, 1990.
21. Bellabona P, Peccoud J, Kappler J, et al: Superantigens interact with MHC class II molecules outside of the antigen groove. Cell 62:1115-1121, 1990.
22. Frelinger JA, Gotch FM, Zweerink H, et al: Evidence of widespread binding of HLA class I molecules to peptides. J Exp Med 172:827-834, 1990.
23. Rudd CE, Anderson P, Morimoto C, et al: Molecular interactions, T-cell subsets and a role of the CD4/CD8: p561ck complex in human T-cell activation. Immunol Rev 111:223-266, 1989.
24. Smith KA: Interleukin-2. Sci Am 262:50-57, 1990.
25. Trinchieri G: Biology of natural killer cells. Adv Immunol 47:187-376, 1989.
26. Weber JN, Weiss RA: HIV infection: the cellular picture. Sci Am 259:101-109, 1988.
27. Rosenberg ZF, Fauci AS: The immunopathogenesis of HIV infection. Adv Immunol 47:377-431, 1989.
28. Redfield RR, Burke DS: HIV infection: the clinical picture. Sci Am 259:90-98, 1988.
29. Leport C, Rousseau F, Perronne C, et al: Bacterial prostatitis in patients infected with the human immunodeficiency virus. J Urol 141:334-336, 1989.
30. Benson MC, Kaplan MS, O'Toole K, Romagnoli M: A report of cytomegalovirus cystitis and a review of other genitourinary manifestations of the acquired immune deficiency syndrome. J Urol 140:153-154, 1988.
31. Randazzo RF, Hulette CM, Gottlieb MS, Rajfer J: Cytomegaloviral epididymitis in a patient with the acquired immune deficiency syndrome. J Urol 136:1095-1097, 1986.
32. Bass JB Jr: The face of TB changes again. Hosp Pract 24:81-85,88,93-95,passim, 1989.
33. Rosengart TK, Coppa GF: Abdominal mycobacterial infections in immunocompromised patients. Am J Surg 159:125-131, 1990.
34. Lowe FC, Lattimer DG, Metroka CE: Kaposi's sarcoma of the penis in patients with acquired immunodeficiency syndrome. J Urol 142:1475-1477, 1989.
35. Palmer MC, Mador DR, Venner PM: Testicular seminoma associated with the acquired immunodeficiency syndrome and acquired immunodeficiency syndrome related complex: 2 case reports. J Urol 142:128-130, 1989.
36. Marks JL, Marks D, Lipshultz LI: Artificial insemination with donor semen: the necessity of frequent donor screening. J Urol 143:308-310, 1990.
37. McNicholas TA, Jones DJ, Sibley GN: AIDS: the contamination risk in urological surgery. Br J Urol 63:565-568, 1989.
38. Krieger JN: The acquired immunodeficiency syndrome: prudent precautions for the practicing urologist. J Urol 139:801-802, 1988.
39. da Silva M, Shevchuk MM, Cronin WJ, et al: Detection of HIV-related protein in testes and prostates of patients with AIDS. Am J Clin Pathol 93:196-201, 1990.
40. Goodnough LT, Radnick S, Price TH, et al: Increased properative collection of autologous blood with recombinant erythropoietin therapy. N Engl J Med 321:1163-1168, 1989.
41. Ueda R, Ogata SI, Morrisey D, et al: Cell surface antigens of human renal cancer defined by monoclonal antibodies: identification of tissue specific kidney glycoproteins. Proc Natl Acad Sci USA 78:5122-5126, 1981.
42. Vesella RL, Moon TD, Chiou R-K, et al: Monoclonal antibodies to human renal cell carcinoma: recognition of shared and retricted tissue antigens. Cancer Res 45:6131-6139, 1985.
43. Liebert M, Jaffe R, Taylor RJ, et al: Detection of SSEA-1 on human renal tumors. Cancer 59:1404-1408, 1987.
44. Tolkoff-Rubin N, Cosimi A, Delmonico F, et al: Diagnosis of renal proximal tubule injury in renal transplant patients by a urinary assay for a proximal tubule antigen, the adenosine-deaminase-binding protein. Transplantation 41:593-597, 1986.
45. Medeiros LJ, Michie SA, Johnson DE, et al: An immunoperoxidase study of renal cell carcinoma: correlation with nuclear grade, cell type, and histologic pattern. Hum Pathol 19:980-987, 1988.
46. Kochevar J, Coffield KS: Differential immunostaining of oncocytic renal tumors with an anti-renal cell carcinoma monoclonal antibody. J Urol 141:625-628, 1989.
47. Bander NH, Finstad CL, Cordon-Cardo C, et al: Analysis of a mouse monoclonal antibody that reacts with a specific region of the human proximal tubule and subsets renal cell carcinomas. Cancer Res 49:6774-6780, 1989.
48. Nanus DM, Pfeffer LM, Bander NH, et al: Antiproliferative and antitumor effects of alpha-interferon in renal cell carcinomas: correlation with the expression of a kidney-associated differentiation glycoprotein. Cancer Res 50:4190-4194, 1990.
49. Ballou B, Jaffe R, Taylor RJ, et al: Tumor radioimmunolocation: differential antibody retention by antigenic normal tissue and tumor. J Immunol 132:2111-2116, 1984.
50. Chiou RK, Vessella RL, Elson MK, et al: Localization of human renal cell carcinoma xenografts with a tumor-preferential monoclonal antibody. Cancer Res 45:6140-6146, 1985.
51. Chiou RK, Vessella RL, Limas C, et al: Monoclonal antibody–targeted radiotherapy of renal cell carcinoma using a nude mouse model. Cancer 61:1766-1775, 1988.
52. Sands H, Jones PL, Shah SA, et al: Correlation of vascular

permeability and blood flow with monoclonal antibody uptake by human Clouser and renal cell xenografts. Cancer Res 48:188-193, 1988.
53. Bander NH: Monoclonal antibodies in urologic oncology. Cancer 60:658-667, 1987.
54. Singh M, Ghose T, Faulkner G, et al: Targeting of methotrexate-containing liposomes with a monoclonal antibody against human renal cancer. Cancer Res 49:3976-3984, 1989.
55. Singh M, Kralovec J, Mezei M, Ghose T: Inhibition of human renal cancer by methotrexate linked to a monoclonal antibody. J Urol 141:428-431, 1989.
56. Coon JS, Weinstein RS: Detection of ABH tissue isoantigens by immunoperoxidase methods in normal and neoplastic urothelium: comparison with the erythrocyte adherence method. Am J Clin Pathol 76:163-171, 1981.
57. Weinstein RS, Alroy J, Farrow GM, et al: Blood group isoantigen deletion in carcinoma in situ of the urinary bladder. Cancer 43:661-668, 1979.
58. Limas C, Lange P: T-antigen in normal and neoplastic urothelium. Cancer 58:1236-1245, 1986.
59. Cintorino M, Del Vecchio MT, Bugnoli M, et al: Cytokeratin pattern in normal and pathological bladder urothelium: immunohistochemical investigation using monoclonal antibodies. J Urol 139:428-432, 1988.
60. Neal DE, Sharples L, Smith K, et al: The epidermal growth factor receptor and the prognosis of bladder cancer. Cancer 65:1619-1625, 1990.
61. Messing EM: Clinical implications of the expression of epidermal growth factor receptors in human transitional cell carcinoma. Cancer Res 50:2530-2537, 1990.
62. Smith NW, Strutton GM, Walsh MD, et al: Transferrin receptor expression in primary superficial human bladder tumours identifies patients who develop recurrences. Br J Urol 65:339-344, 1990.
63. Fradet Y, Cordon-Cardo C, Whitmore WF Jr, et al: Cell surface antigens of human bladder tumors: definition of tumor subsets by monoclonal antibodies and correlation with growth characteristics. Cancer Res 46:5183-5188, 1986.
64. Gauthier J, Fradet Y: Growth-regulated surface glycoproteins of human bladder cancer. Cancer Res 50:293-298, 1990.
65. Okamure K, Miyake K, Koshikawa T, Asai J: Growth fractions of transitional cell carcinomas of the bladder defined by the monoclonal antibody Ki-67. J Urol 144:875-878, 1990.
66. Huland H, Arndt R, Huland E, et al: Monoclonal antibody 486 P 3/12: a valuable bladder carcinoma marker for immunocytology. J Urol 137:654-659, 1987.
67. Lin CW, Young DA, Kirley SD, et al: Detection of tumor cells in bladder washings by a monoclonal antibody to human bladder tumor–associated antigen. J Urol 140:672-677, 1988.
68. Huffman JL, Fradet Y, Cordon-Cardo C, et al: Effect of intravesical bacillus Calmette-Guerin on detection of a urothelial differentiation antigen in exfoliated cells of carcinoma in situ of the human urinary bladder. Cancer Res 45:5201-5204, 1985.
69. Wright GL Jr, Alexander JP, Konchuba AM, et al: Flow cytometric DNA analysis after immunoselection of bladder tumor cells with monoclonal antibody DU83.21. Cancer 66:1242-1252, 1990.
70. Huffman JL, Garin-Chesa P, Gay H, et al: Flow cytometric identification of human bladder cells using a cytokeratin monoclonal antibody. Ann NY Acad Sci 468:302-315, 1986.
71. Oda H, Oda T, Ohoka H, et al: Flow cytometric evaluation of Thomsen-Friedenreich antigen on transitional cell cancer using monoclonal antibody. Urol Res 18:107-111, 1990.
72. Fradet Y, Tardif M, Bourget L, Robert J, Laval University Urology Group: Clinical cancer progression in urinary bladder tumors evaluated by multiparameter flow cytometry with monoclonal antibodies. Cancer Res 50:432-437, 1990.
73. Flam TA, Chopin DK, Leleu C, et al: Immunohistochemical markers defined by monoclonal antibodies and response to bacillus Calmette-Guerin endovesical immunotherapy for superficial bladder tumors. Eur Urol 17:338-342, 1990.
74. Gross MD, Skinner RW, Grossman HB: Radioimmunodetection of a transplantable human bladder carcinoma in a nude mouse. Invest Radiol 19:530-534, 1984.
75. Bubenik J, Kieler J, Perlmann P, et al: Monoclonal antibodies against human urinary bladder carcinomas: selectivity and utilization for gamma scintigraphy. Eur J Cancer Clin Oncol 21:701-710, 1985.
76. Yu DS, Yeh MY, Chen WL, et al: In vivo localisation of human urinary bladder carcinoma xenograft in nude mice using radiolabelled monoclonal antibody. Br J Urol 59:540-546, 1987.
77. Hansson Y, Paulie S, Ben-Aissa H, et al: Radioimmunolocalisation of bladder tumors xenotransplanted in nude mice. Anticancer Res 8:435-441, 1988.
78. Yeh MY, Yu DS, Chang SY, et al: Radioimmunotherapy of xenografted human bladder cancer using monoclonal antibody against blood group A–related antigen. Eur Urol 14:386-390, 1988.
79. Yu DS, Chu TM, Yeh MY, et al: Antitumor activity of doxorubicin-monoclonal antibody conjugate on human bladder cancer. J Urol 140:415-421, 1988.
80. Chopin DK, deKernion JB: Detection of transitional cell carcinoma in bladder by intravesical injection of monoclonal antibodies. Urol Res 14:145-148, 1986.
81. Hasan T, Lin CW, Lin A: Laser-induced selective cytotoxicity using monoclonal antibody-chromophore conjugates. Prog Clin Biol Res 288:471-477, 1989.
82. Thiesen HJ, Juhl H, Arndt R: Selective killing of human bladder cancer cells by combined treatment with A and B chain ricin antibody conjugates. Cancer Res 47:419-423, 1987.
83. Boeckmann W, Baum RP, Schuldes H, et al: Tumour imaging of bladder carcinomas and their metastases with ^{111}indium-labelled monoclonal anti-CEA antibody BW 431/26. Br J Cancer 10(suppl):81-84, 1990.
84. Hetherington JW, Ewing R, Cooper EH: Evaluation of a double monoclonal antibodies radioimmunoassay for the measurement of carcinoembryonic antigen in the urine of patients with bladder cancer. Eur Urol 12:270-273, 1986.
85. Hall RR, Laurence JR, Nevill AM, Wallace DM: Carcinoembryonic antigen and urothelial carcinoma. Br J Urol 45:88-92, 1973.
86. Baker WC, DeVere White R, Rossitto PV, et al: Quantitative analysis of keratin 18 in the urine of patients with bladder cancer. J Urol 140:436-439, 1988.
87. Rossitto PV, Chan R, Strand MA, et al: Characterization of urinary keratin number 18 using a new assay. J Urol 140:431-435, 1988.
88. McCabe RP, Lamm DL, Haspel MV, et al: A diagnostic-prognostic test for bladder cancer using a monoclonal antibody–based enzyme-linked immunoassay for detection of urinary fibrin(ogen) degradation products. Cancer Res 44:5886-5893, 1984.
89. Stock LM, Brosman SA, Fahey JL, Liu BCS: Ras related oncogene protein as a tumor marker in transitional cell carcinoma of the bladder. J Urol 137:789-792, 1987.
90. Niman HL, Thompson AMH, Yu A, et al: Anti-peptide antibodies detect oncogene-related proteins in urine. Proc Natl Acad Sci USA 82:7924-7928, 1985.
91. Grossman HB, Liebert M, Stein J, et al: Two monoclonal antibodies react with a bladder tumor-associated antigen that is shed in vitro and in vivo. Proc Am Assoc Cancer Res 30:354, 1989.
92. Liu BC, Neuwirth H, Zhu LW, et al: Detection of oncofetal bladder antigen in urine of patients with transitional cell carcinoma. J Urol 137:1258-1261, 1988.

93. Zhau HE, Babaian RJ, Hong S-J: a new 180 kDA urine protein marker associated with bladder cancer. J Urol 144:47-52, 1990.
94. Chodak GW, Hospelhorn V, Judge SM, et al: Increased levels of fibroblast growth factor–like activity in urine from patients with bladder or kidney cancer. Cancer Res 48:2083-2088, 1988.
95. Guirguis R, Schiffmann E, Liu B, et al: Detection of autocrine motility factor in urine as a marker of bladder cancer. J Natl Cancer Inst 80:1203-1211, 1988.
96. Wang MC, Valenzuela LA, Murphy GP, Chu TM: Purification of a human prostate specific antigen. Invest Urol 17:159-163, 1979.
97. Hortin GL, Bahnson RR, Daft M, et al: Differences in values obtained with 2 assays of prostate specific antigen. J Urol 139:762-765, 1988.
98. Stamey TA, Yang N, Hay AR, et al: Prostate-specific antigen as a serum marker for adenocarcinoma of the prostate. N Engl J Med 317:909-916, 1987.
99. Oesterling JE, Chan DW, Epstein JI, et al: Prostate specific antigen in the preoperative and postoperative evaluation of localized prostatic cancer treated with radical prostatectomy. J Urol 139:766-772, 1988.
100. Dundas GS, Porter AT, Venner PM: Prostate-specific antigen: monitoring the response of carcinoma of the prostate to radiotherapy with a new tumor marker. Cancer 66:45-48, 1990.
101. Ercole CJ, Lange PH, Mathisen M, et al: Prostatic specific antigen and prostatic acid phosphatase in the monitoring and staging of patients with prostatic cancer. J Urol 138:1181-1184, 1987.
102. Cooner WH, Mosley BR, Rutherford CL Jr, et al: Prostate cancer detection in a clinical urological practice by ultrasonography, digital rectal examination and prostate C-specific antigen. J Urol 143:1146-1154, 1990.
103. Demura T, Kuzumaki N, Oda A, et al: Establishment and characterization of monoclonal antibody against androgen receptor. J Steroid Biochem 33:845-851, 1989.
104. Mobbs BG, Liu Y: Immunohistochemical localization of progesterone receptor in benign and malignant human prostate. Prostate 16:245-251, 1990.
105. Brawer MK, Nagle RB, Pitts W, et al: Keratin immunoreactivity as an aid to the diagnosis of persistent adenocarcinoma in irradiated human prostates. Cancer 63:454-460, 1989.
106. Goldenberg DM, DeLand FH, Bennett SJ, et al: Radioimmunodetection of prostatic cancer: in vivo use of radioactive antibodies against prostatic acid phosphatase for diagnosis and detection of prostatic cancer by nuclear imaging. JAMA 250:630-635, 1983.
107. Leroy M, Teillac P, Rain JD, et al: Radioimmunodetection of lymph node invasion in prostatic cancer. Cancer 64:1-5, 1989.
108. Babaian RJ, Lamki LM: Radioimmunoscintigraphy of prostate cancer. Semin Nucl Med 19:309-321, 1989.
109. Babaian RJ, Murray JL, Lamki LM, et al: Radioimmunological imaging of metastatic prostatic cancer with ^{111}indium-labeled monoclonal antibody PAY 276. J Urol 137:439-443, 1987.
110. Abdel-Nabi HH, Ortman-Nabi JA, See W, et al: Clinical experience with intra lymphatic administration of ^{111}In-labelled monoclonal antibody PAY 276 for the detection of pelvic nodal metastases in prostatic carcinoma. Eur J Nucl Med 16:149-156, 1990.
111. Wright GL Jr, Wilson E, Klinger M, et al: Radiolocalization of human prostate tumor in a mouse subrenal capsule model by monoclonal antibody TURP-27. Prostate 16:81-89, 1990.
112. Lipford GB, Wright GL: Relationship of the prostate carcinoma–associated antigen Turp 27 to HNK 1 and N-CAMs. Proc Am Assoc Cancer Res 31:261, 1990.
113. Ghazizadeh M, Kagawa S, Izumi K, et al: Immunohistochemical detection of carcinoembryonic antigen in benign hyperplasia and adenocarcinoma of the prostate with monoclonal antibody. J Urol 131:501-503, 1984.
114. Mazur MT, Shultz JJ: Prostatic adenocarcinoma: evaluation of immunoreactivity to monoclonal antibody B72.3. Am J Clin Pathol 93:466-470, 1990.
115. Deguchi T, Chu TM, Leong SS, et al: Effect of methotrexate-monoclonal anti-prostatic acid phosphatase antibody conjugate on human prostate tumor. Cancer Res 46:3751-3755, 1986.
116. Deguchi T, Chu TM, Leong SS, et al: Potential therapeutic effect of adriamycin-monoclonal anti-prostatic acid phosphatase antibody conjugate on human prostate tumor. J Urol 137:353-358, 1987.
117. Mann K, Siddle K: Evidence for free beta-subunit secretion in so-called human chorionic gonadotropin–positive seminoma. Cancer 62:2378-2382, 1988.
118. Saller B, Clara R, Spottl G, et al: Testicular cancer secretes intact human choriogonadotropin (hCG) and its free beta-subunit: evidence that hCG (+hCG-beta) assays are the most reliable in diagnosis and follow-up. Clin Chem 36:234-239, 1990.
119. Bellet DH, Ozturk M, Bidart JM, et al: Sensitive and specific assay for human chorionic gonadotropin (hCG) based on anti-peptide and anti-hCG monoclonal antibodies: construction and clinical implications. J Clin Endocrinol Metab 63:1319-1327, 1986.
120. Virji MA, Mercer DW, Herberman RB: Tumor markers in cancer diagnosis and prognosis. CA 38:104-126, 1988.
121. Battifora H, Sheibani K, Tubbs RR, et al: Antikeratin antibodies in tumor diagnosis: distinction between seminoma and embryonal carcinoma. Cancer 54:843-848-1984.
122. Niehans GA, Manivel JC, Copland GT, et al: Immunohistochemistry of germ cell and trophoblastic neoplasms. Cancer 62:1113-1123, 1988.
123. Hitchins RN, Begent RH, Green AJ, et al: Clinical value of imaging using antibody to alpha fetoprotein in germ cell tumours. Nuklearmedizin 28:29-33, 1989.
124. Pectasides D, Vonorta P, Tsialta-Salihou A, et al: Immunoscintigraphy with ^{131}I-labelled H17E2 monoclonal antibody compared with conventional lymphangiography and computed tomography in the detection of metastases in patients with testicular germ cell tumours. Br J Cancer 10(suppl):74-77, 1990.
125. Epenetos AA, Snook D, Hooker G, et al: Indium-111 labelled monoclonal antibody to placental alkaline phosphatase in the detection of neoplasms of testis, ovary, and cervis. Lancet 2:350-353, 1985.
126. Epenetos AA, Carr D, Johnson PM, et al: Antibody-guided radiolocalisation of tumours in patients with testicular or ovarian cancer using two radioiodinated monoclonal antibodies to placental alkaline phosphatase. Br J Radiol 59:117-125, 1986.
127. Takahashi N, Hayano T, Suzuki M: Petidyl-prolyl cis-trans isomerase is the cyclosporin A-binding protein cyclophilin. Nature 337:473-475, 1989.
128. Fischer G, Wittman-Liebold B, Land K, et al: Cyclophilin and petidyl-prolyl cis-trans isomerase are probably identical proteins. Nature 337:476-478, 1989.
129. Siekierka JJ, Staruch MJ, Hung SHY, Sigal NH: FK-506, a potent novel immunosuppressive agent, binds to a cytosolic protein which is distinct from the cyclosporin A-binding protein, cyclophilin. J Immunol 143:1580-1583, 1989.
130. Carpenter CB: Immunosuppression in organ transplantation. N Engl J Med 322:1224-1226, 1990.
131. Thomson AW: Cyclosporin: mode of action and clinical applications. Boston: Kluwer Academic Publishers, 1989.
132. Ortho Multicenter Transplant Study Group: A randomized clinical trial of OKT3 monoclonal antibody for acute rejection of cadaveric renal transplants. N Engl J Med 313:337-342, 1985.
133. Hricik DE, Mayes JT, Schulak JA: Inhibition of anti-OKT3 antibody generation by cyclosporine—results of a prospective randomized trial. Transplantation 50:237-240, 1990.
134. Soulillou JP, Cantarovich D, Le Mauff B, et al: Random-

ized controlled trial of a monoclonal antibody against the interleukin-2 receptor (33B3.1) as compared with rabbit antithymocyte globulin for prophylaxis against rejection of renal allografts. N Engl J Med 322:1175-1182, 1990.
135. Bach J-F: Summary: symposium of lymphocyte activation. Kidney Int 38:381-383, 1990.
136. Smely S, Weschka M, Hillebrand G, et al: Prophylactic use of the new monoclonal antibody BMA 031 in clinical kidney transplantation. Transplant Proc 22:1785-1786, 1990.
137. Dendorfer U, Hillebrand G, Kasper C, et al: Effective prevention of interstitial rejection crises in immunological high risk patients following renal transplantation: use of high doses of the new monoclonal antibody BMA 031. Transplant Proc 22:1789-1790, 1990.
138. Chatenoud L, Ferran C, Legendre C, et al: Immunological follow-up of renal allograft recipients treated with the BMA 031 (anti-TCR) monoclonal antibody. Transplant Proc 22:1787-1788, 1990.
139. Hall BM: Therapy with monoclonal antibodies to CD4: potential not appreciated? Am J Kidney Dis 14:71-77, 1989.
140. Pressman D: The development and use of radiolabelled anti-tumor antibodies. Cancer Res 40:2960-2964, 1980.
141. Ghose T, Norvell ST, Alquino J, et al: Localisation of 131-I-labelled antibodies in human renal cell carcinomas and in a mouse hepatoma and correlation with tumour detection by photoscanning. Cancer Res 40:3018-3031, 1980.
142. Order SE, Klein JL, Ettinger D, et al: Phase I-II study of radiolabelled antibody integrated into the treatment of primary hepatic malignancies. Int J Radiat Oncol Biol Phys 6:703-710, 1980.
143. Goldenberg DM, DeLand FH, Kim E, et al: Use of radiolabelled antibodies to carcinoembryonic antigen for the detection and localisation of diverse cancers by external photoscanning. N Engl J Med 298:1384-1388, 1978.
144. Epenetos AA, Snook D, Durbin H, et al: Limitations of radiolabeled monoclonal antibodies for localization of human neoplasms. Cancer Res 46:3183-3191, 1986.
145. Lotze MT, Rosenberg SA: The immunologic treatment of cancer. CA 38:68-94, 1988.
146. Jain RK: Delivery of novel therapeutic agents in tumors: physiological barriers and strategies. J Natl Cancer Inst 81:570-576, 1989.
147. Dykes PW, Bradwell AR, Chapman CE, Vaughan ATM: Radioimmunotherapy of cancer: clinical studies and limiting factors. Cancer Treat Rev 14:87-106, 1987.
148. Kosmas C, Epenetos AA: Monoclonal antibodies for imaging and therapy. Br J Cancer 59:152-155, 1989.
149. Kosmas C, Man S, Epenetos AA, Courtenay-Luck NS: The role of humoral and cellular immunity in patients developing human anti-murine immunoglobulin antibody responses after radioimmunotherapy. Br J Cancer 10(suppl):85-88, 1990.
150. Lamm DL, Crissmann J, Blumenstein B, et al: Adriamycin versus BCG in superficial bladder cancer: a Southwest Oncology Group Study. Prog Clin Biol Res 310:263-270, 1989.
151. Ratliff TL, Gillen D, Catalona WJ: Requirement of a thymus dependent immune response for BCG-medicated antitumor activity. J Urol 137:155-158, 1987.
152. Bohle A, Gerdes J, Ulmer AJ, et al: Effects of local bacillus Calmette-Guerin therapy in patients with bladder carcinoma on immunocompetent cells of the bladder wall. J Urol 144:53-58, 1990.
153. Bohle A, Nowc C, Ulmer AJ, et al: Elevations of cytokines interleukin-1, interleukin-2, and tumor necrosis factor in the urine of patients after intravesical bacillus Calmette-Guerin immunotherapy. J Urol 144:59-64, 1990.
154. Haaf EO, Catalona WJ, Ratliff TL: Detection of interleukin-2 in the urine of patients with superficial bladder tumors after treatment with intravesical BCG. J Urol 136:970-974, 1986.
155. Netto NR Jr, Lemos GC: A comparison of treatment methods for the prophylaxis of recurrent superficial bladder tumors. J Urol 129:33-34, 1983.
156. Lamm DL, DeHaven JI, Shriver J, et al: A randomized prospective comparison of oral versus intravesical and percutaneous bacillus Calmette-Guerin for superficial bladder cancer. J Urol 144:65-67, 1990.
157. Herr HW, Pinsky CM, Whitmore WF Jr, et al: Long-term effect of intravesical bacillus Calmette-Guerin on flat carcinoma in situ of the bladder. J Urol 135:265-267, 1986.
158. Herr HW, Whitmore WF Jr: Ureteral carcinoma in situ after successful intravesical therapy for superficial bladder tumors: incidence, possible pathogenesis and management. J Urol 138:292-294, 1987.
159. Olsson CA, Chute R, Chadalawada NR: Immunologic reduction of bladder cancer recurrence rate. J Urol 111:173-176, 1974.
160. Jurincic CD, Engelmann U, Gasch J, Klippel KF: Immunotherapy in bladder cancer with keyhole-limpet hemocyanin: a randomized study. J Urol 139:723-726, 1988.
161. Flamm J, Bucher A, Holtl W, Albrecht W: Recurrent superficial transitional cell carcinoma of the bladder: adjuvant topical chemotherapy versus immunotherapy; a prospective randomized trial. J Urol 144:260-263, 1990.
162. Mantovani A, Dejana E: Cytokines as communication signals between leukocytes and endothelial cells. Immunol Today 10:370-375, 1989.
163. Balkwill FR, Burke F: The cytokine network. Immunol Today 10:299-304, 1989.
164. Sporn MB, Roberts AB: Peptide growth factors are multifunctional. Nature 332:217-219, 1988.
165. Quesada JR: Biological response modifiers in the therapy of metastatic renal cell carcinoma. Semin Oncol 15:396-407, 1988.
166. Horoszewicz JS, Murphy GP: An assessment of the current use of interferons in therapy of urological cancers. J Urol 142:1173-1180, 1989.
167. Guadagni F, Witt PL, Robbins PF, et al: Regulation of carcinoembryonic antigen expression in different human colorectal tumor cells by interferon-gamma. Cancer Res 50:6248-6255, 1990.
168. Greiner JW, Fisher PB, Pestka S, Schlom J: Differential effects of recombinant leukocyte interferons on cell surface antigen expression. Cancer Res 46:4984-4990, 1986.
169. Stotter H, Wiebke EA, Tomita S, et al: Cytokines alter target susceptibility of lysis. II. Evaluation of tumor infiltrating lymphocytes. J Immunol 142:1767-1773, 1989.
170. Hawkins MJ, Krown SE, Borden EC, et al: American Cancer Society phase I trial of naturally produced beta-interferon. Cancer Res 44:5934-5938, 1984.
171. Kuebler JP, Goodman PJ, Brown TD, et al: Phase II study of continuous infusion recombinant gamma interferon in renal carcinoma. Invest New Drugs 8:307-309, 1990.
172. de Mulder PH, Debruyne FM, Franssen MP, et al: Phase I/II study of recombinant interferon alpha and gamma in advanced progressive renal-cell carcinoma. Cancer Immunol Immunother 31:321-324, 1990.
173. Torti FM, Lum BL: Superficial bladder cancer: risk of recurrence and potential role for interferon therapy. Cancer 59:613-616, 1987.
174. Glashan RW: A randomized controlled study of intravesical alpha-2b-interferon in carcinoma in situ of the bladder. J Urol 144:658-661, 1990.
175. Old LJ: Tumor necrosis factor. Sci Am 258:59-75, 1988.
176. Akira S, Hirano T, Taga T, Kishimotot T: Biology of multifunctional cytokines: IL6 and related molecules (IL1 and TNF). FASEB J 4:2860-2867, 1990.
177. Mantovani A, Dejana E: Cytokines as communication signal between leukocytes and endothelial cells. Immunol Today 10:370-375, 1989.
178. Chapman PB, Lester TJ, Caper ES, et al: Clinical pharmacology of recombinant human tumor necrosis factor in patients with advanced cancer. J Clin Oncol 5:1942-1951, 1987.
179. Blick M, Sherwin SA, Rosenblum M, Gutterman J: Phase

I study of recombinant tumor necrosis factor in cancer patients. Cancer Res 47:2986-2989, 1987.
180. Bahnson RR, Ballou BT, Ernstoff MS, et al: Toxicity of intravesical recombinant human tumor necrosis factor in cynomolgus monkeys. J Biol Response Mod 9:445-447, 1990.
181. Ostensen MO, Thiele DL, Lipsky PE: Tumor necrosis factor-alpha enhances cytolytic activity of human natural killer cells. J Immunol 138:4185-4191, 1987.
182. Alexander RB, Nelson WG, Coffey DS: Synergistic enhancement by tumor necrosis factor of in vitro cytotoxicity from chemotherapeutic drugs targeted at DNA topoisomerase II. Cancer Res 47:2403-2406, 1987.
183. Donaldson JT, Keane TE, Poulton SH, Walther PJ: Enhanced in vivo cytotoxicity of recombinant human tumor necrosis factor with etoposide in human renal cell carcinoma. Urol Res 18:245-250, 1990.
184. Sondel PM, Hank JA: Prospects for clinical cancer treatment using interleukin-2. Cancer Invest 7:437-442, 1989.
185. Rubin JT, Elwood LJ, Rosenberg SA, Lotze MT: Immunohistochemical correlates of response to recombinant interleukin-2-based immunotherapy in humans. Cancer Res 49:7086-7092, 1989.
186. Pizza G, Severini G, Menniti D, et al: Tumor regression after intralesional injection of interleukin-2 (IL-2) in bladder cancer: preliminary report. Int J Cancer 34:359-367, 1984.
187. Huland E, Huland H: Local continuous high dose interleukin 2: a new therapeutic model for the treatment of advanced bladder cancer. Cancer Res 49:5469-5474, 1989.
188. Mule JJ, Rosenberg SA: Immunotherapy with lymphokine combinations. Important Adv Oncol 1989:99-126, 1989.
189. Redman BG, Flaherty L, Chou T-S, et al: A phase I trial of recombinant interleukin-2 combined with recombinant interferon-gamma in patients with cancer. J Clin Oncol 8:1269-1276, 1990.
190. Krigel RL, Padavic-Shaller KA, Rudolph AR, et al: Renal cell carcinoma: treatment with recombinant interleukin-2 plus beta-interferon. J Clin Oncol 8:460-467, 1990.
191. Rosenberg SA: Immunotherapy of cancer using interleukin-2: current status and future prospects. Immunol Today 9:58-62, 1988.
192. Sondel PM, Hank JA: Prospects for clinical cancer treatment using interleukin-2. Cancer Invest 7:437-442, 1989.
193. Lotze MT, Custer MC, Bolton ES, et al: Mechanisms of immunologic antitumor therapy: lessons from the laboratory and clinical applications. Hum Immunol 28:198-207, 1990.
194. Alexander RB, Isaacs JT, Coffey DS: Tumor necrosis factor enhances the in vitro and in vivo efficacy of chemotherapeutic drugs targeted at DNA topoisomerase II in the treatment of murine bladder cancer. J Urol 138:427-429, 1987.
195. Borden EC, Creekmore SP: Cancer therapy with combinations of biological response modifiers and cytotoxics: an update. Cancer Cells 2:217-220, 1990.
196. Regenass U, Muller M, Curschellas E, Matter A: Antitumor effects of tumor necrosis factor in combination with chemotherapeutic agents. Int J Cancer 39:266-273, 1987.
197. Wadler S, Wersto R, Weinberg V, et al: Interaction and fluorouracil and interferon in human colon cancer cell lines: cytotoxic and cytokinetic effects. Cancer Res 50:5735-5739, 1990.
198. Vuist WMJ, V Buitenen F, Hekman A, Melief CJM: Two distinct mechanisms of antitumor activity mediated by the combination of interleukin 2 and monoclonal antibodies. Cancer Res 50:5676-5772, 1990.
199. Hank JA, Robinson RR, Surfus J, et al: Augmentation of antibody dependent cell mediated cytotoxicity following in vivo therapy with recombinant interleukin 2. Cancer Res 50:5234-5239, 1990.
200. Russell SM, Krauer KG, McKenzie IFC, Pietersz GA: Effect of tumor necrosis factor on the antitumor efficacy and toxicity of aminopterin-monoclonal antibody conjugates: parameters for optimization of therapy. Cancer Res 50:6028-6033, 1990.
201. Smyth MJ, Pietrsz GA, McKenzie IF: Increased antitumor effect of immunoconjugates and tumor necrosis factor in vivo. Cancer Res 48:3607-3612, 1988.
202. Rosenblum MG, Lamki LA, Murray JL, et al: Interferon-induced changes in pharmacokinetics and tumor uptake of In-111-labeled antimelanoma antibody 96.5 in melanoma patients. J Natl Cancer Inst 80:160-165, 1988.
203. Gabrilove JL, Jakubowski A, Scher H, et al: Effect of granulocyte colony–stimulating factor on neutropenia and associated morbidity due to chemotherapy for transitional-cell carcinoma of the urothelium. N Engl J Med 318:1414-1422, 1988.
204. Logothetis CJ, Dexeus FH, Sella A, et al: Escalated therapy for refractory urothelial tumors: methotrexate-vinblastine-doxorubicin-cisplatin plus unglycosylated recombinant human granulocyte–macrophage colony—stimulating factor. J Natl Cancer Inst 82:667-672, 1990.
205. Cosman D: Colony-stimulating factors in vivo and in vitro. Immunol Today 9:97-98, 1988.
206. Bendtzen K, Svenson M, Jonsson V, Hippe E: Autoantibodies to cytokines—friends or foes? Immunol Today 11:167-169, 1990.
207. Rosenberg SA: Adoptive immunotherapy for cancer. Sci Am 262:62-69, 1990.
208. Rosenberg SA, Lotze MT, Muul LM, et al: A progress report on the treatment of 157 patients with advanced cancer using lymphokine-activated killer cells and interleukin-2 or high-dose interleukin-2 alone. N Engl J Med 316:889-897, 1987.
209. West WH, Tauer KW, Yannelli JR, et al: Constant-infusion recombinant interleukin-2 in adoptive immunotherapy of advanced cancer. N Engl J Med 316:898-905, 1987.
210. Fisher RI, Coltman CA, Doroshow JH, et al: Metastatic renal cancer treated with interleukin-2 and lymphokine-activated killer cells. Ann Intern Med 108:518-523, 1988.
211. Robertson CN, Linehan WM, Pass HI, et al: Preparative cytoreductive surgery in patients with metastatic renal cell carcinoma treated with adoptive immunotherapy with interleukin-2 or interleukin-2 plus lymphokine activated killer cells. J Urol 144:614-618, 1990.
212. Belldegrun A, Uppenkamp I, Rosenberg SA: Anti-tumor reactivity of human lymphokine activated killer (LAK) cells against fresh and cultured preparations of renal cell cancer. J Urol 139:150-155, 1988.
213. Phillips JH, Gemlo BT, Myers WW, et al: In vivo and in vitro activation of natural killer cells in advanced cancer patients undergoing recombinant interleukin-2 and LAK cell therapy. J Clin Oncol 5:1933-1941, 1987.
214. Harel W, Shau H, Hadley CG, et al: Increased lysis of melanoma by in vivo–elicited human lymphokine–activated killer cells after addition of antiganglioside antibodies in vitro. Cancer Res 50:6311-6315, 1990.
215. Wang JCL, Walle A, Novogrodsky A, et al: A phase II clinical trial of adoptive immunotherapy for advanced renal cell carcinoma using mitogen-activated autologous leukocytes and continuous infusion interleukin-2. J Clin Oncol 7:1885-1891, 1989.
216. Fisher B, Packard BS, Read EJ, et al: Tumor localization of adoptively transferred indium-111 labeled tumor infiltrating lymphocytes in patients with metastatic melanoma. J Clin Oncol 7:250-261, 1989.
217. Blay J-Y, Favrot MC, Negrier S, et al: Correlation between clinical response to interleukin 2 therapy and sustained production of tumor necrosis factor. Cancer Res 50:2371-2374, 1990.
218. Boccoli G, Masciulli R, Ruggeri EM, et al: Adoptive immunotherapy of human cancer: the cytokine cascade and monocyte activation following high dose interleukin-2 bolus treatment. Cancer Res 50:5795-5800, 1990.

219. Parmiani G: An explanation of the variable clinical response to interleukin 2 and LAK cells. Immunol Today 11:113-115, 1990.
220. Ochoa AC, Hasz DE, Rezonzo R, et al. Lymphokine-activated killer activity in long-term cultures with anti-CD3 plus interleukin 2: identification and isolation of effector subsets. Cancer Res 49:963-968, 1989.
221. Yang SC, Own-Schaub LB, Roth LA, Grimm EA: Characterization of OKT3-initiated lymphokine-activated effectors expanded with interleukin 2 and tumor necrosis factor alpha. Cancer Res 50:3526-3532, 1990.
222. Osband ME, Lavin PT, Babayan RK, et al: Effect of autolymphocyte therapy on survival and quality of life in patients with metastatic renal cell carcinoma. Lancet 335:994-998, 1990.
223. Tomita Y, Nishiyama T, Fujiwara M, Sato S: Immunohistochemical detection of major histocompatibility antigens and quantitative analysis of tumor-infiltrating mononuclear cells in renal cell cancer. Br J Cancer 62:354-359, 1990.
224. Rosenberg SA, Spiess PJ, Lafreniere R: A new approach to the adoptive immunotherapy of cancer with tumor-infiltrating lymphocytes. Science 223:1318-1321, 1986.
225. Cameron RB, Spiess PJ, Rosenberg SA: Synergistic antitumor activity of tumor-infiltrating lymphocytes, interleukin-2, and local tumor irradiation: studies on the mechanisms of action. J Exp Med 171:249-263, 1990.
226. Finke JH, Rayman R, Alexander J, et al: Characterization of the cytolytic activity of CD4+ and CD8+ tumor-infiltrating lymphocytes in human renal cell carcinoma. Cancer Res 50:2363-2370, 1990.
227. Haas GP, Solomon D, Rosenberg SA: Tumor-infiltrating lymphocytes from nonrenal urological malignancies. Cancer Immunol Immunother 30:342-350, 1990.
228. Rosenberg SA, Packard BS, Aebersold PM, et al: Use of tumor-infiltrating lymphocytes and interleukin-2 in the immunotherapy of patients with metastatic melanoma. N Engl J Med 319:1676-1680, 1988.
229. Rosenberg SA, Aebersold P, Cornetta K, et al: Gene transfer into humans—immunotherapy of patients with advanced melanoma, using tumor-infiltrating lymphocytes modified by retroveral gene transduction. N Engl J Med 323:570-578, 1990.
230. Yron I, Wood TA Jr, Spiess PJ, Rosenberg SA: In vitro growth of murine T cells. V. The isolation and growth of lymphoid cells infiltrating syngeneic solid tumors. J Immunol 125:238-245, 1980.
231. Topalian SL, Kasid A, Rosenberg SA: Immunoselection of a human melanoma resistant to specific lysis by autologous tumor-infiltrating lymphocytes: possible mechanism for immunotherapeutic failures. J Immunol 144:4487-4495, 1990.
232. Weber JS, Rosenberg SA: Effects of murine tumor class I major histocompatibility complex expression on antitumor activity of tumor-infiltrating lymphocytes. J Natl Cancer Inst 82:755-761, 1990.
233. Fox BA, Spiess PJ, Kasid A, et al: In vitro and in vivo antitumor properties of a T-cell clone generated from murine tumor–infiltrating lymphocytes. J Biol Response Mod 9:499-511, 1990.
234. Salup PR, Wiltrout RH: Adjuvant immunotherapy of established murine renal cancer by interleukin-2 stimulated cytotoxic lymphocytes. Cancer Res 46:3358-3363, 1986.
235. Stephenson KR, Perry-Lalley D, Griffith KD, et al: Development of antitumor reactivity in regional draining lymph nodes from tumor-immunized and tumor-bearing murine hosts. Surgery 105:523-528, 1989.
236. Chou T, Chang AE, Shu SY: Generation of therapeutic T lymphocytes from tumor-bearing mice by in vitro sensitization: culture requirements and characterization of immunologic specificity. J Immunol 140:2453-2461, 1988.
237. Chou T, Chang AE, Shu S: Generation of therapeutic T lymphocytes from tumor-bearing mice by in vitro sensitization: culture requirements and characterization of immunologic specificity. J Immunol 140:2453-2461, 1988.
238. Shou T, Bertera S, Chang AE, Shu S: Adoptive immunotherapy of microscopic and advanced visceral metastases with in vitro sensitized lymphoid cells from mice bearing progressive tumors. J Immunol 141:1775-1781, 1988.
239. Southern EM: Detection of specific sequences among DNA fragments separated by gel electrophoresis. J Mol Biol 98:503-517, 1975.
240. Hopman AHN, Poddighe PJ, Smeets AWGB, et al: Detection of numerical chromosome aberrations in bladder cancer by in situ hybridization. Am J Pathol 135:1105-1117, 1989.
241. Eisenstein BI: The polymerase chain reaction: a new method of using molecular genetics for medical diagnosis. N Engl J Med 322:178-183, 1990.
242. Slamon DJ: Proto-oncogenes and human cancers. N Engl J Med 317:955-957, 1987.
243. Santos E, Tonic SR, Aaronson SA, et al: T24 human bladder carcinoma oncogene is an activated form of the normal human homologue of Balb- and Harvey-MSV transforming genes. Nature 298:343-347, 1982.
244. Reddy EP, Reynolds RK, Santos E, Barbacid M: A point mutation is responsible for the acquisition of transforming properties by the T24 human bladder carcinoma oncogene. Nature 300:149-152, 1982.
245. Shih C, Weinberg RA: Isolation of a transforming sequence from a human bladder carcinoma cell line. Cell 29:161-169, 1982.
246. McBride OW, Swan DC, Santos E, et al: Localization of the normal allele of T24 human bladder carcinoma oncogene to chromosome 11. Nature 300:773-774, 1982.
247. Fujita J, Srivastava SK, Kraus MH, et al: Frequency of molecular alterations affecting *ras* protooncogenes in human urinary tract tumors. Proc Natl Acad Sci USA 82:3849-3853, 1985.
248. Malone PR, Visvanathan KV, Ponder BAJ, et al: Oncogenes and bladder cancer. Br J Urol 57:664-667, 1985.
249. Visvanathan KV, Pocock RD, Summerhayes IC: Preferential and novel activation of H-*ras* in human bladder carcinomas. Oncogene Res 3:77-86, 1988.
250. Geiser AG, Der CJ, Marshall CJ, Stanbridge EJ: Suppression of tumorigenicity with continued expression of the c-Ha-*ras* oncogene in EJ bladder carcinoma–human fibroblast hybrid cells. Proc Natl Acad Sci USA 83:5209-5213, 1986.
251. Ledwith BJ, Manam S, Kraynak AR, et al: Antisense-*fos* RNA causes partial reversion of the transformed phenotypes induced by the c-Ha-*ras* oncogene. Mol Cell Biol 10:1545-1555, 1990.
252. Kovacs G, Wilkins L, Papp T, de Riese W: Differentiation between papillary and nonpapillary renal cell carcinomas by DNA analysis. J Natl Cancer Inst 81:527-530, 1989.
253. Seizinger BR, Rouleau GA, Ozelius LJ, et al: Von Hippel–Lindau disease maps to the region of chromosome 3 associated with renal cell carcinoma. Nature 332:268-269, 1988.
254. Mikkelsen T, Cavenee WK: Suppressors of the malignant phenotype. Cell Growth Diff 1:201-207, 1990.
255. Fearon ER, Feinberg AP, Hamilton SH, Vogelstein B: Loss of genes on the short arm of chromosome 11 in bladder cancer. Nature 318:377-380, 1985.
256. Olumi AF, Tsai YC, Nichols PW, et al: Allelic loss of chromosome 17p distinguishes high grade from low grade transitional cell carcinomas of the bladder. Cancer Res 50:7081-7083, 1990.
257. McGrath T, Center MS: Mechanisms of multidrug resistance in HL 60 cells: evidence that a surface membrane protein distinct from P-glycoprotein contributes to reduced cellular accumulation of drug. Cancer Res 48:3959-3963, 1988.

258. Deffie AM, Alam T, Seneviratne C, et al: Multifactorial resistance to adriamycin: relationship of DNA repair, glutathione transferase activity, drug efflux, and P-glycoprotein in cloned cell lines of adriamycin-sensitive and -resistant P388 leukemia. Cancer Res 48:3595-3602, 1988.
259. Ueda K, Cornwell MM, Gottesman MM, et al: The *mdr1* gene, responsible for multidrug-resistance, codes for P-glycoprotein. Biochem Biophys Res Commun 141:956-962, 1986.
260. Pastan I, Gottesman MM, Ueda K, et al: A retrovirus carrying an *MDR1* cDNA confers multidrug resistance and polarized expression of P-glycoprotein MDCK cells. Proc Natl Acad Sci USA 85:4486-4490, 1988.
261. Chin JE, Soffir R, Noonan KE, et al: Structure and expression of the human *MDR* (P-glycoprotein) gene family. Mol Cell Biol 9:3808-3820, 1989.
262. van der Bliek AM, Baas F, de Lange TTH, et al: The human *mdr3* gene encodes a novel P-glycoprotein homologue and gives rise to alternatively spliced mRNAs in liver. EMBO J 6:3325-3331, 1987.
263. Kanamaru H, Kakehi Y, Yoshida O, et al: MDR1 RNA levels in human renal cell carcinomas: correlation with grade and prediction of reversal of doxorubicin resistance by quinidine in tumor explants. J Natl Cancer Inst 81:844-849, 1989.
264. Nooter K, Sonneveld P, Janssen A, et al: Expression of the *mdr3* gene in prolymphocytic leukemia: association with cyclosporin-A-induced increase in drug accumulation. Int J Cancer 45:626-631, 1990.
265. Dalton WS, Grogan TM, Meltzer PS, et al: Drug-resistance in multiple myeloma and non-Hodgkin's lymphoma: detection of P-glycoprotein and potential circumvention by addition of verapamil to chemotherapy. J Clin Oncol 7:415-424, 1989.
266. Hofsli E, Nissen-Meyer J: Reversal of multidrug resistance by lipophilic drugs. Cancer Res 50:3997-4002, 1990.
267. Paganelli G, Pervez S, Siccardi AG, et al: Intraperitoneal radio-localization of tumors pre-targeted by biotinylated monoclonal antibodies. Int J Cancer 45:1184-1189, 1990.
268. Morrison SL, Schlom J: Recombinant chimeric monoclonal antibodies. Important Adv Oncol 1990:3-18, 1990.
269. Mayforth RD, Quintans J: Designer and catalytic antibodies. N Engl J Med 323:173-178, 1990.
270. Colcher D, Milenic D, Roselli M, et al: Characterization and biodistribution of recombinant and recombinant/chimeric constructs of monoclonal antibody B72.3. Cancer Res 49:1738-1745, 1989.
271. Colcher D, Bird R, Roselli M, et al: In vivo tumor targeting of a recombinant single-chain antigen-binding protein. J Natl Cancer Inst 82:1191-1197, 1990.
272. Senter PD: Activation of prodrugs by antibody-enzyme conjugates: a new approach to cancer therapy. FASEB J 4:188-193, 1990.
273. Webb KS, Poulton SH, Liberman SN, Walther PJ: Rationale for immunotoxin therapy of metastatic prostate carcinoma formulated as a multi-stage delivery system. J Urol 142:425-432, 1989.
274. Barth RF, Alam F, Soloway AH, et al: Boronated monoclonal antibody 17-1A for potential neutron capture therapy of colorectal cancer. Hybridoma 5:s43-s50, 1986.
275. Sardi A, Workman M, Mojzisik C, et al: Intraabdominal recurrence of colorectal cancer detected by radioimmunoguided surgery (RIGS System). Arch Surg 124:55-59, 1989.
276. Kennedy RC, Melnick JL, Dreesman GR: Anti-idiotypes and immunity. Sci Am 255:48-56, 1986.
277. Kennedy RC, Adler-Storthz K, Henkel RD, et al: Immune response to hepatitis B surface antigen: enhancement by prior injection of antibodies to the idiotype. Science 221:853-855, 1983.
278. Zhou EM, Kennedy RC: Strategies for developing vaccines against acquired immunodeficiency syndrome. Biochim Biophys Acta 989:301-313, 1989.
279. Herlyn D, Wettendorff M, Schmoll E, et al: Anti-idiotype immunization of cancer patients: modulation of the immune response. Proc Natl Acad Sci USA 84:8055-8059, 1987.
280. Kerr L, Huntoon C, Donohue J, et al: Heteroconjugate antibody–directed killing of autologous human renal carcinoma cells by in vitro–activated lymphocytes. J Immunol 144:4060-4067, 1990.

CHAPTER 13

STAPLING DEVICES IN UROLOGY

ANITA N. CASSIS and T. RAND PRITCHETT

The development of stapling devices has added greatly to the armamentarium of the urologic surgeon. Their application was originally limited to bowel anastomoses, but innovations in urology and technical refinements in the instruments and staples have expanded their use to other surgical procedures. This chapter reviews the history and development of surgical stapling devices and the healing and physiology of stapled intestinal wounds. The various metal and absorbable stapling products used in urology are described. The use of staples in small bowel anastomoses, large to small bowel anastomoses, ileal loop, and continent urinary diversion procedures is discussed. For each procedure the technique, potential errors, and precautions are discussed. This comprehensive review should acquaint the urologist with the stapling devices available and provide the information needed to use stapling devices confidently in urologic surgical procedures.

HISTORY AND DEVELOPMENT OF STAPLERS IN SURGERY

The concepts that formed the basis for the development of stapling devices in the early 1900s stemmed from the development of nonstapling mechanical suturing devices in the early 1800s. In 1826 Felix-Nicholas Denans demonstrated a perfectly healed end-to-end iliostomy in a dog. Denans' apparatus consisted of metal rings or ferrules held together by suture that approximated the serous surfaces of the bowel over luminal cylinders.[1] The serosal surfaces of the inverted bowel ends became adherent, and the inverted margins sloughed, resulting in luminal continuity. The rings then passed out in the stool. Variations of Denans' apparatus and technique followed. In 1826 J.H.F. Henroz introduced articulated rings containing alternating pins and holes.[1] The rings were placed outside the bowel with a flange on one everted end, the opposing pins and holes were matched, and the rings were clasped together, creating an end-to-end everting anastomosis. The rings remained permanently in place. Further developments included internal absorbable sutured rings, needle-armed anastomosing blocks and cylinders, and bowel-compressing buttons. The most widely used apparatus was the "Murphy button," which was introduced by John D. Murphy in 1892 and was used in cholecystoduodenal anastomosis.[1] Murphy's button consisted of two metal mushroomlike buttons with hollow stems that telescoped into each other after the mushroom cap of each button was secured in the bowel by a purse-string suture around each of the hollow stems. Compression of the bowel borders between the two mushroom caps resulted in necrosis and reestablished bowel continuity. This implanted device was the basis for many technical and surgical modifications, such as the device for rectocolic anastomoses introduced by Sugarbaker in 1951.[2] His instrument used the principles of retention, via the Henroz mechanism of pins and holes, and of anastomosis, via compression necrosis as in the Murphy button. The literature from the mid-1800s until as late as 1965 included many experimental and clinical reports of nonstapling devices for anorectal anastomoses. Like Sugarbaker's device, most instruments were based on the Murphy button or Henroz principle and resulted in the placement of permanent prostheses. Application of these prostheses required opening the viscus, which led to soilage and contamination.

The use of stapling instruments in bowel sugery was pioneered by Humer Hültl of Budapest, Hungary.[1,3] He recognized the need for a nonmanual surgical device that would allow resection, permit closure of a whole viscus in a clean maneuver without spillage or contamination, and shorten operating time. He challenged Victor Fisher, an engineer and talented manufacturer of surgical instruments, to create such a mechanical suture instrument. In 1908 Fisher presented Hültl with a stapler that could produce staple lines in two lengths, 11 cm for gastric closure and 7 cm for pyloric closure. The instrument was large and had two jaws, one containing slots for the insertion of four rows of steel-wire staples and the other containing curved fixed depressions, or anvils, for forming the staples. When the jaws of the clamp were locked on the viscus, a crank was turned to advance a bar that moved forward and drove the staples sequentially. Manual transection between the two middle rows of staples was then performed, leaving a double staggered row of staples on either side of the divided viscus. This was used only for temporary closure to prevent soiling, and Hültl always inverted the stapled ends with conventional sutures.

Over the subsequent 20 years the Fisher-Hültl stapler underwent several modifications and was the prototype for many staplers. One example was the von Petz stapler, introduced in 1924.[1] This instrument applied two rows of staples of German silver wire and was used for temporary closure of the stomach or intestine before transection. Although the von Petz stapler was popular in its time, Hültl's double staggered row of staples has prevailed in modern devices. The need for the leg of the staple to perforate both walls of the viscus, strike a fixed jaw or anvil, and curve into the tissue to form a B staple closure was also first recognized by Hültl and Fisher and has been a principle of every stapling instrument since theirs.

Two disadvantages of the early staplers were the bulk of the instruments and the complexity of the staple driving mechanism. In 1926 Stefan Sandor presented a new stapling instrument that was lighter and mechanically simpler and that placed the staples obliquely in a simultaneous rather than sequential fashion.[1] The compact instrument had three handles; the lower two closed over the viscus, and the third was a clamp that drove the staples when pressed. This was believed to be a significant advance over the crank and wheel mechanisms that drove the instruments of Hültl and von Petz.

Japanese modifications of the von Petz instrument were introduced by K. Nakayama in 1954.[1] He, like Sandor, removed the wheel and advancing bar, firing the staples with a pair of pliers that pressed down the housings holding the staple drivers. An additional and attractive feature of this instrument was a slot in the slender upper jaws that permitted scalpel division of the tissues between the two staple lines while the clamp was still holding the viscus firmly.

At the Moscow Scientific Research Institute for Experimental Surgical Apparatus and Instruments a program to develop stapling instruments was begun in 1950. Included were instruments for terminal or tangential linear closure of bronchi, pulmonary vessels, and most elements of the gastrointestinal (GI) tract. The greatest contribution was that a preloaded staple cartridge could be placed in these instruments. These metal cartridges were preloaded by hand with fine wire staples, originally of tantalum and then of a steel alloy. The instruments had to be partially disassembled to replace the cartridges. The use of replaceable cartridges and reusable stapling devices was an important concept.

The Russians devised an instrument called the UKL, which applied a single row of staples for linear closure of the lung. For creation of a side-to-side GI anastomosis they created an instrument that included a knife for simultaneous bowel transection and stapling. A single row of staples on each side of the division required manual reinforcement of the staple line, and then the common opening of the bowel was closed with a manually placed purse-string suture to complete a side-to-side bowel anastomosis.

Russian instruments for inverting, end-to-end, circular anastomoses in the GI tract were introduced as early as 1960. Kalinina and Androsov are credited with the early use of these instruments in esophagogastrostomy and colorectal anastomosis.[1]

The Russians also devised an instrument for clipping vessels in continuity, leaving a space for the surgeon to divide the vessel with scissors. They experimented with this instrument in the laboratory and found it unsatisfactory and undependable. The concept of vessel ligation in continuity to allow transection, however, was the basis for a later American instrument that not only ligated but also divided vessels, the ligating and dividing stapler.

All of the Soviet instruments were finished by hand, and their parts were not interchangeable. Replaceable cartridges were available for most instruments, but the cartridges had to be loaded by hand, which was time consuming. Furthermore, the instrument required partial disassembly to replace an expended cartridge. The many fine moving parts created difficulties in usage, cleaning, and maintenance.

As the Soviet literature was carrying reports on the creation of surgical staplers, in America experimental and clinical evaluation of mechanical suturing devices had begun. Dr. Mark Ravitch, a general surgeon (Figure 13–1), pioneered experimental and clinical study of stapling devices in America after he visited the Scientific Research Institute for Experimental Surgical Apparatus and Instruments in Moscow in 1958.[4] He bought a UKL stapler, brought it back to America, and embarked on modifications not only of this instrument, but also of all the instruments available in Russia. From his endeavors came the United States Surgical Corp. (USSC). It took 3 years, from 1964 to 1967, to develop instruments that met American surgical standards. The American goal was to improve mechanical efficiency of the device and to increase its surgical potential and applicability.

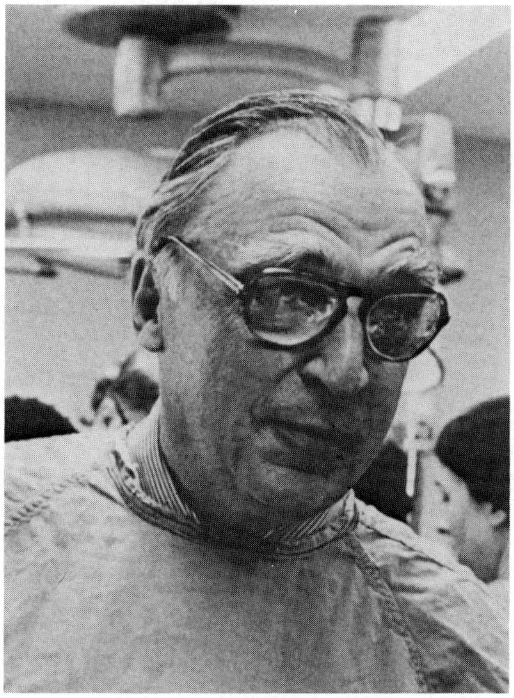

FIGURE 13–1. Dr. Mark Ravitch pioneered the development and use of stapling devices in America.

The principal problem with the Russian staplers was the method of cartridge loading. At the time of surgery the fine staples had to be placed individually in a series of minuscule slots, requiring the use of a magnifying glass. The problem was solved by creating preloaded cartridges that could be slipped into the stapling devices without partial disassembly at the tme of surgery. The cartridges also included a knife blade. From the prototype Russian stapler came the American-made gastrointestinal anastomosis stapling device, the thoracoabdominal stapling device, and the end-to-end anastomosing device. Skin and fascial closure stapling devices, for which no Russian prototypes existed, were manufactured. The successful ligating and dividing stapler, which included a knife blade for dividing vessels in continuity, was another stapling device first made in America.

American instruments were characterized by better balance and by modifications in size and shape. Unlike the Soviet instruments, the American devices did not have a knob that was screwed down to close the jaws of the instrument. Instead they had a single lever that approximated the jaws, eliminating the need to screw down the jaws of the gastrointestinal anastomosis or thoracoabdominal instruments. A wing nut apparatus replaced the knob of the prototype end-to-end anastomosing stapler. In addition, the tissue retention and jaw aligning pin became a part of the instrument and slipped into place as the lever approximated the jaws. All instruments had double staggered rows of staples rather than a single row. The latest development has been disposable units, incorporating a basic unit with its corresponding cartridge, all disposable after a single use. The American stapling instruments followed the principles first developed in the nonstapling anastomotic devices of the 1800s and the original Hültl instrument in that they operated in two stages. In the first stage the instrument jaws are approximated to coapt the tissues with the desired degree of compression, and in the second stage staples are driven through the thick tissues, which are held immobile so that the sharpened staple penetrates without tearing them.

HEALING AND PHYSIOLOGY OF INTESTINAL WOUNDS

The earliest recorded intestinal anastomoses of a hand-sewn and even mechanically approximated type were end-to-end everting anastomoses.[1] In 1826 Antoine Lembert proposed that an inverting, serosa-to-serosa apposition was fundamental in producing bowel adhesions and that everting wounds could not heal, but he recognized that an inverting end-to-end anastomosis might invite excessive inversion, creating obstruction.[1,5] The perception that everting wounds could not heal was supported by Halstead, who in 1887 wrote of inverting anastomoses and made a point of not allowing the suture to penetrate the bowel lumen to preclude contamination of the suture line. Halstead was the first to recognize the cardinal importance of the submucosa as a single layer of strength in the intestinal anastomosis.[5] Initial studies on intestinal healing performed during evaluation of mechanical stapling devices by Ravitch and colleagues suggested that healing occurred without inflammatory changes and thus was an intrinsic process.[6] After these studies interest in the clinical possibilities of mucosa-to-mucosa anastomoses increased markedly because of the obvious advantages and multiple clinical applications of everting end-to-end anastomoses, which could be technically simpler than inverting anastomoses and would avoid the intestinal narrowing produced by inverting anastomoses. Further studies on the healing of intestinal wounds proved that a bowel closed in a mucosa-to-mucosa fashion would heal clinically without adhesion formation that could seal off the bowel or bring new circulation to the end of the bowel.[7] It was concluded that healing depended on the intrinsic circulation of the bowel.[7] Studies on the vascularity of GI staple lines using a silicone rubber injection technique documented noncompromised circulation across GI staple lines.[8] As in almost all of the stapling instruments beginning with Hültl's, the staple for suturing parenchymal organs begins in a squared-off U and ends in a B configuration that is nonstrangulating and nonnecrosing and that permits vessels to pass through the staple loop (Figure 13–2). Although studies on the healing of intestinal wounds in dogs dem-

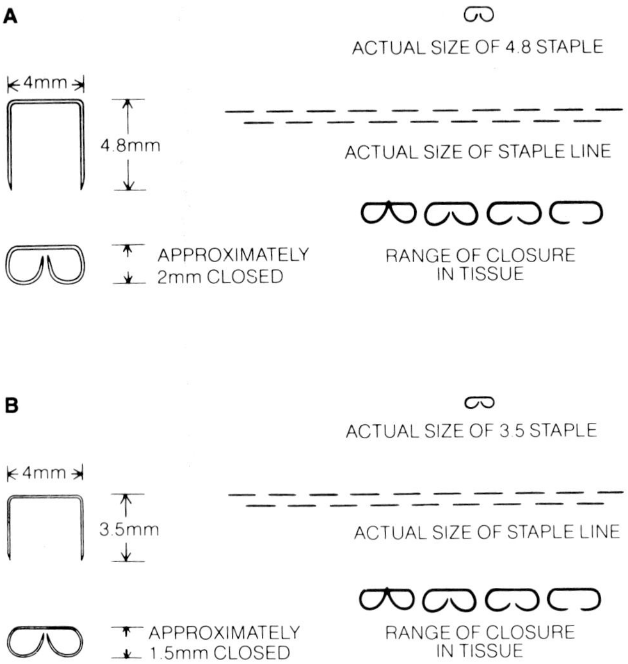

FIGURE 13–2. Staple configuration and size. Staples for suturing parenchymal organs begin in a squared-off U and end in a B configuration. Two staple sizes are represented. **A,** The 4.8 mm leg staples close to approximately 2 mm for thicker tissue. **B,** The 3.5 mm leg staples close to approximately 1.5 mm. Note also the range of closure for the staples. (From U.S. Surgical Corporation, Norwalk, CT, © 1984. Used with permission.)

onstrated that everting hand-sewn anastomoses have a higher incidence of failure than inverting hand-sewn anastomoses,[9] the crossing of the vessels through B configured staples was believed to be the phenomenon that allowed an everted stapled anastomosis to be a safe and reproducible procedure, and presumably, this crossing of vessels might not occur in sutured anastomoses.[8] The vascularity of inverted and everted suture red lines has been studied with inconclusive results.[10] No comparative study on the vascularity between stapled and hand-sewn anastomoses has been performed.

Both prospective and retrospective studies comparing results and complications of sutured and stapled anastomoses confirm that early complications and long-term results are comparable and in some series even decreased in stapled anastomoses.[11–14] The studies also found that stapled anastomoses are constructed with less trauma, better precision, and greater speed than sutured anastomoses.[11,14] Histologic studies suggest that the steel staples used are inert in the tissue and present no foreign body problem. They do not corrode and therefore possess the appropriate physical properties needed for staples: flexibility, durability, and strength.[15] The successful experimental and clinical outcome of stapled anastomoses has encouraged further application.

STAPLERS USED IN UROLOGY

Stapling instruments used in urology include thoracoabdominal (TA) staplers, gastrointestinal anastomosis (GIA) staplers, end-to-end anastomosis (EEA) staplers, ligate-and-divide (LDS) staplers, and skin and fascial staplers. A number attached to an abbreviated designation of the instrument indicates in millimeters the length of the stapled suture line. A description of each instrument, the method of its firing, precautions for its use, and a review of its application follows.

Thoracoabdominal Staplers

The TA instruments are used to place a linear everting mucosa-to-mucosa double line of staggered staples 30, 55, or 90 mm long and are available as standard stainless steel instruments with disposable cartridges and as totally disposable units. For the TA55 and the TA90 instruments, two series of staples are available with legs of 3.5 or 4.8 mm for use with varied tissue thickness. Tissue stapled with 3.5 mm staples can be compressed to 1.5 mm, and tissue stapled with the 4.8 mm staples can be compressed to 2 mm (Figure 13–2). The TA30 has, in addition, a special cartridge loaded with fine, closely spaced staples for closing vessels.

The instrument has an L-shaped frame. A fixed lower jaw accepts a disposable anvil for forming the staples, while the upper jaw holds a disposable staple cartridge. Together, the jaws create a cartridge-anvil assembly (Figure 13–3). Early instruments

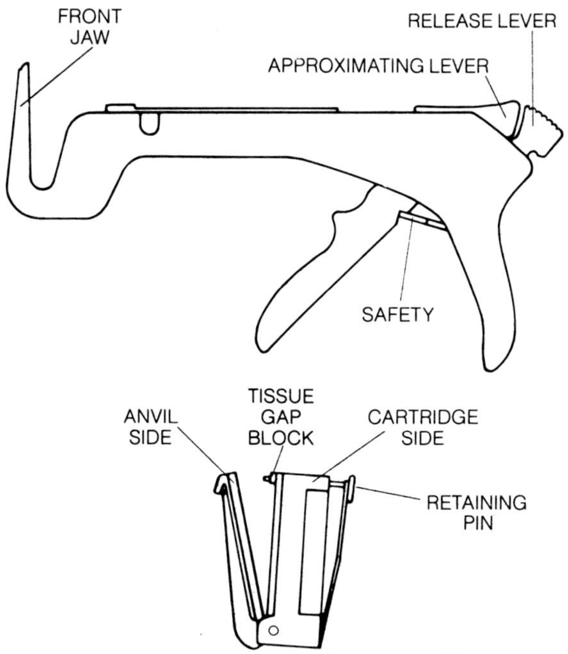

FIGURE 13–3. Schematic view and nomenclature of the TA stapler and disposable cartridge. (From U.S. Surgical Corp. Norwalk, CT, © 1984, 1990. Used with permission.)

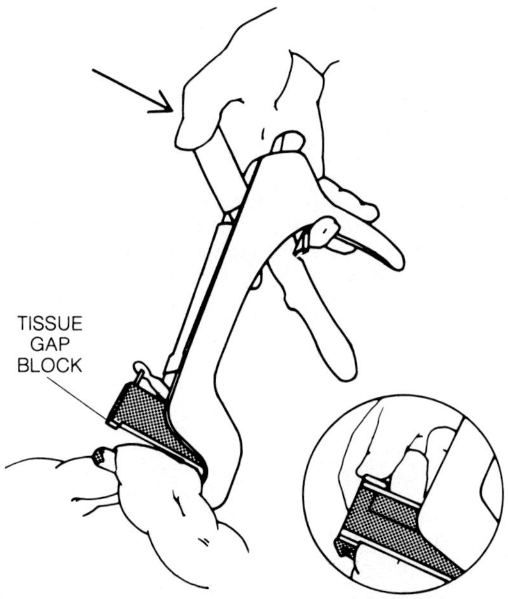

FIGURE 13–4. Firing the TA stapler. Activating a lever *(arrow)* on the vertical shaft of the TA instrument simultaneously advances the tissue-retaining pin, which is an integral part of the cartridge. The tissue secured in the cartridge-anvil assembly is ready to be stapled. (From U.S. Surgical Corporation, Norwalk, CT, © 1984. Used with permission.)

used a wing nut that, when turned, approximated the jaws of the instrument and compressed the tissue. Since 1981 the instrument has been manufactured with jaws that are opened and closed by activating a lever on the vertical shaft. The lever action simultaneously advances the tissue-retaining pin that prevents tissue from being squeezed out of the jaw of the unstapled closure and ensures perfect alignment of the anvil and cartridge assembly for precise closure of the staples (Figure 13–4). Staples are fired when the safety is released and the handles are compressed (Figure 13–5). The bowel being stapled is divided on the edge of the instrument before the instrument is removed. The jaws are opened by firm pressure on the catch on the top of the unit (Figure 13–6).

Careful attention is important during compression of tissue because the tissue has a tendency to slide forward as the cartridge and anvil approximate. Care must also be taken to seat the pin. If it is not seated, staples will not form properly. When any of the staplers are used, the staple line should be checked for hemostasis. Interrupted sutures can be placed on bleeding staple lines. If the tissue selected to be stapled cannot predictably be compressed to 2 mm for 4.8 mm staples, or to 1.5 mm for 3.5 mm staples, serosal cracks of the bowel will form along the stapler jaws and devitalize the tissue. Should this occur, the line of staples can be oversewn with a continuous or interrupted layer of sutures (Figure 13–7).

The TA instruments are used extensively in closure of all parts of the GI tract. They are used most commonly in urologic surgery for closing the opening left when a GIA stapler performs a functional end-to-end bowel anastomosis. This results in overlapping staple lines. Despite initial concerns, clinical and experimental experience demonstrated that intersecting staple lines with the TA and GIA or EEA instruments are safe. The intersecting lines allow a secure anastomosis because the knife of the transecting stapler instrument finds a way through the linear staple line previously applied without disrupting the line.[16]

The TA30-V3 or Roticulator 30-V3 (an Auto Suture product of the United States Steel Corp.), is a vascular stapler for transection of pulmonary vessels and pulmonary surgery. It can, however, be used to control the renal pedicle during nephrectomy or to control the dorsal vein complex during radical retropubic prostatectomy. The Roticulator applies a triple staggered row of staples in a 31 mm line. The staple leg is 2.5 mm long and after closure is 1 mm high. The staple head swivels both around and perpendicular to the axis of the instrument (Figure 13–8).

The clinical use of the Roticulator 30-V3 is limited. For control of the renal pedicle during nephrectomy, the instrument has been tested only in sheep. In one study it was evaluated in nine sheep.[17] The vessels of the sheep pedicles ranged from 3 to

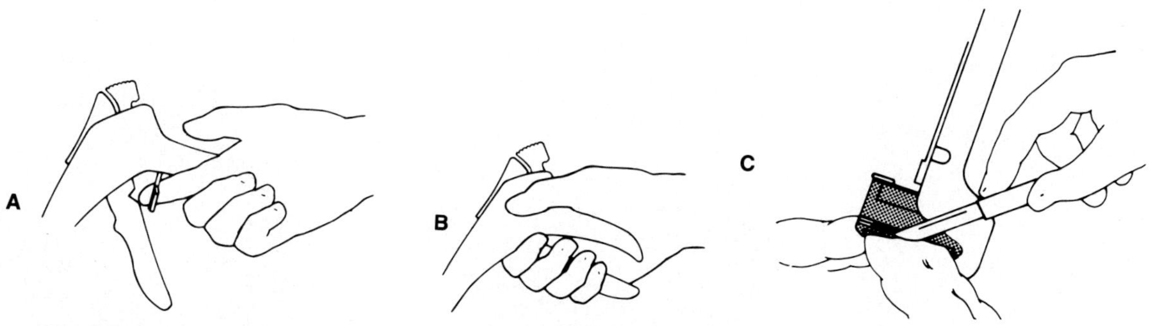

FIGURE 13–5. Firing the TA stapler. Firing is accomplished by, **A,** releasing the safety, **B,** compressing the handles of the instrument, and, **C,** dividing the bowel on the edge of the instrument before the instrument is removed. (From U.S. Surgical Corporation, Norwalk, CT, © 1984. Used with permission.)

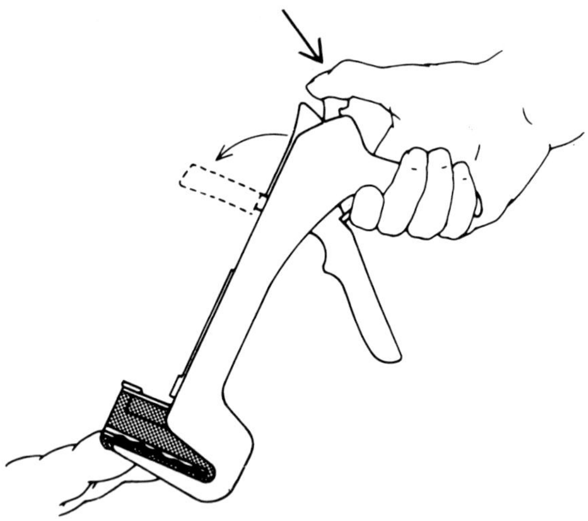

FIGURE 13–6. Firing the TA stapler. Firm pressure on the catch at the top of the unit *(straight arrow)* returns the lever *(curved arrow)* to its original position, simultaneously opening the jaws of the instrument. (From U.S. Surgical Corporation, Norwalk, CT, © 1984. Used with permission.)

12 mm in diameter, similar to the sizes of the human renal vessels. Of the nine pedicles transected with the stapling device, only two had mild hemorrhage. This was thought to result from overstripping of the perivascular tissue. The hemorrhage was controlled by a second triple staggered row of staples placed proximal to the first. Because the animal models presented have vessels similar to human vessels, we can infer that the procedure could control human renal vascular pedicles. However, the stapler probably should be applied twice to ensure a hemostatic pedicle.

The Auto Suture Roticulator 30-V3 has been used to control the dorsal venous complex during radical retropubic prostatectomy.[18] In eight of nine patients the technique was considered successful and less time consuming than control of the dorsal vein complex with conventional ligature. In one patient the staple line was inadvertently excised, leading to hemorrhage and failure. During radical

A

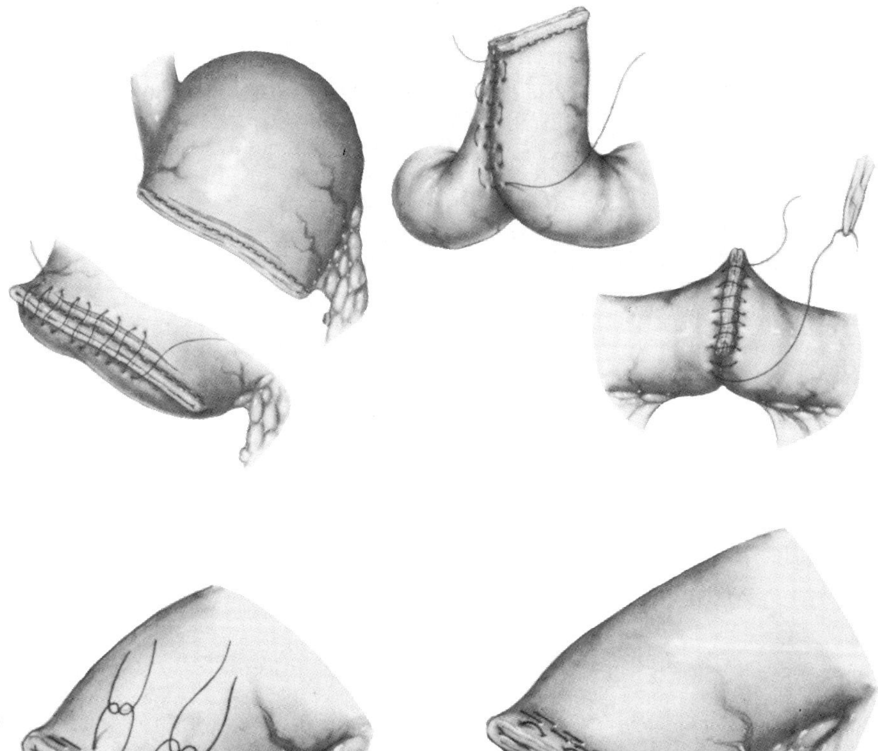

B

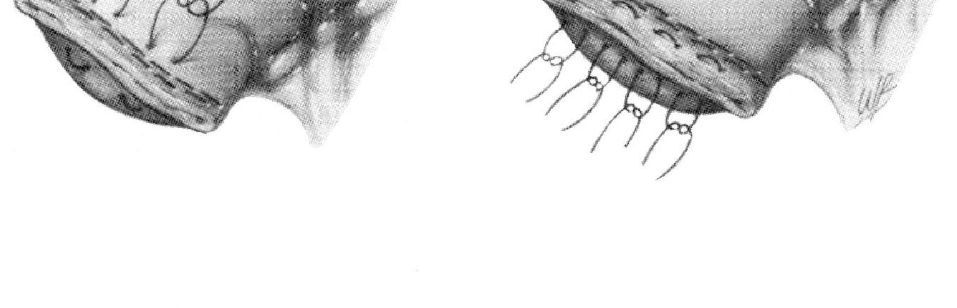

FIGURE 13–7. Suturing serosal cracks. Serosal cracks of thicker walled stomach or bowel can be oversewn in a continuous, **A,** or interrupted, **B,** layer of sutures. (From U.S. Surgical Corporation, Norwalk, CT, © 1979, 1975, 1980. Used with permission.)

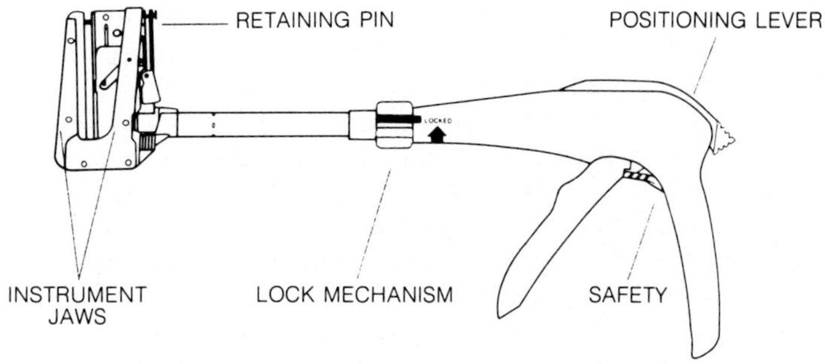

FIGURE 13–8. The TA30-V3 Auto Suture Roticulator. The stapler can be used for vascular control of pedicles. The head swivels both around and perpendicular to the axis of the instrument. A triple row of staples results after firing. Auto Suture is a trademark of the United States Surgical Corp. (From U.S. Surgical Corporation, Norwalk, CT, © 1989. Used with permission.)

retropubic prostatectomy the puboprostatic ligaments are transected and a tunnel is developed by a finger dissection between the prostatomembranous urethra and overlying dorsal vein complex. The Roticulator jaws are passed and are locked over the venal fibrous complex. The triple staggered rows of staples are fired across the complex, which is divided with a knife or electrocautery parallel to the anterior jaw of the Roticulator. The jaws are then unlocked and removed. Clinical experience is limited. However, the instrument appears to produce a hemostatic suture line in less time and therefore may become more popular.

Gastrointestinal Anastomosis Staplers

The GIA instrument places two double staggered rows of minimally inverting serosa-to-serosa staples and in the same maneuver divides the tissue between the two pairs of staggered rows. Two staple leg sizes are available: 3.5 to 4 mm for adults and 3 mm for children. The instrument consists of two interlocking halves that form a flat handle with two straight limbs, one graduated in centimeters. One limb accommodates the staple cartridge, which is slotted to receive a knife. The other limb with a lock lever accepts the anvil (Figure 13–9).

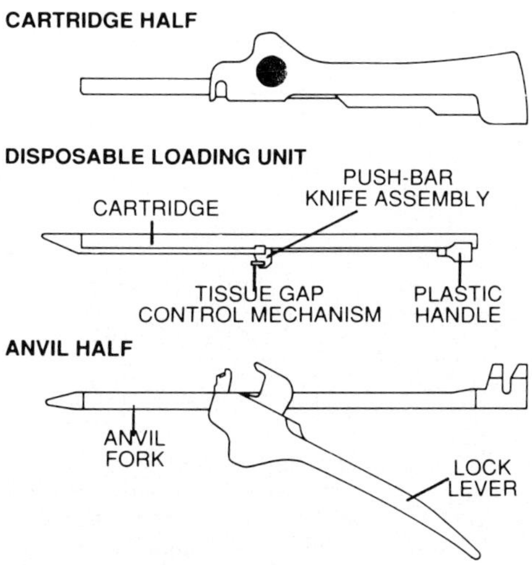

FIGURE 13–9. Schematic view and nomenclature of the GIA stapling device. (From U.S. Surgical Corporation, Norwalk, CT, © 1989. Used with permission.)

Within the cartridge are two double staggered rows of staples that form staple lines 50, 60, or 90 mm long in the tissue, depending on the number of staples in the cartridge. The staple lines in each pair of double staggered rows are 1.2 mm apart, and depending on the stapler the two pairs are 3.5 to 4.4 mm apart after the knife cuts the tissue (Figure 13–10). Pusher bars are seated in the cartridge for driving both the staples and the knife, which is done by advancing a knob to the tip of the stapler and returning it to the original position. The knife stops one or two staples short of the end of the staple line. A special cartridge without a knife, the S-GIA, inserts four rows of staples without tissue division. Thus the instrument can be used for transection or resection, creation of anastomoses, or approximation of tissue when the knifeless cartridge is used. The instrument is available in stainless steel with reusable cartridges or as a totally disposable unit in which the 26 staples are slightly shorter and closer together, so that they leave a 5.3 cm staple line. The GIA Premium is a steel stapler with wider limbs and staples that incorporate a greater cross-sectional area of the tissue.

The GIA stapler can transect all parts of the GI

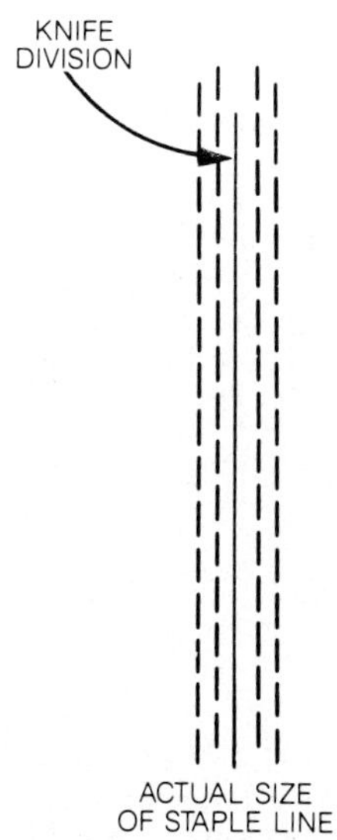

FIGURE 13–10. Schematic view of GIA staple lines. The staple lines in each pair of double staggered rows are 1.2 mm apart. Depending on the stapler, the two pairs are 3.5 to 4.4 mm apart after the knife cuts the tissue. (From U.S. Surgical Corporation, Norwalk, CT, © 1989. Used with permission).

tract and is used for side-to-side, end-to-side, and functional end-to-end anastomoses. Linear staple lines produced with the S-GIA are beneficial in continent diversion procedures to create nipple valves and bowel wall reapproximation after detubularization. When the two limbs of a GIA stapler are slipped into the lumens of separate bowel segments to be connected, mated, locked, and fired, driving the knife divides the bowel and both segments of the bowel are closed in a mucosa-to-mucosa fashion with double staggered rows of staples. Before the instrument is fired, the bowel is centered between the 0 and 6 cm marks where the four rows of staples will be placed. The 1 to 5 cm area is where the knife of the GIA stapling device will cut the bowel. If the bowel is off center, one corner of the ileum may not be stapled or not be incised with the knife. Once the GIA stapling device is closed on the bowel, it will not slip from the stapler jaws. The surgeon places the long and index fingers of the right hand on the shoulders of the GI stapling device, then places the thumb of the right hand on the lever arm that will fire the staples and divide the bowel. Before advancing this lever arm, the surgeon anchors the base of the stapling device with the left hand. The GIA stapling lever arm is fired only once. Firing it a second time could disrupt the staple line, or if the bowel were to slip partially, the advancement of the knife a second time could cut into the staples or disrupt the integrity of the stapled closure on either side of the enterotomy. After firing, the lever arm is slid back and the GIA stapling device is opened (Figure 13–11).

As with the TA staple lines, GIA staple lines should be checked for bleeding, especially when staple lines are intraluminal where bleeding might be concealed. Tissue to be compressed should be perpendicular to the instrument, and no extra tissue should be included in the jaws of the instruments. When bowel anastomoses are performed, whether with staples or suture, linear tension on the anastomosis increases the risk of disruption. Because the diameter of each staple is less than that of a suture, the risk of disruption may be even higher with stapled than with sutured anastomoses when the anastomosis is performed under tension. The limbs of the instrument should be parallel when locked, so that malformed staples do not result, es-

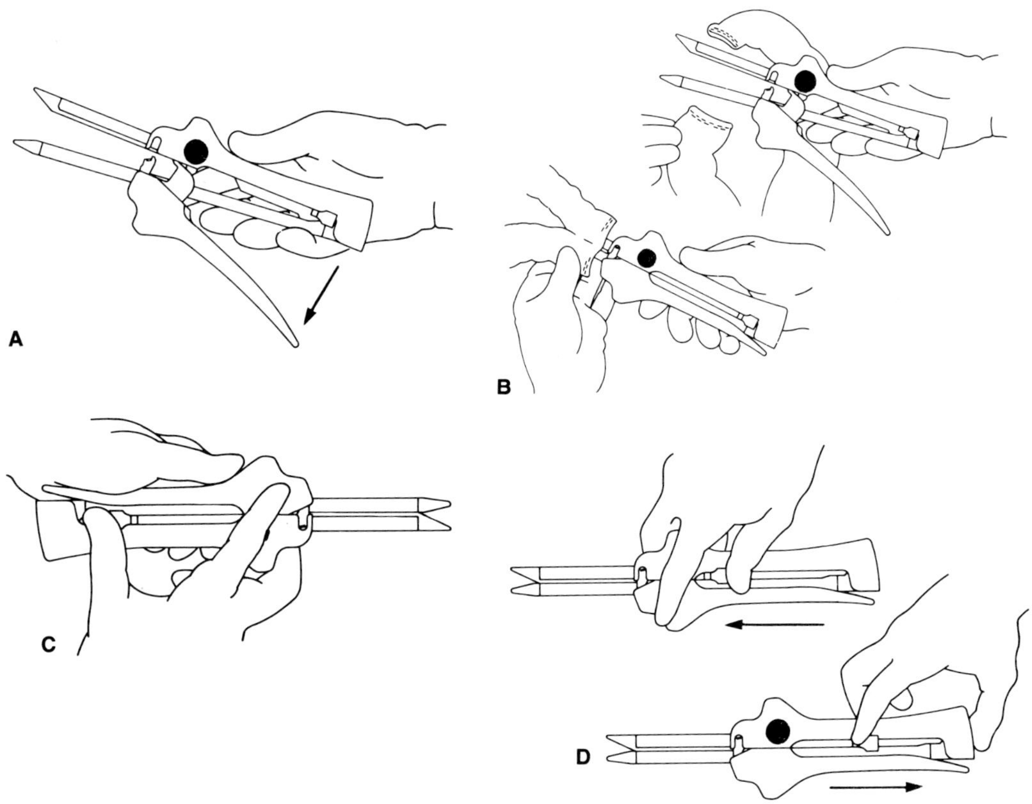

FIGURE 13–11. GIA Stapler firing instructions. **A,** The anvil half and the cartridge half of the instrument are separated by moving the lock lever *(arrow)*. **B,** With the lock lever in the fully open position, the limbs of the instrument are inserted into the lumina of bowel to be stapled or applied across a segment of bowel to be stapled. The limbs are aligned, the rear hinges joined, and the lever lock closed. An audible click signifies that the instrument is ready to fire. **C,** The instrument is steadied in the palm of one hand, and a thumb is placed on the driving knob. **D,** The knob is advanced all the way until it stops and is pulled back. It is not advanced a second time. The lock lever can next be opened as in **A** to remove the instrument. (From U.S. Surgical Corporation, Norwalk, CT, © 1989. Used with permission.)

pecially at the tip of the GIA stapler. The 3.5 mm staples of the GIA stapler compress tissue to 1.5 to 1.75 mm, depending on whether a disposable or a stainless steel reusable unit is used. As with the TA instruments, excessive compression can result in serosal cracks. Tissue that is compressed to less than 1.5 mm thickness will not allow the staples to be tight enough and not ensure hemostasis. The surgeon must always remember to retract the knife blade to its original position before opening the instrument. When the instrument is used repeatedly during the same procedure, the anvil should be checked to make sure it is clean. Tissue or loose staples on the anvil from previous firings may result in obstruction on the anvil and lead to improperly formed staples.

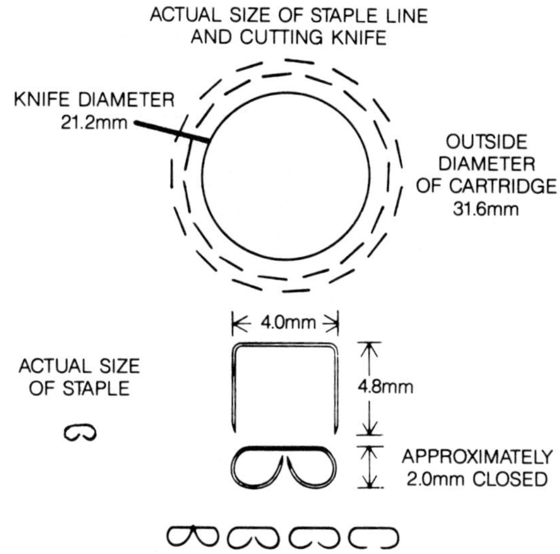

FIGURE 13–12. The EEA 31 staples. The stapler is also available in 28 mm and 25 mm approximate outer diameter, producing anastomoses of approximately 18 mm and 15 mm internal diameter. (From U.S. Surgical Corporation, Norwalk, CT, © 1989. Used with permission.)

End-To-End Anastomotic Staplers

The EEA instrument is a tubular device that can be employed for end-to-end and end-to-side, minimally inverting anastomoses. This is the one stapler that can perform bowel anastomoses honoring the traditional principle of inverting serosa-to-serosa anastomoses that are not end to side but end to end. The instrument has a shaft that can be loaded with a disposable cartridge consisting of a cylinder containing one or two circular rows of staggered staples and a circular knife just inside the inner ring of staples. A dome-shaped nose cone carries the anvil and screws onto the rods that pass through the center of the staple cartridge. Within the nose cone, just inside the inner row of anvil recesses, is a heavy plastic ring against which the circular knife cuts the bowel ends, which are held around the central rods and the nose cone or anvil of the instrument. The staple limbs are 4.8 mm before closure, and the instrument is supplied with cartridges approximately 31, 28, and 25 mm in outer diameter, which produce anastomoses of approximately 21, 18, and 15 mm internal diameter, respectively (Figure 13–12). Disposable instruments are available that come fully assembled with any of the three cartridge sizes. The instrument can be placed through an anastomotic opening in an end-to-end fashion through consecutive yet separated pieces of bowel. Alternatively, because the nose cone or anvil is removable, the cartridge portion of the instrument can be introduced into the bowel lumen with the aid of a trocar that accompanies the EEA device or be passed through a colotomy or other opening of a viscus into the lumen of a segment of a GI tract to be anastomosed. The central rod then emerges through the lumen of the segment and is capped with the anvil, over which a segment of bowel to be anastomosed has already been secured with a purse-string suture. A wing nut separates or approximates the anvil and cartridge portions of the instrument. Once the wing nut is tightened for approximation, the handles of the instrument are compressed and a minimally inverting anastomosis is created (Figure 13–13).

Applications in urology include creation of an end-to-side anastomosis as is performed between large and small bowel during creation of an Indiana pouch or other ileocolonic continent diversion. In addition, because the instrument can be passed through any natural orifice, it may be used to develop a stoma, for example, during a Brooke ileostomy.

A point to remember with the EEA instruments is that using too large a cartridge risks tearing the bowel or devascularization and using too small a cartridge risks relative stenosis. Tight closure of the purse-string suture around the central rod is basic to securing any anastomosis. If the suture is not tight enough, the circular knife fails to surround the entire opening. If the suture is placed too far back from the cut edge of the bowel to be anastomosed, too much tissue is placed in the anvil portion or cartridge portion around the central rod, which creates tissue-destroying pressure. In addition, the instrument must be opened wide before attempts to remove it, and it should always be withdrawn gently. The rings stamped out by the circular knife should always be checked to see that they remain intact.

Intersecting circular EEA and linear TA or GIA stapling lines occur in low rectal anastomoses and at times when an end-to-side anastomosis is performed. As mentioned in the section on TA staplers, initial concerns that intersecting staple lines would lead to leak, fistula, or stricture formation proved invalid.

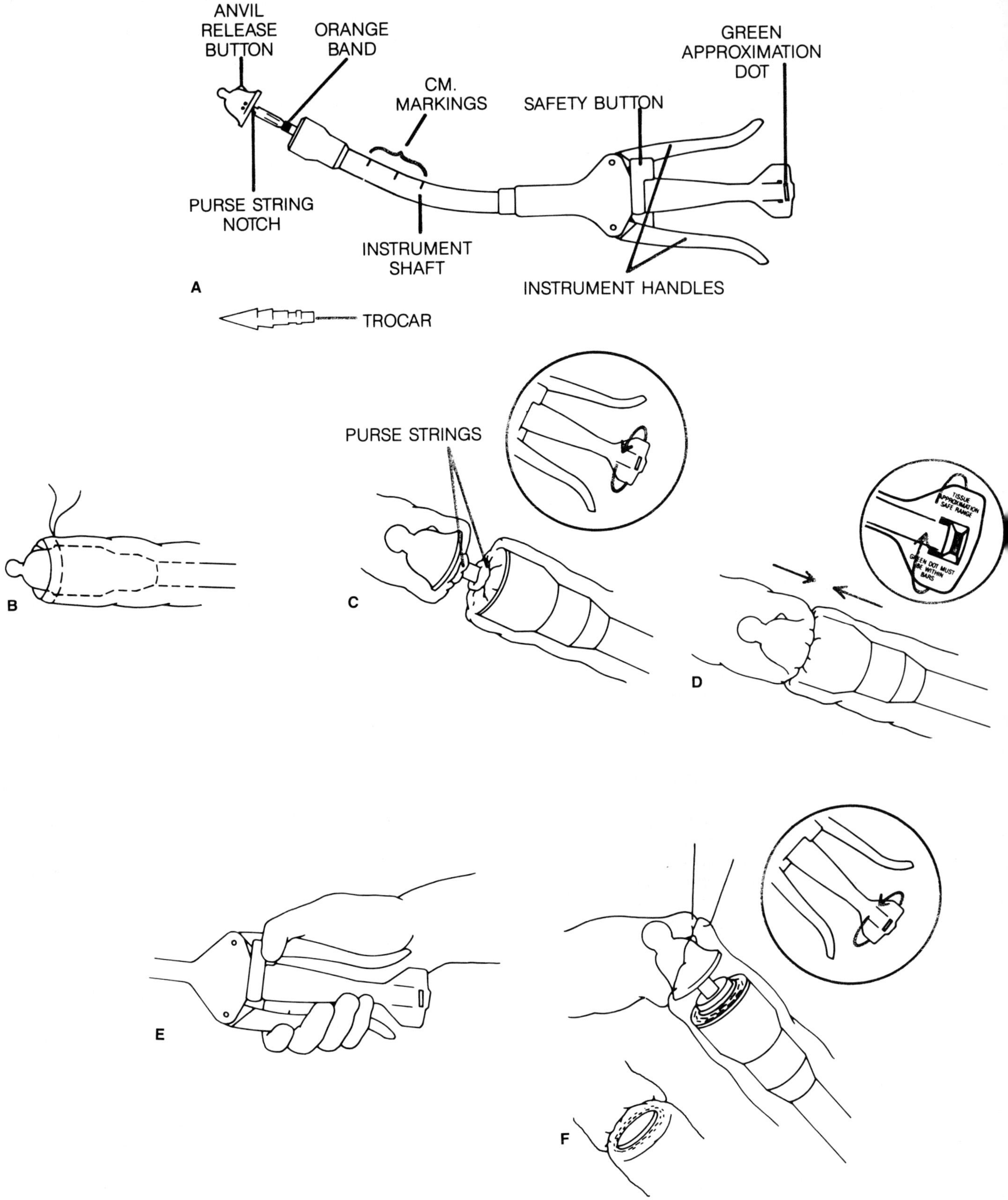

FIGURE 13–13. Schematic view, nomenclature, and firing instructions for the EEA stapler. **A,** Labeled parts of the stapler. **B,** Purse-string sutures are placed no more than 2.5 mm from the edge of both ends of bowel to be anastomosed, and then the instrument is introduced into the bowel until the tip of the anvil protrudes. **C,** The instrument is opened by turning the wing nut counterclockwise until sufficient space is available between the cartridge and the anvil. The anvil portion is introduced into the consecutive piece of bowel to be anastomosed. The distal purse-string suture is tied around the central rod to secure the tissue over the cartridge, and the proximal purse-string suture is tied into the purse-string notch, securing the bowel over the anvil. **D,** The wing nut is turned clockwise until the green dot in the tissue approximation indicator is partially visible within the black markings. **E,** The instrument is fired by simultaneously holding the safety release and squeezing the handles as far as they go. **F,** The instrument is removed by turning the wing nut counterclockwise no more than three full turns. If the wing nut is rotated more than this, the anvil rotates freely, which may prevent easy removal of the instrument through the anastomosis. A portion of the anterior staple line can be lifted over the anvil with the aid of a suture through the staple line. (From U.S. Surgical Corporation, Norwalk, CT, © 1989. Used with permission.)

Ligate, Divide, and Suture Staplers

The LDS stapler places two metal clips of fine stainless steel on either side of the dividing blade, simultaneously suturing and dividing the tissue and vessels in continuity within the curved end of the instrument. A steel preloadable and a totally disposable preloaded model are available. The preloadable, disposable cartridges contain 6 to 15 pairs of U-shaped staples of 5 or 7.3 mm closed width. At the end of the cartridge is a J-shaped jaw within which the structure to be ligated and divided is placed, hooked, and held. A handle is squeezed to fire the U-shaped staple on each side and to close it in a crescent around the tissues, which are divided between the staples with a knife powered by the same squeeze of the handle. The totally disposable model employs a light-pressure button, which causes an integral cartridge to release a notable pulse of specially formulated nontoxic gas that fires the staples (Figure 13–14).

Although the LDS stapler was designed to ligate vessels, it is commonly used in urology for mesenteric division during bowel surgery. It also can be used to ligate and divide the appendix, vas deferens, and omentum.

The main precautionary measure in use of the LDS stapler is that no more tissue should be placed in the J-hook part of the stapler than it will easily accommodate because this could result in a nonhemostatic ligation. Also, if there is tension on the instrument when fired, the vessels that are under tension will recoil elastically and not remain occluded with the metal staples of the LDS stapling device. Should this occur and bleeding result, a horizontal mattress or figure-of-8 suture of 3-0 silk can be applied in the mesentery. Immediately applying pressure on the mesentery with the thumb and index finger to occlude bleeding vessels prevents formation of a large intramesenteric hematoma. The stapler should not be applied across previous staples because this blunts the knife.

Skin and Fascial Staplers

Skin and fascial staplers are available as cartridge-loaded or totally disposable instruments. Like the LDS stapler, some of the totally disposable instruments are powered by a gas-containing cartridge. In addition, some instruments have a swiveling head that allows changes in staple direction and permits direct vision as a staple line is created in any direction. The staples do not close in a B configuration but in a rectangular fashion. The staple cartridges can be interchanged between the fascial and skin stapling devices, but fascial staplers are larger than skin staplers.

The fascial stapler allows a fast and reliable closure of midline incisions; however, because of the ubiquity of computerized tomographic (CT) scanners and the production of artifacts on CT scans by the steel alloy of the staples, they are not commonly used for this purpose. On both CT scans[19] and magnetic resonance images,[20] minimal artifact is observed when titanium clips are used and absorbable copolymer staples produce even less artifact. Greater availability of titanium staples may increase the use of fascial staplers.

In stapling the fascia or the skin, the surgeon applies the end of the stapler firmly against the two edges of the everting tissue to be stapled and fires the staples with a squeeze of the handle. During fascial stapling a narrow malleable retractor or a long knife handle can be placed posterior to the fascia to provide resistance, although this is not necessary.

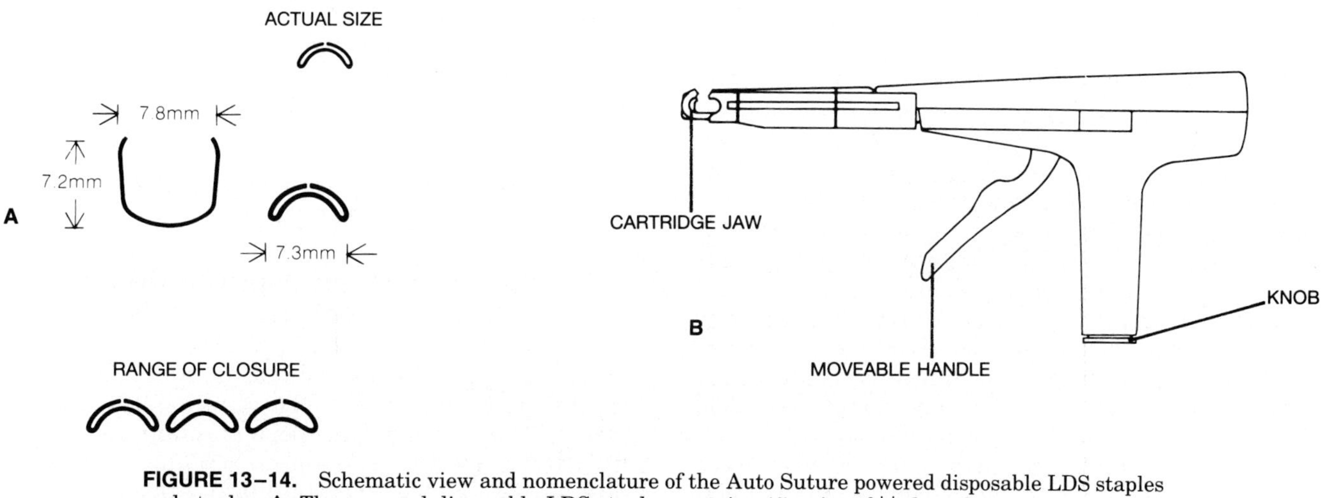

FIGURE 13–14. Schematic view and nomenclature of the Auto Suture powered disposable LDS staples and stapler. **A,** The powered disposable LDS stapler contains 15 pairs of U-shaped staples of 5 mm or 7.3 mm closed width. The 7.3 mm staples are illustrated. **B,** Auto Suture Powered LDS Stapler. Each time it is activated, two staples are placed approximately 9.3 mm apart and the knife blade contained in the cartridge cuts between the two staples after they are formed. (From U.S. Surgical Corporation, Norwalk, CT, © 1988. Used with permission.)

Absorbable Staples

The formation of stones around foreign bodies, such as steel staples, in the urinary tract is a well-described phenomenon.[21–23] From the stapling devices used in the pelvis and from absorbable sutures used in the urinary tract and vagina, absorbable staples evolved. A lactide-glycolic copolymer absorbable staple was introduced in 1982. It was fitted to a TA55 stapler and labeled the Polysorb 55 Lactomer Copolymer stapler (United States Surgical Corp.). It allowed the use of staples in areas such as the vagina and the urinary tract, where steel wire could not be used. Glycolide and lactide, the monomers chosen for the first absorbable staples, were not new. Two widely used suture materials, polyglycolic acid and polygalactin 910, incorporate either pure glycolic acid or both glycolic and lactide acid, and their reliability in tissue closure has been well documented. Like the conventional suture materials, the copolymer staples were found to be degraded by nonenzymatic hydrolysis. Initial in vitro and in vivo testing of a prototype compound at the United States Surgical Corp. by Steckel and associates indicated that the copolymer hydrolyzed back to lactic acid and glycolic acid at a predictable, temperature-dependent rate.[24] Steckel and associates published data from animal experiments evaluating tensile strength, histologic tissue reaction, and efficacy of absorbable staples in vaginal cuff closure. The tensile strength of absorbable staples was retained in rat tissues for 2 weeks after implantation, and loss thereafter was rapid. The friability, or tensile strength loss, was believed to be directly related to the rate of hydrolysis or absorption that occurred at 3 to 6 weeks, depending on the chemical variant of the copolymer used. The copolymer material was found to be histopathologically inert, evoking a minimal early inflammatory response that was replaced by noninflammatory fibrous connective tissue 6 weeks postoperatively. A stable vaginal cuff closure was observed.

Experiments were designed to test the efficacy and the risk of stone formation with absorbable and steel staples in mucosa-to-mucosa closures in sterile, acutely infected, and chronically infected bladders. The investigators found that both the absorbable and steel staple closures were secure and healed without clinical evidence of leaks in all cases.[25] Because of mucosal regeneration, steel staples rarely surfaced to offer a site for stone formation. The authors concluded that bladder closure with absorbable and even stainless steel staples carries a low risk for stone formation and that stone formation is more often associated with states such as chronic infection and acid urine. Others have confirmed the efficacy of absorbable staples in closure of the proximal end of an ileal loop.[26]

Because of the rigidity of the elastomer, the Polyabsorb staples are made on a different principle from the B configuration of the stainless steel staples. The staple is composed of a perforated retainer bar that accepts fastener or staple. When fired, the fastener is forced through tissue and locked into the retainer (Figure 13–15). In an everted closure the fastening bar of the Polysorb staple necroses the compressed tissue at a rate slow enough to permit secure healing of the tissue, as has been documented both experimentally and clinically.[27,28]

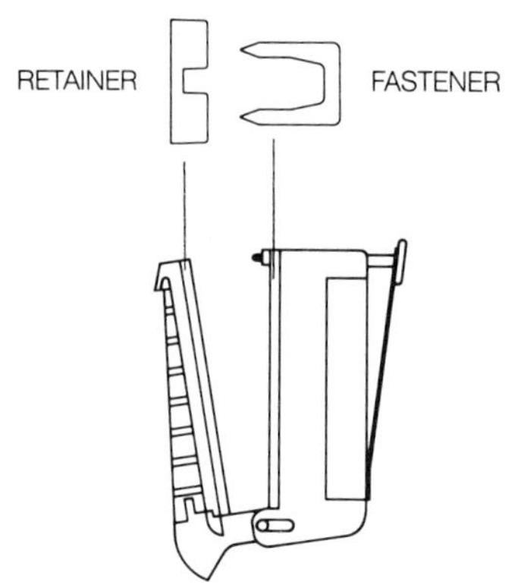

FIGURE 13–15. Auto Suture Polysorb 55 Disposable Loading Unit. The unit comes in four sizes for use with different tissue thicknesses. Closed width ranges from 1.5 to 5 mm. The distance between the bottom of the staple fastener and the top of the retainer on closure corresponds to the different sizes and also to the compressed tissue thickness. (From U.S. Surgical Corporation, Norwalk, CT, © 1987. Used with permission.)

Specific indications for the use of absorbable staplers are in the closure of the proximal end of the urinary conduit, such as an ileal loop, or in the proximal closure of any urinary continent diversion pouch. The detubularized bowel in the creation of continent urinary reservoirs has been closed routinely with absorbable sutures but has also been anastomosed side to side fashion with absorbable staples.[29] In nine patients whose incisions were closed with absorbable staples, no leaks or prolonged urinary fistulas were demonstrated. Absorbable staples can also be applied to cystotomy and vaginal closure and reconstruction.[25,26]

STAPLERS IN UROLOGIC OPERATIONS

Construction of an Ileal Conduit with a Small Bowel Anastomosis

For a stapled bowel anastomosis and construction of an ileal conduit, three GIA stapling devices 6 cm in length and a 4.8 mm TA55 stapling device are used to isolate the loop and to complete the anastomosis. A Polysorb 55 stapling cartridge is used to close the base of the ileal conduit. An LDS stapler may be used to take down the mesenteric windows on either side of the ileal conduit. Also needed are several segments of quarter-inch Penrose drains,

4-0 GI silk marking sutures, and a 3-0 chromic GI suture to close the mesenteric trap.

In the avascular plane of Treves, approximately 10 to 15 cm proximal to the ileal cecal valve, is the vascular arcade that represents the collateralization between the distal branches of the right colic artery and the ileal colic artery. The peritoneal surface of the mesentery at the avascular plane of Treves can be incised with scissors for approximately 10 cm from the mesenteric border of the small bowel toward the root of the small bowel mesentery. This is easier if a small Penrose drain is placed around the ileum at this site and through the mesentery at the most proximal part of its incision. Once the peritoneal surface has been incised on both sides of the mesentery, a curved Crile hemostat can be used to separate the mesentery into vascular bundles approximately 1 cm in length. If the mesentery is thickened because of obesity or reaction, these should be separated into small bundles. If the LDS stapling device is used to divide the small bowel mesentery at the avascular plane of Treves, the nose of the instrument is passed through the small bowel mesentery and then brought back though the second hiatus created with the Crile hemostat. A toothed Adson forceps used by the first assistant is helpful in delivering the nose of the LDS stapling device through the mesenteric window. Usually five to eight firings of the LDS stapler are required to complete the division of the small bowel mesentery at the avascular plane of Treves. A large artery always found in the mesentery approximately 3 cm in from the mesenteric border of the bowel represents the main collateralization between the ileal colic artery and the right colic artery. Careful attention to the presence of this artery is necessary to ensure adequate hemostasis and to prevent mesenteric hematoma formation.

Following mesenteric division the ileum is cleared of mesenteric fat for approximately 1 cm to allow placement of the 6 cm GIA stapling device. An assistant using Adson forceps grasps the fat as it is being trimmed off sharply. Small vessels can be cauterized or ligated with 3-0 silk. The right-handed surgeon holds the proximal aspect of the ileum in the left hand between the thumb and index finger. The assistant holds the antimesenteric border of the terminal ileum just distal to the proposed stapling and dividing site. This places the bowel on a gentle stretch so that no excess thickness of the bowel is in the jaws of the stapler when it is fired. The stapling instrument is applied across the tissue, and the jaws are aligned, mated, and locked. The antimesenteric and mesenteric border of the ileum should be inspected within the jaws of the stapling device. The base of the stapling device is anchored, and the lever is advanced to fire the staples and divide the tissue. The GIA stapling lever arm is advanced forward only once and then returned to its original position. Firing the arm a second time could disrupt the staple line or, if the bowel were to slip, advancing the knife a second time could cut into the staples or disrupt the integrity of the staple closure on either side of the enterotomy. Once the lever arm has been returned to its original position, the GIA stapling device is opened; each end of the bowel should have two rows of staples in place and the entire lumen should be closed (Figure 13–16).

A tape is used to measure out the ileal conduit segment for urinary diversion. For a standard ileal conduit a length of 15 to 30 cm is appropriate. The segment should be longer if a Turnbull loop stoma is to be used, if the left ureter has been shortened toward the renal pelvis to achieve a negative margin during the cancer resection, or if the patient is obese. Before a commitment is made on the length of the segment, the bowel can be positioned up to the selected stoma site and over to both ureters to assess for length. At the proximal end of the measured segment a ¼-inch Penrose drain is passed. The segment is then measured 6 cm proximal to this and a second ¼-inch Penrose drain is passed. The mesentery between these two Penrose drains is divided and the 6 cm piece of bowel is discarded. This affords a good distance between the base of the ileal conduit and the small bowel anastomosis, so that they are not in contact with each other. In addition, mobility is provided without cutting into the mesentery, which eliminates the risk of undercutting the mesenteric blood supply to the ileal conduit. The remaining staples in the LDS cartridge can be used to divide the mesentery from this discarded piece of small bowel. Once the mesentery is divided at this location, the most proximal aspect of the ileum is stapled with a GIA stapling device. The most distal division of this 6 cm piece to be

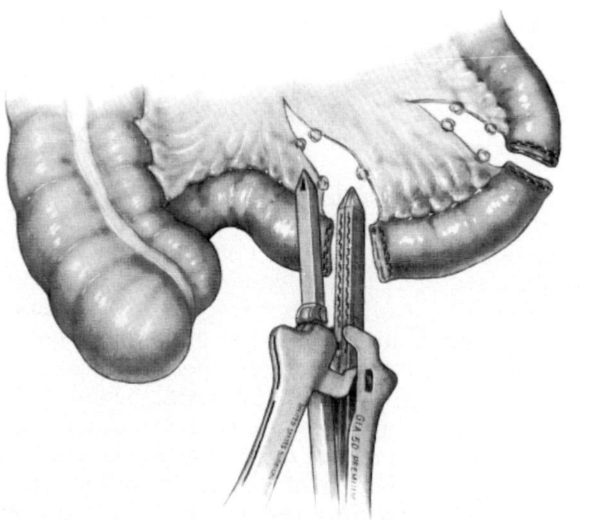

FIGURE 13–16. Construction of an ileal conduit. Isolated ileal segment is shown. The most distal or stomal end of bowel has been transected with the GIA stapler 10 to 15 cm proximal to the ileal cecal valve. (From U.S. Surgical Corporation, Norwalk, CT, © 1988. Used with permission.)

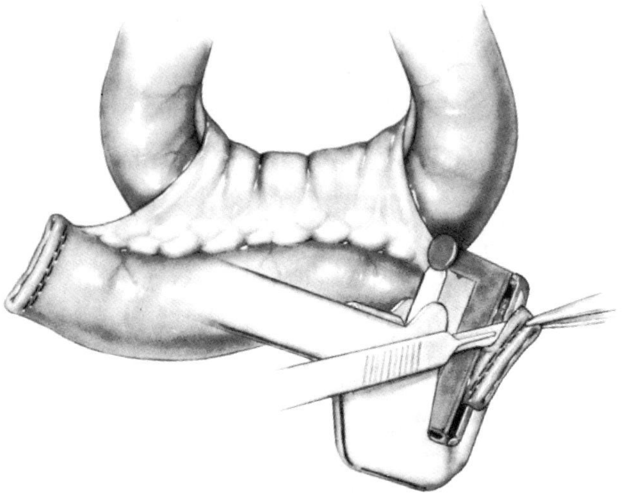

FIGURE 13–17. Construction of an ileal conduit. The proximal end of the conduit is closed using the Auto Suture Polysorb 55 absorbable stapling cartridge in a TA instrument. The absorbable staples prevent metal staple exposure to urine and subsequent stone formation within the conduit. (From U.S. Surgical Corporation, Norwalk, CT, © 1974, 1980, 1988. Used with permission.)

discarded will be the proximal end of the ileal loop. For this division the Polysorb 55 absorbable stapling cartridge in a TA instrument is used to divide the bowel and then the 6 cm bowel segment can be discarded. The stapling device is positioned across the bowel from the mesenteric to the antimesenteric border of the bowel (Figure 13–17). Once the device is fired, the staples are inspected. With the Polysorb cartridge, frequently extra staples extend beyond the limits of the small bowel closure. These should be trimmed off with scissors. However, at least one extra staple is left on each side of the bowel border. Sometimes the Polysorb cartridge remains stuck in the jaws of the TA55 stapler and the surgeon must grasp the entire bowel snugly at the jaw of the stapling device and lift upward with steady, gentle pressure to remove it.

Stapled Small Bowel Anastomosis

For a stapled small bowel anastomosis, the ileal conduit segment is laid caudad and the two ends of the small bowel on either side of the ileal conduit are isolated. The small bowel ends and their orientation with respect to their mesentery are identified. The distal end of the small bowel is held secure with one hand, while with the other hand a square corner is cut off with heavy scissors at the antimesenteric border of the GIA stapling line for a length of approximately 0.5 cm. A 4-0 silk stay suture is placed through the staple line just central to this enterotomy. This suture represents the enterotomy site for the next firing of the stapling device. In a similar fashion the proximal end is secured and an enterotomy at the antimesenteric border is made. Having an assistant grasp the antimesenteric corner with Adson forceps is helpful. A second 4-0 silk suture is placed central to this enterotomy, as well as through the staple line. With the assistant holding both limbs of the small bowel and the mesentery adjacent to each other so that there are no twists of 180 or 360 degrees in the mesentery, each bowel limb is rotated inward to align the antimesenteric borders with each other. A GIA-60 stapling device is opened, the arm containing the staple is passed down one segment of the small bowel, and the anvil arm is passed into the other bowel segment (Figure 13–18). With gentle outward traction on each segment of the bowel, the two arms of the GIA stapling device are closed, compressing the antimesenteric borders of the bowel together over a length of 6 cm (Figure 13–19). The depth to which the calibrated instru-

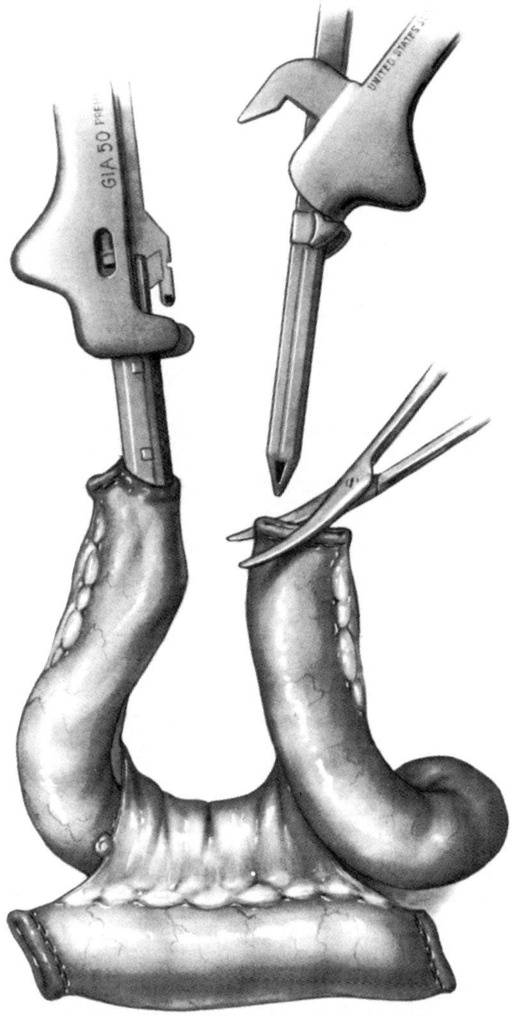

FIGURE 13–18. Stapled small bowel anastomosis. The antimesenteric borders of the bowel are aligned with each other, and a GIA stapling device limb is passed down the two lumina to be anastomosed. The ileal conduit is caudad to the small bowel anastomosis. (From U.S. Surgical Corporation, Norwalk, CT, © 1974, 1980, 1986. Used with permission.)

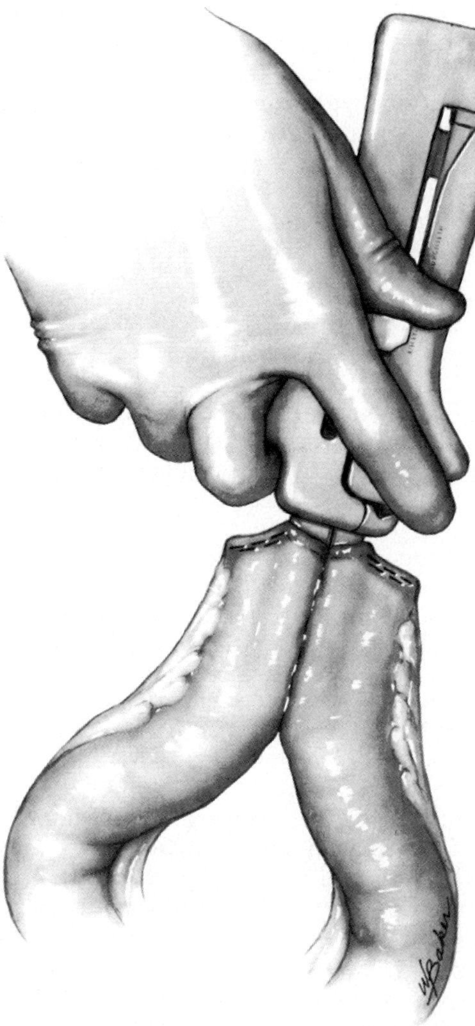

FIGURE 13–19. Stapled small bowel anastomosis. The antimesenteric segments of bowel are compressed within the GIA and stapled. The depth to which the calibrated instrument is inserted determines the size of the anastomosis. The stapler is removed, and the staple line is inspected for hemostasis. (From U.S. Surgical Corporation, Norwalk, CT, © 1974, 1980, 1986. Used with permission.)

ment is inserted determines the size of the anastomosis. At this point, with the stapling device closed, the bowel is inspected again to make sure there are no twists in the mesentery and no compressed areas or kinks within either limb of the two small bowel pieces. With the assistant holding the 4-0 silk stay sutures upward, the lever of the device is slid down the full 6 cm with the thumb and returned to the original position. The stapling device is then unlocked, opened slowly, and withdrawn. As the stapling device is opened, exposure is achieved to the now common luminal crotch of the stapled bowel anastomoses. While the stapling device is being withdrawn, this surface should be carefully inspected for bleeding sites. The outer aspects of the stapled ridge of the small bowel junction on the right and left sides are then secured with Allis clamps. The opening left is an antimesenteric, now common enterotomy that can be closed with a 4.8 mm TA55 stapling device. This opening can be closed in a transverse or longitudinal fashion. For a longitudinal closure the Allis clamps are pulled away from each other and the 4-0 silk stay sutures are brought up together. The opposite is done to perform a transverse closure. With the bowel edges aligned at the same level, the 4.8 mm TA55 stapling device is placed just below the stay sutures and Allis clamps and closed to ensure that all surfaces of the bowel are secured with the stapler (Figure 13–20). The safety of the instrument is released, the instrument is fired, and the assistant trims off the redundant small bowel on free edges of the anastomosis. The anastomosis is again checked for bleeding, which can be controlled with electrocautery or a suture if necessary. The lumen of the anastomosis can be palpated to ensure patency. This represents a 6 cm long anatomic end-to-end small bowel enteroenterostomy.

A 4-0 silk suture is used to reinforce the intersection of the crossing staple lines in a simple or figure-of-8 fashion. The antimesenteric crotch of the anastomoses is identified on the seromuscular surface of the anastomoses, and this is reinforced with a 4-0 silk suture to take the tension off the stapled junction. The small bowel anastomosis is rotated through the mesenteric defect from caudad to cephalad, returning the mesentery to its anatomic location. The mesenteric window is then closed with a running 3-0 chromic suture. The mesentery of the ileal conduit segment should be left as mobile as possible. During closure, care should be taken to avoid injuring the vessels supplying the

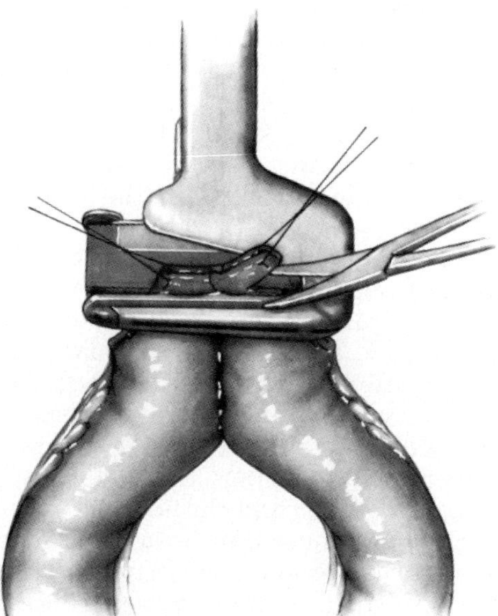

FIGURE 13–20. Stapled small bowel anastomosis. The opening left after the GIA stapler is fired is a common enterotomy, which can be closed with the TA55 stapler. (From U.S. Surgical Corporation, Norwalk, CT, © 1974, 1980, 1986. Used with permission.)

ileal conduit mesenteric pedicle, since this is a potential site for internal hernia.

Once the ureters are connected to the ileal conduit, the stoma can be developed in an end fashion or in a Turnbull loop. If an end stoma is preferred, the two stapled rows of the remaining GIA closure on the distal ileal conduit can be removed with electrocautery. If a Turnbull loop stoma is to be created, the loop portion of the small bowel is delivered through the stomal site and everted in the usual fashion. The remaining staples on the mucosa fistula end of the loop can be left in place because they will not be in contact with urine.

Mistakes and Pitfalls

The most common mistake in the use of staplers for small bowel anastomosis occurs when the two ends of the ileum are aligned and the third GIA stapling cartridge is fired to anastomose and secure the antimesenteric borders of the two limbs of bowel together. The bowel ends can become rotated so that the mesenteries are not opposite each other. This malrotation is easily overlooked. It occurs when the bowel is not twisted in opposite directions, and the result is that the limbs are malaligned with a 180- or 360-degree malrotation. The bowel anastomosis can still be completed with closure of the enterostomy, but once the anastomosis is inspected, a spiral is identified and it is impossible to close the mesenteric window by connecting one mesentery to the other because they do not line up. If this has occurred, taking down the anastomosis with cautery or sharply and performing a hand-sewn bowel anastomosis is recommended. If a repeat stapled anastomosis is attempted, because the antimesenteric border has already been incised 6 cm on either end of the bowel, the common enterotomy is too long for closure with the TA stapler unless a TA90 model is available. To redo a stapled anastomosis with a stapling device, the surgeon must trim off and discard the excess bowel that has already been misconstructed with the prior staple cartridge.

When the enterotomy is closed with the TA55 4.8 mm stapling device, one segment of the bowel can slide out of the jaws of the stapling device before the device is fired. This problem is usually not recognized until after the firing of the device. Inspection reveals an opening in the anastomosis. This is best closed with interrupted 4-0 silk sutures, preferably in two separate layers, the first layer bringing the edges together and the second layer being an imbricated seromuscular closure. Care should be taken not to compromise the lumen of the bowel anastomosis in the attempt to correct this error. If the integrity of the stapled bowel anastomosis becomes a matter of concern, it can be checked by injecting a dilute methylene blue solution into the bowel with a 21- or 23-gauge needle. The assistant can occlude the bowel on both sides of the small bowel anastomosis between the long and index fingers, and the solution can be injected intraluminally into the bowel to distend it. If the bowel anastomosis has been performed correctly, no leakage of blue liquid should be seen.

A practiced surgical team can perform the stapled construction of the ileal conduit and stapled small bowel anastomosis with closures of the mesenteric trap in 10 to 15 minutes.

Stapled Small to Large Bowel Anastomosis

In creating cecoileal reservoirs the operator is left with a small to large bowel or ileocolic anastomosis to reconstitute the fecal stream. The EEA instrument is used to perform the ileocolostomy. The terminal ileum to be reapproximated is prepared by placing a purse-string suture approximately 3 mm from the transected mucosa. The diameter of the lumen is then determined with EEA sizers. A stab wound is made approximately 2 cm from the end of the transected colon on the antimesenteric border. The rod of the instrument, without the anvil, is introduced into the colon lumen through the open transected end and placed through the antimesenteric stab wound. The rod is secured by a purse-string suture. The suture is tied and the anvil placed on the center rod (Figure 13–21, *A*). The anvil is introduced into the lumen of the ileum with the previously placed purse-string suture, the ileum is advanced on the anvil, and the suture is tied (Figure 13–21, *B*). The EEA instrument is closed and the stapler fired (Figure 13–21, *C*). The instrument is opened slightly, and a traction or figure-of-8 suture is placed around the staple line. The edge of the staple is lifted over the edge of the anvil, and simultaneously the instrument is rotated and removed. At this time the anastomotic line for hemostasis is inspected before the closure of the transverse colon. Three stay sutures are placed in a through-and-through mucosa-to-mucosa fashion sequentially to hold the edge of the bowel, and then a TA55 stapler is fired for terminal closure of the anastomosis, completing a functional end-to-side anastomosis (Figure 13–21, *D* and *E*).

An alternative method of approximating the right colon to the small bowel can be performed with the GIA instrument. The bowel segments previously transected with the GIA staplers are brought together in an antimesenteric fashion. The antimesenteric corners of the staple line closure of the ileum and transverse colon are excised. The GIA instrument is inserted into each bowel lumen on the antimesenteric border of each limb of the bowel. The instrument is closed and fired. The anastomosis is checked for hemostasis. The common opening can be closed with a TA55 or TA90 stapler, but because of the discrepancy in the segments of the bowel, the staple lines should be staggered to

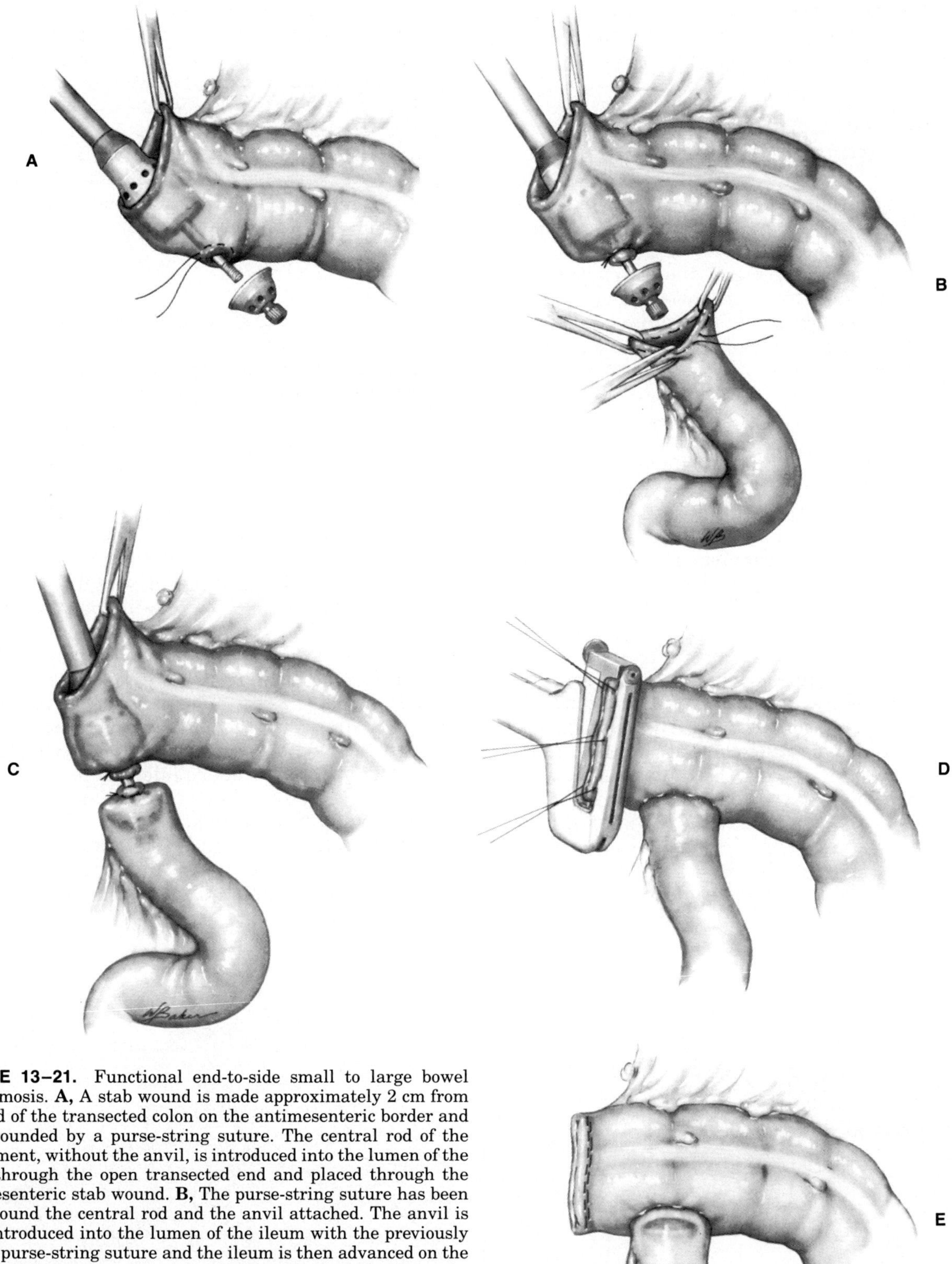

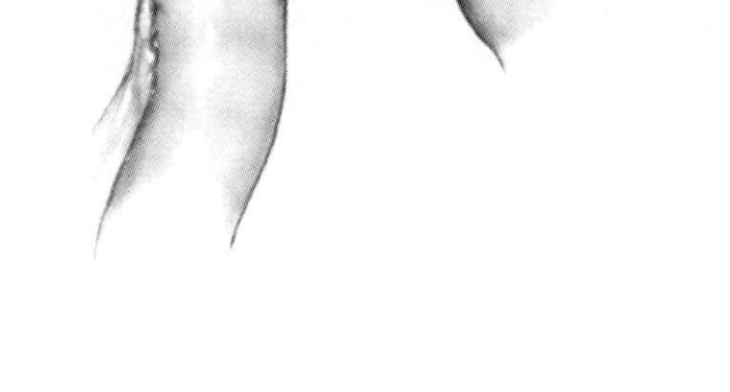

FIGURE 13–21. Functional end-to-side small to large bowel anastomosis. **A,** A stab wound is made approximately 2 cm from the end of the transected colon on the antimesenteric border and is surrounded by a purse-string suture. The central rod of the instrument, without the anvil, is introduced into the lumen of the colon through the open transected end and placed through the antimesenteric stab wound. **B,** The purse-string suture has been tied around the central rod and the anvil attached. The anvil is then introduced into the lumen of the ileum with the previously placed purse-string suture and the ileum is then advanced on the anvil and the suture tied. Allis clamps placed on the ileum facilitate insertion of the anvil. **C,** The EEA stapler is closed and fired. **D,** The transverse colon closure is performed with a TA55 stapler. **E,** Completed functional end-to-side small to large bowel anastomosis. (From U.S. Surgical Corporation, Norwalk, CT, © 1974, 1980, 1986. Used with permission.)

avoid producing three intersecting staple lines. This results in a functional end-to-end anastomosis (Figure 13–22).

Creation of an Indiana Continent Urinary Diversion

In creating an Indiana pouch, or a coloileal reservoir, a coloileal bowel anastomosis is performed to reconstitute the fecal stream, as previously described for using the EEA and the TA55 staplers to construct a small to large bowel anastomosis. The continence mechanism of the Indiana pouch is created by tapering the terminal ileum over a 14F or 16F red rubber catheter. As originally described, this was a sutured plication in which the first layer of sutures was a series of Lembert sutures 8 to 10 mm apart, beginning at the ileocecal valve and extending to the end of the ileal segment.[30] The first row of interrupted or running Lembert sutures was reinforced with a second running suture of 3-0 silk placed in a simple fashion. GIA stapling to reduce the diameter of the ileal segment proved useful for reducing operative time by decreasing the amount of manual sewing required.[31] GIA stapling is performed by placing a 14F or 16F red rubber Robinson catheter into the terminal ileal stoma and placing Allis clamps on the antimesenteric border sequentially to approximate the bowel around the catheter and to provide traction. As the Allis clamps approach the ileocecal valve, they are placed closer to the edge to allow an angled staple line, since a curved staple line cannot be placed. The GIA stapler is then fired sequentially until the final GIA firing occurs, with the tip of the GIA stapler near the ileocecal valve angling off the ileal segment (Figure 13–23). It is important not to overlap the staple lines on consecutive GIA firings because catheters can be caught on the protruding intraluminal staples during intermittent catheterization. Continence has been achieved when either staples or sutures were used to taper the ileum. The use of staples instead of sutures is advocated because staples decrease operative time and produce a more consistent lumen diameter, which promotes a smooth course for the catheter and therefore makes intermittent catheterization easier to perform.

Creation of Nipple Valves

Stapling devices have had a significant role in the evolution of the valve mechanisms for the Kock and Mainz pouch continent urinary reservoirs. The Kock pouch, first described in 1982, is achieved by antimesenteric longitudinal transection of ileum. The pouch is formed from two equal-sized segments of detubularized ileum. Two intussuscepted segments of ileum are sutured into place to create two one-way valves, one to accept the ureters and one for continence, thus allowing flow of urine into but not out of the pouch.[32] The Mainz pouch, first described in 1983, is achieved by antimesenteric longitudinal transection of ileum and cecum with the formation of a pouch from the cecum and two equal-sized ileal loops.[33] This method of bowel reconstruction was first described for augmentation cystoplasty and was then adapted for continent diversion and later for total bladder replacement, with anastomosis of the pouch to the membranous urethra. In each case the ureters are reimplanted into the ascending colon or cecum by a submucosal tunnel technique, which results in an antirefluxing ureterointestinal reimplantation. Alloplastic stomal

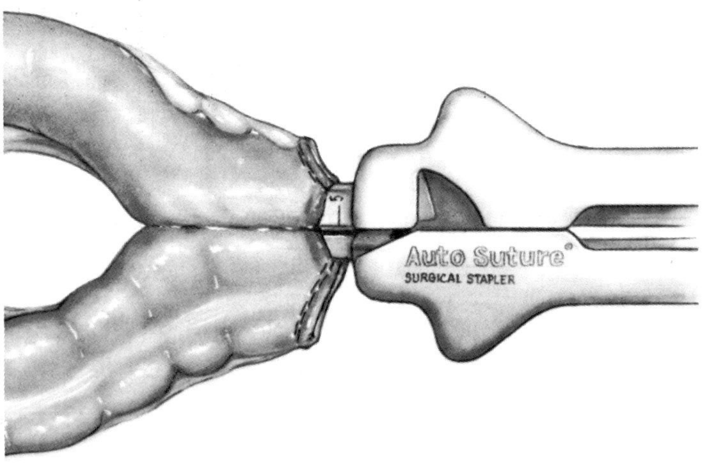

A

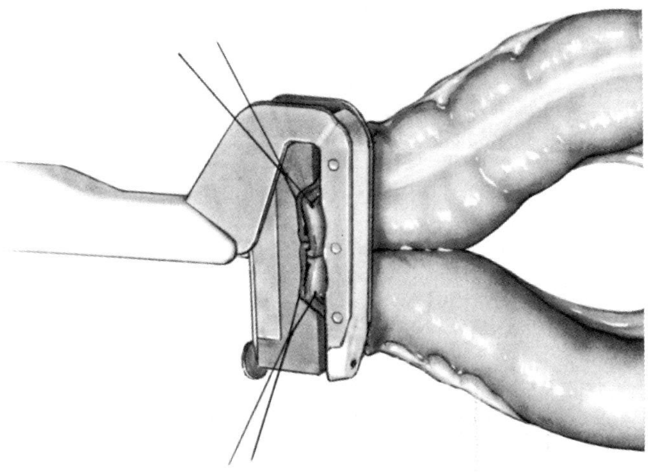

B

FIGURE 13–22. Functional end-to-end small to large bowel anastomosis. **A,** The antimesenteric corners of the staple line closure of the ileum and transverse colon are excised. One limb of the GIA stapler is inserted into each bowel lumen, and the instrument is closed, fired, and removed. **B,** The common opening is closed with a TA55 or TA90 stapler, completing the anastomosis. (From U.S. Surgical Corporation, Norwalk, CT, © 1979, 1980, 1988. Used with permission.)

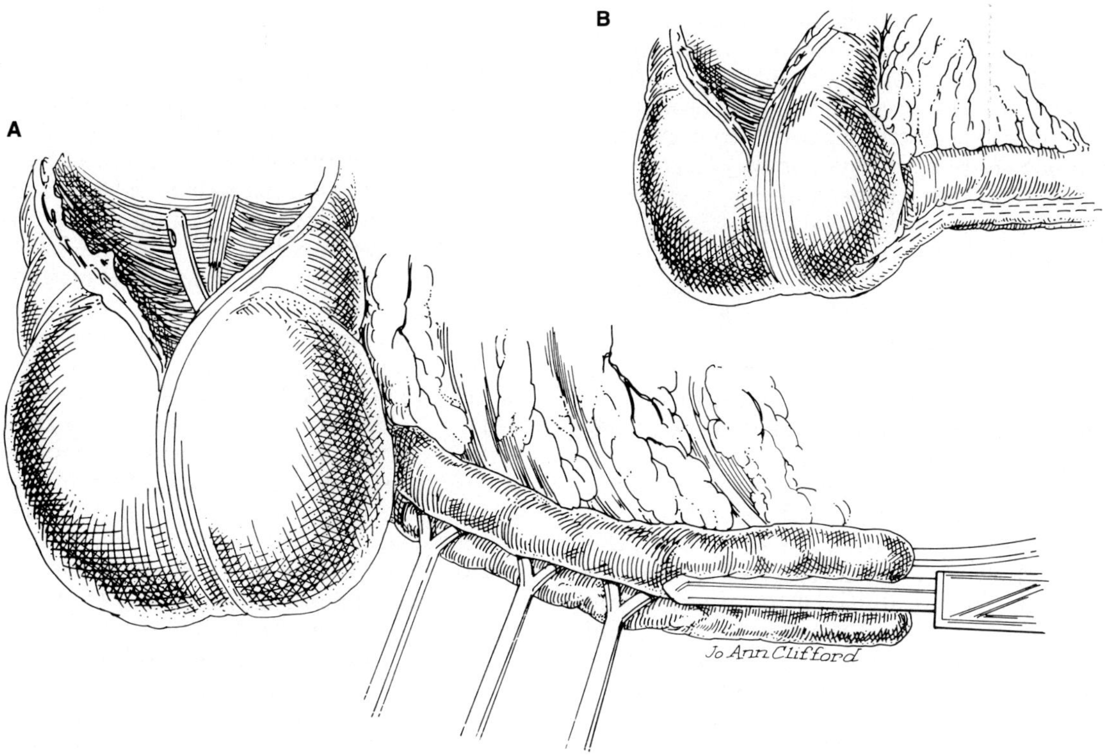

FIGURE 13–23. Stapled tapering of the terminal ileum. **A,** The GIA stapler is fired sequentially between a 14F or 16F red rubber Robinson catheter and Allis clamps placed on the antimesenteric border of the bowel. **B,** Angling off of the ileal segment is necessary near the ileocecal valve. Six to eight plicating sutures are then placed over the cecum itself.

prostheses were used initially to achieve continence, but because of infection and erosion, a technique of ileoileal intussusception through the ileocecal valve was adopted in an attempt to create a continent stoma. In an initial series of eight patients, in whom the ileoileal intussusception was only sutured, seven required surgical revision because of prolapse of the valve.[34] These results, as well as early results with the Kock pouch, showed that the success of the one-way valve in both continent diversions was limited by the difficulty in securing the intussuscepted segment. As a result the use of staplers to construct nipple valves began. Initially ileoileal intussusception was performed with three or four rows of 4.8 mm TA55 staples. The four separate firings of the 4.8 mm TA55 stapling device failed to prevent extussusception when the pouch was filled because the nipple valve was not actually secured to the back wall of the pouch. It became evident that the intussuscepted valve had to be attached to the wall of the reservoir to prevent nipple failure. Several modifications in technique followed. The next modification of the one-way ileal stapled valve was to make a hole in the back wall of the pouch, pass the 4.8 mm TA55 stapling device nose through the hole, and staple the two layers of bowel of the intussuscepted nipple to the back wall of the pouch (Figure 13–24).[35] Therefore the 4.8 mm staples secured three separate layers of ileum together. Although securing the nipple valve to the back wall of the pouch prevented most extussusceptions with pouch filling, a weak point remained because of the alignment pin of the TA55 stapling device.

At the tip of the 4.8 mm TA55 stapling device is a stainless steel alignment pin that must puncture all the layers of bowel to be stapled. If this maneuver is not performed, when the staples are fired, staples near the tip of the stapling device are improperly formed. These exposed and improperly

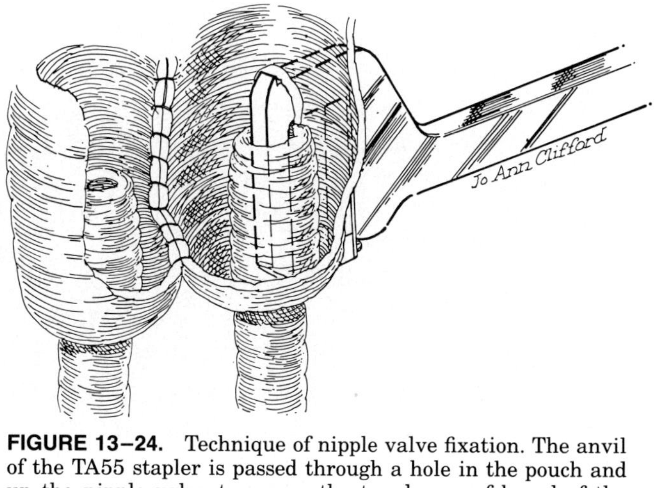

FIGURE 13–24. Technique of nipple valve fixation. The anvil of the TA55 stapler is passed through a hole in the pouch and up the nipple valve to secure the two layers of bowel of the nipple valve to the back wall of the pouch.

closed staples lead to stone formation because intestinal mucosa does not cover them. Nonabsorbable staples, if left exposed to the urinary tract in an intestinal reservoir, incur the risk of stone formation. If, however, the staples are fired correctly, the bowel mucosa grows out over the surface of the staples and the staples do not remain exposed. Nevertheless, stone formation on exposed staples has been reported, as previously discussed in the section on absorbable staples.[21–23] With the alignment pin in place the staples fire securely. Properly formed staples should allow mucosal regeneration, preventing stone formation, but the pinhole tract from the alignment pin must be closed. During one point in the American evolution of the Kock pouch urinary reservoir, the most common cause of failure was the development of a pinhole fistula because of this alignment pin.[36] The fistula developed because the alignment pin, when placed through the nipple valve at the base of the valve, creates an ileoileal fistula. The ileoileal fistula allows urine to pass through the base of the nipple valve into the ileal segment outside the pouch, bypassing the one-way mechanism of the valve. Therefore valves with patent pinhole fistulas have a two-way fistula through which the urine can leak. Although this pinhole tract can be closed in one, two, or three separate layers at the time of one-way nipple valve construction, the frequent passage of a catheter through the continence nipple valve for intermittent drainage of the pouch weakens the valve and may lead to leakage of the continent reservoir at the stomal site.

Two important modifications in stapling devices have been designed to eliminate the problem of pinhole fistulas in stapled one-way nipple valves. The United States Surgical Corp. has developed a two-row 5 cm staple line that does not require an alignment pin. This is a modification of the GIA55 knifeless stapling device, or S-GIA. In this stapling device the inner two rows of the four-row staple cartridge have been removed, and the most proximal six staples from the outer rows have been removed. When this GIA device is passed down the intussuscepted ileum and fired, it leaves two rows of staples approximately 5 mm apart, without staples at the tip of the nipple valve. This special modified S-GIA stapling device has eliminated both the problem with pinhole fistulas and the problem with stone formation at the exposed staples at the tip of the nipple valve.

The other modified stapling instrument that was designed specifically to eliminate pinhole fistulas is the TA55 equivalent instrument developed by the 3M Corp. Because of modification in the construction and firing mechanism, the instrument allows a TA55-type cartridge to be fired without scissoring of the cartridge, even though the alignment pin is eliminated. This instrument is available in the United States only as an experimental prototype, as clinical experience increases, it may prove useful.

A major improvement in the construction of the one-way stapled intussuscepted segment was a modification described by Dr. Rudolf Hohenfellner in Mainz, Germany.[34] In this modification the 4.8 mm TA55 stapling device is used to staple the nipple valve to the back wall of the pouch. However, instead of passing the stapling device from the tip of the nipple valve back toward the base through an enterotomy site, the operator passes the anvil of the stapling device down the serosal surface of the intussuscepted nipple valve. The outer layer of the two-layer nipple valve is next stapled to the back wall of the pouch with one firing of the 4.8 mm TA55 cartridge (Figure 13–25). This places the alignment pinhole at the tip of the nipple valve, where no fistula formation can occur. The staple cartridge staples two layers of bowel together, not three, decreasing the likelihood of ischemic necro-

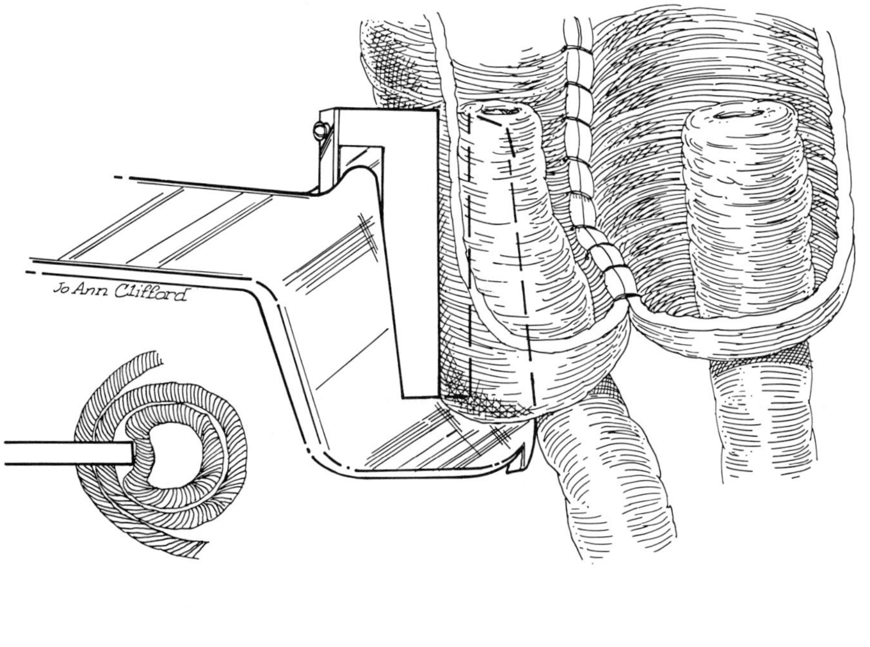

FIGURE 13–25. Hohenfellner technique of nipple valve fixation. The anvil of the TA55 stapler is passed between the two serosal surfaces of the intussuscepted nipple valve. The outer surface of the two-layer nipple valve is next stapled to the back wall of the pouch.

sis from having more layers of bowel in a staple cartridge than the cartridge was designed for. In addition, three staple lines are on each side, preventing asymmetric eversion. Since this technique was adopted, slippage and prolapse have not been problems. The Hohenfellner method can be used for both Kock pouch and Mainz pouch nipple valve construction.

The technique of ileoileal intussusception for creation of a Mainz pouch continent valve begins with the use of cautery or 4-0 silk ties to transect 6 to 8 cm of mesentery from the segment to be intussuscepted. Allis clamps are then used to intussuscept the ileum and pull it through the natural tunnel of the ileocecal valve. Stabilization of the intussuscepted segment is then performed by using the TA-55 to place two rows of 4.8 mm staples at 120-degree angles from each other and from the presumed line of placement of the fixation staple line (Figure 13–26, *A*). Fixation of the ileocecal valve and the intussuscepted segment is accomplished as described by Hohenfellner in creating Kock nipple valves. The stapler is inserted from outside the pouch at the base of the intussusception into the space between the inner and outer walls of the intussusception (Figure 13–26, *B*). In addition, the tip of the intussusception is sutured circumferentially to the cecal opening of the ileocecal valve in an interrupted fashion.

For the construction of the Kock pouch nipple valve, the knifeless S-GIA staple cartridge described previously is fired twice. These two firings are done down the nipple valve approximately 120 degrees apart. Then the 4.8 mm TA55 stapling cartridge is used to staple the outer layer of the intussuscepted bowel to the back wall of the pouch by the Hohenfellner method. The single alignment pinhole that is identified at the tip of the nipple valve can be closed easily with figure-of-8 or horizontal mattress absorbable sutures. A preferred method is to reinforce the seromuscular junction of the stapled one-way ileal segment with a collar of absorbable Dexon mesh, which is sutured into place with 3-0 chromic suture. This method of valve construction has a success rate greater than 90%.

Creation of Urinary Reservoir Stomas

The intraluminal circular stapling device was first used to create intestinal or urinary reservoir stomas when it became apparent that stapling devices reduced operating time. Chung described a technique for using the surgical stapler to make an end colostomy and a Brooke's ileostomy and reported on 26 stomas observed for up to 10 months.[37] The patients in this series had no complications or wound infections, and Chung noted that the cost of the cartridge could be considered recovered because the technique decreased the operating time by an average of 13 minutes. His technique resulted in the creation of a neat, geometric stoma, and he reported not a single instance of prolapse, retraction, necrosis, periostoma herniation, or fistula. Donovan, Winfield, and Williams in 1989 confirmed

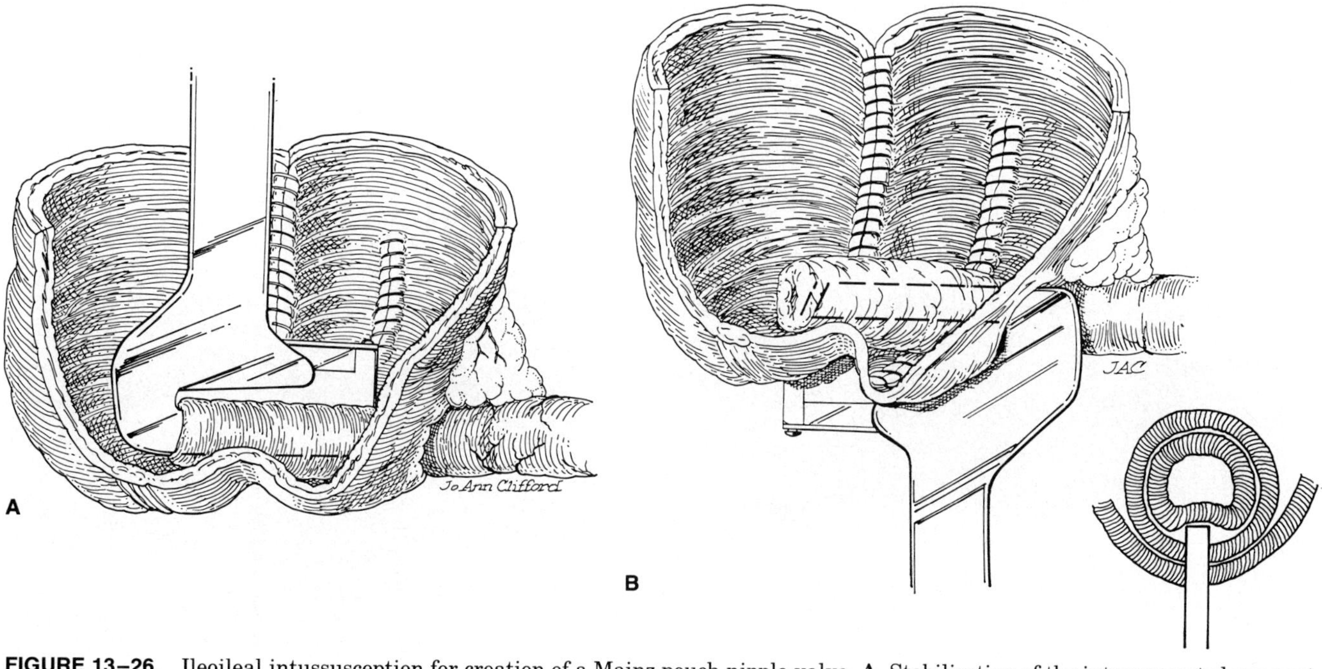

A

B

FIGURE 13–26. Ileoileal intussusception for creation of a Mainz pouch nipple valve. **A,** Stabilization of the intussuscepted segment is performed by using the TA55 stapler to place two rows of 4.8 mm staples at 120-degree angles from one another and the presumed line of placement of the fixating staple line. **B,** Fixation of the ileocecal valve and the intussuscepted segment is accomplished by inserting the anvil between the inner and outer wall of the intussusception from outside the pouch.

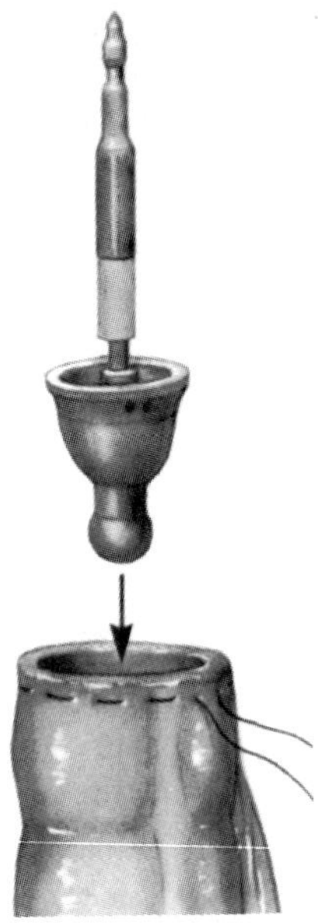

FIGURE 13–27. Colostomy formation with the EEA stapler. From inside the abdomen, the anvil with the anvil shaft is introduced into the open end of the colon, which is then closed around the shaft by drawing up on the previously placed purse-string suture. (From U.S. Surgical Corporation, Norwalk, CT, © 1974, 1980, 1988. Used with permission.)

the reliability and rapidity of the stapled stomal construction technique in eight cases and modified the procedure to include the introduction of ureteral stents.[38] A description of the technique and use of the intraluminal stapling devices for the creation of an end colostomy and urinary ileostomy follows.

A site is chosen for the colostomy. The colon is grasped and the mesentery cleared for 1 to 2 cm, and a purse-string suture of 1-0 silk is inserted circumferentially parallel to the line of transection of the colon. A suitable cartridge for an end colostomy is 29 mm in diameter (21 mm in internal diameter), and the appropriate anvil is chosen. From inside the abdomen the anvil with the anvil shaft is introduced into the open end of the colon, which is then closed around the shaft by drawing up on the previously placed purse-string suture (Figure 13–27). The colon is brought through the abdominal wall by pulling through the anvil shaft until the anvil, now just closed by the colon, sits in the subcutaneous space. The chosen site of the colostomy is prepared from within the abdomen by incising the peritoneum, muscle, and fascia for a zone of 1 to 2 cm or of sufficient size to accommodate the colon. The subcutaneous fat is dissected with electrocautery to the level of the dermis. The anvil shaft is introduced through the incision to the skin, and a knife is used to incise the skin, allowing passage of the shaft through the skin (Figure 13–28). The anvil and colon are directed to just beneath the skin, and the anvil is mounted onto the cartridge of the EEA stapler. The combined thickness of the skin and colon wall is about 2.5 mm, which is the dial setting to be used on instruments that have provision for tissue thickness adjustment, such as the ILS stapler from Ethicon. The instrument is fired and removed (Figure 13–29). The mucosa readily heals to the dermis, and the result is an esthetically acceptable colostomy. With interrupted sutures the colon is secured to the peritoneum from within the abdomen.

An alternative technique for colostomy creation

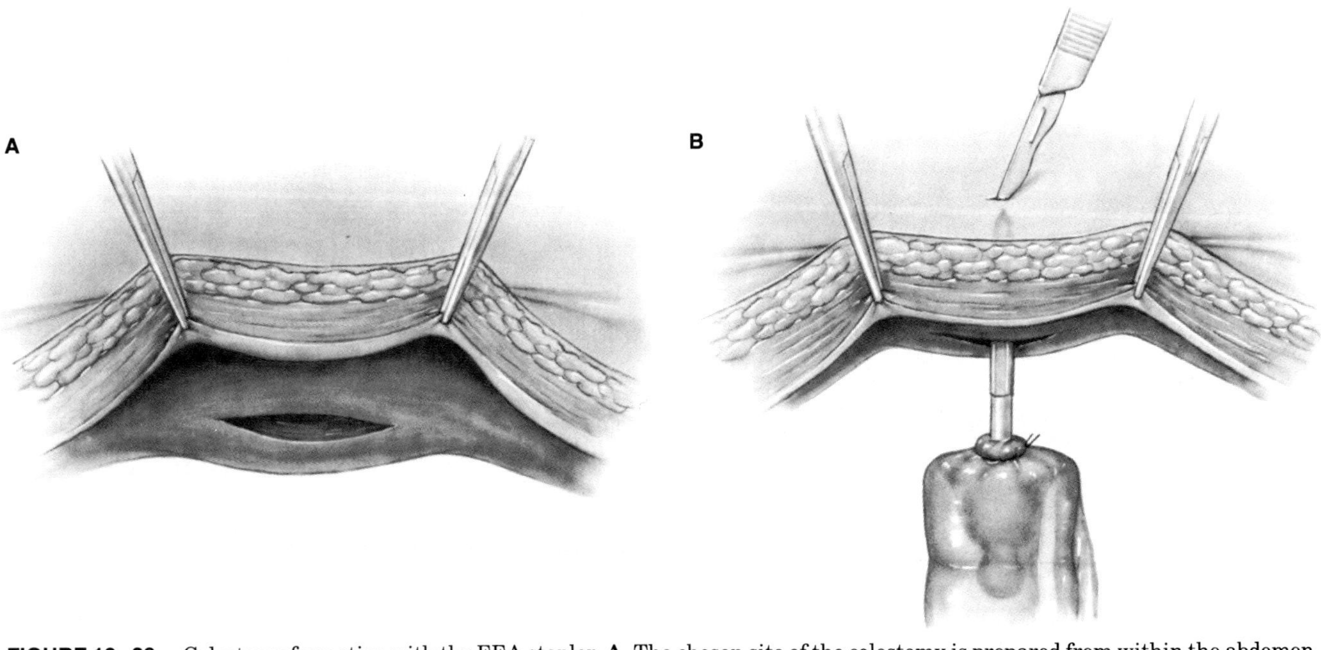

FIGURE 13–28. Colostomy formation with the EEA stapler. **A,** The chosen site of the colostomy is prepared from within the abdomen. **B,** The anvil shaft is introduced to the skin, and a knife is used to incise the skin, allowing passage of the shaft through the skin. (From U.S. Surgical Corporation, Norwalk, CT, © 1974, 1980, 1988. Used with permission.)

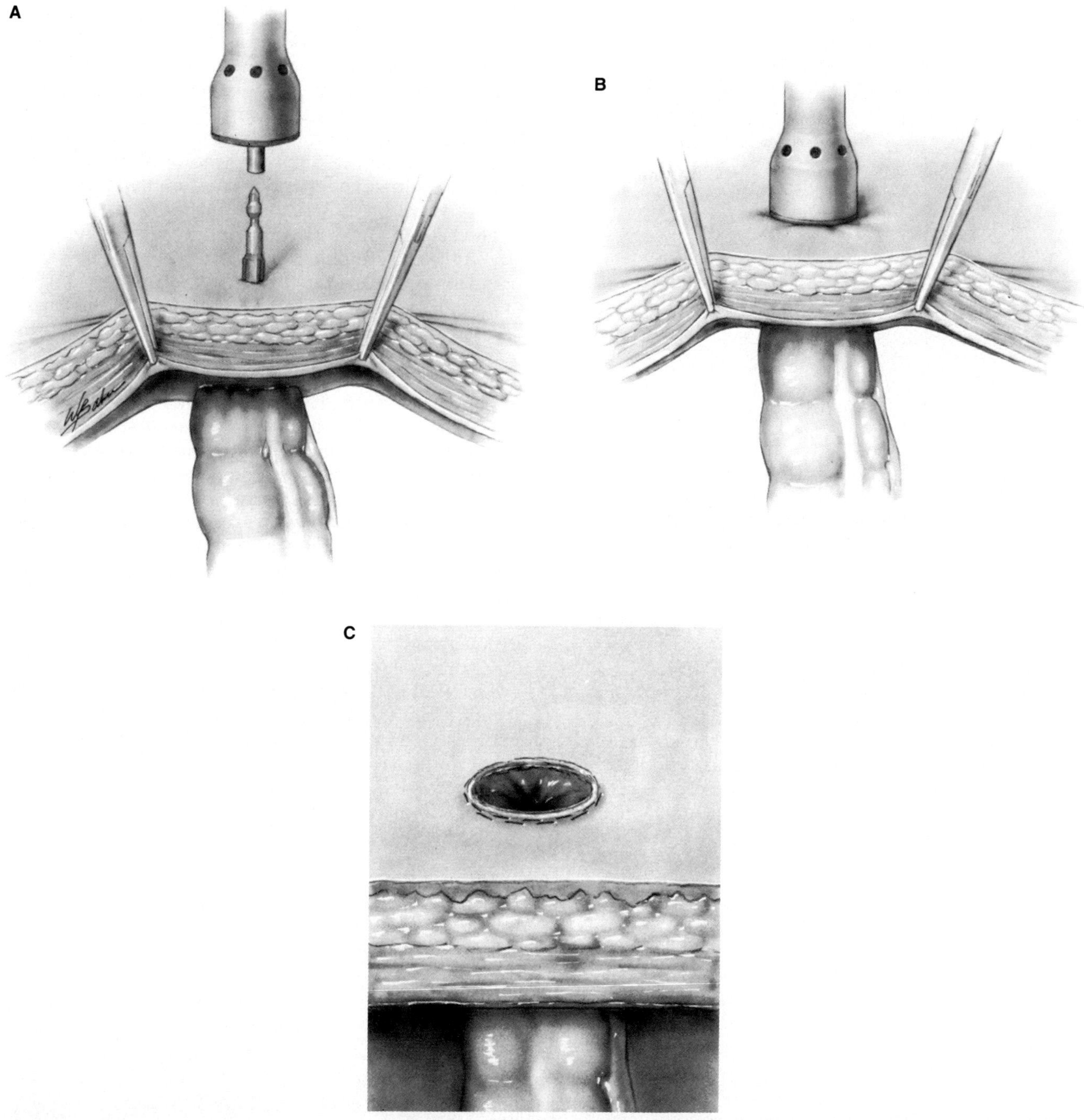

FIGURE 13–29. Colostomy creation using the EEA stapler. **A,** The anvil and colon are positioned just beneath the skin, and the anvil is mounted onto the cartridge. **B,** The anvil-cartridge assembly is approximated and fired. **C,** Completed colostomy. (From U.S. Surgical Corporation, Norwalk, CT, © 1974, 1980, 1988. Used with permission.)

and for stoma development during ileal loop urinary diversion, including the use of ureteral stents, has been described. Following colon or ileum transection, a disk of skin approximately 1 cm for a colostomy or 1.5 to 2 cm for an ileostomy is excised. Too large a defect may cause prolapse, but this larger diameter facilitates drawing the conduit into the subcutaneous space and allows nipple eversion. Once the cruciate incisions are made in the rectus sheath and the transabdominal path through the middle of the rectus muscle has been created, a 2-0 monofilament purse-string suture is placed around the circular skin wound (Figure 13–30). The bowel is drawn through the incision, and a purse-string suture is placed just below the staple line. The distal limb of the conduit can be clamped with a serrated clamp that allows placement of a circumferential purse-string suture with a Keith needle. Once the purse-string suture has been applied, the staples are excised, opening the bowel (Figure 13–31). The anvil is next introduced into the lumen of the bowel and tied around the shaft.

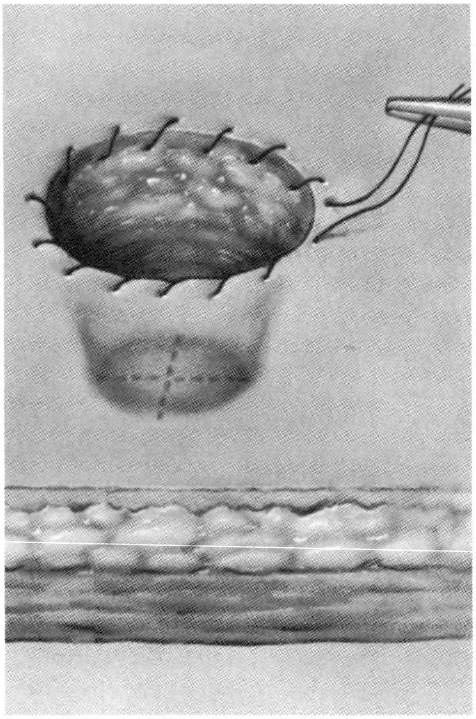

FIGURE 13–30. Colostomy or ileostomy creation with the EEA stapler. A 2-0 monofilament purse-string suture is applied manually to the skin. (From U.S. Surgical Corporation, Norwalk, CT, © 1974, 1980, 1988. Used with permission.)

If ureteral stents have been placed, the stents can be trimmed to 5 cm beyond the distal conduit and then pushed back into the conduit before insertion of the staple anvil into the conduit.[38] Gentle downward traction places the anvil and bowel into the subcutaneous space, and the purse-string suture on the skin is tied. The instrument is closed, fired, and removed (Figure 13–32). Stents can then be retrieved and secured. For ileostomy a nipple is formed by pushing out a suitable length of ileum from inside the abdomen. The ileum is then secured to the peritoneum. This technique allows the operator to adjust the stomal eversion even after the staples have been fired.

The use of the intraluminal stapling device for stomal construction offers distinct advantages over traditional suture techniques. The intercutaneous anastomosis is watertight, eliminating the possibility of continuous contamination of the subcutaneous space by urine. In addition, the stapled enterocutaneous stoma is constructed rapidly, reducing operative time. Eversion of the stoma, achieved by adjusting the length of the distal conduit brought into the subcutaneous compartment, eliminates the need for everting sutures. Only two purse-string sutures are required; in traditional manual construction each stoma skin suture must be tied. Although the first technique described can also be used to create an ileostomy, as was originally described by Chung, Donovan notes that with the second technique, because the conduit is brought out through the skin before being loaded on the anvil, the desired amount of intestine for eversion of the stoma is estimated in a single step. In addition, the second technique allows the use of ureteral stents. When first constructed the stoma is a concentric ring that appears to have been formed with machine precision. With time it becomes somewhat elliptical, reflecting the direction of Langer's lines. The skin between the two rows

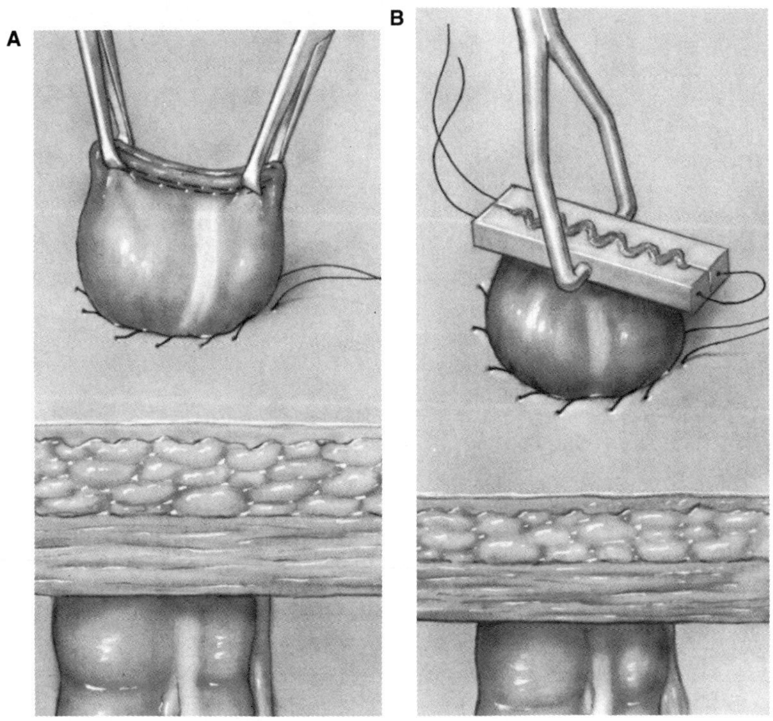

FIGURE 13–31. Colostomy or ileostomy creation with the EEA stapler. **A,** The bowel has been exposed through the incision. **B,** Use of a purse-string device to apply the purse-string suture just below the staple line. (From U.S. Surgical Corporation, Norwalk, CT, © 1974, 1980, 1988. Used with permission.)

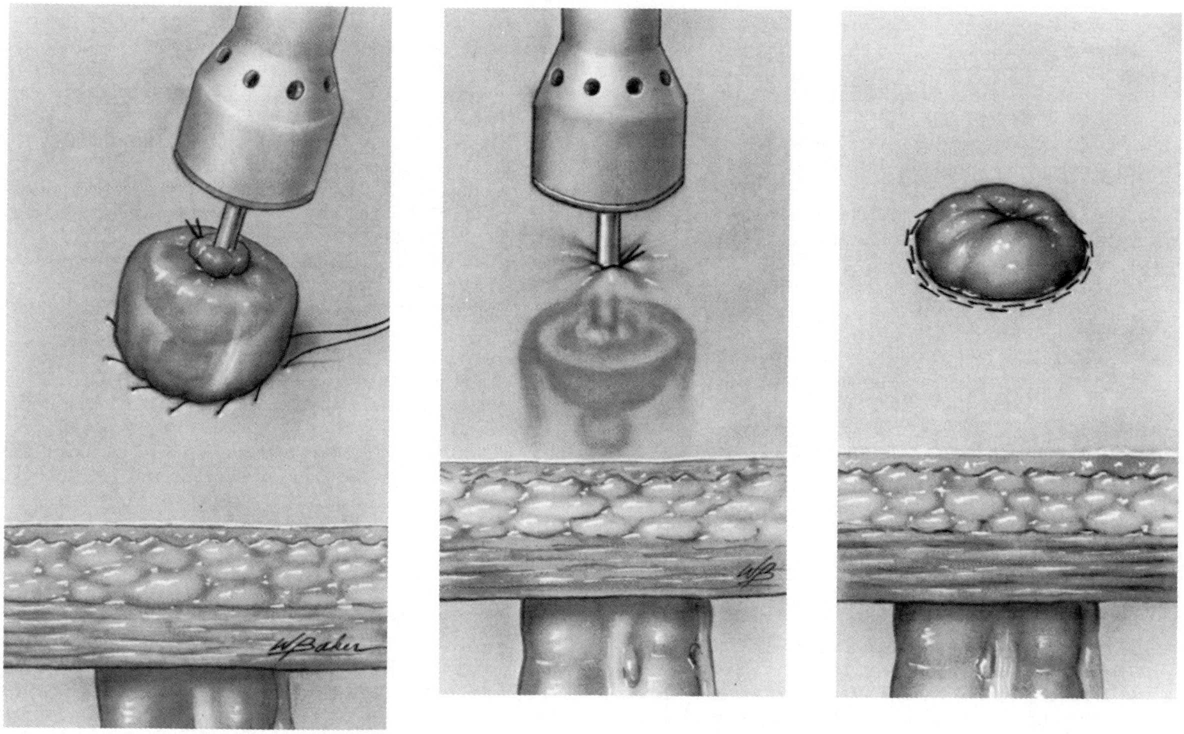

A B C

FIGURE 13–32. Colostomy or ileostomy creation with the EEA stapler. **A,** The anvil has been introduced into the bowel and the purse-string suture tied. **B,** Downward traction places the anvil and bowel into the subcutaneous space, after which the cutaneous purse-string suture is tied. **C,** The instrument has been fired and removed. (From U.S. Surgical Corporation, Norwalk, CT, © 1974, 1980, 1988. Used with permission.)

of staples appears somewhat edematous in the first few days, but this is transient and the staples fall off in a month or two, leaving no scars. In the future this procedure may become preferred, but clinical experience thus far is too small to determine whether it is better.

CONCLUSION

Stapling devices are useful in urologic surgery, and their application is likely to increase. The efficacy of staples has been confirmed, and the urologic surgeon should become familiar with the instruments' technical features and applications. As with suture techniques, tissues to be stapled should demonstrate adequate blood supply, absence of sepsis, and lack of tension across staple lines. With strict adherence to these principles and with adequate fundamental knowledge of stapling, optimal results can be obtained.

REFERENCES

1. Steichen FM, Ravitch MM: History of mechanical devices and instruments for suturing. In Steichen FM, Ravitch MM, (eds): Stapling in surgery. Chicago: Year Book 1984, pp 3-77.
2. Sugarbaker ED, Wiley HM: Rectocolic anastomosis: simplified method. Surg Gynecol Obstel 93:597, 1951.
3. Steichen FM, Ravitch MM: Contemporary stapling instruments and basic mechanical suture techniques. In Steichen FM, Ravitch MM, (eds): The surgical clinics of North America. Philadelphia: Saunders 1984, p 425.
4. Ravitch MM, Hirsch LC: The great Australian staple caper. Surg Rounds, May 1990, p 45.
5. Ravitch MM, Brolin R, Kolter J, Yap S: Studies in the healing of intestinal anastomoses. World J Surg 5:627, 1981.
6. Ravitch MM, Riverola A, VanGrov J: Studies of intestinal healing. I. Preliminary studies of the mechanism of healing of the everting intestinal anastomosis. Johns Hopkins Med J 121:343, 1967.
7. Ravitch MM, Canalis F, Weinshelbaum A, McCormick J: Studies in intestinal healing. III. Observations on everting intestinal anastomoses. Trans Am Surg Assoc 85:368, 1967.
8. Smith CR, Cokelet GR, Adams JT, Schwartz SI: Vascularity of gastrointestinal staple lines demonstrated with silicone rubber injection. Am J Surg 142:563, 1981.
9. Ravitch MM, Brolin RE, Kolter FP Jr, Yap S: Studies in the healing of intestinal anastomoses. World J Surg 5:627, 1981.
10. Ravitch MM, Riverola A, VanGrov J: Studies of intestinal healing. I. Preliminary studies of the mechanism of healing of the everting intestinal anastomosis. Johns Hopkins Med J 121:343, 1967.
11. Chassin JL, Rifkind KM, Sussman B, et al: The stapled gastrointestinal tract anastomosis: incidence of postoperative complications compared with the sutured anastomosis. Ann Surg 188:689, 1978.
12. Relling RB, Relling WA, Bernle WA, et al: Prospective controlled study of gastrointestinal stapled anastomoses. Am J Surg 139:147, 1980.
13. Burbrick MP, Lundeen JW, Hitchcock CR: A comparative

radiographic study of low anterior colon anastomoses in dogs. Surgery 89:454, 1981.
14. Lowden IMR, Gear MWL, Kilby JD: Stapling instruments in upper gastrointestinal surgery: a retrospective study of 362 cases. Br J Surg 69:333, 1982.
15. Schwartzbart G, Lubin J: Experience with Auto Suture surgical stapling instruments: fate of enterically applied staples. Int Surg 63:146, 1978.
16. Ravitch M, Ong TH, Gazzola L: A new precise and rapid technique for intestinal resection and anastomosis with staples. Surg Gynecol Obstet 139:6, 1974.
17. Kirker-Head CA, Steckel RR, Schwartz A, Williams R: Evaluation of surgical staples for ligation of the renal pedicle during nephrectomy. Urol Res 16:63, 1988.
18. Warden WS, Nelson HN, Huley JE: New method to control dorsal vein complexes during radical retropubic prostatectomy. Urology 35:364, 1990.
19. Gross SC, Kowalski JB, Lee SH, et al: Surgical ligation clip artifacts on CT scans. Radiology 156:831, 1985.
20. Kleine LI, Jolesa FA, Patz S: MRI artifacts from surgical clips and staples: effects of imaging method and field strength. Presented at the 1987 annual meeting of the Radiological Society of North America, Chicago.
21. Bisson J, Vinson RK, Leadbetter GW: Urolithiasis from stapler anastomosis. Am J Surg 137:280, 1989.
22. Bergman SM, Sears HF, Javadpour N: Complication with mechanical stapling device in creation of ileal conduit. Urology 12:71, 1978.
23. Assaddia A, Lee CN, Petre JH, et al: Two cases of stone formation in ileal conduits after using staple gun for closure of proximal end of isolated loop. J Urol 108:553, 1972.
24. Steckel MF, Jann MS, Kaplan HW, et al: Experimental evaluation of absorbable copolymer staples for hysterectomy. Obstet Gynecol 68:404, 1986.
25. Julian TB: Closure of the urinary bladder with stainless steel and absorbable staples. Ann Surg 204:186, 1986.
26. Wheeless CR: Use of absorbable staples for closure of proximal end of ileal loops. Obstet Gynecol 67:280, 1986.
27. Wheeless CR: Stapling techniques in operations for malignant disease of the female genital tract. Surg Clin North Am 64:591, 1984.
28. Beresford J: Automatic stapling techniques in abdominal hysterectomy. Surg Clin North Am 64:609, 1984.
29. Penalver MA, Bejany DE, Averette HE, et al: Continent urinary diversion in gynecologic oncology. Gynecol Oncol 34:274, 1989.
30. Rowland RG, Mitchell ME, Bittizle R, et al: Indiana continent urinary reservoir. J Urol 137:1136, 1987.
31. Bejany DE, Politano VA: Stapled and nonstapled tapered distal ileum for construction of a continent colonic urinary reservoir. J Urol 140:491, 1988.
32. Kock NG, Nilson AE, Nilsson LO, et al: Urinary diversion via a continent ileal reservoir: clinical results in 12 patients. J Urol 128:469, 1982.
33. Thüroff IW, Alken P, Engelmann U, et al: The Mainz pouch (mixed augmentation ileum 'n zoecum) applicable for bladder augmentation and continent urinary diversion. Aktuel Urol 16:1, 1985.
34. Thüroff IW, Alken P, Riedmiller H, Engelmann U, et al: The Mainz pouch (mixed augmentation ileal and cecum) for bladder augmentation and continent diversion. J Urol 136:17, 1986.
35. Boyd SD, Skinner DG, Lieskovsky G: The continent ileal reservoir (Kock pouch). Semin Urol 5:15, 1987.
36. Lieskovsky G, Skinner DG, Boyd SD: Complications of the Kock pouch. Urol Clin North Am 15(2):195, 1988.
37. Chung RS: End colostomy and Brooke's ileostomy constructed by surgical stapler. Surg Gynecol Obstet 162:63, 1986.
38. Donovan JF, Winfield HN, Williams RD: Construction of the intestinal stoma with an intraluminal stapling device. J Urol 142:1279, 1989.

CHAPTER 14

UROLOGIC LAPAROSCOPY

DOUGLAS F. MILAM

Urologists have discovered laparoscopy. Once strictly a tool of the gynecologist, laparoscopy has been embraced by many fields. Urologic and general surgical interest in the technique has exploded in the past 2 years. Improved instrumentation and societal pressure for less invasive techniques are driving the development of laparoscopic procedures. Pelvic lymphadenectomy for staging adenocarcinoma of the prostate gland is responsible for most of the recent interest among urologists.

Urologists have used the laparoscope to search for intraabdominal testes, drain lymphoceles, examine the extraperitoneal pelvis, and perform pelvic lymphadenectomy, varicocele ligation, orchiectomy, ureterolithotomy, renal biopsy, and simple nephrectomy. Its use in several other procedures, including ureteroneocystostomy, is contemplated. The indications for these and other procedures are still evolving.

This chapter provides basic information about urologic laparoscopy. The first section traces the development of laparoscopic equipment and techniques. Current laparoscopic equipment is then discussed in some detail. The process of establishing the pneumoperitoneum and placing the trocar is discussed next, followed by descriptions of individual urologic procedures. Finally, the incidence and management of laparoscopic complications are discussed. Successful management of the complications associated with this operative technique will facilitate its acceptance as a safe, minimally invasive procedure.

DEVELOPMENT OF LAPAROSCOPY

The modern era of endoscopy probably began with Phillip Bozzini in 1806.[1] He examined the female urethra with a dual-lumen urethral cannula under candle illumination. After this, little progress occurred for almost 100 years.

Kelling in 1901 used a Nitze cystoscope to perform laparoscopy on a dog.[2] Air was used to create a pneumoperitoneum for better visibility. Also using a Nitze cystoscope, the Stockholm physician Jacobaeus performed diagnostic laparoscopy on a man in 1910.[3] Probably not knowing about others' advances, Ott in 1909 passed a speculum into the abdomen and used a head mirror for illumination.[4]

Interest in diagnostic laparoscopy waxed and waned over the next 20 years. In 1923 Jacobaeus reported performing 10 peritoneoscopic procedures on humans.[5] Results were surprisingly good for the time. Only one patient required laparotomy for bleeding. That paper alone did much to establish the safety of laparoscopy. Steiner[6] and Nadeau and Kampmeier[7] also published reports on diagnostic laparoscopy about that time.

Laparoscopic use and techniques expanded during the 1930s. Fervers in 1933 recommended carbon dioxide as the insufflating agent.[8] Before that time air was commonly used, since the greater safety of carbon dioxide had not been recognized. Goetz pioneered peritoneal insufflation through a small needle before inserting the trocar.[9] Development of the blunt obturator insufflation needle by Veress followed in 1938.[10] With only minor modification, this needle is still in widespread use.*

Most early enthusiasm for the development of laparoscopic equipment occurred in Europe, particularly Germany and France. Ruddock was one of the first American physicians to incorporate laparoscopy into his clinical practice. In 1937 he reported 500 procedures of what he termed peritoneoscopy.[11] His technique was surprisingly similar to that performed today. Most of Ruddock's procedures were for evaluation of malignancy, ascites, or jaundice. He reported eight intestinal perforations and one death, which was due to hemorrhage after liver biopsy.

Steady progress continued for 40 years. The British gynecologist Steptoe published the first atlas of laparoscopy.[12] Kalk, a hepatologist, introduced a dual-trocar technique that facilitated organ retrac-

*The blunt obturator insufflation needle is often spelled Verres. We have chosen to maintain the original spelling consistent with the inventor, J. Veress.

tion and manipulation.[13] Semm developed numerous tools and improved on others.[14] The Roeder loop was modified to facilitate intraabdominal knot tying. Semm also devised an automatic inflation device with continuous monitoring of pressure and flow.

Tremendous improvements in optics occurred in the 1960s. The British optical physicist Hopkins invented the rod lens telescope, which had markedly increased image brightness and enhanced optical clarity. The fiberoptic cold light source was also developed at that time. In this system a fiberoptic cable transfers light from an external source by total internal reflection along a waveguide. Although much of the light was lost, removal of the incandescent bulb from the telescope was a major advance.

Hasson was disturbed by the continued, albeit low, complication rate with blind closed laparoscopy. In 1978 he reported his results in using an open technique.[15] His procedure involved opening the midline fascia and inserting the cannula under direct vision.

The mainstream urologic community did not become involved with laparoscopy until the 1980s. The procedure was initially used for locating the nonpalpable testis. Numerous authors reported laparoscopic findings regarding cryptorchidism.[16-25] Elder in 1989 suggested laparoscopic ligation of the testicular vessels 6 months before Fowler-Stephens orchiopexy.[26] Harrison used laparoscopy to locate high intraabdominal testes before microvascular autotransplantation.[27] All eight testes in seven patients were palpably normal in the scrotum after 7 months' follow-up. Numerous authors have reported internal spermatic vein ligation for varicocele. Figge in 1988 reported a laparoscopically controlled transperitoneal nephrolithotomy in a horseshoe kidney.[28]

The recent surge of interest in urologic laparoscopy began in 1989. This interest is due largely to laparoscopic pelvic lymphadenectomy. The first systematic pelvic lymphadenectomy was performed in 1988 by the French gynecologist Overleu.[29] It was done to stage cervical carcinoma. An increasing number of urologists are performing laparoscopic pelvic lymphadenectomy. Schuessler and associates reported the results of 12 laparoscopic pelvic lymph node dissections.[30] Their paper stressed that laparoscopy had lower morbidity than open pelvic lymphadenectomy and offered similar staging information. Several other papers are either under review or scheduled for presentation.

Recent advances in instrumentation have led to more complex laparoscopic procedures. One particularly interesting development is Clayman's report of laparoscopic nephrectomy.[31] The kidney is visualized by mobilization of the colon along the white line of Toldt. The isolated kidney is then manipulated into a bag and extracted through the abdominal wall with a 10 mm tissue morcellator. Continued improvement of suturing and staple technology is sure to expand the realm of laparoscopic urologic procedures.

LAPAROSCOPIC EQUIPMENT

Urologists are experienced endoscopists, performing not only diagnostic but therapeutic maneuvers through the endoscope. Cystoscopy dates to the latter part of the nineteenth century. More recently, urologists have pioneered rigid and flexible ureteropyeloscopy and nephroscopy. Many of these procedures are performed with a video camera and monitor.

The learning curve for laparoscopic techniques is similar to that for ureteroscopy. Both thorough understanding of the equipment and hands-on experience are required. Recently the range of laparoscopic surgery has widened considerably. This expansion into more complex procedures has hastened the development of new equipment.

Operating Room Layout

Efficient use of operating room space is not difficult. Much of the equipment and one video monitor can be kept on a mobile equipment cart (Figure 14–1). This facilitates setup and protects the equipment when not in use. The equipment cart and monitor are positioned off the foot of the bed to the patient's right, which gives the primary surgeon direct line of sight to the monitor. A second monitor is positioned off the foot of the bed to the left and provides the assistant with line of sight viewing. Emergency laparotomy instruments are set up on a back table. Otherwise, the position of the surgeon, assistant, anesthesiologist, scrub nurse, and frequently used instruments are no different than for an open pelvic procedure.

One additional point should be considered. No industry standard for equipment interchangeability exists. This problem can be lessened by using as much equipment from one manufacturer as possible, which also facilitates service and repair of equipment.

Veress Needle

The blunt obturator insufflation needle was developed by Veress in the late 1930s. No significant modifications have been made since then. This device incorporates a hollow blunt central obturator that retracts into the needle (Figure 14–2). Once the needle has penetrated the fascia and peritoneum, the spring-loaded obturator snaps forward to protect internal structures. The only significant advantage of disposable needles is that they are reliably sharp.

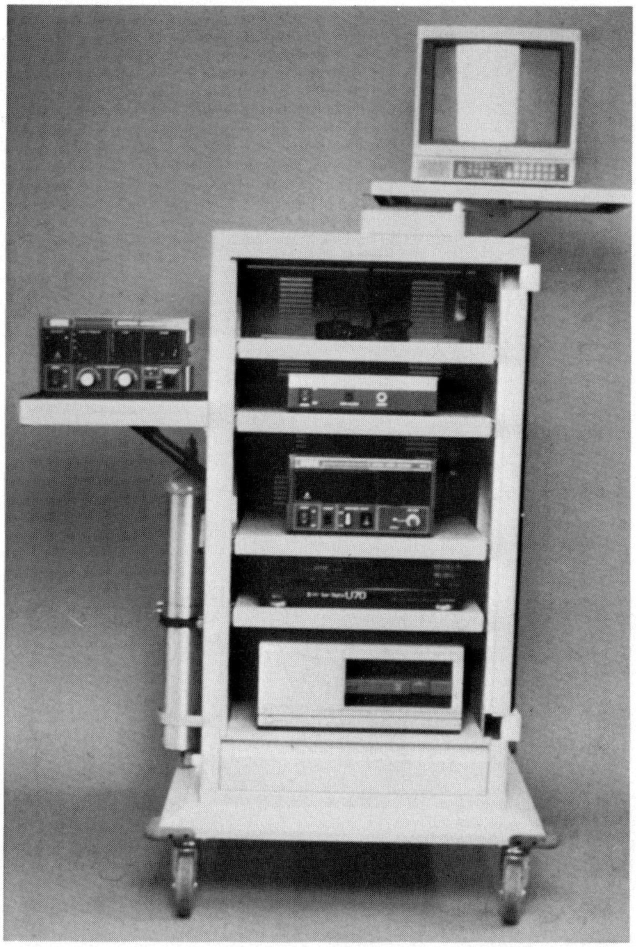

FIGURE 14–1. Mobile equipment cart. The equipment cart can house one monitor and all video and insufflation equipment. (Courtesy of Karl Storz.)

Trocar and Cannula

The peritoneum is entered with a sharp pyramid-tipped trocar surrounded by a cannula (Figure 14–3). This device incorporates both an insufflation port and a channel for instrument placement. Laparoscopic cannulas come in two general size ranges, 10 to 12 and 5 to 6 mm. Reusable stainless steel trocars have a spring-loaded trumpet valve to permit instrument placement but prohibit egress of gas when no instrument is in the channel. Disposable trocars have a flap valve for the same purpose.

Disposable trocars and cannulas have several advantages. First, the trocar is always sharp, which reduces the force required to pierce the abdominal wall. Deep, forceful entry into the peritoneum can result from a dull trocar. Disposable instruments also incorporate a retractable plastic sheath (Figure 14–4). Much like the Veress needle obturator, the sheath snaps foward on passage through the abdominal wall to cover the sharp trocar tip. Threaded gripping devices like that shown on the 5 mm cannula in Figure 14–5 are also useful. They lessen the chance of accidental cannula removal and subsequent loss of pneumoperitoneum.

Insufflation Equipment

The operative space is created by instilling gas into the peritoneal cavity. Once intraperitoneal access is obtained, gas is instilled by a high-volume insufflator. This device must be capable of measuring both flow rate and pressure (Figure 14–6). Gauges or light-emitting diodes should be easily readable, since insufflation pressure is a critical piece of information. A high pressure alarm is helpful.

Older machines had maximum gas flow rates of 3 L/min. This is insufficient for interventional procedures. Multiple cannulas and the passage of instruments cause significant gas leakage. To maintain a constant pneumoperitoneum, the insufflator should have a maximum flow rate of at least 6 and preferably 10 L/min.

Nearly all urologists in the United States use carbon dioxide as the insufflating agent. Air and pure oxygen were used in the past but are now considered unsafe because poor absorption in blood increases the likelihood of gas embolism and because both air and oxygen support combustion. Nitrous oxide is less irritating to the peritoneum than carbon dioxide, which imparts a relative advantage for diagnostic procedures performed under local anesthesia. However, therapeutic or complex diagnostic urologic procedures are performed with general anesthesia, which eliminates the one advantage of nitrous oxide. Also, like air and oxygen, nitrous oxide is poorly absorbed by blood and freely supports combustion.

There is little reason to use anything other than

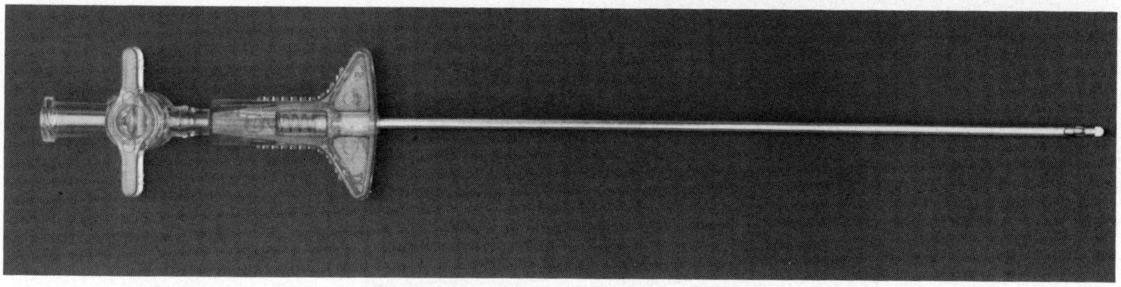

FIGURE 14–2. Veress needle. The spring-loaded blunt obturator shields the needle tip.

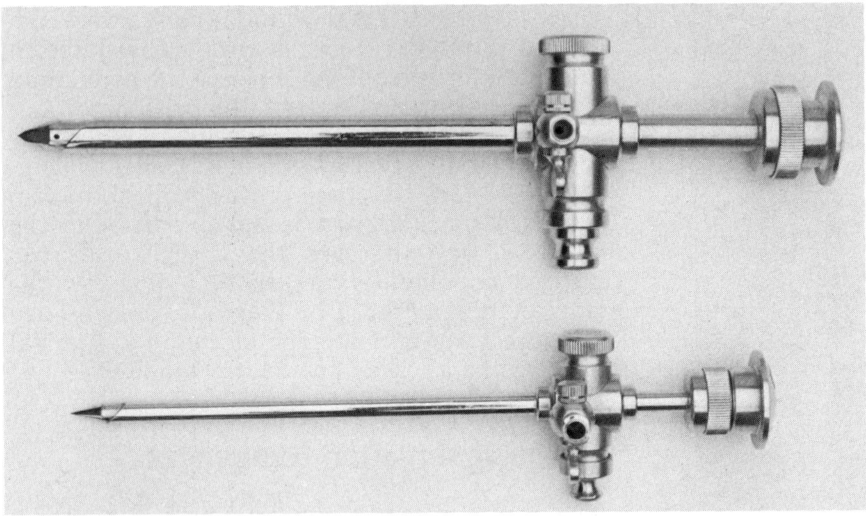

FIGURE 14–3. Reusable stainless steel trocars (5 and 10 mm sizes shown).

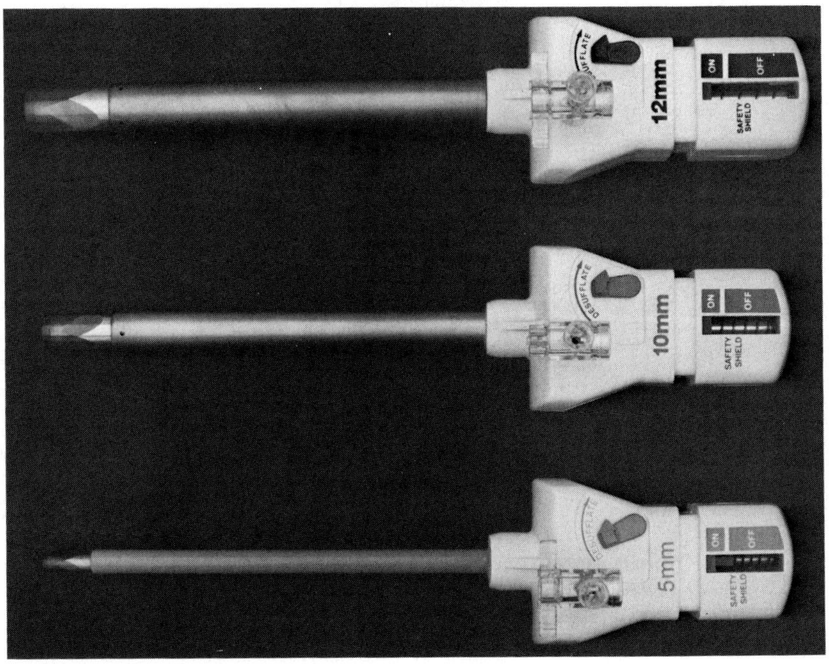

FIGURE 14–4. Disposable trocars. Spring-loaded transparent plastic shields are shown covering the pyramidal trocar tips.

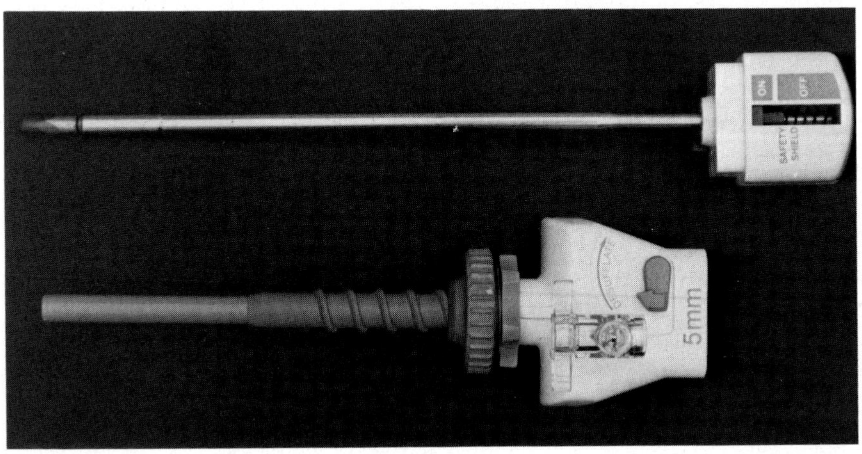

FIGURE 14–5. A 5 mm disposable trocar with a threaded gripping device.

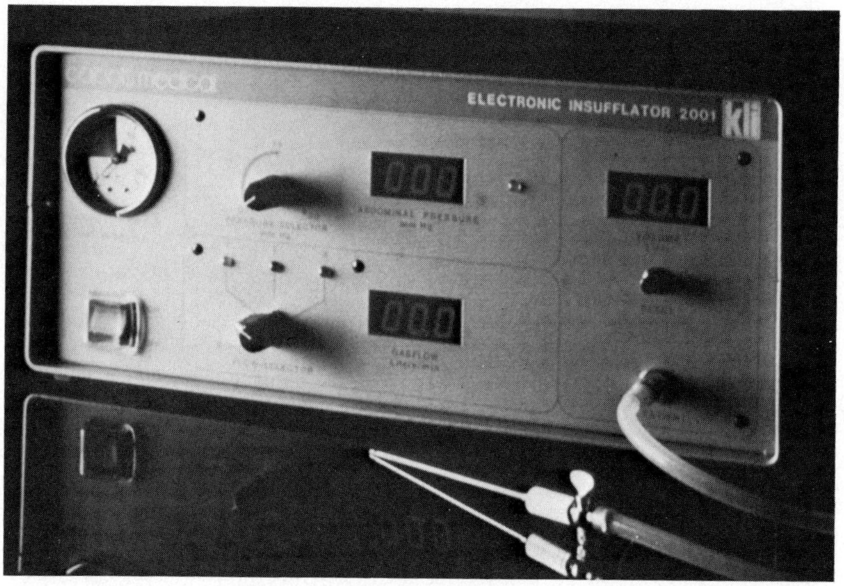

FIGURE 14–6. Automatic high-volume insufflator. (Courtesy of Cabot Medical.)

carbon dioxide as the insufflating agent. It is inexpensive, readily available, and the safest medical gas for laparoscopic use. One side effect of carbon dioxide is profound vasodilation of the peritoneal membrane. This does not significantly increase bleeding during the procedure and resolves quickly following desufflation.

Laparoscopic Telescopes

The laparoscope is similar to the rigid cystoscope (Figure 14–7). They are available in 5 and 10 mm diameters and incorporate a rod lens system similar to that designed by Hopkins.[32] Instead of conventional lenses separated by air, the objective lens and the eyepiece are bridged by a system of fused silica glass rods. The result is a much brighter, sharper image with enhanced field of view.

For most laparoscopic operations a zero-degree forward-looking lens is used. Eye-hand coordination with secondary cannula sites is easier when the zero-degree lens is used. As with cystoscopy, oblique lenses have diagnostic advantages. They are not very useful for therapeutic procedures, however. Flexible instrumentation has yet to find a role in laparoscopy.

Room temperature telescopes quickly fog when placed into the abdominal cavity. This can be prevented by soaking them in warm saline solution before use or placing them in a commercially available telescope warmer. Application of antifogging solution to the objective lens is also helpful. Should the lens fog or acquire debris during the procedure, the tip should not be wiped on a vital structure. Enough heat may be produced by the "cold light" fiberoptic system to cause a tissue burn.

Video Systems

Many urologists use video systems as a part of routine endoscopy. In this technique a split-beam camera allows direct viewing through the cystoscope in addition to the television monitor. Most laparoscopists use an end-viewing camera (Figure 14–8). Removal of the beamsplitter markedly improves optical resolution and image brightness.

Currently available laparoscopy equipment uses a one-chip direct-viewing camera. The limit of resolution is 450 lines per inch. This matches well with medical-grade video monitors that have about 400 lines per inch. Use of a high-end monitor with more than 700 lines per inch would be pointless. Image

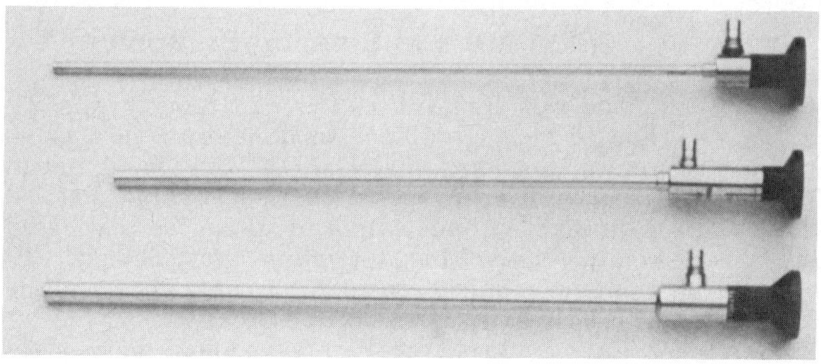

FIGURE 14–7. Rigid laparoscopic telescopes.

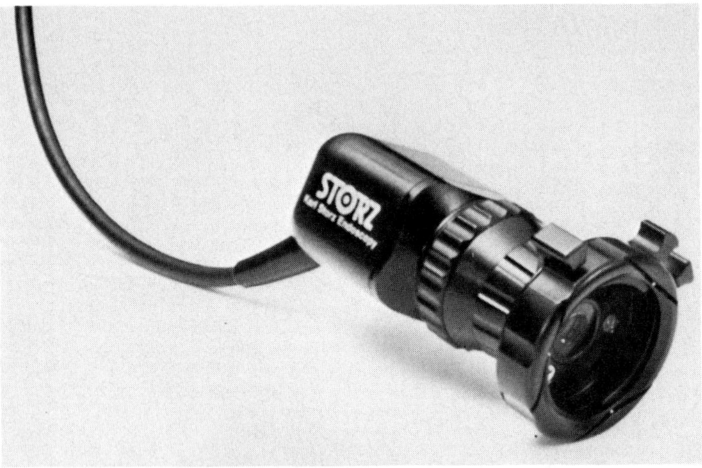

FIGURE 14–8. Single-chip direct-viewing video camera. (Courtesy of Karl Storz.)

quality is only as good as the weakest link, the camera.

Three-chip, 700 lines per inch cameras are in the prototype phase. Such a camera would take full advantage of a high-resolution monitor. Until then, extra expenditure for a high-quality monitor is not justified. High-definition television (HDTV) will certainly be used in future medical video systems. HDTV brings the promise of resolution of well over 1000 lines per inch. Such systems are several years away and will be expensive.

Video cameras have three important features that deserve discussion. The system must be capable of color balancing. When invoked, this feature resets all colors to their natural hues by using a uniform mixture of color, white, as a reference. The second important feature is an automatic iris to adjust incident light intensity. Without this feature, highly reflective surfaces such as the peritoneum appear oversaturated. Ability to focus the camera is also important. This feature is far less important with equipment used in the cystoscopy suite. Cystoscopic telescopes are nearly always used in close approximation to the tissue being viewed. During laparoscopy this is not always true. Withdrawal from the tissue to expand the field of view may exceed the telescope's focal range. When this happens, the camera must be able to correct the image. Most manufacturers build these features into all their laparoscopic systems. A halogen light source with fiberoptic cable is also part of the standard equipment.

Scissors and Grasping Instruments

Tissue cutting through the laparoscope is considerably different than in open surgery. The surgeon is guided only by monocular vision. More important, the surgeon cannot feel what is behind the tissue being cut. All cutting must be performed under direct vision. Past pointing is even more serious than in open surgery. This difference is reflected in instrument design, particularly that of hooked scissors.

Hooked scissor blades first meet at the tip (Figure 14–9). This is especially useful for division of tubular structures or adhesions. Past pointing is essentially impossible. Straight scissors tend to push tissue out of the bite, making past pointing more likely (Figure 14–10). Both types of instruments can be electrically insulated, which allows time-saving electrocoagulation while cutting. Hook scissors are available in only 5 mm diameter. The small size permits easy placement into any size cannula, but small instruments become dull quickly. Straight scissors are available in 5 and 10 mm diameters. Curved instruments of 10 mm diameter will be available shortly.

The choice of grasping forceps is largely one of personal preference. A few points must be considered, however. These instruments are 5 mm in diameter and are the tools of dissection. A ratchet mechanism as shown in Figure 14–9, *B*, is helpful to maintain a grip on the tissue. The bowel should not be grasped with toothed forceps. An atraumatic clamp that performs the same function as a Babcock clamp is available. A sturdy 10 mm dissecting instrument known as the Maryland dissector is useful for separating substantial amounts of tissue. Another 10 mm instrument, the claw forceps, is helpful for removing large bundles of tissue or lymph nodes through an 11 or 12 mm cannula.

Ligature and Stapling Equipment

The first ligature used in laparoscopy was the Roeder knot. This knot, modified by Semm, is essentially a "hangman's noose" that is tightened around an open vessel or tissue bundle. Pretied plain and chromic catgut loops can be purchased commercially. This system has two problems: efficient use requires considerable experience, and the vessel must be divided before ligation.

Endoscopic clip appliers solved both major prob-

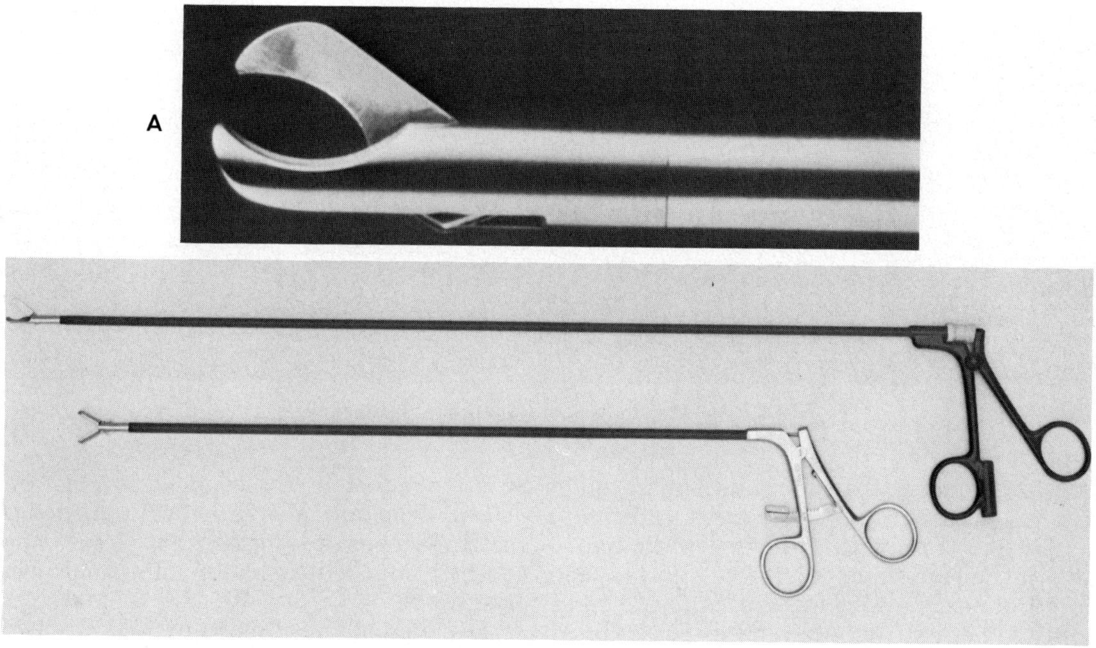

FIGURE 14–9. **A,** Hooked scissors blades. **B,** Hooked scissors instrument.

lems of suture ligation. Reusable clip appliers use 6 mm surgical clips. They are relatively inexpensive to use but must be removed from the abdomen for reloading. An occasional clip becomes dislodged from the jaws of the applier when the instrument is passed through the cannula. Several of the problems of surgical clips can be overcome by using a disposable applier (Figure 14–11). This instrument contains 20 titanium clips of 6 or 9 mm length. It functions exactly like the continuous feeding disposable clip applier used in open surgery.

Laparoscopic suturing has long been difficult. Most surgeons have used a straight needle for this purpose. A curved needle driver is now available that makes intraperitoneal suturing much easier (Figure 14–12).

An endoscopic gastrointestinal anastomosis (GIA) stapler has been developed (Figure 14–13). This device divides the bowel between two triple rows of staples. The stapler is manufactured in 30 and 60 mm lengths. A 12 mm cannula is required to accommodate this instrument. Laboratory and initial clinical trials are reportedly going well, and release of the device is expected soon. In the future the laparoscopic GIA stapler coupled with more advanced suturing techniques may allow construction of urinary diversions through the laparoscope.

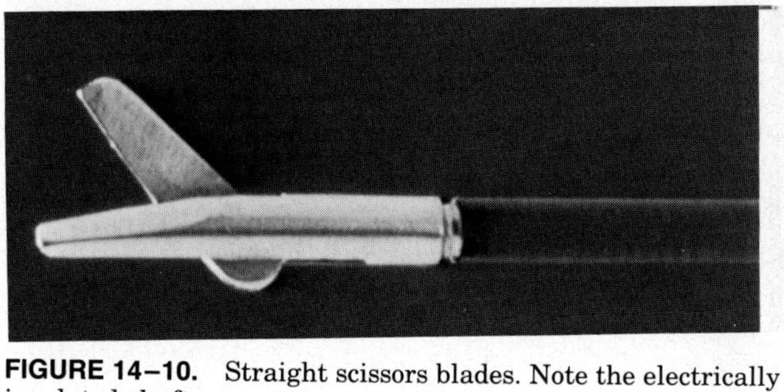

FIGURE 14–10. Straight scissors blades. Note the electrically insulated shaft.

Irrigation and Aspiration Equipment

Irrigation-aspiration probes are 5 mm in diameter. They have either one large common channel or two 2 mm channels. Irrigation pumps generate pressures of nearly 300 mm Hg (Figure 14–14). Even so, the resistance of the long 2 mm channel is great enough to restrict flow significantly. A common channel probe with a thumb-switch control is preferable.

Heparin 1000 to 5000 units/L can be added to the normal saline irrigation fluid to reduce clot formation. This does not produce a significant systemic effect.

Electrosurgical Equipment

Effective electrocoagulation is more important in laparoscopy than in open surgery because direct tissue access is limited. Vessel ligature is more difficult than in open surgery.

Laparoscopic electrosurgical instruments are compatible with existing electrosurgical generators. Frequently known as electrocoagulation or diathermy, this technique involves the application of radiofrequency energy to tissue. An electrosurgical unit is a radiofrequency generator matched not to an antenna but to a hand-held wand or probe. Cutting current is a high-frequency sine wave dis-

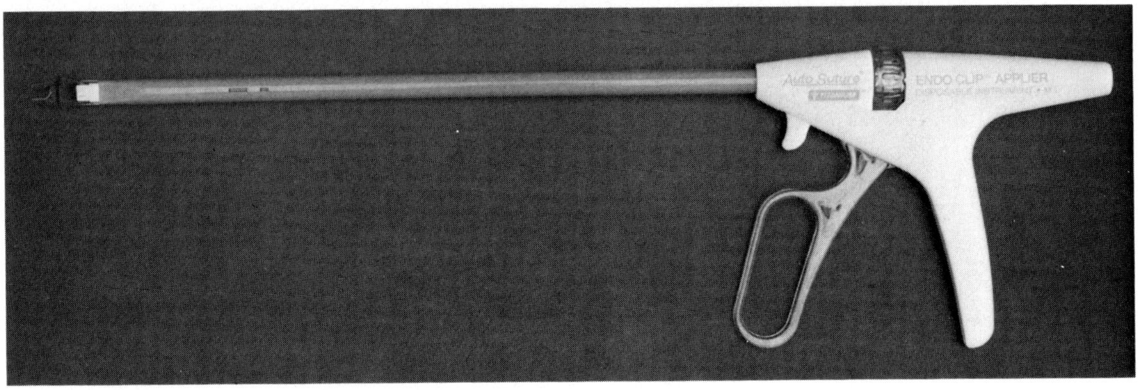

FIGURE 14–11. Disposable laparoscopic clip applier.

charge. The large energy transfer causes intracellular water vaporization and subsequent cellular cleavage. The electrosurgical properties change considerably if the sine wave pulses are allowed to decay before the next pulse. This causes tissue coagulation instead of cutting. Maximum true coagulation effect is achieved at low power settings. Deep, even microwave heating ensues. At higher settings a spark is generated. Tissue injury at that point is markedly greater immediately adjacent to the probe.

Because of the important role of electrosurgery

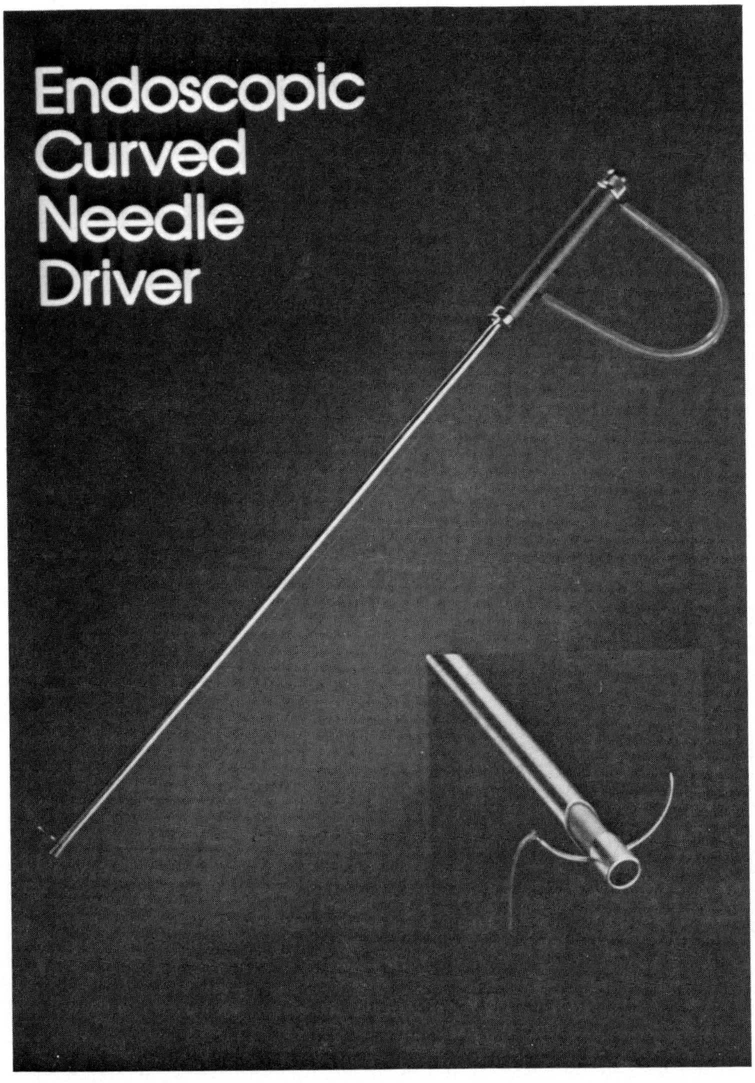

FIGURE 14–12. Reusable curved needle driver. (Courtesy of Cook Urological.)

A

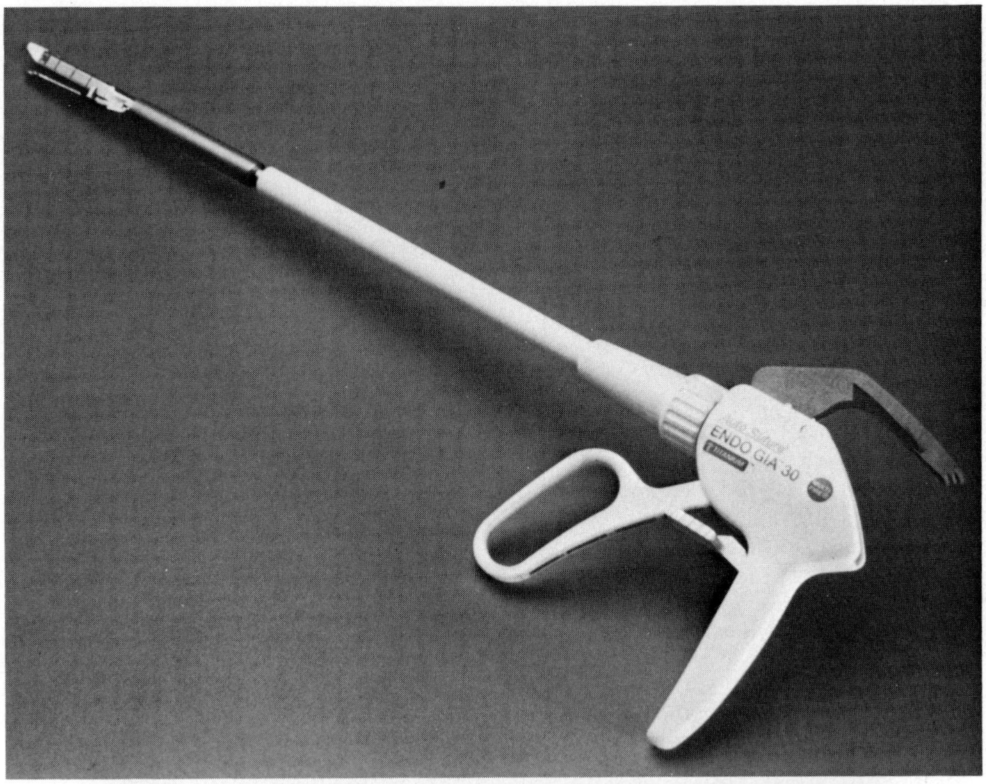

B

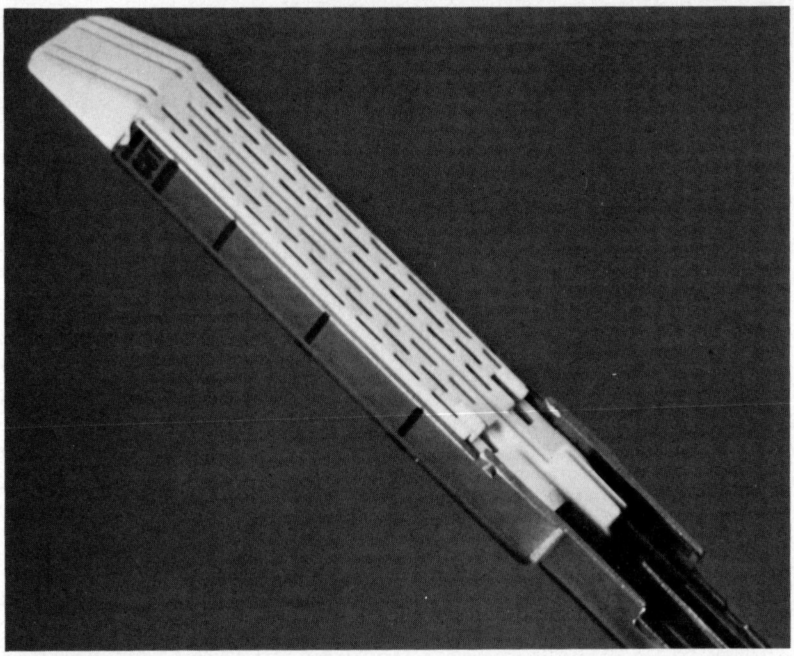

FIGURE 14–13. **A,** Disposable laparoscopic GIA stapler. **B,** GIA stapler. Note the cutting track between triple rows of staples. (Courtesy of U.S. Surgical Corp.)

in laparoscopy, several types of probes have been developed. In general, these are electrically insulated cylindrical probes that fit a 5 mm trocar port. Several different contact area shapes are available (Figure 14–15). The choice of contact head depends largely on personal preference. One important feature is a central channel through the port which allows evacuation of smoke as it is produced so it will not obscure the view of the operative field. The instrument shown in Figure 14–16 provides the convenience of both aspiration and irrigation through the same port.

The instruments mentioned thus far are all monopolar. Current flows between the probe tip and

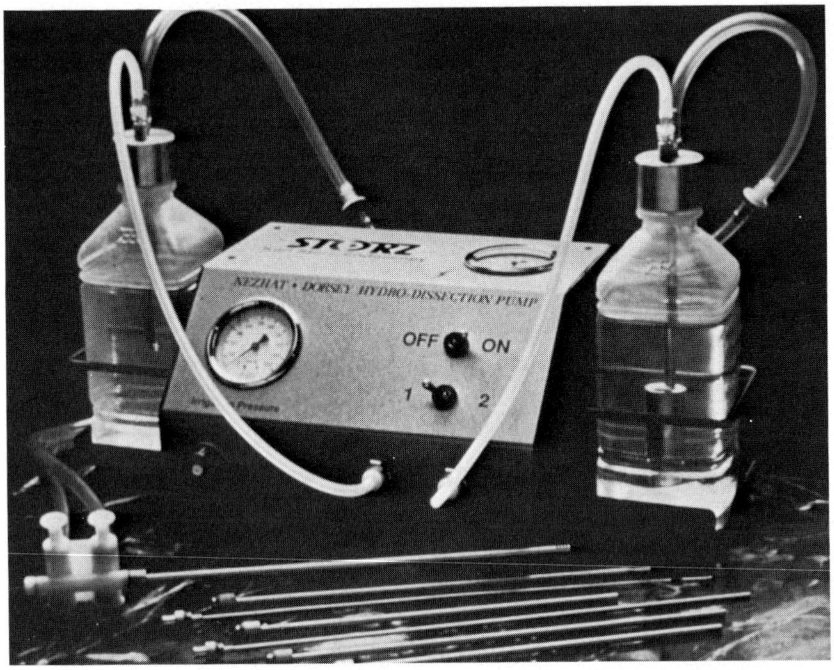

FIGURE 14–14. High-volume irrigation and aspiration equipment. (Courtesy of Karl Storz.)

patient grounding pad. Certain situations, such as electrocoagulation near the bowel, favor bipolar devices. The most useful bipolar instrument is a grasping forceps. Each jaw is electrically insulated from the other. One functions as the active electrode and the other as the ground.

Laser Equipment

The acronym LASER stands for light amplification by stimulated emission of radiation. This type of device generates a coherent beam of monochromatic light. This emerging technology has many potential applications. Laser physics and many applications are discussed in Chapter 3.

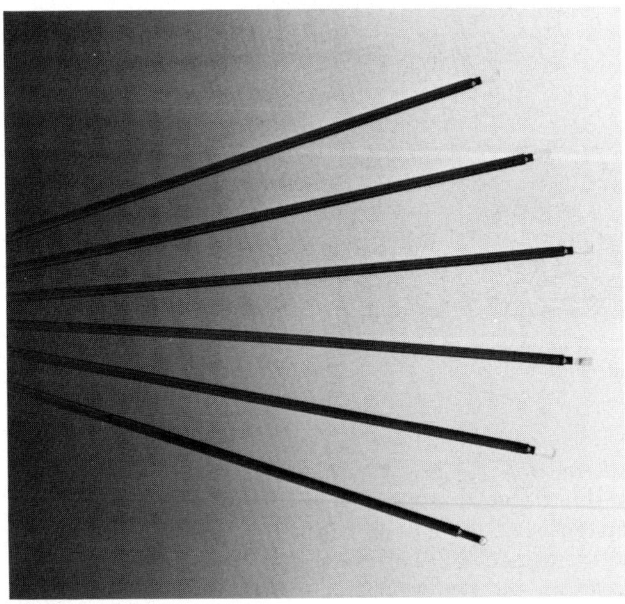

FIGURE 14–15. Insulated electrosurgical probes having various contact head shapes.

The laser's role in urologic laparoscopy is evolving. Current laparoscopic techniques use the laser only for cutting and coagulation. Neodymium/yttrium aluminum garnet (Nd:YAG) and potassium titanyl phosphate (KTP) are the lasers most frequently used. Nd:YAG energy can be delivered by either free beam or contact tip. Laser light is conveyed to the instrument by a fused silica glass waveguide. Free-beam light leaves the waveguide tip and is absorbed within the tissue. Formation of char on the fiber tip can be prevented by not allowing the waveguide to touch the tissue during laser operation. Free-beam Nd:YAG light penetrates approximately 8 mm into tissue. This causes better vascular coagulation than does the KTP laser. No laser coagulates actively bleeding vessels as well as monopolar electrocoagulation, however.

A contact tip facilitates tissue dissection and cutting. The Nd:YAG laser energy penetrates only 1 to 2 mm, which minimizes underlying tissue injury. No definitive data show that this method is superior to conventional cutting and coagulation. Also, all laser equipment, including contact tips, is far more expensive than electrosurgical devices.

The wavelength of the KTP laser is 532 nm, versus 1064 nm for Nd:YAG. Tissue penetration is slightly more than half that of the Nd:YAG. Probably the largest difference for the clinician is that 532 nm light is within the visible spectrum. The green KTP laser light obscures the video image during use. This limitation can be overcome with experience but is annoying.

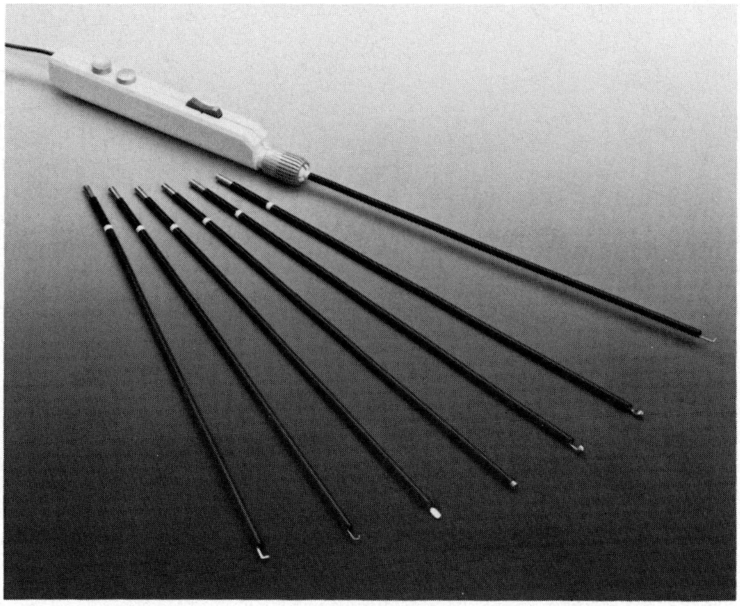

FIGURE 14–16. Electrosurgical equipment. (Courtesy of Valleylab Corp.)

Tissue Morcellator

A 50 mm laparoscopic tissue morcellator-aspirator has been developed. With this instrument large amounts of tissue can be removed through the 11 mm cannula. Clayman used this device to extract the kidney in several patients undergoing laparoscopic nephrectomy.[31]

ESTABLISHMENT OF PNEUMOPERITONEUM

For establishment of a pneumoperitoneum the patient is placed supine on the operating table and secured in place. Routine anesthesia monitoring equipment, including an end-tidal carbon dioxide monitor, is used. Anesthesia, if desired, is then induced. Bladder decompression with either an indwelling Foley urethral catheter or straight catheterization is performed. The choice of method depends on the expected length of the procedure and whether bladder distention would interfere with the operative field. The stomach is decompressed with a nasogastric or orogastric tube. Significant unsuspected gastric distention frequently occurs during induction of general anesthesia. Failure to empty these organs could result in accidental puncture or insufflation. Patients are often given a preoperative mechanical bowel preparation to minimize small and large bowel distention and improve vision of the operative field.

Sterile skin preparation and wide surgical draping are performed as for exploratory laparotomy. For most urologic laparoscopic procedures the inferior aspect of the umbilicus is the initial puncture site. This is the thinnest portion of the abdominal wall. By traversing the linea alba the operator can avoid the thick rectus abdominis musculature and underlying inferior epigastric vessels.

If prior midline laparotomy has been performed, bowel adhesions may underlie the umbilicus. Two options are commonly used. The first and more conservative is to extend the skin incision 2 cm in the midline. The linea alba and peritoneal layers are divided under direct vision. A conventional laparoscope cannula is placed into the peritoneum. Heavy purse-string suture secures an airtight closure of peritoneal and fascial layers around the cannula. Another open technique uses the Hasson cannula. The midline fascia is divided under direct vision. Heavy fascial sutures are placed 1 cm apart. The Hasson cannula is inserted between and secured in place with the fascial sutures. Insufflation through the cannula obviates the need for a blind Veress needle puncture. Zucker and associates reported performing this procedure in 18 patients without complication.[33]

The second option in the case of suspected midline adhesions is to move lateral to the rectus muscle. Needle or trocar insertion through the rectus abdominis muscle risks inferior epigastric vessel injury and subsequent rectus sheath hematoma or hemoperitoneum. These lateral sites, shown in Figure 14–17, are commonly used for paracentesis.

Once the insertion site is selected, the primary surgeon, standing on the patient's left, grasps the insufflation needle between the right thumb and index finger. Most surgeons prefer the Veress needle because the spring-loaded blunt obturator that snaps back to cover the sharp trocar gives an added margin of safety when the parietal peritoneum is punctured. Some surgeons, however, prefer a heavy spinal-type needle. Experienced users of that needle report a comparably low incidence of complications.

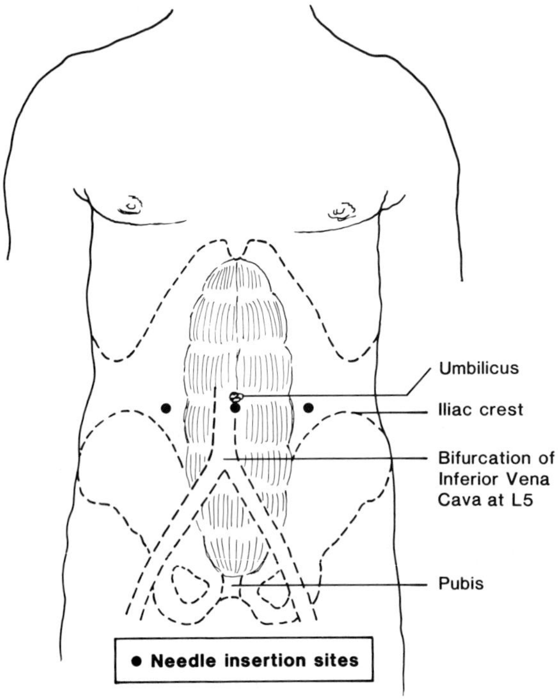

FIGURE 14–17. Veress needle insertion sites.

The surgical assistant everts the inferior aspect of the umbilicus using the thumb and forefinger of each hand. This also raises the anterior abdominal wall somewhat. A 1 cm midline incision is centered on the inferior aspect of the umbilicus. A transverse incision may also be used in the same location for an improved cosmetic result. The insufflation needle penetrates the linea alba on an angle heading toward the hollow of the sacrum. Two points of release are felt: first the fascia and then the parietal peritoneum. The surgeon must be sure the needle is neither in a visceral organ nor anterior to the peritoneum, where subcutaneous emphysema would result.

Several maneuvers have been used to ensure correct intraperitoneal positioning. First, the side hole in the Veress needle trocar allows air to flow through the needle, creating a hiss when anterior traction is placed on the abdominal wall. This hiss is not always audible, however. A second maneuver is to attach a 10 ml syringe filled with about 5 ml of injectable normal saline solution to the Veress needle. Gentle aspiration should not return fluid or gas. Should aspiration return blood, gas, or intestinal content, the needle must be withdrawn and placed in a new site. If aspiration does not return anything, 5 ml of saline solution is injected and aspirated. There should be no resistance to injection or fluid return with aspiration. The third approach is the "hanging drop" test, in which a drop of normal saline solution is placed in the hub of the Veress needle. When the tap on the needle is opened, the negative intraabdominal pressure created by respiration draws the drop into the peritoneum.

Once the Veress needle is correctly positioned in the peritoneum, insufflation can begin. Most laparoscopists use carbon dioxide to create the pneumoperitoneum.[34] Other gases are discussed in detail later. Tubing from the insufflator is connected to the Veress needle. Initial filling should be at 1.5 L/min with gauge pressure less than 5 mm Hg. Filling continues until intraabdominal pressure reaches 10 to 15 mm Hg. Between 3 and 5 L of gas is usually required to reach that pressure. During filling, the anesthesiologist should be particularly attentive to possible respiratory, hemodynamic, or cardiac rhythm disturbances. The surgeon should be certain that subcutaneous emphysema is not developing.

After creation of the initial pneumoperitoneum, the insufflator is turned off and the Veress needle withdrawn. The base of the 11 mm trocar is placed in the palm of the surgeon's right hand, and a fist is made around the instrument. Beginning from the initial subumbilical incision, the trocar is directed toward the hollow of the sacrum. The surgeon's left hand surrounds the cannula and acts as a brake to prevent deeper than desired penetration. The inferior vena cava is the most caudal of the large abdominal vessels and the one most susceptible to injury. The vena cava bifurcates at L5 (Figure 14–17).

A half turn of the wrist is used to penetrate the linea alba. Seven to 14 pounds of force is necessary to enter the abdominal cavity.[35] Once gas is heard escaping, the sharp trocar is removed, leaving the cannula in the peritoneal cavity. The insufflation tubing is connected and the gas flow rate increased to 10 L/min. The insufflator automatically keeps the abdominal pressure at a predetermined value, usually 10 to 15 mm Hg. Insertion of the laparoscope and all further abdominal wall punctures are performed under direct vision.

After completion of the surgical procedure all gas should be removed from the peritoneal cavity. With the patient in the Trendelenburg position the infraumbilical cannula is held parallel to the anterior abdominal wall. The valve is opened and gas is allowed to escape. This step largely eliminates postoperative shoulder pain.

All accessory puncture sites are injected with 0.25% bupivacaine to minimize postoperative pain. Under direct vision with the 11 mm laparoscope in the umbilical position, a wheal of anesthetic is raised immediately anterior to the peritoneum at the site of each accessory trocar puncture. The umbilical site is injected just before placement of one or two fascial sutures. Fascial sutures prevent omental or intestinal herniation. Accessory trocar sites do not require fascial sutures.

LAPAROSCOPIC UROLOGIC OPERATIONS

Urologists initially used the laparoscope to search for nonpalpable testes. Several similar procedures followed, but widespread interest did not develop until 1990. This recent enthusiasm is due to laparoscopic pelvic lymphadenectomy.

Pelvic Lymphadenectomy

Staging laparoscopic pelvic lymphadenectomy appears comparable to open pelvic lymph node dissection, but objective data demonstrating this have yet to be published. However, the margins of dissection are similar. These margins are the lateral pelvic sidewall and external iliac vessels laterally, the bifurcation of the common iliac artery superiorly, the obturator nerve posteriorly, and the confluence of the circumflex iliac vein and the external iliac vein inferiorly.

The indications for laparoscopic pelvic lymphadenectomy are evolving. Currently this is a 90-minute procedure.[30] It is unappealing to embark on a 90-minute endoscopic lymphadenectomy in a patient having a small chance of node positivity if radical retropubic prostatectomy is planned in the same procedure. This is the situation with most patients having low-stage lesions. If, however, radical perineal prostatectomy or radiation therapy is planned, the hospital stay may be decreased by laparoscopic lymphadenectomy. Ileus is uncommon following radical perineal prostatectomy. Consequently, hospital discharge often is possible on the third postoperative morning. Also, laparoscopic lymphadenectomy may provide reliable staging information in patients with markedly elevated PSA, large or high-grade tumors, or before radiation therapy. Laparoscopic pelvic lymphadenectomy is a new procedure in the management of patients with prostatic adenocarcinoma.

Preoperative preparation is similar to that for radical prostatectomy. If the patient is expected to undergo a radical operation immediately after lymphadenectomy, preoperative mechanical and antibiotic bowel preparation is performed. After induction of general anesthesia a towel roll is inserted underneath the buttocks and venous compression stockings are placed on the patient. A Foley catheter is inserted and the stomach is decompressed with an orogastric tube. The operating table is placed in a 15-degree Trendelenburg position.

Trocars are inserted as shown in Figure 14–18. The entire procedure is viewed through a zero-degree laparoscope in the 10 mm infraumbilical cannula. Three 5 mm ports are placed 4 cm above the pubis in the midline and lateral to the rectus muscles.

Figure 14–19 depicts the initial view of the operative field. The medial umbilical ligament or obliterated umbilical artery is a constant landmark. A peritoneal incision is made immediately lateral to this structure with scissors, an electrosurgical probe, or a laser. The vas deferens is clipped and divided. Once the peritoneum is teased

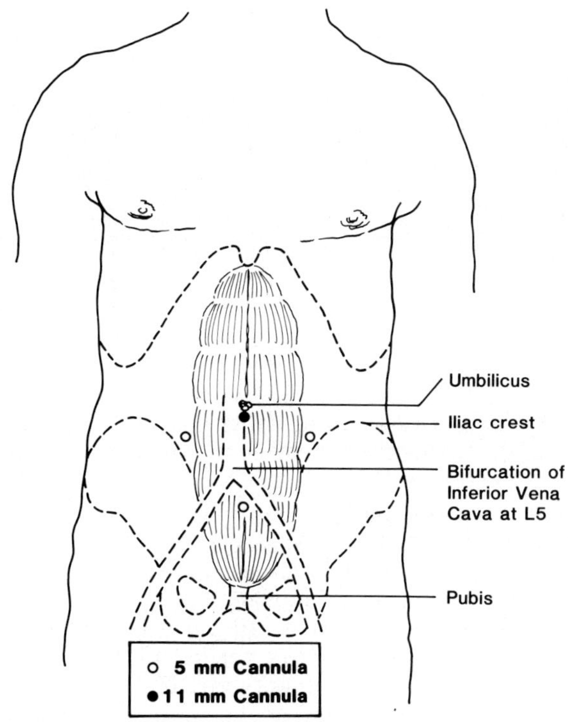

FIGURE 14–18. Trocar placement for pelvic lymphadenectomy.

medially and laterally, the obturator nodal chain and external iliac vessels are exposed (Figure 14–20). Pelvic lymphadenectomy begins immediately cephalad to the circumflex iliac vein and proceeds to the bifurcation of the common iliac artery. As with open lymphadenectomy, blunt and sharp dissection is performed. Small lymphatics are clipped. If frozen section is not planned, the nodal bundle is left in place, instruments are repositioned, and the contralateral side is dissected. After the second side is completed and hemostasis attained, the laparoscope is removed from the 10 mm umbilical cannula. A 5 mm laparoscope is placed in the midline suprapubic port. Ten millimeter claw graspers are used to remove each nodal group through the umbilical cannula. The abdomen is desufflated and the 10 mm fascial opening closed.

Diagnosis of Cryptorchidism

Laparoscopy has been shown to be useful in precisely locating nonpalpable testes.[36,37] The results are superior to medical imaging tests. At this time, however, the role of laparoscopic diagnosis is unclear. If the testis, or blind-ending vessels and vas deferens, are not seen in the inguinal canal, a retroperitoneal exploration is commonly performed. When the testis is located, the usual approach is to proceed with Fowler-Stephens orchiopexy. Results of this technique are good.[38] If the surgeon plans to proceed with Fowler-Stephens orchiopexy, the added benefit of laparoscopic localization is minimal. Laparoscopy may be helpful for first-stage tes-

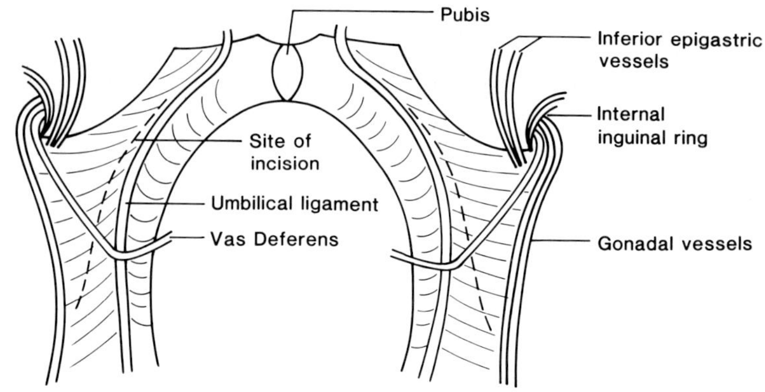

FIGURE 14–19. Wide-angle view of the pelvis showing important landmarks.

ticular vessel ligation as described by Elder or for gonadal harvesting before microvascular autotransplantation.[26,27]

The laparoscopic procedure is straightforward. After induction of anesthesia the patient is placed in a 15-degree Trendelenburg position. The bladder and stomach are decompressed. Pneumoperitoneum is induced and a 10 mm infraumbilical placed. No other access is needed if the intent of the procedure is only diagnostic. If incision of the peritoneum and ligation of the gonadal vessels are planned, two 5 mm trocars are needed. These can be located in the midline and lateral to the contralateral rectus muscle. The normal course of the spermatic vessels is examined. The finding of a blind-ending vas deferens is not proof of anorchia. Locating the spermatic vessels is imperative. The testis is usually found immediately behind the posterior parietal peritoneum. A child's relative lack of fat makes this diagnosis easier.

Varicocele Ligation

The internal spermatic veins can be ligated with use of a laparoscope. The alternative procedures are open inguinal ligation, open high ligation, and percutaneous transvenous embolization. Both open inguinal ligation and percutaneous procedures are easily performed with only local anesthesia. The benefits of laparoscopic varicocelectomy are unproven. Because of the microscopic nature of the technique, however, all veins are properly ligated and the testicular artery and the vasa deferentia are preserved.

The patient is positioned as for pelvic lymphadenectomy. A 10 mm umbilical trocar is placed. Two 5 mm trocars are inserted under direct vision. The spermatic vessels and inguinal ring are identified lateral to the umbilical ligament. The peritoneum covering the spermatic vessels is opened with scissors 2 cm proximal to the internal ring. Blunt and sharp dissection separates the cord vasculature. Veins are individually clipped and divided. Topical papaverine (30 mg/ml) can aid testicular artery identification. Usually only the veins on the left side are divided. Both sides are readily approached with the laparoscope, however, and future investigations may help define the value of bilateral ligation.

MANAGEMENT OF LAPAROSCOPIC COMPLICATIONS

Laparoscopy is a relatively new technique in urology. Because of this, an insufficient number of cases have been reported in the literature to allow meaningful conclusions about the incidence of complications. The only large studies of laparoscopic

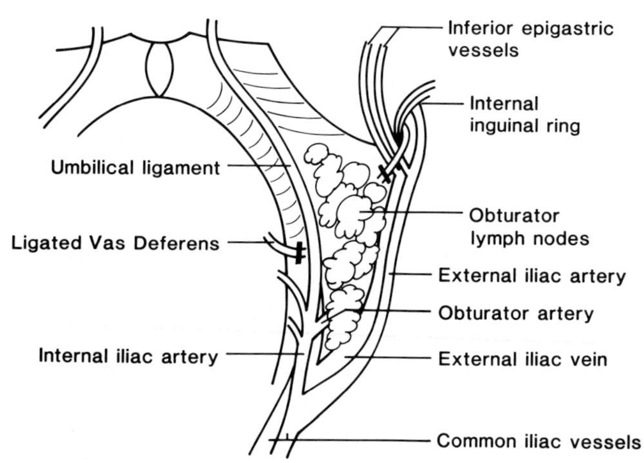

FIGURE 14–20. Laparoscopic pelvic lymphadenectomy. External iliac vessels are readily identified after the peritoneum is incised and teased laterally.

complications are published in the gynecologic literature. Several smaller but important studies have been reported by general surgeons performing laparoscopic cholecystectomy. Since most potential complications are associated with Veress needle and trocar puncture, not the particular operation, complication rates shown in published series may reflect expectations for urologic procedures. One complicating factor is the recent trend to perform increasingly difficult procedures endoscopically.

In 1978 the Royal College of Obstetricians and Gynecologists (RCOG) reported the results of a confidential questionnaire regarding almost 50,000 laparoscopic procedures in Great Britain.[34] This study reported 4 deaths, for a mortality rate of 8 per 100,000 procedures. The causes of death were 1 unrecognized small bowel perforation, 2 cardiac arrests, and 1 fatal gas embolism. The mortality rate for diagnostic laparoscopy was 4.9 per 100,000, whereas that of laparoscopic sterilizations was 10.2 per 100,000 operations. Certainly more difficult procedures are expected to yield more complications.

The American Association of Gynecologic Laparoscopists (AAGL) published a similar study in 1977.[39] This study involved 201,000 sterilization procedures. A major complication rate of 3.7 per 1000 procedures and a mortality rate of 2.5 per 100,000 procedures were reported.

Both the RCOG and AAGL studies were retrospective and probably underestimate the true incidence of complications. Kane and Kreijs reported a recent 7-year prospective study of diagnostic laparoscopy in Dallas.[40] Major and minor complications were 2.3% and 5.1%, respectively. The mortality rate was 0.5%. The authors note that complication rates reported in their study are more than five times higher than in previous retrospective studies. These figures may better represent the true incidence of complications. More involved procedures such as those described in this chapter would probably have higher complication rates.

Many of the potentially serious complications of laparoscopy arise from the establishment of the pneumoperitoneum and initial trocar insertion. However, all potential complications of open operations have endoscopic counterparts.

Abdominal Wall Emphysema

The best way to avoid causing abdominal wall emphysema is by faithful demonstration that the Veress needle is in the proper intraperitoneal location. These techniques are described previously. If the needle tip has not penetrated the anterior parietal peritoneum, either subfascial (preperitoneal) or true subcutaneous emphysema can result. Both, if severe, can force termination of the procedure.

Subcutaneous emphysema is easy to recognize. Initial inflation pressures should be higher than usual. Any early reading during insufflation greater than 5 mm Hg should arouse suspicion of an extraperitoneal needle location. If insufflation is allowed to continue, crepitus of the abdominal wall can be palpated. In extreme cases subcutaneous gas can extend from the neck to the scrotum. Mumford, Bhiwandiwala, and I-Chang reported abdominal wall emphysema in 0.43% of 6976 cases.[41] Postoperative pain is minimized by aspirating as much subcutaneous gas as possible. The large volumes of gas usually trapped within subcutaneous adipose tissue defy aspiration. If subcutaneous emphysema is not severe, the surgeon may attempt repuncture.

Preperitoneal insufflation occurs when the Veress needle penetrates the fascia but not the peritoneal membrane. Inflation dissects the anterior parietal peritoneum from the overlying abdominal wall. No palpable crepitus results, but two changes may be noted: higher than expected inflation pressures and asymmetric abdominal filling. The full round shape of the abdomen may not occur. More frequently, however, this diagnosis is made visually after trocar insertion. A large gas-filled space is seen with intestines underlying the thin peritoneal layer. If an 11 mm cannula was used, aspiration can proceed under direct vision through a secondary port. Placement of a smaller trocar or 18-gauge Angiocath catheter into the insufflated preperitoneal space is usually adequate for aspiration. Once all gas has been aspirated, another needle passage can be attempted. If the preperitoneal space cannot be fully evacuated, laparoscopy should be deferred to another day.

Intestinal Puncture

Again, proper confirmation of Veress needle location should ensure that intestinal puncture is recognized. Aspiration of gas or bowel content confirms an intraluminal location. The Veress needle should then be withdrawn and repuncture attempted with a sterile needle. Simple needle puncture of either small or large intestine is only rarely associated with morbidity. Laparotomy or oversewing of the puncture site is not indicated. Borten described a case of bowel wall emphysema treated by expectant management with good result.[42] Insufflation of the bowel lumen is also not an indication for laparotomy.

Omental and mesenteric emphysema is of little consequence. Endoscopic inspection for hematoma is indicated, but this complication rarely occurs. The best treatment is to allow the carbon dioxide to be absorbed spontaneously, a process that takes several hours. Occasionally, though, the mass effect is great enough to make laparoscopy difficult.

Gas Embolism

Gas embolism is an extremely rare but potentially fatal laparoscopic complication. It is estimated to occur once in 65,000 cases.[43] Most cases have occurred during initial peritoneal insufflation. Previously described aspiration and irrigation techniques assist the surgeon in identifying a vascular puncture before insufflation begins. An 18-gauge vascular puncture alone is of little consequence. Should aspiration yield blood, the needle is simply fully withdrawn and placed in another site. The laparoscopist should remember that the vena cava is only a few centimeters below the fascia and bifurcates at L5. The aortic bifurcation is one lumbar vertebral body higher.

Nearly all therapeutic laparoscopic procedures use carbon dioxide. Complex procedures require general anesthesia, which eliminates the relative advantage of nitrous oxide in procedures using local anesthesia. Because of its high solubility in blood, carbon dioxide is a much safer insufflating agent than nitrous oxide. Two hundred milliliters of carbon dioxide injected directly into the venous system is not lethal in humans.[43] Graff calculated the canine LD_{50} to be 25 ml/kg, five times that of air.[44]

Embolic gas rapidly tracks into the right atrium and ventricle. Gas lock may occur, preventing right atrial inflow and causing a sudden drop in cardiac output. The presence of bubbles produces a loud "mill wheel" heart murmur. Smaller bubbles may disperse into the pulmonary arterial tree, causing pulmonary hypertension and further reduction of cardiac output.

Gas embolism is evidenced by a new onset heart murmur and hypotension. It is caused by high abdominal insufflation pressures (20 to 40 mm Hg). Suspicion of gas embolism should lead to prompt remedial measures. Abdominal desufflation prevents further progression. The patient should be placed in a head-down left lateral decubitus or Durant position to minimize the possibility of right-sided heart obstruction by gas lock.[45] Profound hypotension should prompt insertion of a central venous catheter in the right side of the heart for gas aspiration. Other causes of hypotension must, of course, be excluded.

Trocar Injury

Unlike Veress needle puncture, trocar injuries are usually serious. Large vessel injury is an indication for emergency laparotomy. The patient should have been prepared and draped for this eventuality, and instruments should be immediately available on the back table. A midline intraperitoneal laparotomy incision is made. Intestines are packed out of the way in the upper abdomen after a mechanical retractor is placed. If no discrete bleeding site is seen, the distal aorta and vena cava should be examined before the iliac region. Numerous laparotomy pads and two Yankauer suction cannulas are helpful with profuse bleeding. Venous injuries may be more difficult to control and repair than arterial ones. Vascular clamps are useful on thick-walled arterial vessels such as the aorta or iliac arteries. However, until the vena cava or iliac vein is well mobilized, clamping may prove more injurious than beneficial. Tamponade of the bleeding site with a sponge stick often suffices until proximal and distal control can be established.

Inferior epigastric vessel injury should rarely or never occur during initial trocar placement. The epigastric vessels course superiorly under both bellies of the rectus abdominis muscle anterior to the peritoneum. Initial puncture should be either along the midline or lateral to the rectus muscles (Figure 14–17). Secondary trocars may lacerate the vessels, however. Inferior epigastric vessel injury is suspected when blood is dripping into the peritoneal cavity along a cannula or an extraperitoneal hematoma develops around an accessory cannula. Reddick and Olsen recommend three courses of treatment depending on the severity of bleeding.[46] In all cases the cannula should be left in situ and pneumoperitoneum maintained.

Severe bleeding is treated by making a 2 cm skin incision both medial and lateral to the cannula. All abdominal wall layers except the peritoneum are incised. The peritoneum is clamped cranially and caudally from the site of trocar entry. Suture ligature includes the lacerated vessel. Laparoscopic assessment should tell whether bleeding has stopped.

Moderate bleeding can usually be controlled by laparoscopic electrocoagulation. With a bipolar forceps the anterior perietal peritoneum cranial and caudal to the cannula is coagulated.

Recalcitrant bleeding may require the small open procedure described previously. A hematoma if not bleeding may be managed by placement of deep transverse heavy sutures through the abdominal wall superior and inferior to the cannula. These are tied snugly and left in place for 2 days.

Gonadal vessel injury may occur during surgery for varicocele, cryptorchidism, or rarely pelvic lymphadenectomy. Injury to these small vessels can almost always be managed by endoscopic hemoclip application.

Intestinal or stomach perforation with a trocar of any size, including the 5 mm, necessitates laparotomy. The trocar should be removed, leaving the cannula in place to guide the surgeon to the site of injury. Otherwise, the enterotomy may be surprisingly difficult to locate. The small intestine and transverse colon are the most common sites of injury.

Sharp-edged small bowel perforations may be managed by primary closure in a standard two-layer technique, with an absorbable suture used in the mucosal layer and permanent silk imbricating Lembert suture in the seromuscular layers. Transverse closure minimizes narrowing of the bowel lumen. Ragged edge or large lesions require small bowel resection and primary reanastomosis.

Trocar injuries to the large bowel usually involve the transverse colon. When this occurs, open laparotomy should be performed. Bowel resection with primary reanastomosis is the recommended treatment.[46] Other colonic injuries are handled similarly. Spillage of colonic content is usually minimal, and copious saline lavage should be used. Diverting colostomy is rarely indicated in the acute setting.

Electrosurgical intestinal injury is a relatively common complication. Brief pulses causing serosal blanching can safely be managed expectantly.[47] Deep thermal injuries usually occur during adhesiolysis. Extensive full-thickness electrosurgical injury should be treated by small bowel resection. Thompson reported a 0.3% incidence of delayed gastrointestinal perforation following tubal ligation.[47]

Intestinal injury from exposure to argon or KTP laser energy is significantly shallower than electrosurgical injury. This is true with either free-beam or contact tip delivery.[48,49] If bowel wall blanching (not vaporization) occurs, the injury can be managed expectantly.[50]

Many gynecologists believe that laser cutting is safer than electrosurgical cutting. Little evidence supports this idea, however. Early reports comparing laser with electrosurgical cholecystectomy show no significant safety differences between the two procedures. Laser procedures, however, took longer and were more expensive.[51]

Urinary Bladder Injury

Urinary bladder injury is most commonly caused by failure to decompress the bladder preoperatively. Because the bladder occupies a true intraperitoneal position in infants and young children, failure to empty the bladder in these patients is especially significant. Congenital anomalies such as urachal diverticulum may also predispose the patient to bladder perforation.[51]

Veress needle puncture or insufflation of the bladder is of little consequence. Trocar punctures are more serious. Urine leakage would probably not be recognized while the peritoneum is insufflated and under pressure. Abdominal decompression after the procedure would lead to urine leakage and subsequent peritonitis. If unsure whether bladder injury has occurred, the surgeon should deflate the abdomen and perform cystography on the operating table. Conventional management of large perforations such as an 11 mm trocar puncture involves open primary closure. Cystostomy drainage may or may not be indicated. Smaller trocar punctures may be managed by urethral catheter drainage. Borten reports that 5 mm trocar punctures are adequately treated by 5 days of urethral catheter drainage.[42]

CONCLUSION

Laparoscopic urology is a young discipline. Methods and equipment are evolving rapidly. Unfortunately, as with all new technology, the knowledge of when a particular technique is indicated lags behind the technique's development. In many ways the situation is reminiscent of the introduction of ureteroscopy in the 1980s. Less than 10 years later the original tools and techniques used seem archaic and in some instances dangerous. The same will probably be true of laparoscopy.

Markedly improved video systems will soon be available. Refined tissue extraction techniques may allow safe removal of larger and more vascular organs. An intestinal stapler, currently undergoing laboratory trials, holds the possibility of laparoscopic urinary diversion. Another potential area for improvement is intraabdominal retraction, which may decrease the number of trocar punctures required. These and other new techniques will fuel further advances in urologic laparoscopy and help define its diagnostic and therapeutic capabilities.

REFERENCES

1. Ohlgiswser M, Sorokin Y, Keifetz M: Gynecologic laparoscopy: a review article. Obstet Gynecol Surv 40(7):385-396, 1985.
2. Kelling G: Uber Oesophagoskopie, Gastroskopie and colioskopie. Munch Med Wochenschr 49:21-24, 1901.
3. Jacobaeus HC: Uber die Moglichkeit, die Zystoskopie bie Unterschung Seroser Hohlungen Anzuwenden. Munch Med Wochenschr 57:2090-2092, 1910.
4. Ott D: Die direkte Beleuchtung der Bauchhohle, der Harnblase, des Dickdarms und des Uterus zu diagnostischen Zwecken. Rev Med Tcheque (Prague) 2:27, 1909.
5. Jacobaeus HC: Kurze Ubersicht uber meine Erfahrungen mit der Laparoskopie. Munch Med Wochenschr 58:2017-2019, 1923.
6. Steiner OP: Abdominoscopy. Surg Gynecol Obstet 28:266, 1924.
7. Nadeau OE, Kampmeier OF: Endoscopy of the abdomen. Abdominoscopy 41:624, 1925.
8. Fervers C: Die Laparoscopie Mit dem Zystoskope. Med Klin 29:1042-1045, 1933.
9. Goetze O: Die Rontgendiagnostik die gasgefullter Bauchhohle; eine neue Methode. Munch Med Wochenschr 65:1275-1280, 1918.
10. Veress J: Neues Instrument zur Ausfuhrung von Brust- oder Bauchpunktionen. Dtsch Med Wochenschr 41:1480-1481, 1938.
11. Ruddock JC: Peritoneoscopy. Surg Gynecol Obstet 65:623-639, 1937.
12. Steptoe PC: Laparoscopy in gynecology. Edinburgh: Livingstone, 1964.
13. Kalk H, Bruhl W: Leitfaden der Laparosckopie. Stuttgart: Thieme, 1951.
14. Semm K: History. In Sanfilippo JS, Levine RL (eds): Operative gynecologic endoscopy. New York: Springer-Verlag, 1989.
15. Hassan HM: Open laparoscopy vs. closed laparoscopy: a

comparison of complication rates. Adv Planned Parenthood 13:41-50, 1978.
16. Cortes N, Errar P, Zambarda E, et al: Diagnosis of bilateral abdominal cryptorchidism by laparoscopy. Endoscopy 8:33-34, 1976.
17. Garibyan H: Use of laparoscopy for the location of impalpable testes. Neth J Surg 39(2):68-71, 1987.
18. Weiss RM, Seashore JH: Laparoscopy in the management of the nonpalpable testis. J Urol 138(2):382-384, 1987.
19. Castilho LN, Ferreira V: Laparoscopy in adults and children with nonpalpable testes. Andrologia 19(5):539-543, 1987.
20. Bloom DA, Ayers JW, McGuire EJ: The role of laparoscopy in managment of nonpalpable testes. Urol 94(9-10):465-470, 1988.
21. Das S: Laparoscopy in the management of the nonpalpable testis [Letter]. J Urol 140(6):1556-1557, 1988.
22. Guiney EJ, Corbally M, Malone PS: Laparoscopy and the management of the impalpable testis. Br J Urol 63(3):313-316, 1989.
23. Naslund MJ, Gearhart JP, Jeffs RD: Laparoscopy: its selected use in patients with unilateral nonpalpable testis after human chorionic gonadotropin stimulation. J Urol 142(1):108-110, 1989.
24. Castilho LN: Laparoscopy for the nonpalpable testis: how to interpret the endoscopic findings. J Urol 144(5):1215-1218, 1990.
25. Doig CM: Use of laparoscopy in children with impalpable testes. Int J Androl 12(6):420-422, 1989.
26. Elder JS: Laparoscopy and Fowler-Stephens orchiopexy in the management of the impalpable testis. Urol Clin North Am 16(2):399-411, 1989.
27. Harrison CB, Kaplan AW, Scherz HC, et al: Microvascular autotransplantation of the intra-abdominal testis. J Urol 144(2):506-507, 1990.
28. Figge M: Percutaneous transperitoneal nephrolithotomy. Eur Urol 14(5):414-416, 1988.
29. Querleu D: Laparoscopic pelvic lymphadenectomy. Presented at the Thirteenth International Workshop on Reconstructive Plastic Surgery in Gynecology, Levven, Belgium, Aug. 31–Sept. 2, 1989.
30. Schuessler WW, Vancaillie TG, Reich H, Griffith DP: Transperitoneal endosurgical lymphadenectomy in patients with localized prostate cancer. J Urol 145:988-991, 1991.
31. Clayman RV, Soper N, Kavoussi LR, et al: Lapaproscopic nephrectomy: laboratory and clinical experience. Presented at the Eighty-Sixth Annual Meeting of the American Urological Association, Toronto, Canada, June 6, 1991.
32. Hopkins HH: Neue fortschsitte in der medizineschen endoskopie. 70. Tagung der Deutschen Ges. f. angew. Optik, Lubek, 1969.
33. Zucker KA, Bailey RW, Gadacz TR, Imbembo AL: Laparoscopic guided cholecystectomy. Am J Surg 161:36-44, 1991.
34. Carron Brown JA, Chamberlain AVP, Jordan JA, et al: Gynaecological laparoscopy: the report of the working part of the confidential enquiry into gynaecological laparoscopy: conducted by the Royal College of Obstetricians and Gynaecologists, 1978.
35. Corson SL, Batzer FR, Gocial B, Maislin A: Measurement of the force necessary for laparoscopic trocar entry. J Reprod Med 34(4):282-284, 1989.
36. Lowe DH, Brock WA, Kaplan GW: Laparoscopy for localization of nonpalpable testes. J Urol 131:728-729, 1984.
37. Das S, Amar A: Impact of laparoscopy on modern urological practice. Urol Clin North Am 15(3), 1988.
38. Kogan SJ, Houman BZ, Reda EF, et al: Orchiopexy of the high undescended testis by division of the spermatic vessels: a critical review of 38 selected transections. J Urol 141:1416, 1989.
39. Phillips J, Mulka J, Keith D, et al: Laparoscopic procedures: a national survey for 1975. J Reprod Med 18:219, 1977.
40. Kane MA, Kreijs AJ: Complications of diagnostic laparoscopy in Dallas: a 7-year prospective study. Gastrointest Endosc 30:237-240, 1984.
41. Mumford ST, Bhiwandiwala PP, I-Chang CH: Laparoscopic and minilaparotomy female sterilization compared in 15,176 cases. Lancet 2:1066, 1980.
42. Borten M: Laparoscopic complications: prevention and managment. Toronto: Decker, 1986.
43. Palkmer R: Security in laparoscopy. In Phillips JM, Keith L (eds): Gynecological laparoscopy. Miami: Symposia Specialists, 1974, pp 17-26.
44. Graff TD, Arbegast NR, Phillips OC: Gas embolism: a comparative study of air and carbon dioxide as embolic agents in systemic venous system. Am J Obstet Gynecol 78:259, 1959.
45. Hasnain JU, Matjasko MJ: Practical anesthesia for laparoscopic procedures. In Zucker KA (ed): Surgical laparoscopy. St. Louis: Quality, 1991.
46. Reddick EJ, Olsen DO: Laparoscopy for the general surgeon. Tuttlingen, FRG: Storz, 1990.
47. Thompson BH, Wheeless CR: Gastrointestinal complications of laparoscopic sterilization. Obstet Gynecol 41:669-676, 1973.
48. Hunter JA, Burt RW, Becker JM, et al: Quantitation of colonic injury from argon laser, neodymium:YAG laser and monopolar electrocautery applied to flat mucosa and small sessile polyps of the canine colon. Gastrointest Endosc 35:16-21, 1989.
49. Schroder T, Brackett K, Joffe SN: An experimental study of the effects of electrocautery and various lasers on gastrointestinal tissue. Surgery 101:691-697, 1987.
50. Hunter JA: Laser or electrocautery for laparoscopic cholecystectomy? Am J Surg 161:345-349, 1991.
51. Yong EL, Prabhakaran K, Lee YS, Ratnam SS: Peritonitis following diagnostic laparoscopy due to injury to a vesicouracal diverticulum. Br J Obstet Gynaecol 96:365-368, 1989.

CHAPTER 15

INNOVATIONS IN PEDIATRIC UROLOGY

BRENT W. SNOW and PATRICK C. CARTWRIGHT

The urologic management of infants and children has been greatly influenced by recent technologic advances. Applying this technology innovatively, while maintaining a discerning attitude, holds great potential for significantly improving pediatric patient care. Of the many interesting developments, four have particular promise and are reviewed in this chapter. These are endoscopic subureteric injection, laparoscopy, electrical bladder stimulation, and fetal surgery.

ENDOSCOPIC SUBURETERIC INJECTION FOR REFLUX

The reshaping of tissues by injection is a well-described surgical concept. Otolaryngologists have long injected Polytef (Teflon) paste into vocal cords to treat dysphonia.[1] Plastic surgeons use subdermal collagen injections to modify body contours.[2] The principle has been applied in urology as well, with periurethral injections of Polytef described as therapy for incontinence.[3] The body of literature on endoscopic subureteric injection techniques to correct vesicoureteral reflux is growing.[4-17]

The optimal treatment for vesicoureteral reflux remains in dispute. Low-grade reflux is usually managed with prophylactic antibiotics and observation with the hope for spontaneous resolution. Higher grades of reflux, associated with upper tract dilation, are much less likely to resolve spontaneously and are often treated with open ureteral reimplantation. Although such operations have a high success rate, surgeons continue to seek simpler, less morbid, and more economical ways to manage vesicoureteral reflux. The idea of subureteric injection to correct reflux stems from such efforts.

Matouschek in 1981 first suggested correcting vesicoureteral reflux by injecting Polytef in a subureteric location.[18] The basic concept of this procedure was to place a material under the ureterovesical junction to support the intramural segment. The results of animal trials were first published in 1984 by Puri and O'Donnell.[5] They surgically created reflux in guinea pigs and then corrected it by subureteric injection of Polytef in 75% of the ureters. During and after these experimental studies, multiple clinical experiences have been reported. The pseudoacronym STING (*S*ubureteric *T*eflon *In*jection) was coined by O'Donnell to describe the technique.

Surgical Technique

The patient is placed in a lithotomy position and prepared and draped for cystoscopy. Three variations on the basic instrumentation needed for the STING procedure have been described: (1) a Puri catheter (Storz) with the 21-gauge needle tip, which is used through a 14F cystoscope; (2) the "Stinger" (Wolf), designed specifically for this procedure, with a rigid 20-gauge needle at the tip; and (3) a flexible 21-gauge needle through an 11F cystoscope attached to a high-pressure injector (Storz). The Johns Hopkins group, who used bovine collagen, described a catheter with a 25-gauge needle tip.[17] The collagen is less viscous and easier to inject through a small needle.

With the bladder relatively empty, the orifice is approached endoscopically (Figure 15–1). The needle is inserted bevel up at the 6 o'clock position, 3 to 5 mm distal to the orifice. It is then advanced in the submucosal plane, and care is taken not to perforate mucosa. The practitioner advances the tip until it is 4 to 5 mm proximal to the ureteral orifice and confirms its submucosal position by gently lifting the ureteral catheter and observing the tip. O'Donnell and Puri report performing this needle placement after a 3F or 4F ureteral catheter has been passed up the ureter.[19]

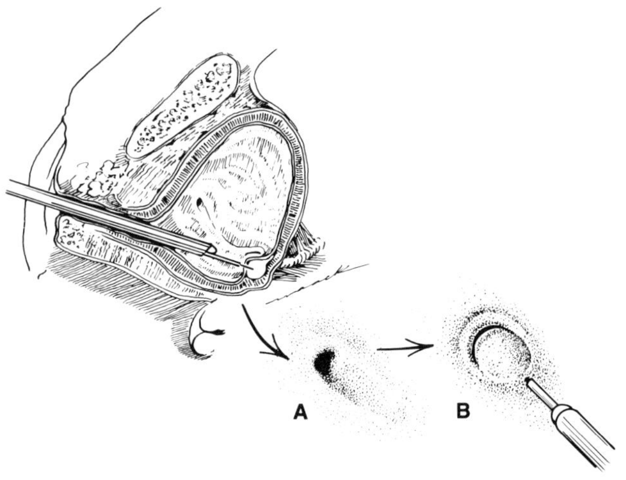

FIGURE 15–1. Subureteric injection to prevent vesicoureteral reflux. **A,** Ureteral orifice before injection. **B,** Desired inverted crescent appearance of orifice after injection.

While the orifice is watched, a glass or metal high-pressure injector and a 1 ml syringe are used to inject small increments of the material. This creates a small elevation under the orifice so that the orifice appears as an inverted crescent (Figure 15–1). The needle is left in place for 30 to 60 seconds to prevent extrusion after its removal. Generally 0.2 to 0.8 ml of the solution is required. To ensure adequacy of injection, the Johns Hopkins group fills the bladder and observes the orifice for maintenance of the inverted crescent configuration.[17] An intraoperative cystogram to document reflux resolution is beneficial.

As a point of technique, several authors report that poor injections are most often placed lateral or distal to the orifice.[7,16] If the injection is judged to be poor at the time of surgery, a second injection should be attempted. Prophylactic antibiotics are generally continued until a follow-up cystogram confirms resolution of the reflux. Some surgeons use anticholinergic agents to prevent excessive bladder spasms.[4] Bleeding and infection are not generally problems. Ureteral obstruction is unusual and only transient.

Clinical Experience

Many medical centers have reported their results with subureteric injections for reflux. Benefits realized from the procedure include short operative time (15 to 45 minutes), no incision, minimal discomfort, and outpatient management.

Deciphering the results of the STING procedure can be confusing. Some authors report downgrading of reflux as "success," whereas others consider only complete cessation as success. Furthermore, the duration of follow-up varies. Because in some cases reflux resumes after initial cessation, the length of follow-up is an important issue in determining the true success rate.

The results with subureteric Polytef (STING) are generally good in patients with primary reflux of all grades. Puri reported that of 143 patients with primary reflux, 79% had resolution of reflux after a single injection.[14] After two to four injections the success rate rose to 95%. However, after follow-up of 2 to 5½ years recurrences were found, and the eventual success rate was 88%. Farkas, Moriel, and Lupa reported on 115 ureters treated with the STING procedure.[16] They achieved 94% initial success with a single injection in primary reflux. With multiple injections the success rate increased to 98%. Interestingly, their success rate for stopping reflux in duplex systems was 82%. Prior experience with duplex systems had been less favorable. In yet another study, Gelet and associates described overall success with Polytef in 80% to 90% of 101 ureters injected.[20] In an interesting variation the STING was used to stop reflux in seven of nine ureters in preparation for renal transplant.[11] Kaplan, Dalton, and Firlit have shown a 71% success rate in treating reflux in patients with neurogenic bladder by the STING technique, although follow-up was short.[9] Politano and Molina also reported 70% to 80% success in patients with failed reimplants and with neurogenic bladders.[21] Kaminetsky and Hanna recently confirmed this, reporting a 70% success rate with the STING in children with neurogenic bladder dysfunction.[22] While several other reports in the literature have less successful percentages, the STING technique clearly stops reflux. The major question is whether Polytef is safe for use in this fashion.[23]

Polytef particles injected locally may cause a granulomatous reaction with giant cell formation.[24,25] With time such a reaction might induce fibrosis and ureteral obstruction. In addition, concern has been expressed that a reoperation for ureteral reimplantation would be much more difficult after a STING. This has not been borne out clinically in the first few years of follow-up, although occasional complaints of difficult post-STING surgeries have been made.

Serious concern about the potential for migration of Polytef particles remains.[24-26] Malizia and associates have documented significant migration of Polytef particles to various organs in an experimental model.[24] Although problems with migration have been minimal in adults injected periurethrally with Polytef, children's longer life expectancy and thus longer exposure time may make them less suitable candidates.[23] This issue has been the subject of lively debate.[27]

Alternative materials for subureteric injection have been sought.[17,28,29] An ideal substance would be easily injected, maintain its volume, cause little inflammatory or immune response, and remain local without migration. Among the substances suggested are polyvinyl alcohol foam, silicone, autologous fat, cultured fibroblasts, and glutaraldehyde cross-linked bovine collagen. Polyvinyl foam has been used experimentally in rabbits with reasonable success, but it induced occasional neoplastic growth.[28]

The Johns Hopkins group has reported results of an investigation approved by the Food and Drug Administration, in which glutaraldehyde cross-linked bovine dermal collagen was injected subureterally to correct reflux.[17] The patients were carefully monitored; a summary of initial causes of the reflux and results appears in Table 15–1. For primary reflux in nonduplex systems, the cure rate was 78% at 1 month but diminished to 62% at 1 year. Although collagen is an easy substance to work with, it is partially degraded and loses bulk in time, which probably accounts for the recurrence of reflux.[29] In addition, grade IV and V reflux seemed to respond better to subureteric Polytef injection than to collagen injection. The search for an ideal substance continues.

TABLE 15–1. Results of Trial of Bovine Collagen Injected Subureterally for Vesicoureteral Reflux

Cause of Reflux	No. of Ureters	Reflux Cured on Follow-up: 1 Month	1 Year
Primary	63	47/60 (78%)	29/47 (62%)
Primary with Duplex System	12	6/12 (50%)	8/12 (67%)
Reimplant Failures	17	10/12 (83%)	7/9 (78%)

Data from Leonard MP, Canning DA, Peters CA, et al: J Urol 145:115-119, 1991.

Summary

The technique of subureteric injection to correct vesicoureteral reflux is well described. Success rates are moderate to high depending on the material used and the practitioner's experience with the technique. Although Polytef paste is the most often used material, its long-term safety when used in children has been a cause for concern.

Correction of reflux with subureteric injection is an excellent concept. If an appropriately safe and durable substance for injection can be found, this innovative technique will have a major role in the management of vesicoureteral reflux.

LAPAROSCOPY

Laparoscopy is a commonly applied diagnostic procedure. Gynecologists have used it extensively to diagnose and manage pelvic diseases. Recently, general surgeons have gathered impressive experience with laparoscopic cholecystectomy.[30] In pediatric surgery, laparoscopy has been used to evaluate a variety of conditions, including abdominal masses, appendicitis, hepatomegaly, and recurrent abdominal pain.[31,32]

The laparoscope seems to be a natural instrument for urologists, considering their sizable experience in diagnosis and treatment by endoscopic means. Recent reports have described pelvic node dissection[33] and even nephrectomy[34] performed with the laparoscope. In pediatric patients, laparoscopy has been used primarily for localization and management of the impalpable testis[35-48] and for evaluation of intersex states.[42,49]

Technique of Pediatric Laparoscopy

The first step in laparoscopy is the safe creation of a pneumoperitoneum. Next a sheath is placed through the abdominal wall into which the laparoscope can be inserted for peritoneal inspection. The equipment needed is relatively simple. A Veress needle is used to create the pneumoperitoneum. A trocar and a 4.5 to 5.5 mm sheath are next inserted to accommodate the laparoscope. A carbon dioxide insufflator along with its tubing connections is also required. Contraindications to laparoscopy are prior abdominal surgery, bleeding disorders, and the prune belly syndrome.

In preparation, the patient is placed supine and the entire abdomen and the genitalia are prepared and draped into the sterile field. A small curved incision is made with a No. 11 blade in the inferior crease of the umbilicus and carried down just through the fascia. Traction sutures are placed at each end of the incision to assist with instrument manipulation. A right-handed surgeon standing on the patient's left side grasps the suprapubic skin with the left hand and elevates it, drawing the abdominal wall away from the intraabdominal contents (Figure 15–2). The Veress needle is introduced through the small incision and angled at 45 degrees so that it points toward the pelvis. The needle is pushed sharply through the abdominal wall. Resistance is met at the fascia and the peritoneal level. The Veress needle has a spring-loaded inner cannula that is pushed back into the barrel of the needle as it is advanced through the abdominal wall (Figure 15–2, *A*). Once the needle gains access to the intraabdominal space, the cannula quickly pops forward, shielding the abdominal contents from injury (Figure 15–2, *B*). With the needle in place, 5 ml of saline solution is irrigated through the port and aspiration is attempted. If the saline solution flows in easily and none can be withdrawn by aspiration, proper placement of the needle is presumed. If the needle tip is still extraperitoneal,

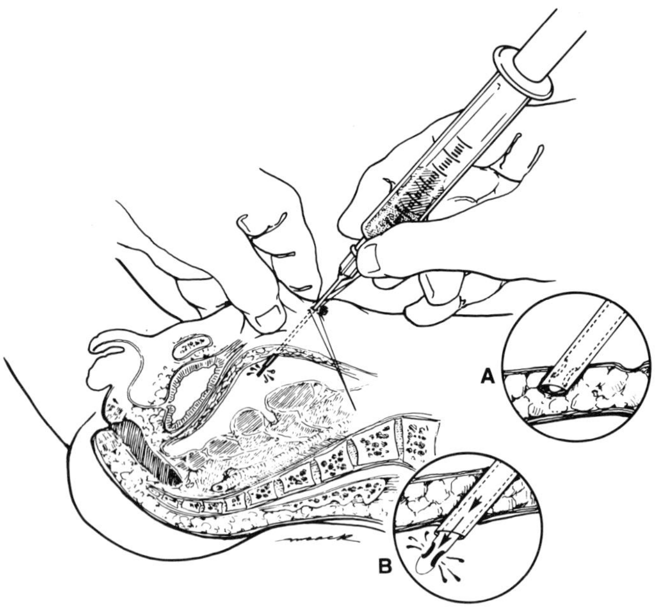

FIGURE 15–2. Veress needle insertion (and saline test) for laparoscopy. **A,** The needle passing through the abdominal wall with cannula retracted. **B,** As the needle enters the peritoneum the cannula springs forward to protect the viscera from puncture.

difficulty in irrigation is encountered and generally some saline solution can be aspirated back.

Once in position, the carbon dioxide insufflator is connected with a Luer-Lok stopcock to the Veress needle. Insufflation is begun and the pressure monitor is observed. Filling pressures greater than 20 mm Hg indicate either that the needle is extraperitoneal or that the needle tip is abutting bowel or omentum. Simple repositioning of the needle often improves the filling pressure. Extraperitoneal insufflation should be managed by stopping the insufflation immediately and allowing carbon dioxide to leak back out through the needle before removing it and attempting a second pass to the intraperitoneal space.

In children, less than 1.5 L of carbon dioxide is generally needed to create a sufficient pneumoperitoneum. Intraperitoneal pressures should remain less than 20 mm Hg. With a sufficient pneumoperitoneum created, the trocar and sheath are inserted in the same orientation as the Veress needle. The same resistance at fascia and peritoneum is generally encountered, and the lower abdomen is retracted upward as the trocar is placed. The inserting hand must be carefully braced on the abdominal wall so that a quick thrust will not insert the trocar too deeply and cause intraperitoneal or retroperitoneal injury. The audible exit of carbon dioxide from the instrument confirms intraperitoneal positioning. The trocar is removed, and a thumb is used to cover the sheath so that carbon dioxide is not lost. A zero- or 30-degree laparoscopic lens is inserted, and inspection of the peritoneum is begun. A 20-degree Trendelenburg position helps during pelvic inspection.

After laparoscopy is completed, the carbon dioxide is allowed to escape via the sheath unless intraabdominal exploration is planned. The fascia and skin are closed with absorbable suture in a standard fashion. The procedure usually takes 15 to 30 minutes.

The most common complications of laparoscopy are bleeding at the site of sheath insertion and extraperitoneal carbon dioxide insufflation. Less common complications include bowel perforation, bladder perforation, major vessel injury, and insufflation of the mesentery or omentum. The gynecologic literature estimates that viscus perforation occurs in 1 to 2.7 cases per 1000.[50]

Management of the Impalpable Testis

Approximately 20% of undescended testes are impalpable.[51] The reported percentages of impalpable testes that are intraabdominal, canalicular, ectopic, or absent vary widely. Cortesi and associates reported the first diagnostic laparoscopy for an impalpable testis in 1976.[52] Since then, experience with impalpable testes has shown that laparoscopy is useful in diagnosis, in planning the surgical approach, and in initiating treatment.

Laparoscopic inspection of the peritoneal cavity is not difficult, but accurate assessment of the anatomy involves a learning curve. The normal descended side should be inspected first to observe the vas deferens and internal spermatic vessels coursing downward through the internal inguinal ring. Once these are identified, the involved side may be evaluated.

Several findings may be anticipated. If laparoscopy reveals the vas and vessels coursing through the internal ring beside a patent processus vaginalis, a testicle will often be found distally and inguinal exploration is indicated. If the vas and vessels are seen coursing into the internal ring but no patent processus vaginalis is present, inguinal exploration is still advisable. In this case the testis may be absent, atrophic, or ectopic. Interestingly, Weiss and Seashore note that in their experience with 15 such patients, inguinal exploration revealed absence of the testicle in each case.[47] Thus they are comfortable with omitting exploration in this subgroup of patients.

Most experienced laparoscopists believe that if the vas and vessels end together just inside the internal ring with no apparent testicular tissue, the patient has the vanishing testis syndrome and no further exploration is required. If instead the vas and vessels lead to a testis just inside the internal ring, options for therapy are considered. In this situation many urologists make a high inguinal incision, enter the peritoneum, and assess the length of the internal spermatic vessels to determine whether a standard orchiopexy is feasible or division of the vessels and a Fowler-Stephens procedure are needed. Bloom has reported passing instruments through the laparoscope to place vessel clips on the internal spermatic vessels well above the testis.[48] This permits the development of collateral vasculature via the artery of the vas deferens. Several months later a Fowler-Stephens orchiopexy can be performed to improve testicular viability. Occasionally the vas deferens or internal spermatic vessels cannot be found with laparoscopy. If blind-ending spermatic vessels cannot be confirmed, intraabdominal exploration is required for definitive diagnosis.

The results of laparoscopy for impalpable testis are found in several series as depicted in Table 15–2.[40-47] In general, laparoscopy obviates the need for exploration in one third of the patients, although this figure varies depending on the surgeon's experience and treatment philosophy. Nonpalpable testes more frequently prove to be absent on the left side than on the right. Thus a left-sided situation has a greater chance of needing laparoscopy only.[53] In a review of the pediatric literature only one instance of viscus perforation (bladder) during laparoscopy was found, and this was of minor clinical significance.[54] The difficulties encountered in each of the series are summarized in Table 15–2.

Laparoscopy for Intersex Disorders

Laparoscopy may be useful for the inspection of internal genital structures and for identification and biopsy of gonads. Lowe, Brock, and Kaplan reported that in a patient with gonadal dysgenesis, laparoscopy revealed unilateral fallopian tube development.[42] Wolfman reported his experience in laparoscopic examination of 13 patients with intersex disorders.[49] Biopsy of gonads may be performed with a standard biopsy needle placed in a separate abdominal location but directly observed with the laparoscope.[55] This may obviate the need for open exploration and biopsy in some patients. A recent report even describes laparoscopic gonadectomies in a patient with dysgenetic gonads.[56]

Summary

Laparoscopy is a safe, relatively quick procedure in pediatric urology. It can be used to locate intraabdominal testes and may alter the incision for some surgeons. Furthermore, the finding of blind-ending spermatic vessels within the abdomen may obviate the need for further surgical intervention. In Duckett's practice, however, laparoscopy has not greatly altered surgical decision making.[57] He reserves it for unusual cases or at times for evaluating intersex disorders. The development of laparoscopy as a procedure in pediatric urology will be interesting to follow.

ELECTRICAL BLADDER STIMULATION

The improperly innervated bladder is a major problem in urologic practice. Estimates suggest that more than 1 million people in the United States have bladder dysfunction. The problem has a traumatic or neoplastic origin in many adults, whereas in childhood congenital anomalies are more frequently the cause.

TABLE 15–2. Summary of Literature on Laparoscopy for Nonpalpable Testis

Reference	No. of Testes	Location of Testes		
		Absent	*Intraabdominal*	*Canal (or distal)*
Bloom (1988)[40]	28	10	11	7
Boddy (1985)[41]	55	29	19	7
Lowe (1984)[42]	36	10	14	12
Guiney (1989)[43]	103	39	53	11
Manson (1985)[44]	17	1	5	11
Naslund (1989)[45]	21	18	2	1
Scott (1982)[46]	24	12	10	2
Weiss (1987)[47]	33	21	5	7
TOTAL	317	140 (44%)	119 (38%)	58 (18%)

Laparoscopic difficulties included the following: unable to see spermatic vessels (2), omental insufflation (1), gonadal dysgenesis (1), poor visualization (4), no vessels seen (14), no vessels or vas seen (2), inconclusive (1), and extraperitoneal insufflation (1).

As neurophysiology advanced and action potentials were better studied, the electrical nature of nerve stimulation became better understood. Interest in electrical control of bladder function began in the 1950s and 1960s. Several aspects were studied, including direct electrical stimulation using implantable electrodes in the spinal cord,[58-62] direct detrusor stimulation,[59,63-66] stimulation of pelvic nerves,[59,63,67] and sacral nerve stimulation.[68-70]

Extravesical Electrical Stimulation

The history of electrical stimulation of the bladder has been extensively reviewed by Tanagho and Schmidt.[71] Skin surface electrodes were tried initially. First, generalized stimulation with a low-level stimulus activated the sphincteric musculature, and then increased stimulation activated the detrusor. Unfortunately, the sphincteric activity often outweighed the bladder contractions, which made synergistic voiding unlikely.

Direct detrusor stimulation has the advantage of high organ specificity. Such stimulation has not proved successful clinically because of problems with electrode malfunction and displacement, fibrosis around the electrode, erosion into the bladder, and the need for abnormally high current densities. Direct pelvic nerve stimulation, although promising at first, has not been effective because pelvic nerves do not tolerate long periods of stimulation. The pudendal nerves are also activated so that outflow resistance is augmented. Because of the mixed nature of these nerves, pain is a significant problem.

Further studies of sacral roots were performed by stimulating entire intact bilateral roots, intact ventral and dorsal roots separately, the proximal and distal ends of divided roots, and the proximal ends of divided dorsal and ventral roots. Stimulation of the entire sacral root at S2 showed bladder dominance, whereas stimulating S1 and S2 together influenced sphincter closure more. After division of dorsal roots, stimulation of proximal and distal cut ends showed that the response was primarily reflexive. Sphincter reflex contractions were extremely efficient and were eliminated only through subsequent division of all remaining sacral nerves.[70-73]

Further long-term studies were performed by implanting electrodes in male and female dogs, but the success was minimal.[74,75] Satisfactory results in dogs were not obtained until the dorsal fibers were separated and cut, the ventral component was stimulated, and selective neurotomy was performed. This gave adequate emptying, but still control was not perfect.[76-78] Sacral root stimulation was necessary to enhance closure of the bladder neck and sphincter activity. The studies showed that stimulation with low frequency and low voltage can maintain adequate sphincteric activity but that high frequency and low voltage fatigue the external sphincter and block its activity. When high-frequency, low-voltage stimulation is followed by high-voltage stimulation, bladder contraction is induced and voiding follows.

As of 1988, Schmidt and Tanagho had implanted complete bladder pacemakers in 22 patients. Approximately 70% of their patients have had storage function of the bladder restored and can maintain continence. Fifty percent of the patients completely evacuate the bladder with synergistic voiding at low pressure.[71] Further experience should be watched carefully for progress.

Intravesical Electrical Stimulation

The concept of intravesical electrical field stimulation of the bladder was significantly different from direct nerve stimulation, which is reviewed previously. Intravesical stimulation was first practiced in Hungary by Katona.[79-83] The technique involved introducing an electrode catheter into the bladder, which was partially filled with sterile saline solution. An electrical stimulator allowed the voltage, frequency, impulse duration, and later exponential waveforms and intensity to be altered. The electrical stimulation was given in 90-minute sessions daily for 27 to 110 sessions.[82] Of Katona's initial 100 myelomeningocele patients treated in 1958, 71 attained daytime and nighttime continence. This level has not been reliably duplicated but has been sufficiently encouraging for others to try.

In efforts to control urinary incontinence, indirect stimulation of pelvic and sphincter musculature has been tried. Electronic devices placed in the vagina as a pessary have had limited success.[84,85] Others have tried stimulation by anal plug electrode with modest success.[86]

Intravesical stimulation has been popularized in the United States by Dr. William E. Kaplan at Children's Memorial Hospital in Chicago. The current technique for achieving conscious micturitional control is to use intravesical electrical bladder stimulation with visual biofeedback. The patients undergo 90-minute stimulation sessions each day for at least 1 month followed by refresher courses as needed.[87-90] The exponential waveform characteristics include current of 1 to 10 mA, frequency of 60 to 90 Hz, impulse duration of 2 to 6 msec, rise time of 1 to 3.5 seconds, and interval of 2 to 4 seconds. These parameters can be adjusted for each patient as the procedure progresses. The results of treatment vary widely and cannot be well correlated with the level or degree of spinal injury. Although the results are inconsistent, bladder capacity has been shown to increase significantly. This capacity increase has not been at the expense of pressure increase.[91] The success reported by Kaplan is summarized as follows: 72% of the patients have detrusor contractions, 70% have achieved some sensation, 42% void, and 38% void with total control.[98] These results have encouraged approximately 15 other children's treatment centers around the United States to begin intravesical transurethral bladder stimulation. As might be expected, early unpublished reports vary greatly and are somewhat less enthusiastic than Kaplan's reports.

Summary

The future of bladder stimulation is uncertain. It offers hope for controlled voiding to a small percentage of patients. In a larger group of patients, bladder capacity is increased and bladder irritability is reduced so that intermittent catheterization may provide better continence. The place of bladder stimulation in treatment of neurologically impaired patients is still uncertain, but new developments should be watched with interest.

FETAL SURGERY

Since the development of obstetric ultrasonography and amniocentesis, treatment of the fetus as a patient has been considered. This possibility has put a new emphasis on understanding normal antenatal physiology of both the mother and fetus, as well as the postnatal course of diseases diagnosed in the fetus. Many urologic disorders can be diagnosed in utero before clinical signs or symptoms appear and often before renal function deteriorates. The decision of when to intervene depends on knowledge of the natural history of the disease and the outcome of the disease process with early or delayed intervention. Furthermore, the risks to the mother and fetus posed by the various options must be carefully evaluated.

Fetal surgical intervention has been considered for several problems, including hydronephrosis, hydrocephalus, and diaphragmatic hernia.[92] Intervention has been pondered for other diseases, but for the most part treatment has yet to be instituted. Probably the best studied of these diseases is obstructive uropathy.[93]

Antenatal surgery in obstructive uropathy would relieve obstruction, allowing free urine flow and therefore better nephrogenesis and kidney function. However, few cases of antenatally diagnosed hydronephrosis require or are amenable to treatment. Unilateral ureteropelvic junction obstruction, ureterovesical junction obstruction, multicystic kidney, prune belly syndrome, posterior urethral valves, vesicoureteral reflux, and bilateral ureteral pelvic junction obstruction are among the diagnoses that can be made by antenatal ultrasound. Of these, only posterior urethral valves and bilateral ureteral pelvic junction obstruction would benefit from antenatal intervention. The other diseases do not require urgent neonatal intervention and may not require surgical intervention at all.

A brief review of embryogenesis and antenatal physiology helps in understanding the formidable problems of antenatal intervention. Organogenesis is thought to be completed by the 12th week of gestation. Most obstructive uropathies develop several weeks before this time. The earliest an ultrasound examination can determine hydronephrosis is around the 16th to 17th week. Often, serial ultrasound studies are necessary to be certain of the diagnosis, and these are usually performed 1 to 2 weeks apart. Thus obstructive uropathy is difficult to diagnose before midpregnancy.

Animal studies, mostly of sheep, have shown that obstruction in the second trimester often leads to renal dysplasia. Reversal of this obstruction after a period of 4 to 6 weeks may relieve the hydronephrosis and possibly prevent dysplasia.[94-97] However, in our unpublished sheep studies, in which ureteral obstruction was produced in the second trimester, in utero decompression 4 to 6 weeks later did not reverse the renal dysplasia.

The preceding facts indicate that when hydronephrosis is diagnosed in the second trimester, months after the obstruction has developed, antenatal relief of the obstruction may be unrewarding because irreversible renal changes have already occurred. In attempts to confirm the diagnosis and predict recoverability following intervention, fetal urine osmolarity, and electrolytes have been studied.[98] Although exceptions have been found, hypotonic fetal urine (sodium <100 mmol/ml, chlorine <90 mmol/ml, osmolarity <210 mmol/L) indicates preserved glomerular and tubular function and a favorable prognosis.[99] Other variables such as beta$_2$-microglobulins, ammonia, and creatinine have been studied.[93] The best ultrasonographic indicator of fetal renal dysfunction is diminished amniotic fluid before 20 weeks of gestation, which suggests a poor prognosis.

At present a fetus with bilateral hydronephrosis and diminishing amniotic fluid may be a candidate for antenatal intervention. Chromosome studies should be done before intervention to search for the often associated abnormalities. As mentioned previously, urinary electrolytes obtained by aspiration of the bladder may be useful in evaluation. The most common intervention is a vesicoamniotic shunt placed percutaneously under ultrasonic guidance. Reliable shunt function has been a problem because the shunts often become occluded or displaced, necessitating replacement. For this reason some investigators favor open surgical decompression by bilateral ureterostomies or vesicostomy.[98,100-102]

A fetal surgery registry was established to chronicle attempts at fetal surgical intervention.[92] As of July 1, 1989, the registry showed 87 cases of fetal obstructive uropathy with intervention and 35 survivors (40.2%). In 13 of the 87 cases the woman had elective pregnancy termination after shunt placement (14.9%). The fetal death rate attributable to vesicoamniotic shunting is 4.7% (4 of 85 cases).[93]

In the late 1980s interest in open fetal surgery increased as more effective tocolytic agents were developed to prevent premature labor, which had been a major problem during surgery. In one series twelve carefully selected patients underwent in utero surgery. Five of the fetuses underwent urinary diversion operations, and all have survived with variable renal function.[102] A recent review of maternal outcome after open fetal surgery found no mortality or decrease in future fertility. However, a significant number of women had preterm labor requiring tocolytic agents and early confinement.[103]

Fetal surgery is a recent innovation that holds great promise. Of all the surgical advances in recent years, fetal surgery seems to have the greatest requirement for careful scientific investigation, both into aspects of fetal physiology that would influence the success of intervention and into the actual risks and benefits to the fetus and the mother when intervention is undertaken. Enthusiasm should be tempered by a high-quality scientific approach involving special expertise and a highly trained team. The fruits of this research endeavor hold great possibilities.

REFERENCES

1. Arnold GE: Further experiences with intrachordal Teflon injection. Laryngoscope 74:802, 1964.
2. Webster RC, Kattner MD, Smith RC: Injectable collagen for augmentation of facial areas. Arch Otolaryngol 110(10):652-656, 1984.
3. Vorstman B, Lockhart J, Kaufman M, Politano V: Polytetrafluoroethylene injection for urinary incontinence in children. 133:248-250, 1985.
4. Walker RD: The injection of Teflon paste to correct urinary incontinence and vesicoureteral reflux. AUA Update Series, Lesson 20, Vol VIII, 1989.
5. Puri P, O'Donnell B: Correction of experimentally produced vesicoureteric reflux in the piglet by intravesical injection of Teflon. Br Med J 289:5-7, 1984.
6. O'Donnell B, Puri P: Endoscopic correction of primary vesicoureteric reflux: results in 94 ureters. Br Med J 293:1404-1406, 1986.
7. Puri P, O'Donnell B: Endoscopic correction of grades IV and V primary vesicoureteric reflux: six to 30 month follow-up in 42 ureters. J Pediatr Surg 22(12):1087-1091, 1987.
8. Schulman CC, Simon J, Pamart D, Avni F: Endoscopic treatment of vesicoureteral reflux in children. J Urol 138:950-952, 1987.
9. Kaplan WE, Dalton DP, Firlit CF: The endoscopic correction of reflux by polytetrafluoroethylene injection. J Urol 138:953-955, 1987.
10. Brown S: Open versus endoscopic surgery in the treatment of vesicoureteral reflux. J Urol 142:499-500, 1989.
11. Jackson CL, Kay R, Bretan P, et al: Endoscopic correction of vesicoureteral reflux in the renal transplant candidate. J Urol 142:710-711, 1989.
12. Saslawsky M, Niederberger C, Schacht M, et al: Ureterocutaneous fistula: a case report of treatment by subtrigonal infection of polytetrafluoroethylene (STING procedure). J Urol 142:1310-1311, 1989.
13. Yachia D: Submeatal injection of polytetrafluoroethylene paste for the endoscopic treatment of vesicoureteric reflux in adults. Br J Urol 64:552-555, 1989.
14. Puri P: Endoscopic correction of primary vesicoureteric reflux by subureteric injection of polytetrafluoroethylene. Lancet 335:1320-1322, 1990.
15. Giuliano CT, Cohen HL, Haller JO, Glassberg KI: The STING procedure and its implications: sonographic evaluation. J Clin Ultrasound 18:415-420, 1990.
16. Farkas A, Moriel EZ, Lupa S: Endoscopic correction of vesicoureteral reflux: our experience with 115 ureters. J Urol 144:534-536, 1990.
17. Leonard MP, Canning DA, Peters CA, et al: Endoscopic injection of glutaraldehyde cross-linked bovine dermal collagen for correction of vesicoureteral reflux. J Urol 145:115-119, 1991.
18. Matouschek E: Die Behandlung des vesikorenalen Refluxes durch transurethrale Einspritzung von Teflonpast. Urologe 20:263, 1981.
19. O'Donnell B, Puri P: Technical refinements in endoscopic correction of vesicoureteral reflux. J Urol 140:1101-1102, 1988.
20. Gelet A, Martin X, Salas M, et al: Endoscopic treatment of vesico-ureteral reflux. Presented at the annual meeting of the American Urological Association, Boston, June 1988.
21. Politano V, Molina L: Correction of vesicoureteral reflux with Polytef paste. Presented at the annual meeting of the American Urological Association, Boston, June 1988.
22. Kaminetsky JC, Hanna MK: Endoscopic treatment of vesicoureteral reflux in children with neurogenic bladders. Urology 37(3):244-247, 1991.
23. Peters CA: Why use Teflon® in children? Dialogues in Pediatric Urology, vol 14, no 2, Feb 1991.
24. Malizia AA, Reiman HM, Myers RP, et al: Migration and granulomatous reaction after periurethral injection of Polytef (Teflon). JAMA 251:3277, 1984.
25. Mittleman RE, Marraccini JV: Pulmonary Teflon granulomas following periurethral injection for urinary incontinence. Arch Pathol Lab Med 107:611, 1983.
26. Claes H, Stroobants D, Van Meerbeek J, et al: Pulmonary migration following periurethral polytetrafluoroethylene injection for urinary incontinence. J Urol 142:821-822, 1989.
27. Politano VA: Migration of polytetrafluoroethylene—Polytef. JAMA 254(14):1902-1903, 1985.
28. Merguerian PA, McLorie GA, Khoury AE, et al: Submucosal injection of polyvinyl alcohol foam in rabbit bladder. J Urol 144:531-533, 1990.
29. Canning DA: New implants for endoscopic correction in the nineties and beyond. Dialogues in Pediatric Urology, vol 14, no 2, Feb 1991.
30. Zucker JA, Bailey RW, Gadacz TR, Imbemlos AL: Laparoscopic guided cholecystectomy. Am J Surg 161(1):36-42, 1991.
31. Gans SL, Berci G: Peritoneoscopy in infants and children. J Pediatr Surg 8:399, 1975.
32. Leape LL, Ramenofsky ML: Laparoscopy in children. Pediatrics 66:215, 1980.
33. Clayman RV, Kavoussi LR, Long SR, et al: Laparoscopic nephrectomy: initial report of pelvioscopic organ ablation in the pig. J Endourol 4(3):247-252, 1990.
34. Meaney JT, Schuessler WW, Vancaille TH, et al: Initial results of endoscopic pelvic lymph node dissection as compared with open pelvic lymph node dissection. AUA Abstract No 840, Toronto, June 1991.
35. Silber SJ, Cohen R: Laparoscopy for cryptorchidism. J Urol 123:928-929, 1980.
36. Malone PS, Guiney EJ: The value of laparoscopy in localizing the impalpable undescended testis. Br J Urol 56:429-431, 1984.
37. Das S, Amar AD: The impact of laparoscopy on modern urologic practice. Urol Clin North Am 15(3):537-540, 1988.

38. Elder JS: Laparoscopy and Fowler-Stephens orchiopexy in the management of the impalpable testis. Urol Clin North Am 16(2):399-411, 1989.
39. Gearhart JP, Jeffs RD: Diagnostic maneuvers in cryptorchidism. Semin Urol 6(2):79-83, 1988.
40. Bloom DA: The Ann Arbor experience with laparoscopy. Dialogues in Pediatric Urology, vol 11, no 7, July 1988.
41. Boddy SM, Corkery JJ, Gornall P: The place of laparoscopy in the management of the impalpable testis. Br J Surg 72:918-919, 1985.
42. Lowe DH, Brock WA, Kaplan GW: Laparoscopy for localization of nonpalpable testes. J Urol 131:728-729, 1984.
43. Guiney EJ, Corbally M, Malone PS: Laparoscopy and the management of the impalpable testis. Br J Urol 63:313-316, 1989.
44. Manson AL, Terhune D, Jordan G, et al: Preoperative laparoscopic localization of the nonpalpable testis. J Urol 134:919-920, 1985.
45. Naslund MJ, Gearhart JP, Jeffs RD: Laparoscopy: its selected use in patients with unilateral nonpalpable testis after human chorionic gonadotropin stimulation. J Urol 142:108-110, 1989.
46. Scott JES: Laparoscopy as an aid in the diagnosis and management of the impalpable testis. J Pediatr Surg 17:14, 1982.
47. Weiss RM, Seashore JH: Laparoscopy in the management of the nonpalpable testis. J Urol 138:382-384, 1987.
48. Bloom DA: Celiopelviscopy in the nonpalpable testicle. Dialogues in Pediatric Urology, vol 13, no 9, Sept 1990.
49. Wolfman WL, Kreutner K: Laparoscopy in children and adolescents. J Adolesc Health Care 5:261-265, 1984.
50. De Cherney A: Complications in laparoscopy. Dialogues in Pediatric Urology, vol 11, no 7, July 1988.
51. Scorer G, Farrington GH: Congenital deformities of the testis and epididymis. New York: Appleton-Century-Crofts, 1971.
52. Cortesi N, Ferrari P, Zambarda E, et al: Diagnosis of bilateral abdominal cryptorchidism by laparoscopy. Endoscopy 8:33-34, 1976.
53. Scherz HC, Kaplan GW: Pediatric laparoscopy. Dialogues in Pediatric Urology, vol 11, no 7, July 1988.
54. Kogan SJ, Gill G, Bennett B, et al: Human monorchism: a clinico-pathological study of unilateral absent testes in 65 boys. J Urol 135:758, 1986.
55. Portuondo JA, Neyro JL, Barral A, et al: Management of phenotypic female patients with an XY karyotype. J Reprod Med 31:611, 1986.
56. Droesch K, Droesch J, Chumas J, Bronson R: Laparoscopic gonadectomy for gonadal dysgenesis. Fertil Steril 53(2):360-361, 1990.
57. Duckett JW: Laparoscopy for cryptorchidism. Dialogues in Pediatric Urology, vol 11, no 7, July 1988.
58. Hald T: Neurogenic dysfunction of the urinary bladder: an experimental and clinical study with special reference to the ability of electrical stimulation to establish voluntary micturition. Danish Med Bull 16(suppl 5):1, 1969.
59. Bradley WE, Timm GW, Chou SN: A decade of experience with electrical stimulation of the micturition reflex. Urol Int 26:283, 1971.
60. Nashold BS, Friedman H, Glenn JF, et al: Electro micturition in paraplegia: implantation of spinal neuro-prosthesis. Arch Surg 104:195, 1972.
61. Jonas U, Heine JP, Tanagho EA: Studies on the feasibility of urinary bladder evacuation by direct spinal cord stimulation. I. Parameters of most effective stimulation. Invest Urol 13:142, 1975.
62. Jonas U, Tanagho EA: Studies on the feasibility of urinary bladder evacuation by direct spinal cord stimulation. II. Post stimulus voiding: a way to overcome outflow resistance. Invest Urol 13:151, 1975.
63. Ingersoll EH, Jones LL, Heggre ES: Effect on urinary bladder of unilateral stimulation of pelvic nerves in the dog. Am J Physiol 189:167, 1957.
64. Hald T, Agrawal G, Kantrowitz A: Studies in stimulation of bladder and its motor nerves. Surgery 60:848, 1966.
65. Timm GW, Bradley WE: Electro-stimulation of the urinary detrusor to affect contraction and evacuation. Invest Urol 6:562, 1969.
66. Jonas U, Jones LW, Tanagho EA: Spinal cord versus detrusor stimulation: a comparative study in 6 acute dogs. Invest Urol 13:171, 1975.
67. Holmquist B: Electro-micturition by pelvic nerve stimulation in dogs. Scand J Urol Nephrol 2(suppl):1, 1968.
68. Stenberg CC, Burnette HW, Bunts RC: Electrical stimulation of human neurogenic bladders: experience with 4 patients. J Urol 97:79, 1967.
69. Habib HN: Experience and recent contributions in sacral nerve stimulation for voiding in both humans and animal. Br J Urol 39:73, 1967.
70. Heine JP, Schmidt RA, Tanagho EA: Intra-spinal sacral route stimulation for controlled micturition. Invest Urol 15:78, 1977.
71. Tanagho EA, Schmidt RA: Electrical stimulation in the clinical management of neurogenic bladder. J Urol 140:1331, 1988.
72. Schmidt RA, Burschini H, Tanagho EA: Urinary bladder and sphincter responses to stimulation of dorsal and ventral sacral roots. Invest Urol 16:300, 1979.
73. Schmidt RA, Burschini H, Tanagho EA: Sacral root stimulation in controlled micturition: peripheral somatic neurotomy in stimulated voiding. Invest Urol 17:130, 1979.
74. Thuroff JW, Bazeed MA, Schmidt RA, et al: Functional pattern of sacral root stimulation in dogs. I. Micturition. J Urol 127:1031, 1982.
75. Thuroff JW, Bazeed MA, Schmidt RA, et al: Functional pattern of sacral root stimulation in dogs. II. Urethral closure. J Urol 1927:1034, 1982.
76. Schmidt RA, Tanagho EA: Feasibility of controlled micturition through electrical stimulation. Urol Int 34:199, 1979.
77. Tanagho EA, Schmidt RA: Bladder pacemaker: scientific basis and clinical future. Urology 20:614, 1982.
78. Tanagho EA: Induced micturition via intraspinal sacral root stimulation: clinical implications. In Hambrecht FT, Reswick JB (eds): Functional electrical stimulation. New York: Marcel Dekker, 1977, p 157.
79. Katona F: Intravesicalis elektromos ingerles a hugyholyagbenulasok diagnosticajaban es therapiajaban. Ideggyogy Szle 11:165, 1959.
80. Katona F, Pasztor E, Tomka I: Untersuchungen uber die kortikale Afferentation der Harnblasentatigkeit. Acta Physiol Hung 18(suppl):24, 1961.
81. Katona F: Intravesikale Elektrotherapie bei Myelodysplasic bedingter Lahmungsblase. Z Kinderchir 13:114, 1973.
82. Katona F: Stages of vegetative afferentation in reorganization of bladder control during intravesical electrotherapy. Urol Int 30:192, 1975.
83. Katona F, Berenyi M: Intravesical transurethral electrotherapy in meningomyelocele patients. Acta Paediatr Hung 16:363, 1975.
84. Alexander S, Rowan D, Millar W, Scott SR: Treatment of urinary incontinence by electric pessary: a report of 18 patients. Br J Urol 42:184, 1970.
85. Harrison NW, Paterson PJ: Urinary incontinence in women treated with an electronic pessary. Br J Urol 42:41, 1970.
86. Godec CJ, Cass AS: Electrical stimulatioı for incontinence in myelomeningocele. J Urol 120:729, 1978.
87. Katona F, Berenyi M: Ideggyogyaszati szempontok a hugyholyagbenulasok transurethralis, intravesicalis elektroterapiajagban. Ideggyogy Szle 28:299, 1975.
88. Madersbacher H, Pauer W, Reiner E: Rehabilitation of micturition by transurethral electrostimulation of the bladder in patients with incomplete spinal cord lesions. Paraplegia 20:191, 1982.
89. Madersbacher H: Intravesical electrotherapy—a useful

help in the (re)habilitation of micturition in children with a lazy voider syndrome [Abstract 577]. J Urol 137:248, 1987.

90. Kaplan WE, Richards I: Intravesical bladder stimulation and myelodysplasia. J Urol 140:1282, 1988.

91. Kaplan WE, Richards TW, Richards I: Intravesical transurethral bladder stimulation to increase bladder capacity. J Urol 142:600, 1989.

92. Manning FA, Harrison MR, Rodeck C: Catheter shunts for fetal hydronephrosis and hydrocephalus. N Engl J Med 315:336-340, 1986.

93. Evans MI, Drugan A, Manning FA, Harrison MR: Fetal surgery in the 1990s. Am J Dis Child 143:1431-1436, 1989.

94. Harrison MR, Ross NA, Naoll R, deLorimier AA: Correction of congenital hydronephrosis in utero. I. The model: fetal urethral obstruction produces hydronephrosis and pulmonary hypoplasia in fetal lambs. J Pediatr Surg 18:247-256, 1983.

95. Harrison MR, Nakayama DK, Noall R, et al: Correction of congenital hydronephrosis in utero. II. Decompression reverses the effects of obstruction on the fetal lung and urinary tract. J Pediatr Surg 17:965-974, 1982.

96. Glick PL, Harrison MR, Noall RA, Villa RL: Correction of congenital hydronephrosis in utero. III. Early mid-trimester urethral obstruction produces renal dysplasia. J Pediatr Surg 18:681-687, 1983.

97. Glick PL, Harrison MR, Adzick NS, et al: Correction of congenital hydronephrosis in utero. IV. In ureteral decompression prevents renal dysplasia. J Pediatr Surg 19:649-657, 1984.

98. Bond SJ, Harrison MR: Obstructive uropathy: when to intervene. Contemp Obstet Gynecol, Special Issue, 1987, pp 64-74.

99. Golbus MS, Filly RA, Callen PW, et al: Fetal urinary tract obstruction: management and selection of treatment. Semin Perinatol 9:91-97, 1985.

100. Harrison MR, Golbus MS, Filly RA, et al: Management of the fetus with congenital hydronephrosis. J Pediatr Surg 17:728-742, 1982.

101. Glick PL, Harrison MR, Adzick NS, et al: Management of the fetus with congenital hydronephrosis. II. Prognostic criteria and selection for treatment. J Pediatr Surg 20:376-387, 1985.

102. Crombleholme TM, Harrison MR, Langer JC, et al: Early experience with open fetal surgery for congenital hydronephrosis. J Pediatr Surg 23:1114-1121, 1988.

103. Longaker MT, Golbus MS, Filly RA, et al: Maternal outcome after open fetal surgery: a review of the first 17 human cases. JAMA 265:737-741, 1991.

INDEX

Note: Numbers in *italics* refer to illustrations; numbers followed by t refer to tables.